SLEEP DISORDERS MEDICINE:
Basic Science, Technical Considerations, and Clinical Aspects

SLEEP DISORDERS MEDICINE:
Basic Science, Technical Considerations, and Clinical Aspects

EDITED BY

Sudhansu Chokroverty, M.D.

PROFESSOR OF NEUROLOGY AND CHIEF OF CLINICAL NEUROPHYSIOLOGY
UNIVERSITY OF MEDICINE AND DENTISTRY OF NEW JERSEY
ROBERT WOOD JOHNSON MEDICAL SCHOOL AND UNIVERSITY HOSPITAL
NEW BRUNSWICK, NEW JERSEY
CHIEF, NEUROLOGY SERVICE, VETERANS ADMINISTRATION MEDICAL CENTER
LYONS, NEW JERSEY

WITH 39 CONTRIBUTING AUTHORS

Butterworth–Heinemann

Boston London Oxford Singapore Sydney Toronto Wellington

I devote this book to my wife Manisha and our
daughters, Linda and Keka.

ISBN: 0-7506-9002-X

Butterworth–Heinemann
80 Montvale Avenue
Stoneham, MA 02180

10 9 8 7 6 5 4 3 2 1

Printed in the United States of America

Contents

Contributing Authors

BARBARA G. BIGBY, M.A., R.R.T.
Clinical Research Specialist, Division of Sleep Disorders, Scripps Clinic and Research Foundation, La Jolla, California

ROGER J. BROUGHTON, M.D., PH.D., F.R.C.P.
Professor, Department of Medicine, University of Ottawa, Medical Director, Sleep Disorders Clinic, Division of Neurology, Ottawa General Hospital, Ottawa, Ontario, Canada

RAFAEL DE JESUS CABEZA, PH.D.
Department of Psychiatry, University of California, San Diego, La Jolla, California

MINDY B. CETEL, M.D.
Director, Sleep Disorders Center, University of California, Irvine, Orange, California

WILLIAM C. DEMENT, M.D., PH.D., A.C.P.
Professor of Psychiatry and Behavioral Sciences, Stanford University School of Medicine, Palo Alto, California

NORMAN H. EDELMEN, M.D.
Professor of Medicine and Dean, UMD—Robert Wood Johnson Medical School, Piscataway, New Jersey

C. WILLIAM ERWIN, M.D.
Duke University Medical Center, Durham, North Carolina

MILTON G. ETTINGER, M.D.
Department of Neurology, University of Minnesota Medical School, Department of Neurology, Minnesota Regional Sleep Disorders Center, Hennepin County Medical Center, Minneapolis, Minnesota

RICHARD FERBER, M.D.
Assistant Professor, Department of Neurology, Harvard Medical School, Director, Center for Pediatric Sleep Disorders, Children's Hospital, Boston, Massachusetts

J. CHRISTIAN GILLIN, M.D.
Department of Psychiatry, University of California, San Diego, La Jolla, California

CHRISTIAN GUILLEMINAULT, M.D.
Professor, Sleep Disorders Center, Stanford University School of Medicine, Stanford, California

PAUL HARTMAN, PH.D.
Research Psychologist, Sleep Disorders and Research Center, Deaconess Hospital, St. Louis, Missouri

WAYNE A. HENING, M.D., PH.D.
Assistant Professor, Department of Neurology, UMDNJ—Robert Wood Johnson Medical School, New Brunswick, New Jersey; Clinical Investigator, Department of Neurology, Veterans Affairs Medical Center, Lyons, New Jersey

MAX HIRSHKOWITZ, PH.D.
Associate Professor, Department of Psychiatry, Baylor College of Medicine; Director, Sleep Research Laboratory, Research Service, Veterans Affairs Medical Center, Houston, Texas

ISMET KARACAN, M.D., D.SC.
Professor, Department of Psychiatry, Director, Sleep Disorders Center, Baylor College of Medicine, Houston, Texas

SHARON A. KEENAN, R. EEG T., R. PSG T.
Director, The School of Sleep Medicine, Stanford, California

JOHN B. KOSTIS, M.D.
Professor of Medicine and Pharmacology, Chairman, Department of Medicine, UMDNJ—Robert Wood Johnson Medical School; Chief of Cardiology, Robert Wood Johnson University Hospital, New Brunswick, New Jersey

JAMES KOWALL, M.D.
Staff Physician, Sleep Disorders and Research Center, Deaconess Hospital, St. Louis, Missouri

MARK W. MAHOWALD, M.D.
Department of Neurology, University of Minnesota Medical School; Department of Neurology, Minnesota Regional Sleep Disorders Center, Hennepin County Medical Center, Minneapolis, Minnesota

GAIL R. MARSH, PH.D.
Associate Professor of Medical Psychology, Psychiatry Department, Duke University, Durham, North Carolina

W. VAUGHN MCCALL, M.D.
Medical Director, Sleep Laboratory, Assistant

Professor, Department of Psychiatry, Bowman Gray School of Medicine, Winston-Salem, North Carolina

ROBERT W. MCCARLEY, M.D.

Professor of Psychiatry, Director, Neuroscience Laboratory, Department of Psychiatry, Harvard Medical School; Medical Investigator, Research Service, Brockton/West Roxbury Veterans Affairs Medical Center, Brockton, Massachusetts

MERRILL M. MITLER, PH.D.

Clinical Professor of Psychiatry, University of California at San Diego, San Diego, California; Director of Research, Division of Sleep Disorders, Scripps Clinic and Research Foundation, La Jolla, California

KEVIN A. O'CONNOR, M.D.

Department of Psychiatry, University of Minnesota Medical School; Department of Psychiatry, Minnesota Regional Sleep Disorders Center, Hennepin County Medical Center, Minneapolis, Minnesota

RICHARD A. PARISI, M.D.

Associate Professor of Medicine, Department of Medicine, UMDNJ—Robert Wood Johnson Medical School; Assistant Medical Director, Comprehensive Sleep Disorders Center, Robert Wood Johnson University Hospital, New Brunswick, New Jersey

J. STEPHEN POCETA, M.D.

Clinical Director of the Sleep Laboratory, Division of Sleep Disorders, Scripps Clinic and Research Foundation, La Jolla, California

TIMOTHY A. ROEHRS, PH.D.

Adjunct Associate Professor, Department of Psychology, Wayne State University, Director of Research, Sleep Disorders and Research Center, Henry Ford Hospital, Detroit, Michigan

LEON D. ROSENTHAL, M.D.

Staff Clinician/Researcher, Sleep Disorders and Research Center, Henry Ford Hospital, Detroit, Michigan

THOMAS ROTH, PH.D.

Clinical Professor, Department of Psychiatry, University of Michigan School of Medicine, Ann Arbor, Michigan; Division Head, Sleep Disorders and Research Center, Henry Ford Hospital, Detroit, Michigan

MARK H. SANDERS. M.D.

Associate Professor of Medicine and Anesthesiology, University of Pittsburgh School of Medicine, Director, Pulmonary Sleep Evaluation Center; University of Pittsburgh Medical Center, Pittsburgh, Pennsylvania

TEODORO V. SANTIAGO, M.D.

Professor, Division of Pulmonary and Critical Care Medicine, UMDNJ—Robert Wood Johnson Medical School, Medical Director, Comprehensive Sleep Disorders Center, Robert Wood Johnson University Hospital, New Brunswick, New Jersey

DANIEL M. SHINDLER, M.D.

Associate Clinical Professor of Medicine, Robert Wood Johnson Medical School, Director, Electrocardiography and Echocardiography, Robert Wood Johnson University Hospital, New Brunswick, New Jersey

RONALD A. STILLER, M.D., PH.D.

Assistant Professor of Medicine and Anesthesiology, University of Pittsburgh School of Medicine; Associate Director, Medical Intensive Care Unit, Presbyterian University Hospital, Pittsburgh, Pennsylvania

MICHAEL J. THORPY, M.D.

Associate Professor of Neurology, Albert Einstein College of Medicine, Director, Sleep-Wake Disorders Center, Montefiore Medical Center, Bronx, New York

THADDEUS S. WALCZAK, M.D., A.C.P.

Assistant Professor, Director, Epilepsy Monitoring Unit, Department of Neurology, Columbia University College of Physicians and Surgeons and The Neurological Institute; Attending Physician, Department of Neurology, Columbia Presbyterian Medical Center, New York, New York

JAMES K. WALSH, PH.D.

Clinical Associate Professor, St. Louis University School of Medicine; Director, Sleep Disorders and Research Center, Deaconess Hospital, St. Louis, Missouri

ARTHUR S. WALTERS, M.D.

Department of Neurology, UMDNJ—Robert Wood Johnson Medical School, New Brunswick, New Jersey; Department of Neurology, Veterans Affairs Medical Center, Lyons, New Jersey

VIRGIL WOOTEN, M.D.

Clinical Associate Professor, Department of Psychiatry, University of Arkansas for Medical Sciences; Medical Director, Sleep Disorders Center for Adults and Children, St. Vincent Infirmary Medical Center, Little Rock, Arkansas

REBECCA K. ZOLTOSKI, PH.D.

Department of Psychiatry, University of California, San Diego, La Jolla, California

Foreword

In January 1993, when the Report of the National Commission on Sleep Disorders Research was released, it became evident that practitioners involved in the diagnosis and treatment of sleep disorders must be ready to provide a new level of service to the American public. The report emphasizes that as many as 40 million Americans suffer from chronic disorders of sleep and wakefulness. The vast majority of these disorders, though often severely disabling and, indeed, life threatening, go unrecognized by the medical community, and the annual cost to society is measured in tens of billions of dollars.

Dr. Chokroverty and his collaborators have approached this challenge by developing a comprehensive textbook, one that deals with the underlying scientific concepts, clinical approaches, and technical considerations. The organization of the text, as well as the list of outstanding contributors, confirms for me the very important precept that the most complete and sophisticated approach to the diagnosis and management of sleep disorders is a multidisciplinary one. Those with special interests in the pathophysiology of sleep, from the fields of neurology, psychiatry, psychology, adult and pediatric pulmonary medicine, the surgical subspecialties and even dentistry, all have important contributions to make, and in the ideal setting, provide interactive and complementary input into management of patients and the conduct of research.

In my opinion, it is essential for the maintenance of the sophistication of this field that we do not succumb to the temptation of viewing sleep medicine as a primary specialty. Rather we should preserve the advantages of the multidisciplinary approach.

Readers of this volume who are new to the field will be surprised by the level of technologic advance and the depth of the knowledge base. Readers who are familiar with sleep disorders will be impressed by the rapidity with which advances are being made.

We are off to a good start in helping society to awaken.

Norman H. Edelman, M.D.

Preface

Sleep, that gentle tyrant,[1] has aroused the interest of mankind since time immemorial, as reflected in the writings of the Eastern and Western religions and civilizations (e.g., Upanishads,[2] circa 1000 B.C. wrote about "the dreaming" and "a deep dreamless sleep"; see Chapter 2). Even though there are many poetic, philosophical, and religious references to the phenomenon, and to the mystical nature of sleep, the science of sleep was very slow to evolve. In the last 40 years, however, an explosive growth took place in the basic and clinical aspects of sleep research. Recent major discoveries and advances include the discovery of REM sleep and the cyclic pattern of non-REM–REM sleep stages throughout a human being's night sleep; the standardized sleep-scoring technique; the discovery of the mechanism of sleep apnea and better management of this disorder; better understanding of the nature of narcolepsy; an awareness of the parasomnias, their treatment, and their differentiation from epilepsy; phototherapy for circadian rhythm and other sleep disorders; pharmacotheraphy for insomnias; and better understanding of the treatment of sleep apnea and hypoventilation related to neuromuscular disorders. Other significant recent developments include the formation of the Association of Sleep Disorders Centers, growing numbers of sleep disorders centers, formal certification for accreditation of such centers, formation of the American Board of Sleep Medicine to test practitioners' competency in sleep disorders medicine, publication of the scientific journal *Sleep*, and incorporation of the subject of sleep in other subspecialty board examinations (e.g., American Board of Clinical Neurophysiology; Added Qualifications in Clinical Neurophysiology). Growing awareness in the medical profession of the importance of sleep is reflected in the development of training programs in sleep disorders medicine, approval by the American Academy of Neurology for a section on sleep, and the formation of the National Commission on Sleep Disorders Research (NCSDR). The latter is significant because experts in the sleep field are now voicing their concerns in the political arena. The study of sleep has come a long way, and in this Decade of the Brain it is hoped that sleep medicine will find its rightful place as an independent specialty in the broad field of medicine.

Dement[3] defined sleep disorders medicine as the branch of medicine that deals with the sleeping brain and all manifestations and pathologies deriving therefrom. Sleep disturbances affect as many as one-third of all American adults, and about 40 million Americans suffer from chronic disorders of sleep and wakefulness. The majority of those affected remain undiagnosed and untreated (executive summary and findings NCSDR).[4] Therefore, education in sleep disorders medicine is urgently needed. This book aims to provide clinicians in many disciplines who have an interest in sleep and sleep disorders with a comprehensive scientific basis for understanding sleep, as well as to present information on the diagnosis and treatment of a wide variety of sleep disorders, which are, increasingly, being recognized. The purpose, therefore, is to produce a comprehensive treatise on sleep disorders medicine, not only for beginners but also for those who are already engaged in the art and science of sleep medicine. Thus, it is meant to be a practical exposition of the subject that also provides an appropriate foundation in the basic science. With these objectives in mind the monograph is divided into three sections: basic aspects of sleep; sleep technology; and the clinical science of sleep. The monograph is directed to all who are interested in sleep disorders medicine and should, therefore, be useful to neurologists, internists (particularly those subspecializing in pulmonary,

[1]Webb WB. Sleep: The Gentle Tyrant. Bolton, Mass.: Anker Publishing, 1992.

[2]Wolpert S. A New History of India. New York: Oxford University Press, 1982; 48.

[3]Dement WC. A personal history of sleep disorders medicine. J Clin Neurophyisol 1990;7:17–47.

[4]National Commission on Sleep Disorders Research. Report of the National Commission on Sleep Disorders Research. DHHS Pub. No. 92-XXXX. Washington, D.C.: U.S. Government Printing Office, 1992.

cardiovascular, or gastrointestinal medicine), psychiatrists, psychologists, pediatricians, otolaryngologists, neurosurgeons, general practitioners dealing with many apparently undiagnosed sleep disorders patients, and neuroscientists with an interest in sleep research.

I must express my gratitude to all the contributors, who are investigators in the forefront of sleep research, for finding time to write the scholarly chapters for this monograph. Special thanks are due to William C. Dement, M.D., Ph.D., one of the foremost sleep researchers of our time, for writing the Introduction, and to Christian Guilleminault, M.D., a giant in the field of sleep disorders medicine, for agreeing to contribute two chapters.

I should like to express my gratitude and appreciation to Norman Edelman, M.D., Dean of Robert Wood Johnson Medical School and a member of the National Commission on Sleep Disorders Research, for his thoughtful Foreword.

I must thank Peter McGregor and Michael Thorpy, M.D., also a contributor in this volume, for making available the tracings for two figures used in the text. Wayne Hening, M.D., Ph.D., in addition to being a contributor, made helpful suggestions for several of my own chapters.

I wish to thank all those authors, editors, and publishers who allowed me to reproduce illustrations that were first published in other books and journals. Specific permission is acknowledged in the appropriate figures.

I am also grateful to the American Sleep Disorders Association for giving me permission to reproduce the Glossary of Terms that appeared in the International Classification of Sleep Disorders in 1990.

It is a pleasure to acknowledge my appreciation to Lena DiMauro for her splendid support and for typing and retyping the manuscripts during all stages of preparation and to James Cummings for help with making numerous copies of the chapters.

I wish also to thank Debbie MacDonald, Assistant Editor, and Susan Pioli, Publisher, Medical Division, and others of the Butterworth-Heinemann publishing company for their excellent help.

Finally, it is my utmost pleasure to acknowledge my wife, Manisha Chokroverty, M.D., for her support, patience, tolerance, and caring throughout the arduous, long process of preparation for publication.

1

Introduction

W.C. Dement

The existence of sleep disorders medicine is based primarily on the fact that there are really two fully functioning brains—the brain awake and the brain in sleep. The cerebral activity of wakefulness and the cerebral activity of sleep have contrasting consequences. In addition, the brain's two major functional states influence each other. Problems during wakefulness affect sleep, and disordered sleep or disordered sleep mechanisms impair the functions of wakefulness. Perhaps, the most important clinical symptom in sleep disorders medicine is an awareness of sleep-related impaired alertness, in other words, a complaint of excessive sleepiness.

The fundamental concept of sleep disorders medicine is that some function (e.g. breathing) may appear normal in the waking state and pathological in sleep. In addition, there are a host of non-sleep disorders that are, or may be, modified by the sleeping state. It should no longer be necessary to argue that health issues in human beings must include the organism in sleep as an equal partner to health issues concerning the organism awake. Patient care is therefore a 24-hour commitment. This latter statement enhances one aspect of sleep medicine, circadian regulation of sleep and wakefulness. It is worth noting that, of all the 24-hour professions whose clocks should be shifted to promote full alertness and optimal performance at night, it is the medical profession who holds human lives in the palm of their hands.

WHAT IS SLEEP DISORDERS MEDICINE?

"Sleep disorders medicine is a clinical specialty which deals with the diagnosis and treatment of patients who complain about disturbed nocturnal sleep, excessive daytime sleepiness, or some other sleep-related problem."[1] The spectrum of disorders and problems in this area is extremely broad, ranging from merely troublesome ones such as a day or two of mild jet lag to the catastrophic ones such as sudden infant death syndrome (SIDS), fatal familial insomnia, or a tragic accident involving a patient with sleep apnea who falls asleep at the wheel. The dysfunctions may be primary, apparently involving the basic neural mechanisms of sleep and arousal, or

secondary, in association with other medical, psychiatric, or neurologic illnesses. This young field has not yet established that sleep mechanisms play a causal role in a number of possibly related illnesses, such as endogenous depression, but progress is being made.

The final fundamental principle that must be mentioned is that the sleep disorders specialist must examine the sleeping patient in one way or another and must take into account and evaluate the impact of sleep on waking functions. Sleep disorders medicine also, in common with other specialties, has an enormous responsibility for the societal implications of its illnesses, particularly impaired alertness due to inadequate sleep or sleep problems. Physicians should always be sensitive to the level of alertness in their patients and the potential consequences of a sleep-related accident.

A BRIEF HISTORY

Well into the nineteenth century, the phenomenon of sleep escaped systematic observation, in spite of the fact that it occupies a third of a human lifetime. (For newborn infants this aphorism must be restated: rapid eye movement (REM) sleep occupies one-third of their days, non-REM (NREM) sleep occupies a third, and wakefulness, barely established, is utilized by the organism mainly for feeding.) All other things being equal, we may assume that there were a wide variety of reasons for preferring not to study sleep, one of which was the unpleasant necessity for staying awake at night. For other discussions of this historical puzzle see Dement.[2]

Although in the 1960s there were hints (e.g., a fee-for-service narcolepsy clinic at Stanford University and research on non–sleep-related illnesses like asthma and hypothyroidism at UCLA[3,4] sleep disorders medicine can quite clearly be identified as having begun at Stanford University in 1970, with the routine utilization of respiration and cardiac sensors together with the time-honored continuous electroencephalography (EEG), electrooculography (EOG), and electromyography (EMG) in all-night polygraphic recordings. Continuous all-night recordings utilizing this array of data gathering was finally

1

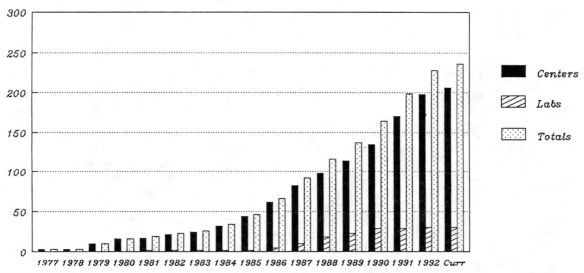

FIGURE 1-1.   *Shown graphically is the rapid growth of the number of sleep disorders centers accredited by the American Sleep Disorders Association (ASDA). Reproduced with permission from ASDA (APSS Newsletter 1993; 8(2)).*

named *polysomnography* by Holland and coworkers,[5] and patients paid for the tests as part of a clinical fee-for-service.

The Stanford model included responsibility for medical management and care of patients beyond mere interpretation of the test and an assessment of daytime sleepiness. After several false starts, the latter effort culminated in the development of the Multiple Sleep Latency Test,[7,8] and the framework of the discipline of sleep medicine was essentially complete.

The comprehensive evaluation of sleep in patients who complained about their daytime alertness led rapidly to a series of discoveries and clarifications, which included the high prevalence of obstructive sleep apnea in patients complaining of sleepiness, the role of periodic limb movement in insomnia, the sleep misperception syndrome, first called pseudoinsomnia, and so on. As in the beginning of any medical practice, though for most specialties that goes back almost before recorded history, the case series approach, wherein patients were evaluated and carefully tabulated, was very important.[8,9]

increased both in breadth and in depth, and in order to document sufficient knowledge and skills, the American Board of Sleep Medicine was incorporated in 1990. Before that, the American Sleep Disorders Association offered certifying examinations and the successful candidates became Accredited Clinical Polysomnographers. The professional societies and their annual meetings have increased in size, and the organized body of knowledge, as presented herein and elsewhere, has increased dramatically.

It was the assimilation of this body of knowledge and several years' experience in diagnosing and treating any and all patients with a sleep-related problem or complaint that produces the sleep specialist. Their number, however, is far too small to bring the benefits of sleep disorders medicine to the 50 million Americans who have sleep problems. There is a continuing need for effective presentation of the organized body of knowledge of sleep medicine, and this book fulfills that need. Any field worth its salt has several different textbooks, and sleep medicine should be no exception.

THE PRESENT

Although it got a late start, the field of sleep disorders medicine has grown very rapidly. The number of sleep disorders centers has increased almost exponentially (Figure 1-1). The number of practitioners has also increased rapidly. The amount of material for which a sleep specialist must be responsible has

REFERENCES

1. Walsh J. Sleep Disorders Medicine. Rochester, MN: Association of Professional Sleep Societies, 1986.
2. Dement W. A personal history of sleep disorders medicine. Clin Neurophysiol 1990;7:17–47.
3. Kales A, Beall GN, Bajor GF, et al. Sleep studies in asthamatic adults: Relationship of attacks to sleep stage and time of night. J Allergy 1968;41:164–173.

4. Kales A, Heuser G, Jacobson A, et al. All night sleep studies in hypothyroid patients, before and after treatment. J Clin Endoctrinol Metab 1967;27:1593–1599.

5. Holland V, Dement W, Raynal D. Polysomnography responding to a need for improved communication. Presented at annual meeting of Sleep Research Society, Jackson Hole, Wyoming, 1974.

6. Carskadon M, Dement W. Sleep tendency: An objective measure of sleep loss. Sleep Res 1977;6:200.

7. Richardson G, Carskadon M, Flagg W, et al. Excessive daytime sleepiness in man: Multiple sleep latency measurement in narcoleptic and control subjects. Electroencephalogr Clin Neurophysiol 1978;45:621–627.

8. Dement W, Guilleminault C, Zarcone V. The pathologies of sleep: A case series approach. In: Tower D, ed. The Nervous system, vol 2. The Clinical Neurosciences. New York: Raven Press, 1975;501–518.

9. Guilleminault C, Dement W. 235 Cases of excessive daytime sleepiness. Diagnosis and tentative classification. J Neurol Sci 1977;31:13–27.

I

Basic Aspects of Sleep

2

An Overview of Sleep

Sudhansu Chokroverty

HISTORICAL PERSPECTIVE

Since the dawn of civilization and the creation of the world, the mysteries of sleep have intrigued poets, artists, philosophers, and mythologists alike. This intrigue, awe, and delight are reflected in literature, folklore, religion, and medicine. *Upanishad*[1,2] (circa 1000 B.C.), the famous ancient Indian textbook of philosophy, sought to divide human existence into four states: the waking, the dreaming, the deep dreamless sleep, and the superconscious ("the very self"). One finds the description of pathologic sleepiness (possibly a case of Kleine-Levin syndrome) in the mythologic character Kumbhakarna in the great Indian epic *Ramayana*[3,4] (circa 1000 B.C.). Kumbhakarna would sleep for months at a time and would get up to eat and drink voraciously before falling asleep again.

The definition of sleep and its functions have baffled scientists since the beginning. Moruzzi,[5] while describing the historical development of the deafferentation hypothesis of sleep, quoted the concept Lucretius articulated 2000 years ago that sleep is the absence of wakefulness. A variation of the same concept was expressed by Hartley[6] in 1749, and then in 1830 by Macnish.[7] Macnish[7] defined sleep as suspension of sensorial power in which the voluntary functions are in abeyance but the involuntary powers, such as circulation or respiration, remain intact.

Throughout the literature, a close relationship between sleep and death has been perceived, but the rapid reversibility of sleep episodes differentiates it from coma and death. There are myriad references to sleep, death, and dream in poetic and religious writings: "The deepest sleep resembles death" (the *Bible*, I Samuel 26:12); "sleep and death are similar . . . sleep is one-sixtieth [i.e., one piece] of death." (the *Talmud*, Berachoth 576); "There she [Aphrodite] met sleep, the brother of death" (Homer's *Iliad*, circa 700 B.C.); "To sleep perchance to dream . . . . For in that sleep of death what dreams may come?" (Shakespeare's *Hamlet*); "How wonderful is death; Death and his brother sleep" (Shelley).

Sleep and wakefulness, the two basic processes of life, are like two different worlds, with independent controls and functions. Borbely,[2] in his monograph

Secrets of Sleep, gives an interesting historical introduction to sleep, and the reader is referred there.

What is the origin of sleep? The word *sleep* or *somnolence* is derived from the Latin word *somnus,* the German words *sleps, slaf,* or *schlaf,* and the Greek word *hypnos.*[2] Hippocrates,[2] the father of medicine, postulated a humoral mechanism for sleep and stated that it was caused by the retreat of blood and warmth into the inner regions of the body, whereas the Greek philosopher Aristotle[2] thought sleep was related to food, which generates heat and causes sleepiness. Paracelsus,[2] a sixteenth-century physician, wrote that "natural" sleep lasted 6 hours, which would eliminate tiredness and would refresh the sleeper. He also spoke about the length of sleep and suggested people not sleep too much or too little but wake when the sun rises and to go to bed at sunset. These views of Paracelsus' are strikingly similar to modern teachings about sleep. The views about sleep in the seventeenth and eighteenth centuries were expressed by Alexander Stuart,[2] the British physician and physiologist, and by the Swiss physician, Albrecht von Haller.[2] According to Stuart,[2] sleep was due to a deficit of the "animal spirits"; von Haller[2] wrote that the flow of the "spirits" to the nerves was cut off by the thickened blood in the heart. Nineteenth-century scientists used principles of physiology and chemistry to explain sleep. Both Humboldt[2] and Pfluger[2] thought that sleep resulted from a reduction or lack of oxygen in the brain. None of the suggestions are based on solid scientific experiments, which were not conducted until the twentieth century. Ishimori,[8] in 1909, and Legendre and Pieron,[9] in 1913, observed sleep-promoting substances in the cerebrospinal fluid of animals during prolonged wakefulness.

The discovery of the EEG waves in dogs by the English physician Caton[10] in 1875 and of the alpha waves from the surface of the human brain by the German physician Hans Berger[11] in 1929 initiated contemporary sleep research. It is interesting to note that Kohlschutter,[2] a nineteenth-century German physiologist, thought sleep was deepest in the first few hours and became lighter as time went on. Modern sleep laboratory studies generally confirmed these observations. The golden age of sleep research began with the discovery in 1937, by the American

7

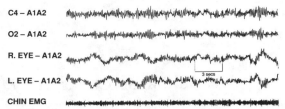

FIGURE 2-1.   *PSG recording shows wakefulness. Note 9 to 10 Hz alpha activity in the EEG (C4-A1A2; 02-A1A2: International nomenclature) mixed with some low-amplitude beta activity. Chin EMG shows much tonic activity. Waking eye movements are seen in the EOGs (right eye [R] and left eye [L] are referred to linked ear—A1A2). Paper speed, 10 mm/sec. (Timer: 3 sec) Calibration: 50 μV for EEG and eye channels, and 20 μV for EMG channel.*

physiologist Loomis[12] and coworkers of different stages of sleep reflected in EEG changes. The discovery by Aserinsky and Kleitman,[13] in the laboratory of the University of Chicago, of rapid eye movement (REM) sleep electrified the scientific community and propelled sleep research to the forefront. This was followed by the now famous Rechtschaffen and Kales[14] technique of sleep scoring based on Electroencephalography (EEG), Electromyography (EMG), and Electrooculography (EOG), which has become the gold standard for sleep scoring throughout the world.

SLEEP ARCHITECTURE
AND SLEEP PROFILE[15–17]

The beginning of stage I non-REM (NREM) sleep in adults is heralded by the diminution of the alpha waves of wakefulness (Figure 2-1) in the EEG to

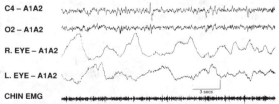

FIGURE 2-2.   *PSG shows stage 1 NREM sleep. EEGs (top 2 channels) show a decrease of alpha activity to less than 50% and low-amplitude mixed-frequency activities in the range of 3 to 7 Hz. Note vertex sharp waves in the midportion of the EEGs. EOGs (right eye and left eye) show slow, rolling eye movements (SEMs). Tonic EMG persists. Timer: 3 sec. Calibration: 50 μV for EEG and eye channels, 20 μV for EMG channel.*

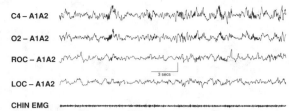

FIGURE 2-3.   *Stage 2 NREM sleep. Note 14-Hz sleep spindles in the EEG channels. No eye movements are seen. Tonic EMG persists though EMG activity is less than in wakefulness and stage 1. Timer: 3 sec. Calibration: 50 μV for EEG and eye channels, 20 μV for EMG channel.*

fewer than 50% in an epoch (Figure 2-2) which are replaced by the theta (and some beta) waves, accompanied by slow, rolling eye movements demonstrated in the EOG recordings. Muscle tone in the EMG decreases slightly. Within a few minutes, the hypnogram shows bursts of 12- to 16-Hz sleep spindles intermixed with K complexes. The vertex sharp waves are noted toward the end of stage I and are also present in stage II NREM sleep (Figure 2-3), which is dominated by the spindles. The EOG does not register eye movements at this stage, and EMG tone is less than in wakefulness or stage I sleep. The EEG contains theta and (fewer than 20%) delta waves. Stage II sleep lasts about 30 to 60 minutes. Sleep next progresses to the stages of slow-wave sleep (stages III and IV NREM sleep) characterized by the delta waves, which constitute 20% to 50% in stage III (Figure 2-4) and more than 50% in stage IV (Figure 2-5). Toward the end of the deep sleep (delta sleep), body movements are registered as artifacts in the polysomnographic recordings. Stage III and IV NREM sleep is briefly interrupted by stage II NREM sleep, which is followed by the first REM sleep about 60 to 90 minutes after sleep onset. REM sleep (Figure 2-6) is characterized by rapid eye movements, desynchronization of the EEG, often accompanied by "sawtooth" waves, and marked reduction or absence of

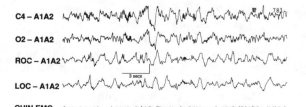

FIGURE 2-4.   *PSG shows stage 3 NREM sleep. EEG (top 2 channels) shows 20% to 50% of the epoch occupied by waves of 2 Hz or less with amplitudes greater than 75 μV from peak to peak. Timer and calibration are as in Figure 2-1.*

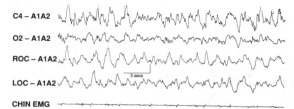

FIGURE 2-5. *Stage 4 NREM sleep. More than 50% of the epoch in the EEG (top 2 channels) now consists of 2 Hz or slower waves having an amplitude greater than 75 μv. EOGs (third and fourth channels from top) are contaminated with EEG waves. Timer and calibration are as in Figure 2-1.*

muscle tone in the EMG recording. The first REM period lasts only a few minutes and is followed by progression to stage II, and then stage III and IV, NREM sleep before the second REM sleep begins. Thus, a full sleep cycle consists of a sequence of NREM and REM, and each cycle lasts about 90 to 110 minutes. Generally, 4 to 6 such cycles are observed during a night's sleep. The first two cycles are dominated by the slow-wave sleep (stages III and IV NREM sleep), and subsequently these stages are noted only briefly, sometimes not at all. On the other hand, the REM sleep cycle increases from the first to the last cycle, and the longest REM cycle, toward the end of the night, may last as long as an hour. Thus, the slow-wave sleep is dominant in the first third of the night and REM sleep is dominant in the last third. This characteristic sleep cycling is noted in both humans and animals.

THE ONTOGENY OF SLEEP

Newborns have a polyphasic sleep pattern and spend about two-thirds of their time sleeping in the first few days of life. This multiphasic sleep pattern gradually changes into the monophasic adult pattern later in life.[16,18–20] On falling asleep, a newborn baby goes immediately into REM sleep or active sleep, which is accompanied by restless

movements of the arms and legs and the facial muscles. In premature babies it is often difficult to differentiate REM from wakefulness. By the age of about 3 months, the usual NREM-REM cyclic pattern is evident. Polyphasic sleep changes to biphasic sleep in preschool children, and finally to monophasic sleep in adults. It reverts to bi- or multiphasic sleep in elderly persons. During the first few months of an infant's life REM sleep decreases. By 2 to 3 years of age REM sleep occupies only about 20% of the total sleep time. The EEG begins to show adult sleep pattern with the appearance of spindles around age 3 months,[21] and K complexes at 6 months.[22] Although a NREM-REM cycle is noted in children, it is shorter lived than in adults. At age 1 year the cycle may last 45 to 50 minutes, whereas at age 5 to 10 years it increases to 60 to 70 minutes. Around age 10 years adult REM sleep cycle (90 to 110 minutes) and REM percentage (20% to 25%) are observed. In older people delta waves are less pronounced but the percentage of REM sleep remains relatively constant. Older adults have difficulty sleeping and often awaken frequently and in the early morning. Elderly persons often complain increasingly about poor sleep. The evolution of sleep stage distribution in newborns, infants, children, adults, and elders is shown schematically in Figure 2-7. Figure 2-8 shows night sleep histograms of a child, a young adult, and an elderly person.

Sleep Habits

Sleep specialists sometimes divide people into two groups, "evening types" and "morning types."[2] The morning types feel rested and fresh, and wake up early and work efficiently in the morning. These people get tired soon and they go to bed early. In contrast, evening types have difficulty getting up early and they feel tired in the morning; they feel fresh and energetic toward the end of the day. These people perform best in the evening and they go to sleep late and wake up late. The body temperature

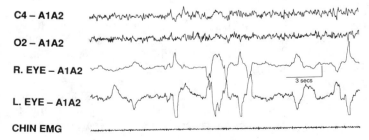

FIGURE 2-6. *REM sleep stage is shown in the PSG. EEG (top 2 channels) shows low-amplitude, mixed-frequency theta, including some alpha activity without any sleep spindles or K complexes. REMs are seen in the EOGs (third and fourth channels from above). EMG shows marked reduction or absence of tonic activities. Timer and calibration are as in Figure 2-1.*

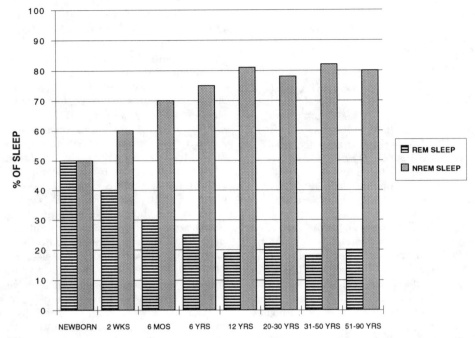

FIGURE 2-7. *Graphic representation of percentages of REM and NREM sleep in different ages. Note the dramatic changes in REM sleep in the early years. Adapted and modified from Roffwarg HP, Muzzio JN, Dement WC. Ontogenic development of the human sleep-dream cycle. Science 1966, 152 604–619.*

rhythm shows two different curves in these two types of people.[2] The body temperature reaches the evening peak an hour earlier in morning types than in evening types. What determines morning or evening type is not known but heredity may play a role.

Need for and Quantity of Sleep

The average adult's sleep requirement is about 7 to 8 hours, regardless of environmental or cultural differences.[20,23–25] Webb and Friel[26] observed that about 1.1% of college students sleep less than 5½ hours and 3.2% sleep 9½ hours.

The most important epidemiologic study to determine a relationship between the length of sleep and the health of the individual was conducted by Kripke and coworkers.[27] They found that the chances of death from coronary artery disease, cancer, or stroke are greater for those who sleep less than 4 hours or more than 9 hours than for those who sleep an average of 7 to 8 hours. No personality trait or other psychological factor has been found that might differentiate "long" or "short" sleepers from average sleepers.

Taub and Berger[28] have clearly shown that our efficiency decreases if we sleep too much. These authors have also drawn attention to the fact that

sometimes exhaustion and irritability may follow excessive sleep, which they refer to as the *Rip Van Winkle effect.*[29]

The study by Benoit and colleagues[30] showed that long sleepers spend more time asleep but have fewer stages III and IV and more stage II sleep than short sleepers.

Dream and Sleep

Humankind has been fascinated by dreams since time immemorial, and since the discovery of REM sleep by Aserinsky and Kleitman[13] dream research has taken a new direction. It is now believed that most dreams occur on awakening from REM sleep, but dreams also occur on awakening from NREM sleep.[2,20] There are some differences, however. REM sleep dreams appear to be more highly emotionally charged, complex, and bizarre, whereas NREM dreams are characterized by more realistic and rational fact. In this connection it should be remembered that, people on awakening from REM sleep are generally oriented but on awakening from NREM sleep subjects generally are somewhat disoriented and confused.

What is the significance of dreams? The most significant contemporary dream research has been

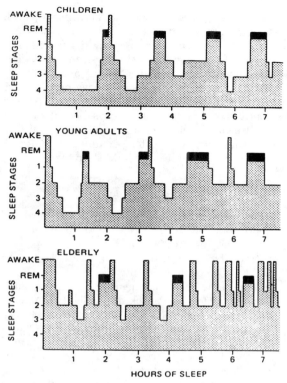

FIGURE 2-8. *Night sleep histogram from a child, a young adult, and an elderly person. Note significant reduction of stage 4 NREM sleep as one grows older. (Reproduced with permission from Kales A, Kales JD. Sleep disorders: Recent findings in the diagnosis and treatment of disturbed sleep. N Engl J Med 1974;290:487.)*

conducted by Hobson and McCarley,[31] who suggested that dreams result from activation from the neural networks in the brain. According to Koukkou and Lehmann[32] dreams result from restructuring and reinterpretation of data stored in memory. This resembles Jouvet's[33] hypothesis of REM sleep relating to recently acquired information. According to molecular biologists Crick and Mitchison,[34] the function of dream is to unlearn, that is, to remove unnecessary and useless information from the brain. In conclusion, the biologic significance of dreams at present remains unknown.

PHYLOGENY OF SLEEP

Studies have been conducted to find out if, like humans, other mammals have sleep stages.[2,35–38] The EEG recordings of mammals resemble the EEG sleep stages of humans. Similarly, both REM and NREM sleep stages can be differentiated by recording EEG, EMG, and EOG in these animals. Dolphins and Australian spiny anteaters [the monotremes, or egg-laying mammals, echidna] show no REM sleep.[2,39,40] Like humans, also, mammals can be short or long sleepers. There are considerable similarities between sleep length and length of sleep cycles in small and large animals. Small animals with a high metabolic rate have a shorter life span and sleep longer than larger animals with lower metabolic rates.[41] Similarly, smaller animals have a shorter REM-NREM cycle than larger animals.

A striking finding in dolphins is that during sleep half the brain shows the characteristic EEG features of sleep while the other half shows the EEG features of waking.[42] Each sleep episode lasts some 30 to 60 minutes, then the roles of the two halves of the brain reverse.

Both vertebrates and invertebrates display sleep and wakefulness.[43] Most animals also show the basic rest-activity rhythms during a 24-hour period.

In conclusion, the purpose of studying the phylogeny of sleep is to understand the neurophysiologic and neuroanatomic correlates of sleep as one ascends the ladder of phylogeny from inframammalian to mammalian species.

CIRCADIAN SLEEP-WAKE RHYTHM

The existence of circadian rhythms has been known since the eighteenth century, when the French astronomer de Mairan[2,44] noted in a heliotrope plant a diurnal rhythm manifested by closing of the leaves at sunset and opening at sunrise, even when the plants were kept in darkness, shielded from direct sunlight. These findings of 24-hour rhythm in the movements of plant leaves suggested to de Mairan an "internal clock" in the plant. Experiments by chronobiologists Pittendrigh[45] and Aschoff[46] clearly proved the existence of 24-hour rhythms in animals.

The term *circadian rhythm*, coined by chronobiologist Halberg[2] and coworkers, is derived from the Latin *circa*, which means *about*, and *dian*, which means *day*. Experimental isolation from all environmental time cues (German *Zeitgebers*), as in a cave or underground bunkers to study free-running rhythms in humans has clearly demonstrated the existence of a circadian rhythm independent of environmental stimuli.[2,20] This cycle lasts approximately 25 hours (range 24.7 to 25.2 hour) instead of the 24 hours of a day-night cycle.[2] Normally, environmental cues of light and darkness would synchronize or entrain the rhythms to the night-day cycle; however, the existence of environment-independent, autonomous rhythm suggests that the human body also has an internal biologic clock.[2]

The experiments in rats in 1972 by Stephan and Zucker[47] and by Moore and Eichler[48] clearly demonstrated the site of the biologic clock in the suprachiasmatic nucleus in the hypothalamus, above the optic chiasm. Experimental stimulation, ablation, and lesion of these nuclei altered circadian rhythms. The existence of the suprachiasmatic nucleus in humans was recently confirmed.[49] We do not know enough of the neuroanatomical connections, except that there is a retinohypothalamic pathway[50] that sends the environmental cues of light to the suprachiasmatic nucleus. We also do not know enough about the neurotransmitters involved in this nucleus. Daily rhythms are noted in several other human physiologic processes. Body temperature rhythm is sinusoidal; cortisol and growth hormone secretion rhythms are pulsatile.[20] It is well-known that plasma levels of prolactin, growth hormone, and testosterone are all increased during sleep at night[20] (see Chapter 5). Sleep decreases body temperature whereas activity and wakefulness increase it. It should be noted that during free-running experiments there is internal desynchronization, and body temperature rhythm dissociates from the sleep rhythm as a result of that desynchronization.[2,20] This raises the question of whether there is more than one circadian or internal clock or circadian oscillator.[2] The existence of two oscillators was postulated by Kronauer and coworkers.[51] They suggested a 25-hour rhythm for temperature, cortisol, and REM sleep and observed that the second oscillator is somewhat labile and consists of the sleep-wake rhythm. Other authors,[52] however, suggested that one oscillator could explain both phenomena. It is important to have an idea about circadian rhythms, because several sleep disturbances are related to alterations in them, such as those associated with shift work and jet lag. The circadian rhythms can be manipulated to treat certain disorders, and thus was born chronotherapy. Examples are phase advance or phase delay of sleep rhythms and application of bright light at certain periods of the evening and morning.

THE FUNCTIONS OF SLEEP

Neither humans nor animals can do without sleep, although the amount of sleep necessary to individual persons or species varies much. A lack of sleep leads to sleepiness, but we do not know the exact functions of sleep. One way to study the functions of sleep is to observe the effects of sleep deprivation. Experiments in rats using the carousel device by Rechtschaffen and coworkers[53] have provided evidence that sleep is essential for survival. All rats deprived of sleep for 10 to 30 days died after having lost weight, despite increasing their food intake. At the same time, they lost temperature control. It took longer for rats deprived of REM sleep to die.

Total Sleep Deprivation

What are the effects on physical and mental health of deprivation of NREM sleep, REM sleep, and all sleep? Sleep deprivation, whether in shift workers or in travelers who cross several time zones, impairs the ability to function optimally.

One of the early experiments in sleep deprivation was conducted by Patrick and Gilbert in 1896,[54] who studied the effects of a 90-hour period of sleep deprivation on three healthy young men. One of them reported sensory illusions, which disappeared completely when at the end of the experiment he was allowed to sleep for 10½ hours. All subjects had difficulty staying awake, but they felt totally fresh and rested after they were allowed to sleep.

A spectacular experiment in this century was conducted in 1965.[55] A 17-year-old California college student named Randy Gardner tried to set a new world record for staying awake. Dement and associates observed him during the later part of the experiment. He went 264 hours and 12 minutes without sleep and then slept 14 hours and 40 minutes. On waking, he recovered fully. Thus, the conclusion of the experiment is that it is possible to deprive people of sleep for a prolonged period without causing serious mental impairment. An important observation is the loss of performance with long sleep deprivation, and this is due to the loss of motivation—and the frequent occurrence of microsleep.

In another experiment, Johnson and MacLeod[56] showed that it is possible to intentionally reduce the total amount of sleeping time by 1 to 2 hours without suffering any adverse effect. The recent experiment by Carskadon and Dement[57,58] showed that sleep deprivation increases the daytime tendency to sleep. This has been conclusively proven by the multiple sleep latency test in such subjects.[58,59]

Following sleep deprivation during the recovery sleep period, the percentage of slow-wave sleep (stages III and IV NREM) increases considerably.[2] Similarly, after a long period of sleep deprivation, the

REM sleep percentage increases during the recovery sleep. (This increase was not shown after short period of sleep deprivation, up to 4 days.[2]) Thus, these experiments suggest that different mechanisms regulate NREM and REM sleep.[2]

Partial Sleep Deprivation

Measurements of mood and performance after partial sleep deprivation (e.g., restricting sleep to 4.5 to 5.5 hours for 2 to 3 months) showed minimal deficits in performance, which may have been related to decreased motivation. Thus, both total and partial sleep deprivation produced minimal deleterious effects in humans.[2,20,60,61]

Selective REM Sleep Deprivation

Dement[62] performed REM deprivation experiments (awakening the person for 5 minutes at the moment the polysomnographic [PSG] recording demonstrated onset of REM sleep). PSG showed increased REM pressure (i.e., earlier and more frequent onset of REM sleep during successive nights) and REM rebound (i.e., quantitative increase of REM percentage during recovery nights). These findings were subsequently replicated by Borbely[2] and others,[63,64] but Dement's third observation—a psychotic reaction following REM deprivation—proved to be inaccurate in subsequent investigations.[63]

Stage IV Sleep Deprivation

Agnew and coworkers[65] reported that following stage IV NREM sleep deprivation for two consecutive nights there was an increase in stage IV sleep during the recovery night. Two important points were raised by this groups' later experiments[64]: (1) REM rebound was more significant than stage IV rebound during recovery nights, and (2) it was more difficult to deprive a person of stage IV than of REM sleep.

It should be noted that the effects of total sleep deprivation, as well as REM sleep deprivation, are similar in animals and humans, suggesting that the sleep stages and the fundamental regulatory mechanisms for controlling sleep are also the same in all mammals.

Theories of Sleep's Function

Several theories of the functions of sleep[20] have been proposed, and these are described briefly below.

The restorative theory. Proponents of this theory[66-69] ascribed body tissue restoration to NREM and brain tissue restoration to REM sleep. The findings of increased anabolic[70-72] hormone (e.g., growth hormone, prolactin, testosterone, luteinizing hormone) secretion and decreased levels of catabolic[73] hormones (e.g., cortisol) during sleep, along with the subjective feeling of being refreshed after sleep, may support such a contention.[20] Increased slow-wave sleep[2] following sleep deprivation further supports the role of NREM sleep in restoring the body. The critical role of REM sleep for the development of the central nervous system of young organisms, and increased protein synthesis in the brain during REM sleep, are cited as evidence of restoration of brain functions by REM sleep.[74]

The Energy Conservation Theory. Zepelin and Rechtschaffen[41] found that animals with a high metabolic rate sleep longer than those with slower metabolism, suggesting that energy is conserved during sleep. Also, during sleep, metabolism in general is reduced, which helps conserve energy.

The Adaptive Theory. In both animals and humans, sleep is an adaptive behavior that allows the creature to survive under a variety of environmental conditions.[75,76]

The Instinctive Theory. This theory views sleep as an instinct,[66,77] which relates to the theory of adaptation and energy conservation.

The Theory of Memory Reinforcement and Consolidation. This theory applies particularly to REM sleep, which is thought to facilitate memory and learning. In fact, McGaugh and coworkers[78] suggested that sleep-waking-related fluctuations of hormones and neurotransmitters may be modulating memory processes. Crick and Mitchison[34] proposed that REM sleep would remove undesirable data from the memory. According to Hobson[79] these two theories are not necessarily incompatible.

Horne[80] summarized the following conclusions about the functions of sleep:

1. Sleep deprivation does not cause any permanent behavioral, psychological, or physical illnesses.
2. Contrary to the general belief, human sleep does not necessarily cause restitution. It is misleading to conclude tissue restitution increases during human sleep. Rodents may exhibit increased tissue restitution during sleep, but sleep is not the stimulus for such restitution.
3. Cerebral hemisphere is always in a state of readiness during wakefulness and cannot relax without sleep. Thus, the cerebrum needs sleep for

recovery and restitution. The human cerebrum needs a portion—not 8 hours—of sleep. He termed this portion *core* sleep, which characteristically occupies the first three sleep cycles.

4. Core sleep of Horne refers to the EEG delta activity and consists of slow-wave sleep (stages III and IV NREM sleep). This also includes REM sleep within the first three sleep cycles. Horne termed the remaining half of the REM sleep, along with the stage II sleep, *optional sleep*, which is dispensible and has a circadian rhythm. Following sleep deprivation the core sleep is restituted but the optional sleep is lost. Short sleepers have less optional sleep than core sleep. When people adapt to sleeping 5.5 to 6 hours from their normal 7 to 8 hours they do so by reducing the optional sleep.

5. Slow-wave sleep, but not REM sleep, is related to cerebral recovery.

6. There are two types of sleep*iness*, core sleepiness resulting from the loss of core sleep, which impairs cerebral functioning, and optional sleepiness secondary to the loss of optional sleep, which may affect motivation. Human sleep centers around slow-wave sleep, not REM sleep. Horne[80] further suggested that a better way to classify sleep would be as core and optional instead of REM and NREM.

7. REM sleep is not necessary for memory consolidation, and the experimental findings in animals could represent the artifacts of experiments.

REFERENCES

1. Wolpert S. A New History of India. New York: Oxford University Press, 1982;48.
2. Borbely A. Secrets of Sleep. New York: Basic Books, 1984.
3. Mazumdar S. Ramayana. Calcutta: Deva Shahittya Kutir, 1979.
4. Parkes JD. Sleep and Its Disorders. Philadelphia: WB Saunders, 1985;314.
5. Moruzzi G. The historical development of the deafferentation hypothesis of sleep. Proc Am Philosoph Soc 1964;108:19–28.
6. Hartley D. Observations on Man, His Frame, His Duty, and His Expectations. London: Leake and Frederick, 1749.
7. Macnish R. The Philosophy of Sleep. Glasgow: E M'Phun, 1830.
8. Ishimori K. True causes of sleep—a hypnogenic substance as evidenced in the brain of sleep-deprived animals. Igakkai Zasshi (Tokyo) 1909;23:429–457.
9. Legendre R, Pieron H. Recherches sur le besoin de sommeil consecutif a une veille prolongee. Z Allg Physiol 1913;14:235–262.
10. Caton R. The electric currents of the brain. Br Med J 1875;2:278.
11. Berger H. Uber das Elektroenkephalogramm des Menschen. Arch Psychiatr Nervenber 1929;87:527–570.
12. Loomis AL, Harvey EN, Hobart GA. Cerebral states during sleep, as studied by human brain potentials. J Exp Physiol 1937;21:127–144.
13. Aserinsky E, Kleitman N. Regularly occurring periods of eye motility and concomitant phenomena during sleep. Science 1953;118:273–274.
14. Rechtschaffen A, Kales A. A Manual of Standardized Terminology, Techniques and Scoring Systems for Sleep Stages of Human Subjects. Los Angeles: UCLA Brain Information Service/Brain Research Institute, 1968.
15. William RL, Agnew HW Jr, Webb WB. Sleep patterns in young adults: An EEG study. Electroencephalogr Clin Neurophysiol 1964;17:376–381.
16. Williams RL, Karacan I, Hursch CJ. Electroencephalography (EEG) of Human Sleep: Clinical Applications. New York: John Wiley, 1974.
17. Chokroverty S. Sleep and breathing in neurological disorders. In: Edelman NH, Santiago TV, eds. Breathing Disorders of Sleep. New York: Churchill Livingstone, 1986;225–264.
18. Roffwarg HP, Muzzio JN, Dement WC. Ontogenetic development of the human sleep-dream cycle. Science 1966;152:604–619.
19. Anders TF. Maturation of sleep patterns in the newborn infant. In: Weitzman ED, ed. Advances in Sleep Research. New York: Spectrum, 1975;43–66.
20. Anch AM, Browman CP, Mitler MM, et al. Sleep: A Scientific Perspective. Englewood Cliffs, NJ: Prentice Hall, 1988.
21. Metcalf DR. The effects of extrauterine experience on the ontogenesis of EEG sleep spindles. Psychosomat Med 1969;31:393–399.
22. Metcalf DR, Mondale J, Burler FK. Ontogenesis of spontaneous K complexes. Psychophysiology 1971; 8:340–347.
23. Kleitman N. Sleep and wakefulness, rev. ed. Chicago: University of Chicago Press, 1963.
24. White RM Jr. The Lengths of Sleep. Washington, DC: American Psychological Association, 1975.
25. Browman CP, Gordon GC, Tepas DI, et al. Reported sleep and drug use of workers: A preliminary report. Sleep Res 1977;6:111.
26. Webb WB, Friel J. Sleep stages and personalities characteristics of "natural" long and short sleepers. Science 1971;171:587–588.
27. Kripke DF, Simons RN, Garfinkel L, et al. Short and long sleep and sleeping pills: Is increased mortality associated? Arch Gen Psychiatr 1979;36:103–116.
28. Taub JM, Berger RJ. Effects of acute sleep pattern alteration depend upon sleep duration. Physiol Psychol 1976;4:412–420.

29. Taub JM, Berger RJ. Extended sleep and performance: The Rip Van Winkle effect. Psychonom Sci 1969;16:204–205.

30. Benoit O, Foret J, Bouard G. The time course of slow-wave sleep and REM sleep in habitual long and short sleepers: Effect of prior wakefulness. Hum Neurobiol 1983;2:91–96.

31. Hobson JA, McCarley RW. The brain as a dream state generator: An activation synthesis hypothesis of the dream process. Am J Psychiatr 1977;134:1335–1348.

32. Koukkou M, Lehmann D. Psychophysiologie des Traumens und der Neurosentherapie: Das Zustands-Wechsel-Modell, eine Synopsis. Fortschr Neurol Psychiatr 1980;48:324–450.

33. Jouvet M. Le sommeil paradoxal, est-il responsable d'une programmation genetique de cerveau? Soc Seances Soc Biol Fil 1978;172:9–30.

34. Crick F, Mitchison G. The function of dream sleep. Nature 1983;304:111–114.

35. Zepelin H. Mammalian sleep. In: Kryger MH, Roth T, Dement WC, eds. Principles and Practice of Sleep Medicine. Philadelphia: WB Saunders, 1989:30–49.

36. Tauber ES. Phylogeny of sleep. In: Weitzman ED, ed. Advances in Sleep Research, vol I, Flushing, NY: Spectrum, 1974:133–172.

37. Tobler I, Horne J. Phylogenetic approaches to the functions of sleep. In: Koella WP, ed. Sleep 1982. Basel: S Karger, 1983:126–146.

38. Tobler I. Evolution of the sleep process: A phylogenetic approach. In: Borbely AA, Valatx JL, eds. Sleep Mechanisms: Experimental Brain Research. Heidelberg: Springer-Verlag, 1984; 8 (Suppl):227–238.

39. Allison T, Van Twyver H, Goff WR. Electrophysiological studies of the echidna, *Tachyglossus aculeatus*. I. Waking and sleep. Arch Ital Biol 1972;110:145–184.

40. Mukhametov LM. Sleep in marine mammals. Exp Brain Res 1984; 8 (Suppl):227–238.

41. Zepelin H, Rechtschaffen A. Mammalian sleep, longevity and energy metabolism. Brain Behav Evol 1974;10:425–470.

42. Mukhametov LM, Supin AY, Poliakova IG. Interhemispheric asymmetry of the electroencephalographic sleep patterns in dolphins. Brain Res 1977;124:581–584.

43. Hartse KM. Sleep in insects and nonmammalian vertebrates. In: Weitzman ED, ed. Advances in Sleep Research. Flushing, NY: Spectrum, 1989;64–73.

44. de Mairan JJD. Observation Botanique. Histoire de l'Academie Royale des Sciences. Paris: Imprimerie Royale, 1731;35–36.

45. Pittendrigh CS. Circadian rhythms and the circadian organization of living systems. Cold Spring Harb Symp Quant Biol 1960;25:159–184.

46. Aschoff J. Exogenous and endogenous components in circadian rhythms. Cold Spring Harb Symp Quantit Biol 1960;25:11–28.

47. Stephan FK, Zucker I. Circadian rhythms in drinking behavior and locomotor activity of rats are eliminated by hypothalamic lesions. Proc Natl Acad Sci USA 1972;69:1583–1586.

48. Moore RY, Eichler VB. Loss of a circadian adrenal corticosterone rhythm following suprachiasmatic lesion in the rat. Brain Res 1972;42:201–206.

49. Lydic R, Schoene WC, Czeisler CA, et al. Suprachiasmatic region of the human hypothalamus: Homolog to the primate circadian pacemaker? Sleep 1980;2:355–361.

50. Moore RY, Lenn NJ. A retinohypothalamic projection in the rat. J Comp Neurol 1972;146:1–14.

51. Kronauer RE, Czeisler CA, Pilato SF, et al. Mathematical model of the human circadian system with two interacting oscillators. Am J Physiol 1982;242:R3–R17.

52. Daan S, Beersma DGM, Borbely AA. The timing of human sleep: Recovery process gated by a circadian pacemaker. Am J Physiol 1984;246:R161–R178.

53. Rechtschaffen A, Gilliland MA, Bergmann BM, et al. Physiological correlates of prolonged sleep deprivation in rats. Science 1983;221:182–184.

54. Patrick GT, Gilbert JA. On the effects of loss of sleep. Psychol Rev 1896;3:469–483.

55. Dement WC. Some Must Watch while Some Must Sleep. San Francisco: WH Freeman, 1974.

56. Johnson LC, MacLeod WL. Sleep and awake behavior during gradual sleep reduction. Percept Motor Skills 1973;36:87–97.

57. Carskadon MA, Dement WC. Effects of total sleep loss on sleep tendency. Percept Motor Skills 1979;48:495–506.

58. Carskadon MA, Dement WC. Cumulative effects of sleep restriction on daytime sleepiness. Psychophysiology 1981;18:107–113.

59. Dement WC, Carskadon MA. An essay on sleepiness. In: Baldy-Moulinier M, ed. Actualites en Medecine Experimentale, en Hommage au Professeur P Passouant. Montpellier: Euromed, 1981;47–71.

60. Webb WB, Agnew HW Jr. The effects of a chronic limitation of sleep length. Psychophysiology 1974;11:265–274.

61. Friedmann JK, Globus G, Huntley A, et al. Performance and mood during and after gradual sleep reduction. Psychophysiology 1977;14:245–250.

62. Dement W. The effect of dream deprivation. Science 1960;131:1705–1707.

63. Kales A. Hoedemaker FS, Jacobson A, et al. Dream deprivation: An experimental reappraisal. Nature 1964;204:1337–1338.

64. Agnew HW Jr, Webb WB, Williams RL. Comparison of stage 4 and 1-REM sleep deprivation. Percept Motor Skills 1967;24:851–858.

65. Agnew HW Jr, Webb WB, Williams RL. The effects of stage 4 sleep deprivation. Electroencephalogr Clin Neurophysiol 1964;17:68–70.

66. Moruzzi G. The sleep-waking cycle. Ergeb Physiol 1972;64:1–165.

67. Hartmann E. The Functions of Sleep. New Haven: Yale University Press, 1973.

68. Oswald I. Sleep. Harmondsworth, Middlesex: Penguin, 1974.

69. Adam K, Oswald I. Sleep is for tissue restoration. J R Coll Phys 1977;11:376–388.

70. Takahashi Y, Kipnis D, Daughaday W. Growth hormone secretion during sleep. J Clin Invest 1968;47:2079–2090.

71. Sassin JF, Frantz AG, Kapen S, et al. The nocturnal rise of human prolactin is dependent on sleep. J Clin Endocrinol Metab 1973;37:436–440.

72. Boyar RM, Rosenfeld RS, Kapen S, et al. Human puberty: Simultaneous augmented secretion of luteinizing hormone and testosterone during sleep. J Clin Invest 1974;54:609–618.

73. Weitzman ED, Hellman L. Temporal organization of the 24-hour pattern of the hypothalamic-pituitary axis. In: Ferin M, Halberg F, Richart RM, et al. eds. Biorhythms and Human Reproduction. New York: John Wiley, 1974; 371–395.

74. Drucker-Colin R. Protein molecules and the regulation of REM sleep: possible implications for function. In: Drucker-Colin R, Shkurovich M, Sterman MD, eds. The Functions of Sleep. New York: Academic Press, 1979; 99–112.

75. Meddis R. The Sleep Instinct. London: Routledge and Kegan Paul, 1977.

76. Webb WB, Sleep: The Gentle Tyrant. Bolton, Mass, Anker, 1992.

77. McGinty DJ, Harper TM, Fairbanks MK. Neuronal unit activity and the control of sleep states. In: Weitzman E, eds. Advances in Sleep Research, vol I. New York: Spectrum, 1974;173–212.

78. McGaugh JL, Gold PE, Van Buskirk RB, et al. Modulating influences of hormones and catecholamines on memory storage processes. In Gispen WH, van Wimersma-Gridanus TB, Bohus B, et al., eds. Hormones, Homeostasis and the Brain. Amsterdam: Elsevier, 1975;151–162.

79. Hobson JA. Sleep. New York: Scientific American Library, 1989;189–203.

80. Horne J. Why We Sleep. New York: Oxford University Press, 1988.

3

Neurophysiology of Sleep: Basic Mechanisms Underlying Control of Wakefulness and Sleep

Robert W. McCarley

This chapter presents an overview of the current state of the art of knowledge of the neurophysiology and cellular pharmacology of sleep mechanisms. This field is at the beginning of a Golden Age of learning about sleep mechanisms, owing to the capability of current cellular neurophysiologic techniques to provide focused, detailed, and replicable studies that will enrich and extend the knowledge of sleep phenomenology and pathology derived from electroencephalography (EEG) analysis. Because this chapter has a cellular and neurophysiologic focus, much of the emphasis is on mechanisms relevant to rapid eye movement (REM) sleep, because more is known about the cellular physiology and pharmacology of this state than about non-REM (NREM) sleep, though an important series of recent studies bear on the mechanisms for spindle and delta wave generation. A more detailed treatment of most of the topics outlined here is available in a recent book,[1] which also contains extensive references to the research literature. For readers interested in an update on the terminology and techniques of cellular physiology, one of the standard neurobiology texts could be consulted (e.g. Kandel and Schwartz[2]), or one of the many brief overviews (e.g. McCarley[3]; that overview also covers sleep neurophysiology, and this chapter draws from this account but also presents more recent developments). This chapter does not survey in any detail the literature on humoral factors in sleep, and the reader is referred to recent reviews.[4,5]

This chapter begins with brief and elementary overviews of sleep architecture and phylogeny/ontogeny, to provide a basis for the later mechanistic discussions. Next is a discussion of REM sleep and the relevant anatomy and physiology. Neural mechanisms of EEG desynchronization during waking and REM sleep and of spindles and delta waves during NREM sleep are treated in the final section.

SLEEP ARCHITECTURE

Sleep may be divided into two phases. *REM sleep* is most often associated with vivid dreaming and a high level of brain activity. The other phase of sleep, *NREM sleep* or slow-wave sleep, is usually associated with reduced neuronal activity; thought content during this state in humans usually is nonvisual and consists of ruminative thoughts.

As shown in Figure 3-1, as one goes to sleep the low-voltage fast EEG of waking gradually gives way to a slowing of frequency and, as sleep moves toward the deepest stages, an abundance of *delta waves*, high amplitude EEG waves with a frequency between 0.5 and 4 Hz. The first REM period usually occurs about 70 minutes after the onset of sleep. REM sleep in humans is defined by the presence of low-voltage fast EEG activity, suppression of muscle tone (usually measured in the chin muscles), and the presence, of course, of rapid eye movements. The first REM sleep episode in humans is short. After this first episode, the sleep cycle repeats itself with the appearance of NREM sleep, and then about 90 minutes after the start of the first REM period another REM episode. This rhythmic cycling persists throughout the night. The REM sleep cycle is 90 minutes long in humans, and the duration of each REM episode after the first is approximately 30 minutes. This time course is schematized in Figure 3-2, together with a representation of the intensity of REM-related neuronal activity. Over the course of the night, delta wave activity tends to diminish and NREM sleep has waves of higher frequencies and lower amplitude.

Sleep Ontogeny and Phylogeny

Periods of immobility and "rest" are present in many lower animals, including insects and lizards. Because they lack a cortical brain structure like that of

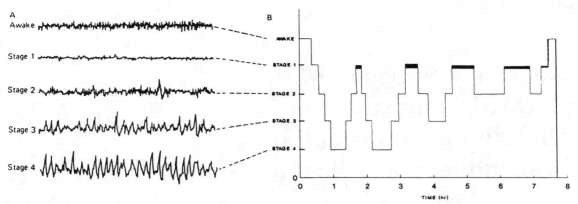

FIGURE 3-1.   (Left) *Examples of EEG patterns associated with the stages of sleep and the time course of sleep stages. During wakefulness there is a low-voltage fast EEG pattern, often with alpha waves. Stage 1 descending (i.e., occurring before deeper sleep) has a low-voltage fast EEG. As sleep deepens the EEG wave frequency slows. During stage 3, delta waves (0.5 to 4 Hz) appear, and in stage 4 they are present more than 50% of the time. Often, stages 2, 3, and 4 are lumped together as NREM sleep. Note that during REM sleep the EEG pattern returns to a low-voltage fast pattern. The percentage of time spent in REM sleep increases with successive sleep cycles, whereas the percentage of stages 3 and 4 decreases. (EEG is recorded from the vertex, Cz, and each trace is about 30 seconds long.) (Adapted from Kandel E, Schwartz JH, Jessel TM, eds. Principles of Neural Science. New York: Elsevier, 1991.)*

humans, it is difficult to say whether the absence of slow waves in these animals means they are not having the equivalent of human slow-wave sleep or whether this is present but expressed in a form not detectable with EEG recordings. REM sleep is present in all mammals except the egg-laying mammals (monotremes) such as the echidna (spiny anteater). Birds have very brief bouts of REM sleep. REM sleep cycles vary in duration according to the size of the animal, elephants having the longest cycle and

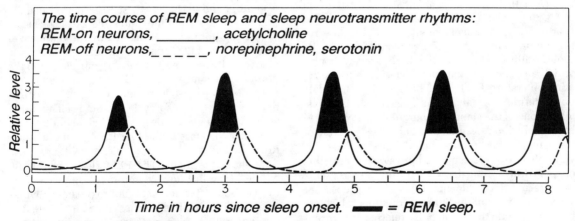

FIGURE 3-2.   *Schematic diagram of a night's course of REM sleep in humans depicts the occurrence and intensity of REM sleep as depending on the activity of populations of REM-on (REM-promoting) neurons (solid line). As the REM-on neuronal activity reaches a certain threshold, the full set of REM signs occurs (black areas under curve indicate REM sleep). Note, however, that, unlike the steplike EEG pattern of stage in Figure 3-1, the underlying neuronal activity is a continuous function. The first REM episode is of short duration and less intense because of circadian modulation of the REM sleep oscillator. As I will discuss later, the neurotransmitter acetylcholine is important in REM production, acting to excite populations of brain stem reticular formation neurons to produce the set of REM signs. Other neuronal populations, that utilize the monoamine neurotransmitters serotonin and norepinephrine, are REM-suppressive; the time course of their activity is sketched by the dotted line. These curves were generated by a mathematical model, the limit cycle reciprocal interaction model,[32] which rather accurately models the time course and percentage of REM sleep and is discussed further in the text.*

smaller animals having shorter cycles. For example, a cat's sleep cycle is approximately 22 minutes long, whereas a rat's is about 12 minutes.

In utero, mammals spend a large percentage of time in REM sleep—some 50% to 80% of a 24-hour day. At birth, animals born with an immature nervous system spend a much larger percentage of sleep time in REM sleep than adults of the same species. For example, sleep in the human newborn occupies two-thirds of any day, and REM sleep accounts for half of the total sleep time or about a third of the entire 24-hour period. The percentage of REM sleep declines rapidly during early childhood, so that by approximately age 10 years the percentage of REM sleep is the same as for adults, 20% of total sleep time. The predominance of REM sleep in young animals suggests an important function in promoting nervous system growth and development.

Delta sleep is minimally present in newborns but increases over the first years of life, reaching a maximum at about age 10 years and declining thereafter. Feinberg and coworkers[6] have noted that the first three decades of this delta-activity time course fit a gamma probability distribution and that approximately the same time course obtains for synaptic density and positron emission tomographic (PET) measurements of metabolic rate in human frontal cortex. They speculate that the reduction in these three variables may reflect a "pruning" of redundant cortical synapses, a key factor in cognitive maturation, allowing greater specialization and sustained problem solving.

REM SLEEP PHYSIOLOGY AND RELEVANT BRAIN ANATOMY: REM-PROMOTING SYSTEMS

Transection Studies

Lesion studies performed by Jouvet and coworkers in France demonstrated that the brain stem contains the neural machinery of the REM sleep rhythm. As illustrated in Figure 3-3, a transection made just above the junction of the pons and midbrain produced a state in which periodic occurrence of REM sleep was observed in recordings made in the isolated brain stem, while, in contrast, recordings in the isolated forebrain showed no signs of REM sleep. Thus, while forebrain mechanisms (including those related to circadian rhythms) modulate REM sleep, the fundamental rhythm-generating machinery is in the brain stem, and it is there that anatomic and physiologic studies have focused. The anatomic sketch provided by Figure 3-3 also shows the cell groups important in REM sleep; the reader's attention is called to the cholinergic neurons, which act as

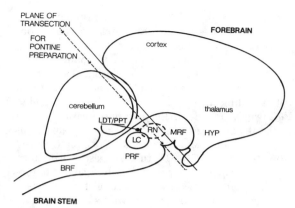

FIGURE 3-3. *Schematic diagram of a sagittal section of a cat's brain shows the plane of transection that preserves REM sleep signs caudal to the transection but abolishes them rostral to the transection. (Key: BRF, PRF, MRF, bulbar, pontine, and mesencephalic reticular formation; LDT/PPT, laterodorsal and pedunculopontine tegmental nucleus.) LDT/PPT is the principal site of cholinergic (acetylcholine-containing) neurons important for REM sleep and EEG desynchronization. (These nuclei are more extensive than indicated on this sketch — see Figure 3-6.) Key: LC, locus ceruleus, where most norepinephrine-containing neurons are located; RN, dorsal raphe nucleus, the site of serotonin-containing neurons; HYP, hypothalamus. (Adapted from McCarley RW. The biology of dreaming sleep. In: Kryger M, Roth T, Dement W, eds. Principles and Practices of Sleep Medicine. Philadelphia: WB Saunders, 1989.)*

promoters of REM phenomena, and to the monoaminergic neurons, which may act to suppress most components of REM sleep. Note that Figure 3-3 shows that the Jouvet transection spared these essential brain stem zones.

Effector Neurons for Different Components of REM Sleep Are Present Principally in Brain Stem Reticular Formation

By *effector neurons* we mean those neurons directly in the neural pathways leading to the production of different REM components, such as the rapid eye movements. A series of physiologic investigations conducted over the past three decades have shown that the "behavioral state" of REM sleep in nonhuman mammals is dissociable into different components that are under control of different mechanisms and different anatomic loci. Readers familiar with pathology associated with human REM sleep will find this concept easy to understand, as much pathology consists of inappropriate expression or suppression of individual components of REM sleep. As in humans, the cardinal signs of REM sleep in nonhuman mammals are muscle atonia. EEG desynchronization (low-voltage fast pattern), and rapid eye movements.

PGO waves are another important component of REM sleep found in recordings from deep brain structure in many animals. (They are visible in the cat recording in Figure 3-4.) PGO waves are spiky EEG waves that arise in the *pons* and are transmitted to the thalamic lateral *geniculate* nucleus (a visual system nucleus) and to the visual *occipital* cortex (thus the name *PGO*). There is suggestive evidence that PGO waves are present in humans, but the depth recordings necessary to establish their existence have not been done. PGO waves are EEG signs of neural activation; they index an important mode of brain stem activation of the forebrain during REM sleep. It is worth noting that they are also present in nonvisual thalamic nuclei, though their timing is linked to eye movements. The first wave of the usual burst of three to five waves occurs just before an eye movement.

Most of the physiologic events of REM sleep have effector neurons located in the brain stem reticular formation, with important neurons especially concentrated in the *pontine reticular formation (PRF)*. Thus, PRF neuronal recordings are of special interest because they contain information on mechanisms of production of these events. Intracellular recordings of pontine reticular formation neurons (see Figure 3-4) show that these effector neurons have relatively hyperpolarized membrane potentials and generate almost no action potentials during NREM sleep. As illustrated in Figure 3-4, PRF neurons begin to depolarize even before the first EEG sign of the

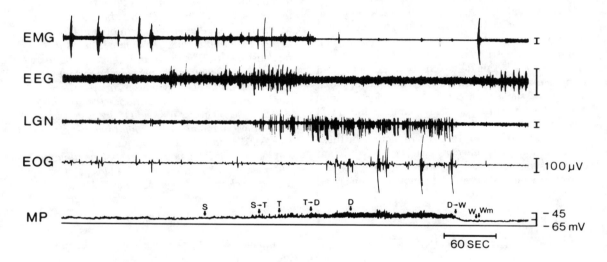

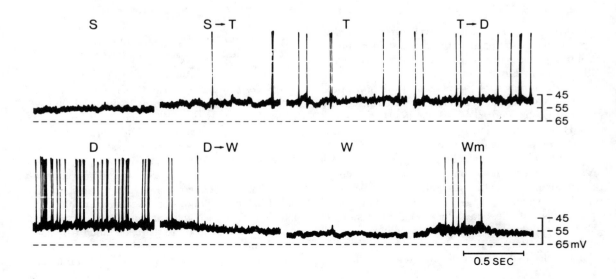

approach of REM sleep, the PGO waves that occur 30 to 60 seconds before the rest of the EEG signs of REM sleep. As PRF neuronal depolarization proceeds and the threshold for action potential is reached, these neurons begin to discharge (generate action potentials). Their discharge rate increases as REM sleep is approached, and the high level of discharge is sustained throughout REM sleep, owing to the maintenance of this membrane depolarization.

Throughout the entire REM sleep episode almost the entire population of PRF neurons remains depolarized. The resultant increased action potential activity leads to the production of those REM sleep components that have their physiologic bases in activity of pontine reticular formation neurons. Figure 3-5 provides a schematic overview of REM sleep as arising from increases in activity of the various populations of reticular formation neurons that are important as effectors of REM sleep phenomena. Pontine reticular formation neurons are important for the rapid eye movements (the generator for saccades is in PRF) and the PGO waves (a different group of neurons), and a group of dorsolateral PRF neurons controls the muscle atonia of REM sleep (these neurons become active just before the onset of muscle atonia). Neurons in midbrain reticular formation (MRF, see Figure 3-3) are especially important for EEG desynchronization, for the low-voltage fast EEG pattern. These neurons were originally described as making up the *ascending reticular activating system* (ARAS), the set of neurons responsible for EEG de-

synchronization. Subsequent work has enlarged this original ARAS concept to include cholinergic neurons, with contributions in waking to EEG desynchronization also coming from monoaminergic systems, neurons utilizing serotonin and norepinephrine as neurotransmitters.

Cholinergic Mechanisms Are Important for Initiation and Coordination of REM Sleep

Work during the last few years has led to an appreciation of the importance of the neurotransmitter acetylcholine for REM sleep. Current data suggest that cholinergic influences act by increasing the excitability of brain stem reticular neurons important as effectors in REM sleep and that cholinergic neurons may directly mediate PGO wave transmission from brain stem to forebrain. There is now rather widespread agreement among physiologists about the importance of cholinergic mechanisms, and the essential data supporting this conclusion are outlined below.

Production of a REM-like state by direct injection of acetylcholine agonists into the pontine reticular formation

It has been known since the mid-1960s that cholinergic agonist injection into the pontine reticular formation produces a state that very closely mimics natural REM sleep (for review and detailed literature citations

FIGURE 3-4. *Changes in action potential frequency and membrane potential (MP) of an intracellularly recorded medial pontine reticular formation neuron in cat over a sleep-wake cycle. The top panel is a set of inkwriter records defining behavioral state and a record of MP with action potentials filtered out. The lower panel shows cathode ray oscilloscope photographs taken at the indicated points in the inkwriter record. The record begins in waking (W): note, there is eye movement activity in the EOG record, low-voltage fast EEG activity, and transient bursts of high-amplitude activity in the EMG record indicating somatic movement. In W, the membrane potential was about − 60 mV and remained at approximately the same level with the onset of S (note EEG slow-wave activity). Postsynaptic potential (PSP) activity in S was low. Even before the onset of the first PGO wave in the lateral geniculate nucleus (LGN) record, the MP showed a gradual onset of MP depolarization. By the time of the first LGN PGO wave (labeled S-T), the PSP activity increased and there was one action potential. With the advent of more PGO waves (segment T, transition period), and the onset of REM sleep (here D, for desynchronized, or REM, sleep), there was further MP depolarization and an accompanying increase in action potentials and PSPs (bottom, T and T→D); the increase in PSPs is visible as the thickening of the inkwriter MP trace. With the onset of full REM sleep (D), and during runs of the phasic activity of PGO waves and REMs, there were storms of depolarizing PSP activity and corresponding action potentials (D). The MP remained tonically depolarized at about − 50 mV throughout REM sleep, with further phasic depolarizations. With the end of REM sleep and the onset of W (D-W), there was membrane repolarization to about the same tonic − 57-mV level seen in the initial W episode. At point Wm, there was a somatic movement that was accompanied by increased PSPs, a transient (phasic) membrane depolarization, and a burst of action potentials, before the MP returned to its baseline W polarization level. Key: EMG, nuchal electromyogram; EEG, sensorimotor cortex EEG; LGN, EEG record from lateral geniculate nucleus; EOG, electrooculogram. (Adapted from Steriade M, McCarley RW. Brainstem Control of Wakefulness and Sleep. New York: Plenum Press, 1990.)*

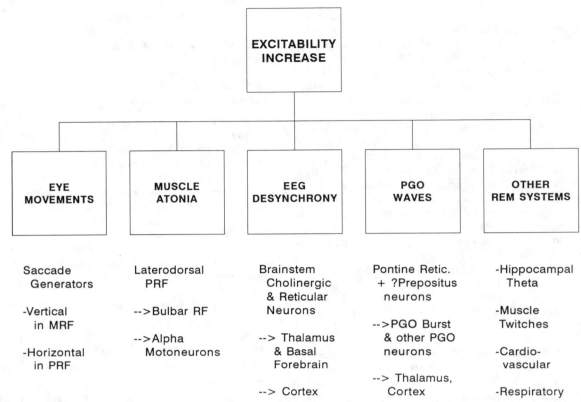

FIGURE 3-5.   *Schematic diagram of REM sleep control. Increasing the excitability (activity) of brain stem neuronal pools subserving each of the major components of the state causes the occurrence of this component. For example, the neuronal pool important for the REMs is suggested to be the brain stem saccade-generating system whose main machinery is in paramedian pontine reticular formation. Although vertical saccades are fewer in REM, their presence suggests similar involvement of the mesencephalic reticular formation. Information under the other system components sketches the major features of the anatomy and projections of neuronal pools important for muscle atonia, EEG desynchronization, and PGO waves. The last part of the diagram lists other components of REM sleep.*

for this section, see Steriade and McCarley[1]). The latency to onset and duration are dose dependent; within pontine reticular formation, most workers have found the shortest latencies to come from injections in dorsorostral pontine reticular sites, though recent work suggests a ventral site is equally effective,[7] or more so. Muscarinic cholinergic receptors appear to be of major importance; nicotinic receptors play a less important role. Thus, this series of studies suggest that cholinergic pharmacologic manipulations can produce REM sleep. The obvious follow-up question is whether cholinergic mechanisms are important in natural REM sleep. Current anatomic, lesion, and physiologic data strongly sug-

gest the answer is yes, and the next sections summarize this evidence.

LDT and PPT cholinergic projections to reticular formation neurons

Cholinergic projections in brain stem and to brain stem sites arise from two nuclei at the pons-midbrain junction that contain cholinergic neurons, the laterodorsal tegmental nucleus (LDT) and the pedunculopontine tegmental nucleus (PPT). A sagittal schematic drawing of their location in Figure 3-3, and Figure 3-6, a coronal view, shows their projections to critical pontine reticular formation zones, as first shown by Mitani and coworkers[8] and confirmed repeatedly. A recent study has found extensive LDT and PPT innervation of both pontine and bulbar reticular formation, as well as cranial nerve nuclei, by projections that are often bilateral, indicating the relatively global nature of their projection, as one would expect for pathways important in behavioral state control.[9] A similar series of studies has documented the extensive rostral projections of cholinergic neurons to thalamus and basal forebrain, where their actions are important for EEG desynchronization, a topic discussed under REM Sleep Control Model.

Direct excitation of pontine reticular formation neurons by cholinergic agonists

Injections of cholinergic agonists in vivo, have several intrinsic limitations in testing hypotheses about cholinergic effects. Fortunately, these can be overcome by use in vitro of a pontine brain stem slice preparation. This preparation allows investigators to apply agonists and antagonists in physiologic concentrations, which are usually in the low micromolar range, whereas effective in vivo injection concentrations are a thousandfold greater, in the millimolar range, and thus raise the possibility of mediation of effects by nonphysiologic mechanisms. That cholinergic excitation is effected by physiologic mechanisms is implied by experiments in vitro, where application of micromolar amounts of cholinergic agonists in vitro produces excitation of a majority (80%) of reticular formation neurons (Figure 3-7[10]). Another advantage of the in vitro preparation is the ability to use a sodium-dependent action potential blocker, tetrodotoxin; these experiments show that the excitatory effects of cholinergic agonists on PRF neurons are direct (see review in Greene and McCarley[11]). Furthermore, the depolarizing, excitatory effects of cholinergic agonists (see Figure 3-7) mimic the changes seen in PRF neurons during natural REM sleep (see Figure 3-4).

Effects of lesion

Extensive destruction of the cell bodies of LDT and PPT neurons by local injections of excitatory amino acids leads to a marked reduction of REM sleep.[12]

Discharge activity of LDT and PPT neurons over the REM cycle

A subset of these neurons has been shown to discharge selectively during REM sleep, and the onset of increased discharges precedes the onset of REM sleep[13] (see Figure 3-2). This LDT-PPT discharge pattern and the presence of excitatory projections to the PRF suggest that LDT-PPT cholinergic neurons

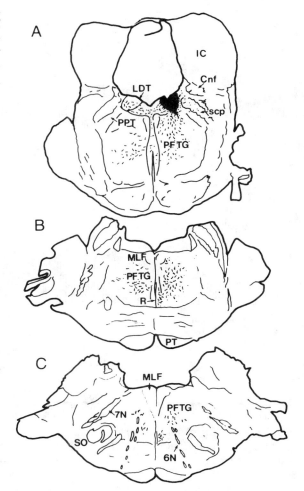

FIGURE 3-6. *(A) Frontal section of the brain stem at the pons-midbrain junction showing the location of the acetylcholine-containing neurons most important for REM sleep, those in the LDT/PPT nuclei. In this anatomic study, phaseolous leukoaglutin has been injected into the LDT; this substance is transported anterograde from LDT neuronal somata down the axons. Transport and terminal boutons are observed (A) in pontine reticular formation and (B,C) in more caudal sections. Other experiments used a combination of retrograde labeling from PRF injections with labeling for the synthetic enzyme for acetylcholine, choline acetyltransferase (ChAT), to demonstrate that LDT projections to PRF are cholinergic. Key: PFTG, giant cell portion of PRF; IC, inferior colliculus; Cnf, cuneiform nucleus; scp, superior cerebellar peduncle. (Adapted from Mitani A, Ito K, Hallanger AH, et al. Cholinergic projections from the laterodorsal and pedunculopontine tegmental nuclei to the pontine gigantocellular tegmental field in the cat. Brain Res 1988; 451:397–402.)*

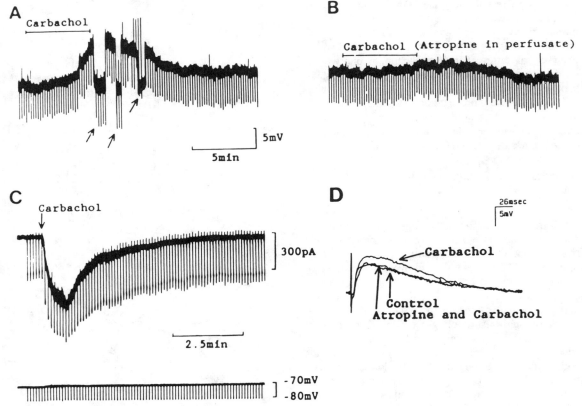

FIGURE 3-7.   *The cholinergic agonist carbachol depolarizes and increases the postsynaptic potential (PSP) responsiveness of medial PRF (mPRF) neurons recorded in vitro. (A) Chart record of a typical depolarizing response of medial PRF neuron to bath application of 0.5 μM carbachol. Downward deflections are due to intracellular current pulses (pA = picoamps) applied to assess input resistance. At arrows, membrane potential was returned to the baseline potential; the increased amplitude of voltage deflections indicates increased input resistance. (B) Atropine (0.5 μM) blocks the depolarizing response to carbachol (same neuron as in A). (C) Decreased membrane conductance during micropipette pressure application (arrow, 1 sec, 3 psi) of carbachol (1 mM) is indicated by the decreased amplitude of downward deflections in the upper current record in response to 10-mV, 400-msec membrane potential shift commands (lower record) in a neuron under voltage clamp control. (D) Three superimposed oscilloscope traces from medial PRF neuron of a PSP elicited by stimulation of the contralateral medial PRF (stimulation artifact is the first biphasic positive-negative deflection). Topmost trace made during bath perfusion with carbachol (0.5 μM), and bottom traces made during the control condition and during bath perfusion with both carbachol and atropine (0.5 μM). Note the 20% increase of PSP amplitude in the presence of carbachol compared to control and carbachol-atropine conditions. (Adapted from Greene RW, Gerber U, McCarley RW. Cholinergic activation of medial pontine reticular formation neurons in vitro. Brain Res. 1989; 476:154–159).*

may be important in producing the depolarization of reticular effector neurons, leading to production of the events that characterize REM sleep. The group of LDT-PPT and reticular formation neurons that become active in REM sleep are often referred to as *REM-on neurons*. Subgroups of PRF neurons may show discharges during waking motor activity, ei-ther somatic or oculomotor, but a sustained depolarization (see Figure 3-4) throughout almost all of the population occurs only during REM sleep.

Cholinergic neurons are important in production of the low-voltage fast or "desynchronized" EEG pattern of both REM sleep and waking

Rostral projections of another subgroup of LDT and PPT neurons are important for the EEG desynchronization of both REM sleep and waking. This topic is discussed in a later section.

Peptides "colocalized" with acetylcholine. Many peptides are colocalized with the neurotransmitter acetylcholine in LDT and PPT neurons; this colocalization likely also means they have synaptic corelease with acetylcholine. The peptide substance P is found in about 40% of LDT and PPT neurons, and, overall, more than 15 different colocalized peptides have been described. The role of these peptides in modulating acetylcholine activity relevant to wakefulness and sleep remains to be elucidated, but it should be emphasized that the colocalized vasoactive intestinal peptide (VIP) has been reported by several different investigators to enhance REM sleep when it is injected into the ventricular system.

Summary of Neurotransmitter Palette
Affecting Pontine Reticular
Formation Neurons

At this point it is useful to present a summary of the neurotransmitters that affect reticular formation neurons, which we have characterized as the "effector neurons" for REM phenomena. It is important to emphasize that these data come primarily from stud-

ies on medial PRF neurons and that other reticular neurons may have different response profiles, though there is no reason now to suspect that populations in other areas are strikingly different. It is also important to note that the list of neurotransmitters, receptor types, and ion mechanisms is incomplete.

Knowledge of neurotransmitter effects is useful not only from a basic science point of view but also in terms of predicting what kinds of effects will be produced by pharmacologic agents. Figure 3-8 summarizes effects in terms of excitation and inhibition and describes the various ion currents that mediate neurotransmitter effects. An important consideration in interpreting Figure 3-8 is that different neurons may have different sets of receptors and be involved in different behavioral systems. For example, the set of neurons that are excited in response to serotonin apparently includes a class that may mediate rapid reticulospinal excitatory responses such as those in startle and that are not so important for sleep. For the neurons that are important in REM sleep, it is a reasonable first approximation to predict that pharmacologic agents that excite will promote REM sleep phenomena while those that inhibit will have the opposite effect. This is clearest with cholinergic compounds, which have excitatory actions on about 80% of PRF neurons; this 80% includes those important in REM sleep. This

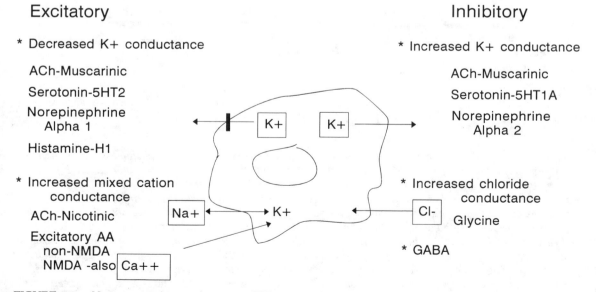

FIGURE 3-8. *Neurotransmitter actions on mPRF neurons in vitro.*

figure is based on work, too extensive to cite here, of members of the Harvard-Brockton group, including Greene, Stevens, Gerber, Haas, Luebke, Birnstiel, and myself. (Recent papers by Stevens[14] and Gerber[15] and their respective coworkers, as well as the Steriade and McCarley book,[1] provide pointers to the literature.)

Muscle Atonia

Muscle atonia is an important REM feature from a clinical point of view, because disorders of this system are present in many patients who present to sleep disorders clinicians. We shall consider three important zones for atonia, which we list according to their projections (as indicated by arrows):

pontine reticular formation → bulbar reticular formation → motoneurons.

Motoneurons

The target of the muscle inhibition system is the alpha motoneuron. REM sleep effects on motoneurons have been principally investigated at the cellular level by Chase and coworkers,[16-18] both in trigeminal motoneurons and spinal alpha motoneurons. Figure 3-9 illustrates the phenomenon

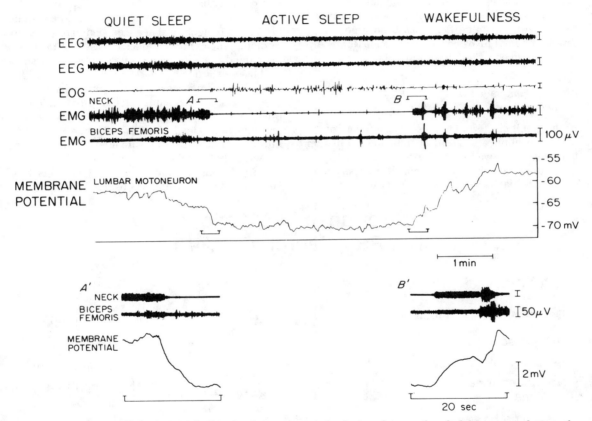

FIGURE 3-9.   *Intracellular record from a lumbar motoneuron during sleep and wakefulness: correlation of membrane potential and behavioral state. This figure highlights the membrane hyperpolarization that accompanies active (REM) sleep. Hyperpolarization commenced prior to the cessation of muscle tone, which was accompanied by a further and rather sharp increase in membrane polarization A, and shown oscilloscopically at higher gain and expanded time base in A'. At the termination of active sleep the membrane depolarized coincident with the resumption of muscle tone and behavioral awakening (B,B';). Note the brief periods of depolarization during active sleep and wakefulness, which were accompanied by phasic increases in muscle activity (i.e., muscle twitches during active sleep and leg movement during wakefulness). Spike potentials often occurred during these periods of depolarization but are not evident in this high frequency–filtered record. The first and second polygraph traces are those of EEG activity recorded from left and right frontal-parietal cortex, respectively. (Adapted from Morales FR, Chase MH. Intracellular recording of lumbar motoneuron membrane potential during sleep and wakefulness. Exp Neurol 1978; 62:821–827.)*

of membrane hyperpolarization of motoneurons that accompanies REM sleep. Morales and Chase[16,17] recorded antidromically identified lumbar motoneurons in naturally sleeping cats using the chronic intracellular recording techniques pioneered by them. Mean resting potential in waking (W) was −65 mV, and there was a slight hyperpolarization from active W to slow-wave sleep. During the passage from slow wave sleep to REM there was marked membrane hyperpolarization, averaging 6.7 mV (range 4 to 10 mV); this hyperpolarization was temporally coincident with the loss of nuchal EMG activity. On transition to W, the level of polarization decreased. Chase and colleagues[18] found that the microiontophoretic application of strychnine (but not picrotoxin or bicuculline) onto lumbar motoneurons was effective in abolishing the large-amplitude spontaneous inhibitory postsynaptic potentials IPSPs of REM sleep, suggesting that glycine is the principal neurotransmitter mediating these potentials in lumbar motoneurons. Other data suggest that the projections providing this inhibitory input ultimately arise from the bulbar reticular formation, with perhaps an intermediate synapse in spinal cord.

Pontine reticular formation and bulbar reticular formation.

Jouvet and colleagues in Lyon, France reported that bilateral lesions of the pontine reticular region just ventral to the locus ceruleus (LC), termed by this group the *peri-LC alpha*, and its descending pathway to the bulbar reticular formation abolished the muscle atonia of REM sleep (Figure 3-10[19,20]). It is to be emphasized that this zone is a reticular zone, not one containing noradrenergic neurons like the LC proper, and that the name refers only to proximity to the LC. The Lyon group also reported that not only was the nuchal muscle atonia of REM suppressed, but that cats so lesioned exhibited "oneiric behavior," including locomotion, attack behavior, and behavior with head raised and with horizontal and vertical movements "as if watching something." Morrison and collaborators[21] confirmed the basic

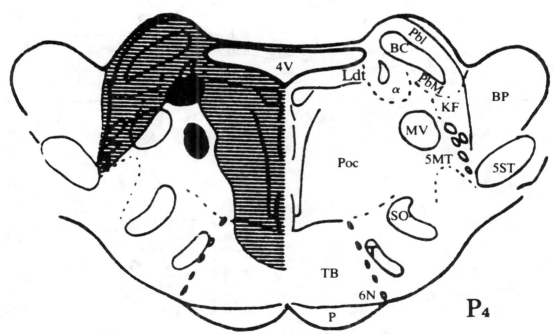

FIGURE 3-10. *Frontal section of the pons of the cat. The solid areas indicate the localization of the lesions, which, according to Jouvet and coworkers, suppress postural atonia during REM. These lesions coincide with the reticular formation zone termed locus ceruleus alpha (α) or its descending pathway. The horizontal hatching corresponds to lesions that do not suppress postural atonia. Key: Pbl, n. parabrachialis lateralis; Ldt, n. lateralis tegmenti dorsalis; PbM, n. parabrachialis medialis; KF, n. Kolliker-Fuse; Poc, n. pontis caudalis; BP, brachium pontis; MV and 5MT, motor nucleus and mesencephalic tract of trigeminal nerve; 5ST, sensory nucleus of trigeminal nerve; BC, brachium conjunctivum; 4V, fourth ventricle. (Reprinted from Jouvet M. What does a cat dream about? Trends Neurosci 1979; 2:15–16, with permission).*

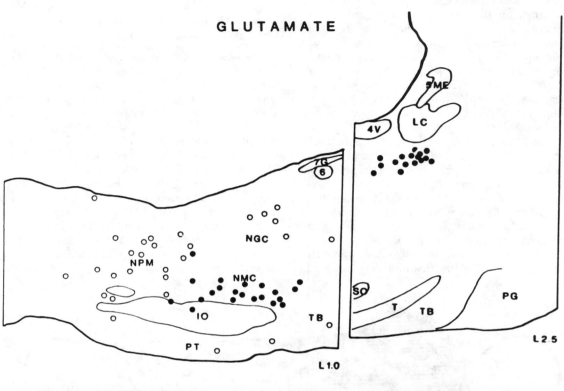

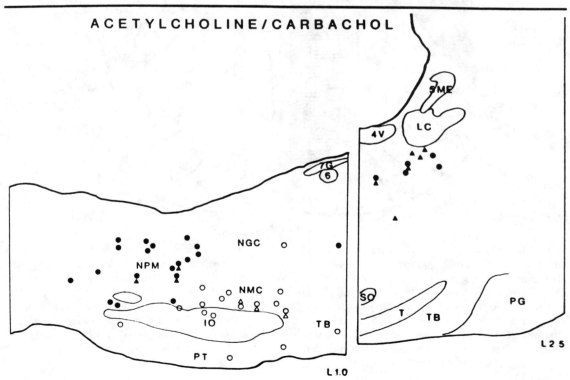

finding of REM without atonia with bilateral pontine tegmental lesions but report that lesions extending beyond the LC alpha region and its efferent pathway to bulb were necessary for more than a minimal release of muscle tone and to produce the elaborate oneiric behaviors. They found particular lesion locations were associated with particular sets of behaviors (e.g., attack behavior with lesions that extended into midbrain and interrupted amygdalar pathways, locomotion with lesions near the brainstem stem locomotor region, and orienting-like behavior with small, symmetric dorsolateral pontine lesions). Finally, the presence of attack and locomotion behaviors in REM without atonia was reported to be associated with an increased incidence of these behaviors during wakefulness, leading to the inference that the lesions may have done more than simply counteract behaviorally nonspecific muscle inhibition during REM: they may have released the particular behaviors appearing during both REM and wakefulness. Still another zone of neurons and neuronal projection pathways associated with muscle suppression has been reported to be in the midline (Ohta and coworkers).[22] The exact location and numbers of inhibitory pathways are still matters of some controversy, though all investigators agree on the important, if not exclusive, role of the peri-LC alpha, or, as it is often termed, *the dorsolateral small cell reticular group.*

An overview of reticular areas important in muscle atonia, and evidence about important neurotransmitters is provided by Figure 3-11,[23] which shows sites where in decerebrate cats, injection of glutamate or cholinergic agonists induced atonia. The strong data implicating acetylcholine in REM phenomena were described above. Precise in vitro evidence for glutamatergic reticular formation neurotransmission has been obtained by the Brockton group.[24] Lai and Siegel[25] recently obtained evidence that the glutamate effective sites show muscle atonia to non–N-methyl-d-aspartate (NMDA) agonists, whereas NMDA agonists produced increased muscle tone and locomotion, suggesting that REM-related activation and inhibition of muscle activity might be mediated by different receptors responding to glutamate.

REM SLEEP PHYSIOLOGY AND RELEVANT BRAIN ANATOMY: REM-SUPPRESSING SYSTEMS

We have defined *REM-on neurons* as those that become active during REM sleep, as opposed to slow-wave sleep or waking, and that presumably have a protagonist role in production of REM sleep phenomena. Neurons with reciprocal discharge time course that become inactive as REM sleep is approached and entered are called *REM-off neurons* (see schematic of discharge time course in Figure 3-2). REM-off neurons are most active during wakefulness, have discharge activity that declines in slow-wave sleep, and are virtually silent in REM until they resume discharge toward the later portion of the REM sleep episode. Electrophysiologic data suggest REM-off neurons include the following classes of aminergic neurons (see Figure 3-3 for anatomy): (1) *Norepinephrine-containing neurons* are located principally in the LC, called the *blue spot* because of its appearance in unstained brain tissue (first demonstrated to be REM-off by Hobson and associates.[26] (2) *Serotonin-containing neurons* are located in the *raphe system* of the brainstem, the midline collection of neurons that extends from the bulb to the midbrain, and are present in higher concentrations in the more rostrad neurons (REM-off neurons in the dorsal raphe, the midbrain nucleus, were first recorded by McGinty and Harper[27]). (3) *Histamine-containing neurons* are located in the posterior hypothalamus, and recording experiments suggest they are REM-off (see English summary in Lin and colleagues[28]). This histaminergic system has been conceptualized as one of the wakefulness-promoting systems; antihistamines, it will be noted, have drowsiness as a common side effect. Transection studies indicate, however, that the histaminergic neurons are not essential for the REM sleep oscillation.[29]

A strikingly inverse time course over the REM sleep cycle between PGO-wave activity and the discharge activity of dorsal raphe neurons (presumptively serotonergic) has been demonstrated by Lydic and colleagues.[30] A similar inverse pattern of activity

FIGURE 3-11.   *Pontobulbar inhibitory areas on sagittal section. In decerebrate cats, electrical stimulation produced atonia at all indicated points. Filled symbols indicate points where muscle atonia was produced by injections of glutamate (top, 0.2 M) or cholinergic agonists (bottom, either 1.1 M acetylcholine [circles] or 0.01 M carbachol- [triangles]). Key: open symbols, no effect; IO, inferior olive; LC, locus ceruleus; 7G & 6, genu of 7th nerve and 6th nucleus; NGC, bulbar nucleus gigantocellularis, NMC, nucleus magnocellularis; NPM, nucleus paramedianus; PG, pontine gray; PT, pyramidal tract; SO, superior olivary nucleus; TB, trapezoid body; Adapted from Lai YY, Siegel JM. Medullary regions mediating atonia. J. Neurosci 1988; 8:4790–4796.)*

of REM-off neurons in the LC with REM-on neurons led to the hypothesis that REM-off neurons may be REM suppressive and interact with REM-on neurons to control the REM sleep cycle, a topic discussed in the next section.

REM SLEEP CONTROL MODEL: INTERACTION OF REM-OFF AND REM-ON NEURONS

In 1975, McCarley and Hobson[31] hypothesized that the REM sleep cycle rhythm resulted from interaction of REM-on and REM-off neurons, and presented a mathematical and structural model based on this hypothesis, termed the *reciprocal interaction model*. A mathematically more sophisticated version[32] rather accurately predicted the timing and amount of REM sleep in a human's night's sleep and its variation with the circadian temperature rhythm. That is the basis for the time course curves of Figure 3-2. A more extensive presentation of this model is in Chapter 12 of the book by Steriade and McCarley. Here I provide an overview of my current version of this model (Figure 3-12).

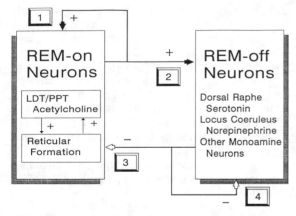

FIGURE 3-12.   *Reciprocal interaction model of REM sleep control. Cholinergic neurons activate reticular formation neurons in a positive-feedback interaction to produce the onset of REM sleep. REM sleep is terminated by the inhibitory activity of REM-off aminergic neurons (right box), which become active at the end of a REM sleep period owing to their recruitment by REM-on activity. REM-off neuronal activity decreases in slow-wave sleep and becomes minimal at the onset of REM sleep owing to self-inhibitory feedback. This decreased REM-off activity disinhibits REM-on neurons and allows the onset of a REM sleep episode. The cycle then repeats itself.*

A simplified verbal account of the model's dynamics is: REM-on, REM-promoting, neurons in the cholinergic mesopontine nuclei LDT and PPT activate reticular formation effector neurons in a positive-feedback interaction (Figure 3-12, label 1) to produce the onset of REM sleep. This also slowly excites (Figure 3-12, label 2) REM-off, REM-suppressive neurons in the dorsal raphe and LC (Figure 3-12, right box). As the REM-off neurons become active at the end of a REM sleep period owing to recruitment by REM-on activity, they terminate REM sleep by inhibiting REM-on neurons (Figure 3-12, label 3). REM-off neuron activity is maximal just after REM sleep and then decreases in the following NREM period and becomes minimal at the onset of REM sleep, owing to self-inhibitory feedback (Figure 3-12, label 4). This decreased REM-off activity disinhibits REM-on neurons and allows the onset of a REM sleep episode. The cycle then repeats itself.

The label numbers in Figure 3-12 provide a useful guide for discussion of the evidence bearing on each of its postulates.

1. Positive feedback of REM-on neurons.   Reticular neurons have excitatory interconnections (reviewed in reference[1]). Within the REM-on neuronal box is sketched a further positive-feedback interconnection between cholinergic and reticular neurons. In this chapter I have already reviewed data supporting projections from the LDT and PPT to pontine reticular formation and the predominantly excitatory effect of cholinergic agonists. Preliminary data in vitro indicate excitatory effects of the excitatory amino acids (EAAs) on LDT and PPT neurons,[33,34] and there is strong evidence that EAAs are the principal excitatory transmitter of RF.[24] Indirect evidence of RF excitation of LDT and PPT is provided by the data of Lydic and coworkers,[35] indicating that excitation of RF neurons increases the release of brain stem acetylcholine, presumably from LDT and PPT. It is of interest that cholinergic LDT and PPT neurons are inhibited by cholinergic agonists[36,37]; thus, the population coupling for the positive feedback has to be through other connections, and the latest version of the model suggests it is through reticular neurons.

2. Excitation of REM-off neurons by REM-on neurons. There is anatomic evidence (reviewed in references 1 and 38) for cholinergic projections to both LC and dorsal raphe. In vivo data indicate excitatory effects of acetylcholine on LC neurons, but new data from my laboratory do not indicate such clear excitatory effects on dorsal raphe (Birnstiel, personal communication). There is evidence in vitro for EAA excitatory effects on both LC and dorsal raphe neurons, and anatomic data[39] suggest that brain stem RF neurons may be the source of much of this input.

3. Inhibition of REM-on neurons by REM-off neurons. For many years, this aspect of the reciprocal interaction model has been the most controversial, since the indirect evidence from data in vivo, though generally supportive, was subject to alternative explanations. (An example of the supporting data in vivo is the production of REM sleep from cooling (inactivating) the dorsal raphe and LC, nuclei where REM-off neurons are found.[40,41]) New data in vitro[42] provide important direct evidence that most cholinergic neurons in the LDT are inhibited by serotonin. LDT neurons are inhibited by serotonin (Figure 3-13).

Inhibition is especially consistent for the population of LDT neurons that fire in bursts; such burst firing has been shown in extracellular recordings in vivo to be tightly correlated with lateral geniculate nucleus PGO waves, which other data indicate are cholinergically mediated. The action potential burst itself is caused by a particular calcium current, the *low-threshold spike (LTS)*, which provides sufficient calcium influx for depolarization to a level that produces a burst of sodium-dependent action potentials. Some nonburst cholinergic neurons are also hyperpolarized by serotonin. Effects of norepinephrine on LDT and PPT are currently under investigation, and preliminary data suggest this substance is also inhibitory to cholinergic neurons.

4. Inhibitory feedback of REM-off neurons. There is strong in vitro physiologic evidence that norepinephrine inhibits LC neurons and serotonin inhibits DR neurons, and anatomic studies indicate the presence of recurrent collaterals (review reference in 1). These recurrent collaterals, which have been demonstrated to be inhibitory, could be the source of suppression of raphe activity, the prolonged silence during REM resulting from long duration neurotransmitter effects, perhaps from coupling with second or third messengers. However, there may be an unconventional mode of serotonin release during REM sleep that leads to increased extracellular serotonin and thus to inhibition. In vivo voltammetry data from Cespuglio and coworkers in the Jouvet laboratory[43] suggest that, even though action potential activity in dorsal raphe neurons during REM

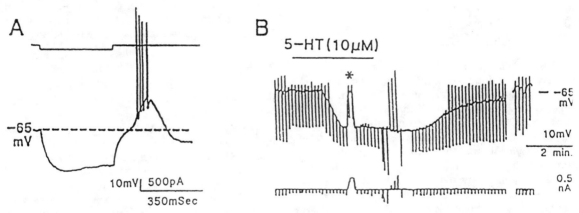

FIGURE 3-13.   *Serotonin (5-HT) inhibits cholinergic low-threshold burst neurons in the laterodorsal tegmental nucleus. Intracellular recordings from in rat in vitro preparation. (A) With the membrane potential held at −65 mV, a hyperpolarizing current step results in a rebound low-threshold burst, the likely mechanism for the production of bursts seen in extracellular recordings of PGO burst neurons in vivo (see text). (B) Application of 10 μM (5-HT) to a cholinergic bursting neuron results in a hyperpolarization of the membrane potential (top trace), a response that other experiments showed persisted in the presence of tetrodotoxin, indicating the inhibition was a direct serotoninergic effect. The voltage deflections in the top trace are responses to constant current pulses used to measure input resistance; repolarization of the membrane to resting levels (at asterisk) demonstrated a decrease in input resistance that was independent of the change in membrane potential, and thus was due to a direct drug action. The same current that was effective in producing a burst in A did not result in a burst during the application of 5-HT (not shown in this figure). Other experiments indicated a 5-HT1A receptor mediated these effects. (Modified from Luebke JI, Greene RW, Semba K, et al. Serotonin hyperpolarizes cholinergic low threshold burst neurons in the rat laterodorsal tegmental nucleus in vitro. Proc Natl Acad Sci USA 1992; 89:743–747.)*

sleep is low, the levels of serotonin metabolites increase. This suggests release of serotonin not coupled with soma depolarization. While this might be viewed as a highly improbable mechanism, Pan and Williams[44] have obtained in vitro data compatible with such an unconventional release of serotonin in dorsal raphe neurons. However, recent in vivo microdialysis data from Portas and McCarley indicate that the extracellular concentration of serotonin in the dorsal raphe parallels that of neuronal discharge: W > non-REM > REM.

In summary, the basic structure of the reciprocal interaction model, as described in 1986,[32] still appears to be plausible, although it remains a model in need of empirical verification. The major experimental advances of the past 5 years have been the recognition of the importance of acetylcholine and the very recent documentation of serotoninergic inhibition of cholinergic neurons. Several important areas for future physiologic investigation include the mechanisms of coupling between circadian and REM sleep control systems and the mechanisms of REM sleep rebound.

IMPORTANCE OF CHOLINERGIC ACTIVITY IN SUPPRESSION OF EEG SYNCHRONIZATION AND OF SLOW-WAVE ACTIVITY

One of the major recent advances has been the growing understanding of the importance of a cholinergic activating system in EEG desynchronization. This is likely a major component of the ARAS, a concept that arose before methods were available for labeling of neurons by specific neurotransmitters. We now know that a subset of the cholinergic LDT-PPT neurons has high discharge rates during waking and REM sleep and low discharge rates during slow-wave sleep; this group is anatomically interspersed with the physiologically distinct REM-selective cholinergic neurons (see review in reference 1). There is also extensive anatomic evidence that these cholinergic neurons project to thalamic nuclei important in EEG desynchronization and synchronization. Neurophysiologic studies in vivo and in vitro have indicated that the target neurons in the thalamus respond to cholinergic agonists in a way consistent with EEG activation; this is detailed below.

Cholinergic systems are not the only substrate of EEG desynchronization; brain stem reticular formation projections to thalamus (utilizing EAA) may also play an important role, and norepinephrine projections from LC may be relevant during wakefulness (LC neurons are silent in REM sleep). In addition to brain stem cholinergic systems, cholinergic input to

thalamus from the basal forebrain cholinergic nucleus basalis of Meynert is also important for EEG desynchronization.

Slow-Wave Sleep at the Cellular Level in the Thalamus: The "Burst Mode" of Relay Cell Discharge and Failure of Information Transmission

Extracellular recordings by myself and coworkers[45] demonstrated that dorsal lateral geniculate relay neurons discharged in stereotyped bursts during non-REM sleep but not during wakefulness or REM. Intracellular investigations in vivo[46] and in vitro[47] indicate the bursting occurs on a background of membrane hyperpolarization. This hyperpolarization removes the inactivation of particular Ca^{++} channels and enables the production of a "low-threshold calcium spike" (LTS) and a burst of sodium-mediated action potentials, as discussed above for LDT neurons. Cholinergic input from LDT and PPT abolishes the burst mode: the relay neuron is depolarized by a muscarinically mediated reduction of a potassium current while the hyperpolarizing GABA-ergic influence of interneurons is lessened by muscarinically mediated hyperpolarization of the interneuron. The net result of relay neuron depolarization is to inactivate the LTS and to permit faithful following of high-frequency retinal input.

Spindles

Spindles occur during stage two of human sleep and in the light slow-wave sleep phase of animals; they are composed of waves of approximately 10 to 12 Hz frequency whose amplitudes waxes and wanes over the spindle duration of 1 to 2 seconds. Wave frequency varies with species and is higher in primates. Spindles are relatively well-understood at the cellular level. Studies by Steriade and coworkers (reviewed in reference 1) indicate spindle waves arise as the result of interactions of spindle pacemaker GABA-ergic thalamic nucleus reticularis (RE) neurons and thalamocortical neurons. Spindle waves are blocked by cholinergic brain stem–thalamus projections, which act to hyperpolarize the RE neurons, likely through a muscarinically mediated potassium conductance increase. The forebrain nucleus basalis also provides cholinergic and hyperpolarizing GABA-ergic input to RE that assists brain stem input in disrupting the spindles.

Delta EEG Activity

The cellular basis of delta waves (between 0.5 and 4 Hz) is now an area of intensive investigation. Figure 3-14 is a schematic drawing of mechanisms proposed

Model for Generation of Delta Waves by Thalamocortical Neurons
"Rhythmic Burst Mode", Hyperpolarized Membrane Potential (MP)

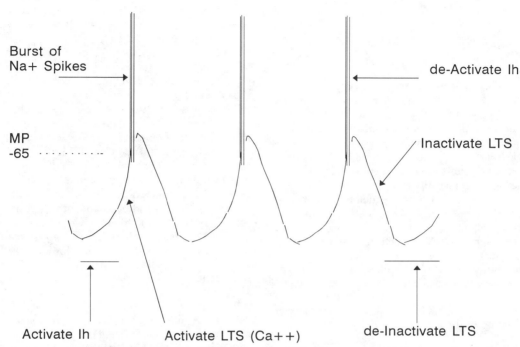

FIGURE 3-14. *Schematic drawing of mechanisms proposed for generation of delta waves by thalamocortical neurons. The sequence of events is as follows: As the membrane becomes hyperpolarized a particular cation current, Ih, is activated. The in rush of positive ions depolarizes the neuron to the point where another current, the low-threshold spike (LTS) current, a calcium-dependent current, is activated. (This current and burst of action potentials is like that shown for the LDT low-threshold burst neuron in Figure 3-13.) The in rush of calcium further depolarizes the neuron, to the point where the firing threshold of the sodium action potential is crossed. As sketched in the right portion of the figure, Ih is deactivated at depolarized potentials and, with a slower time course, the LTS current gates are inactivated. Once the neuron's MP is hyperpolarized, the inactivation of the LTS is removed and the MP is set for the next cycle of oscillation. The time course of activation, deactivation, inactivation, and deinactivation, as well as the time course of thalamocortical population interactions determine the timing of this rhythm. Many aspects of this process, especially the interaction of thalamocortical neuronal populations, remain to be determined, but the necessity of a hyperpolarized membrane potential in both cortical and thalamocortical neurons if delta waves are to occur seems firmly established. This figure and the mechanisms described are based on in vitro data of McCormick and Pape[47,50] and in vivo data of Steriade and coworkers.[48]*

for generation of delta waves by thalamocortical neurons. This sketch portrays intracellularly recorded events in a thalamocortical neuron during delta wave generation and is based on studies in vivo by Steriade and associates[48] and work in vitro by McCormick and Pape.[47] The basic concept is that a hyperpolarized membrane potential permits the occurrence of delta waves in thalamocortical circuits. Any factors that depolarize the membrane block delta waves. During waking input, the cholinergic forebrain nucleus basalis is important for suppression of slow-wave activity, as shown by lesion studies.[49] Also, brain stem norepi-

nephrinergic and serotonergic projections may disrupt delta activity[50] in waking, although they are inactive during REM sleep. During REM sleep, cholinergic input from brain stem is a major factor in producing membrane depolarization; reticular formation input, likely utilizing EAA neurotransmission, also plays an important role. This membrane depolarization leads to suppression of delta wave activity. Thus, delta waves during sleep may be seen to represent oscillations occurring in the absence of activating inputs. From the standpoint of the cellular physiologist, the relative intensity of cortical desynchronization correlates well with the intensity of cholinergic input to thalamus; conversely, the relative intensity of cortical synchronization, including delta waves, correlates well with the relative absence of cholinergic activity.

CONSEQUENCES OF REM SLEEP: FUNCTIONAL QUESTIONS

Perhaps the major unanswered question in sleep research is the function(s) of sleep. There are many plausible theories about, for example, REM sleep. Its prominence in the developing animal implies a possible functional role in promoting development. A reasonable extension postulates that REM sleep "exercises" neural circuits in adults, keeping functionally fit the many neural pathways heavily encephalized higher animals do not use on a regular basis. However, we would suggest that, without the development of knowledge about the deeper consequences of REM sleep for neuronal biology, such theories will remain speculative.

The consequences of REM-like states for cellular biology are now beginning to be explored, and the effect of these states on immediate early genes is now a topic of considerable interest. I first present a brief introduction to the topic.

Immediate Early Genes

Neurotransmitters may activate mechanisms that regulate the transcription of DNA, the genetic material. The induction of the immediate early genes (IEG), such as c-*fos* and *jun*, is one example of this mechanism. The term *fos* was first used to describe the oncogene (cancer gene) encoded by the Finkel-Biskis-Jenkins murine osteogenic sarcoma virus. The normal cellular sequences from which the viral oncogene (v-*fos*) was derived are referred to as the *fos* proto-oncogene or c-*fos*. In normal cells the level of the protein product of the c-*fos* gene, Fos, is highly regulated; many stimuli, some associated with cellular differentiation and some linked with neuronal excitation, lead to transient induction of c-*fos* mRNA. The name for the immediate early gene, *jun*, was derived in similar fashion from the oncogene carried by the avian sarcoma virus ASV17; *ju-nana* is Japanese for *seventeen*. An extensive recent discussion of stimulus-transcription coupling can be found in Morgan and Curran.[51] Schematically, with successive steps in the cascade indicated by arrows:

Neurotransmitter/binding at receptors
- → change in second messenger levels
- → induction of transcription of the genes c-*fos* and *jun*
- → c-*fos* and *jun* mRNAs present in cytoplasm for 1 to 2 hours
- → translation of Fos and Jun proteins
- → possible alterations in posttranslational modification (e.g., phosphorylation) of Fos by stimuli
- → translocation to nucleus and formation of a Fox/Jun dimer (Fos half-life about 2 hours)
- → Fos/Jun dimer complex binds to DNA regulatory element (*AP1* site)
- → increase in transcription of DNA
- → increase in production of a particular protein

This area is one of intensive current work, and thus of much flux in defining (1) which neurotransmitters and stimuli lead to the IEG production and (2) which proteins are regulated by this transcriptional control (a much more difficult question).

Neurotransmitters and receptors reported to modulate c-*fos* expression include EAAs (especially NMDA but also kainate), dopamine, opioids, cholecystokinin, progesterone, interleukin 1, and nicotine. Stimuli and conditions known to activate c-*fos* include heat shock, dehydration, electrical stimulation, seizures (especially in hippocampus), manipulation of internal calcium concentration, treadmill locomotion, and stimulation with light (for further information see, for example, the list of published studies furnished by Morgan and Curran[51]). While this list is long, it should not be assumed that all cellular activation leads to c-*fos* production and that c-*fos* production is nonspecific.

There appears to be relatively specific production of c-*fos* in the hypothalamic suprachiasmatic nucleus (SCN). The SCN contains the basic mechanisms of the circadian clock, which regulates the circadian oscillations of many body systems, including temperature and sleep. This clock may be reset to an earlier time (this kind of reset is called *phase advancing*) in response to a light stimulus applied just before the expected onset of light in the environment. Several groups of investigators have found that light stimuli applied at this time—but not at other times that do not induce the same phase reset — have the capability of inducing c-*fos*. While it has been hypothesized that the transcriptional regulation of DNA is important in resetting the circadian clock, this has not yet been proven.

The induction of immediate early genes may be very important for REM sleep function, since this process may mediate long-term alterations. Initial studies[52] have used as a model cholinergic induction of a REM-like state. Compared with vehicle control, induction of REM-like state by carbachol microinjections in the medial PRF led to a marked increase in Fos-like immunoreactivity (Fos-LI) in cells in several brain stem areas thought to be important in REM sleep. Longer REM-like episodes were associated with more Fos-LI cells than the shorter-lived ones. Fos-LI increases were found in the lateral dorsal tegmental (LDT) and pedunculopontine tegmental

(PPT) nuclei, where some Fos-LI cells were immunohistochemically identified as cholinergic; the LC, where some of the Fos-LI cells were identified to be catecholaminergic; the dorsal raphe; and the pontine reticular formation. These findings suggest immediate early gene activation is associated with the carbachol-induced REM-like sleep state. More studies are needed to explore the induction of other IEGs and the association of IEG induction with natural REM sleep. This line of investigation, while in its infancy, appears to offer the potential of answering questions about the functional consequences of REM sleep.

REFERENCES

1. Steriade M, McCarley RW. Brainstem Control of Wakefulness and Sleep. New York: Plenum, 1990.
2. Kandel E, Schwartz JH, Jessel TM, eds. Principles of Neural Science. New York: Elsevier, 1991.
3. McCarley RW. Human electrophysiology: Basic cellular mechanisms and control of wakefulness and sleep. In Yudofsky S, ed. Handbook of Neuropsychiatry. New York: American Psychiatric Press, 1992.
4. Borbely AA, Tobler I. Endogenous sleep-promoting substances and sleep regulation. Physiol Rev 1989;69:605–70.
5. Krueger JM. Somnogenic activity of immune response modifiers. Trends Pharmacol Sci 1990; 11:122–126.
6. Feinberg I, Thode HC, Chugani HT, et al. Gamma function describes maturational curves for delta wave amplitude, cortial metabolic rate and synaptic density. J Theoret Biol 1990;142:149–161.
7. Reinoso-Suarez F, Rodrigo-Angulo ML, Rodriquez-Veiga E, et al. Thalamic connections of the oral pontinetegmentum sites whose cholinergic stimulation produces enhancement of paradoxical sleep signs. In: Mancia M, Marini G, eds. The Diencephalon and Sleep. New York: Raven, 1990.
8. Mitani A, Ito K, Hallanger AH, et al. Cholinergic projections from the laterodorsal and pedunculopontine tegmental nuclei to the pontine gigantocellular tegmental field in the cat. Brain Res 1988;451:397–402
9. Yanagihara M, Ito K, Dauphin L, et al. Multiple brainstem projection targets of laterodorsal tegmental (LDT) and pedunculopontine tegmental (PPT) nucleus cholinergic neurons in the rat. Soc Neurosci Abstr 1991;17:1163.
10. Greene RW, Gerber U, McCarley RW. Cholinergic activation of medial pontine reticular formation neurons in vitro. Brain Res 1989;476:154–159.
11. Greene RW, McCarley RW. Cholinergic neurotransmission in the brainstem: Implications for behavioral state control. Steriade M, Biesold D, eds. Brain Cholinergic Systems. Oxford: Oxford University Press, 1990.
12. Webster HH, Jones BE. Neurotoxic lesions of the dorsolateral pontomesencephalic tegmentum-cholinergic area in the cat. II. Effects upon sleep-waking states. Brain Res 1988;458:285–302.
13. Steriade M, Datta S, Pare D, et al. Neuronal activities in brainstem cholinergic nuclei related to tonic activation processes in thalamocortical systems. J Neurosci 1990;10:2541–2559.
14. Stevens DR, McCarley RW, Greene RW. 5HT$_1$ and 5HT$_2$ receptors hyperpolarize and depolarize separate populations of medial pontine reticular neurons in vitro. Neuroscience 1992;47:545–553.
15. Gerber U, Stevens DS, McCarley RW, et al. A muscarinic-gated conductance increase in medial pontine reticular neurons of the rat in vitro. J Neurosci 1991; 11:3861–3867.
16. Morales FR, Chase MH. Intracellular recording of lumbar motoneuron membrane potential during sleep and wakefulness. Exp Neurol 1978;62:821–827.
17. Morales FR, Chase MH. Postsynaptic control of lumbar motoneuron excitability during active sleep in the chronic cat. Brain Res 1981;225:279–295.
18. Chase MH, Soja PJ, Morales FR. Evidence that glycine mediates the postsynaptic potentials that inhibit lumbar motoneurons during the atonia of active sleep. J Neurosci 1989;9:743–751.
19. Sastre JP, Jouvet M. Le comportement onirique du chat. Physiol Behav 1979;22:979–989.
20. Jouvet M. What does a cat dream about? Trends Neurosci 1979;2:15–16.
21. Hendricks JC, Morrison AR, Mann GL. Different behaviors during paradoxical sleep without atonia depend on pontine lesion site. Brain Res 1982;239:81–105.
22. Ohta Y, Mori S, Kimura H. Neuronal structures of the brainstem participating in postural suppression in cats. Neurosci Res 1988;5:181–202.
23. Lai YY, Siegel JM. Medullary regions mediating atonia. J Neurosci 1988;8:4790–4796.
24. Stevens DR, Greene RW, McCarley RW. Pontine reticular formation neurons: Excitatory amino acid receptor–mediated responses. In: Horne J, ed. Sleep '90. 1990: Pontenagel Press, 1990.
25. Lai YY, Siegel JM. Pontomedullary glutamate receptors mediating locomotion and muscle tone suppression. J Neurosci 1991;11:2931–2937.
26. Hobson JA, McCarley RW, Wyzinski PW. Sleep cycle oscillation: Reciprocal discharge by two brain stem neuronal groups. 1975;189:55–58.
27. McGinty DJ, Harper RM. Dorsal raphe neurons: Depression of firing during sleep in cats. Brain Res 1976;101:569–575.
28. Lin JS, Sakai K, Vanni-Mercier G, et al. Involvement of histaminergic neurons in arousal mechanisms demonstrated with H$_3$-receptor ligands in the cat. Brain Res 1990;523:325–330.
29. Jouvet M. Recherches sur les structures nerveuses et les mecanismes responsables de differentes phase du sommeil physiologique. Arch Ital Biol 1962;100:125–206.
30. Lydic R, McCarley RW, Hobson JA. Serotonin neurons and sleep: I. Long-term recordings of dorsal raphe discharge frequency and PGO waves. Arch Ital Biol 1987:125:317–343.
31. McCarley RW, Hobson JA. Neuronal excitability modulation over the sleep cycle: A structural and mathematical model. Science 1975;189:58–60.

32. McCarley RW, Massaquoi SG. A limit cycle mathematical model of the REM sleep oscillator system. Am J Physiol 1986;251:R1011–R1029.

33. Leonard CS, Sanchez R. Synaptic potentials in mesopontine cholinergic neurons evoked by local stimulation in vitro. Soc Neurosci Abstr 1991;17:1042.

34. Sanchez R, Khateb A, Muhlethaler M, et al. Glutamate and NMDA actions on mesopontine cholinergic neurons in vitro. Soc Neurosci Abstr 1991;17:256.

35. Lydic R, Baghdoyan HA, Zorinc Z. Microdialysis of cat pons reveals enhanced acetylcholine release during state-dependent respiratory depression. Am J Physiol (Reg. Integ. Comp. Physiol. 30). 1991;261:R766–770.

36. Leonard CS, Llinas RR. Electrophysiology of mammalian pedunculopontine and laterodorsal tegmental neurons in vitro: Implications for the control of REM sleep. In: Steriade M, Biesold D, eds. Brain Cholinergic Systems. Oxford University Press, York: 1990.

37. Muhlethaler M, Khateb A, Serafin M. Effects of monoamines and opiates on pedunculopontine neurons. In: Mancia M, and Marini G, eds. The Diencephalon and Sleep. New York: Raven, 1990.

38. Jones BE. Paradoxical sleep and its chemical/structural substrates in the brain. Neuroscience 1991;40:637–656.

39. Higo S, Ito K, Fuchs D, et al. Anatomical interconnections of the peduculopontine tegmental nucleus and the nucleus prepositus hypoglossi in the cat. Brain Res 1990;536:79–85.

40. Cespuglio R, Gomez ME, Walker E, et al. Effets du refroidissement et de la stimulation des noyaux du systeme du raphe sur les etats de vigilance chez le chat. Electroencephalogr Clin Neurophysiol 1979;47:289–308.

41. Cespuglio R, Gomez ME, Faradji H, et al. Alterations in the sleep-waking cycle induced by cooling of the locus coeruleus area. Electroencephalogr Clin Neurophysiol 1982;54:570–578.

42. Luebke JI, Greene RW, Semba K, et al. Serotonin hyperpolarizes cholinergic low threshold burst neurons in the rat laterodorsal tegmental nucleus in vitro. Proc Natl Acad Sci USA 1992;89:743–747.

43. Cespuglio R, Sarda N, Gharib A, et al. Voltammetric detection of the release of 5-hydroxyindole compounds through the sleep-waking cycle of the rat. 1990; 80:121–128.

44. Pan ZZ, Williams JT. Differential actions of cocaine and amphetamine on dorsal raphe neurons in vitro. J Pharmacol Exp Ther 1989;251:56–62.

45. McCarley RW, Benoit O, Barrioneuvo G. Lateral geniculate nucleus unitary discharge in sleep and waking: State and rate specific aspects. J Neurophysiol 1983;50:798–818.

46. Hirsch JC, Fourment A, Marc ME. Sleep-related variations of membrane potential in the lateral geniculate body relay neurons of the cat. Brain Res 1983;259:308–312.

47. McCormick DA, Pape HC, Properties of a hyperpolarization-activated cation current and its role in rhythmic oscillation in thalamic relay neurons. J Physiol 1990;431:291–318.

48. Steriade M, Curro Dossi R, Nunez A. Network modulation of a slow intrinsic oscillation of cat thalamocortical neurons implicated in sleep delta wave: Cortically induced synchronization and brainstem cholinergic suppression. J Neurosci 1991;11:3200–3217.

49. Buzsaki G, Bickford RG, Ponomareff G, et al. Nucleus basalis and thalamic control of neocortical activity in the freely moving rat. J Neurosci 1988;8:4007–4026.

50. McCormick DA, Pape H-C. Noradrenergic and serotonergic modulation of a hyperpolarization-activated cation current in thalamic relay neurons. J Physiol 1990;431:319–342.

51. Morgan TJ, Curran T. Stimulus-transcription coupling in the nervous system: Involvement of the inducible proto-oncogenes *fos* and *jun*. Annu Rev Neurosci 1991;14:421–452.

52. Shiromani PJ, Kilduff TS, Bloom FE, et al. Cholinergically induced REM sleep triggers *Fos*-like immunoreactivity in dorsolateral pontine regions associated with REM sleep. Brain Res 1992;580:351–357.

53. McCarley RW. The biology of dreaming sleep. In: Kryger M, Roth T, Dement W, eds. Principles and Practices of Sleep Medicine. Philadelphia: WB Saunders, 1989.

4

Biochemical Pharmacology of Sleep

Rafael de Jesus Cabeza
Rebecca K. Zoltoski
J. Christian Gillin

What is sleep and what purpose does it serve? These questions have been the topic of philosophical, psychological, and physiologic inquiry for centuries. Although the epiphenomena of sleep, dreaming, and wakefulness were described centuries ago, it was not until this century, after the advent of the polygraph and the discovery of the electroencephalogram (EEG), that the basic architecture of sleep was characterized.[1,2] Speculation about the function of sleep has been, and remains, based on the ideas of circadian rhythmicity and homeostasis. The first idea emphasizes the daily cycles of rest and activity, with the implication that the survival of the species is facilitated by appropriate timing of sleep and wakefulness over the 24-hour day. The second idea regards sleep as important for necessary repair or the maintenance of homeostasis; that is, following wakefulness and activity, sleep in some way has a restorative purpose. Unfortunately for these hypotheses, no specific physiologic repair or homeostatic process has yet been shown to occur during sleep. Though we have a better idea of how sleep and wakefulness are structured and generated, the functions of sleep remain an enigma.

Various theoretical models have been proposed to account for the regulation of sleep and wakefulness. One model, which takes into account both circadian and homeostatic considerations, is the two-process model developed by Borbely and associates.[3] It postulates two processes: *process S* is a homeostatic process: the longer the organism is awake, the greater will be its propensity to sleep and have a more "intense" sleep, specifically measured as the power density in the delta frequency (0.25 to 3 Hz) EEG band during slow-wave sleep. Because a positive correlation exists between the length of time a creature spends awake and its propensity for sleep, the model hypothesizes the existence of an endogenous sleep factor that is synthesized or accumulated exponentially during waking and is catabolized or dissipated exponentially during sleep. *Process C*, the second component, reflects an oscillatory process that determines the threshold of sensitivity to the homeostatic factor and thus affects the propensity for sleep and waking. Process C is hypothesized to

entrain or be entrained with other oscillators responsible for biologic rhythms, such as temperature, cortisol secretion, and rapid eye movement (REM) sleep.

The two-process model of sleep regulation has important implications for clinicians as well as basic scientists. In evaluating and treating patients with sleep-wake disorders, the clinician must evaluate not only how much the patient sleeps but also the history, timing, and duration of sleep-wake episodes. Normal sleep architecture and duration are generally promoted when sleep is preceded by a long period of wakefulness and when it occurs at the appropriate phase of the circadian sleep-wake cycle. Two peaks of normal sleep propensity—presumably reflecting process C—have been identified in humans entrained to the customary sleep-wake schedule, and these occur at nighttime and at midafternoon.

Two behavioral states exist in mammals and birds: wakefulness and sleep. Thus, animals can be awake and conscious of their environment or they can be asleep and responsive only to strong stimuli. Sleep itself is composed of two very different states: non-REM (NREM) sleep, a state characterized by global slowing of brain metabolism, and REM sleep, characterized by a level of brain metabolism comparable to waking.[4–6] In the quiet waking state, the EEG contains low-amplitude waves called alpha activity (8 to13 Hz) and beta activity (14 to 35 Hz). Four stages can be identified in the NREM sleep of humans and higher primates.[1] The first stage, considered to be a transition stage from waking to sleep, is characterized by a mixture of low-amplitude, mixed-frequency EEG waves, including beta activity and some theta activity (4 to 7 Hz). As sleep deepens, the EEG shows mostly theta activity, punctuated periodically by either high-amplitude biphasic waves called K complexes or fast, rhythmic waves called spindles (12 to 14 Hz). This stage, designated stage 2, is considered to be part of true sleep. Stages 3 and 4 are characterized by delta EEG waves, high-amplitude (75 μV in humans), slow waves (0.5 to 2 Hz), stage 3 having 20% to 50% of an epoch (usually 20 to 30 seconds) as delta waves and stage 4 more than 50% in delta waves. Together, these two stages have been named delta sleep because of the EEG characteristics used to classify them. In lower mammals commonly used in research, NREM sleep is normally divided into light and deep stages only. REM sleep is defined by the appearance of tonic and phasic events. Tonic events include a desynchronized EEG (high-frequency, low-amplitude waves), persistent atonia of antigravity muscles, and hippocampal theta activity. Phasic events include rapid eye movements, periodic twitches of skeletal muscles, variability of autonomic function (such as heart rate and respiration), and the presence of pontine-geniculate-occipital (PGO) spikes. In human studies, the "intensity" of REM sleep is often measured by the amount of ocular activity per minute of sleep, sometimes referred to as *REM density*. Under normal circumstances, NREM sleep always precedes REM sleep. These two sleep states alternate in a cyclic, ultradian (i.e., more than one cycle per 24 hours) cycle, which in humans is about 90 minutes.

Whether an animal be nocturnal or diurnal, most species entrain their wake-sleep cycle to the daily light-dark periods. In the case of homeotherms, the entrainment of the circadian wake-sleep cycle to the daily light-dark period requires a small group of oscillatory cells located within the floor of the third ventricle directly above the optic chiasm, the suprachiasmatic nucleus (SCN). The SCN receives information about environmental lighting conditions via pathways leading from the retina (the retinal-hypothalamic pathway) and from the intrageniculate leaflet.[7,9] The light-dark cycle provides the major *Zeitgeber*, or time giver, which entrains the phase position of the SCN endogenous oscillations to the environment. One important output eventually reaches the pineal gland (via the superior cervical ganglia) that times the circadian release of melatonin, which occurs only during the dark period.[10] Ablation of this nucleus disrupts the entrainment of the sleep-wake cycle to the light-dark cycle and the circadian organization of sleep and wakefulness as well as the circadian changes in body temperature, cortisol secretion, and REM sleep.[7-11] Animals whose SCN has been lesioned exhibit a succession of short bouts of sleep and activity distributed randomly over the 24 hour day, with neither having circadian predominance over the other. Nevertheless, SCN-lesioned animals show rebound compensation in sleep following sleep deprivation, suggesting that the physiologic mechanisms regulating the homeostasis of sleep and wakefulness can be physiologically isolated from those responsible for the circadian organization of sleep and wakefulness.[12] These observations also suggest that basic mechanisms generating sleep and wakefulness do not reside in the SCN. The SCN, however, may well be the anatomic site for process C, which was previously described. A major function is to provide temporal organization over the 24-hour day to a variety of circadian processes, including sleep and wakefulness.

An implication of the two-process model is that duration of wakefulness is positively correlated with the increased sleep propensity, perhaps induced by an endogenous sleep-promoting compound.[3] An interesting implication is that many so-called hypnotic agents may promote sleep by unmasking a prior "sleep debt," in addition to (or instead of) exerting inherent sleep-inducing or wakefulness-suppressing properties. For example, alcohol's sleep-promoting properties probably depend on a sleep debt.[13] Likewise, Edgar and coworkers [14] have reported that triazolam, a benzodiazepine hypnotic, does not induce sleep in SCN-lesioned rats; since SCN animals sleep frequently around the clock, in short bursts, it is assumed that it does not develop a sleep debt that could be unmasked by triazolam.

Though the two-process model has been useful in the search for factors or processes that affect sleep, it does not address the regulation of NREM versus REM sleep with the same rigor. The length of the NREM-REM cycle is species dependent and in humans has a period of about 90 minutes. According to the reciprocal interaction model of REM sleep,[15,16] the ultradian cycle of REM and NREM sleep results from the reciprocal interactions between cholinergic, REM facilitatory neurons and REM inhibitory neurons, possibly noradrenergic and serotonergic cells.

It is important at this juncture to mention two points that should be kept in mind throughout the reading of this chapter. The models we have described, the two-process model and the reciprocal interaction model, have predictive and heuristic value but are not yet firmly supported by anatomic, physiologic, and neurochemical evidence. Furthermore, the models described above were developed in an effort to describe sleep, so the physiologic mechanisms of wakefulness are not considered in depth. Thus, it is hoped that a discussion of the pharmacology of all three states, not just those of sleep, will be helpful in gaining a better understanding and appreciation of the interesting pharmacology of sleep.

THE PHARMACOLOGY OF WAKEFULNESS AND SLEEP

As proposed by Koella,[17] the sleep-organizing and regulation apparatus (SORA) may comprise a coordinating center with two programs, one sustaining wakefulness and the other sleep. The output of these processes is controlled by the various neurotransmitters, such as acetylcholine (ACh), dopamine (DA), norepinephrine (NE) and serotonin (5-HT for 5-hydroxytryptamine), with the assistance of inhibitory neurotransmitters, in coordination with the excitatory and inhibitory flow as processed through the SORA. The overall net output of this apparatus determines the state of alertness of the organism.

Wakefulness

Wakefulness is maintained by the tonic activity of neurons distributed throughout the brain stem reticular formation, which project to the thalamus, the hypothalamus, and the basal forebrain.[2] The major neurotransmitter systems that appear to regulate wakefulness are the dopaminergic and noradrenergic neurons of the pontomesencephalic tegmentum, and the posterior hypothalamic histaminergic neurons, which all project diffusely to and through the forebrain to subcortical and cortical areas.

Dopamine

The effects of amphetamine[18] and cocaine[19] on sleep suggests a role for DA and other amines in promoting wakefulness. Amphetamine and stimulants increase wakefulness and decrease REM sleep, while withdrawal from these stimulants in long-term users increase both total sleep and REM sleep.[20] The effect of amphetamine on sleep can be largely blocked by pretreatment with pimozide, a dopaminergic receptor antagonist.[21] Additionally, in narcoleptic dogs, an animal model of the REM sleep disorder, a decrease in DA turnover has been suggested, as evidenced by elevated catecholamines in a number of brain stem and forebrain regions in brains obtained from these affected canines.[22] The mechanisms of the observed phenomena are still unclear.

Studies using intracranial injections of DA[23,24], treatment with the precursor L-dopa,[25] and lesion of the ventral tegmentum and substantia nigra, which are dopaminergic,[26,27] suggested that DA is important in the maintenance of wakefulness. Biochemical and electrophysiologic studies also suggest that DA activity is associated with waking rather than sleep. DA content is high during waking,[28] and its turnover decreases during the transition from waking to sleep.[29] Thus, pharmacologic, biochemical, and electrophysiologic studies on DA suggest that dopamine maintains behavioral waking.

In rats and dogs, moderate to large doses of apomorphine, a DA agonist, increase wakefulness at the expense of sleep, REM sleep being more sensitive to its effects than NREM sleep[30,31]; administration of

pimozide, a DA antagonist, causes the opposite to occur.[32] In humans, following intravenous infusion of apomorphine in moderate to large doses, complete abolition of REM sleep, severe reduction in stage 2, and marked increase in stage 4 were noticed.[53] Interestingly, small doses of apomorphine have been reported to increase sleep, possibly by exerting a preferential effect on presynaptic, as opposed to postsynaptic, dopaminergic receptors, thus reducing presynaptic release of dopamine. Further studies with D2 receptor antagonists, haloperidol and sulpiride, suggested that these effects were mediated via the D2 receptor.[54] In summary, drugs that increase availability of DA also increase wakefulness and decrease sleep, which appears to be mediated through the D2 receptor. Despite these observations implicating DA in the regulation of sleep and wakefulness, its role remains unclear. Single cell recordings, for example, of dopaminergic neurons in the substantia nigra show only minor changes across the sleep-wake cycle.[35] Therefore, it is possible that DA plays a role in maintaining wakefulness in narcolepsy or other hypersomnolent states, or under the influence of powerful stimulants, but it is not involved in the normal sleep-wake cycle.

Norepinephrine

Recordings of unit activity or noradrenergic neurons in the locus ceruleus (LC) have shown that the firing rate of these cells is state dependent: most cells exhibit a high firing rate during wakefulness which then decreases over NREM sleep until they are virtually silent during REM sleep.[36]

Pharmacologic studies have shown an important interaction of α-adrenergic and β-adrenergic receptors that mediate the components of the wake-sleep cycle. Peripheral administration of clonidine, an α_2-adrenoceptor agonist, increased drowsiness while decreasing sleep in rats, cats, and humans.[37-41] In addition, local administration of clonidine into the LC increases wakefulness an suppresses REM sleep.[40,42] Administration of an α_1-adrenoceptor antagonist, phenoxybenzamine, also increases wakefulness while reducing REM sleep.[43] In rats, systemic administration of the β-adrenergic receptor antagonist propranolol, which may decrease noradrenergic activity, increases wakefulness and inhibits REM sleep,[40] whereas in cats, localized administration into the medial pontine reticular formation had no effect on wakefulness but increased REM sleep.[44] The nature of this adrenergic interaction still needs to be analyzed, owing to the confusing nature of these observations.

One of the most significant side effects of propranolol is drowsiness. The mechanism of this side effect is not known, but it may involve peripheral sympathomimetic receptors, as this drug does not penetrate the blood-brain barrier easily.

Histamine

The proposal that histamine (HA) plays a neuroregulatory role in sleep and waking derived mainly from pharmacologic studies in which the arousing effect of HA and the sedative and sleep-inducing actions of some H_1-receptor antagonists were described.[45,46] In humans, H_1 antihistamines impair vigilance,[47–49] shorten latency to drowsy sleep, but have little or no effect on nocturnal sleep.[50] H_2 antihistamines, on the other hand, do not appear to impair vigilance[51] but cause an increase in the amount of slow-wave sleep and the number of movements in and out of NREM sleep.[50] Schwartz and colleagues have proposed an ascending histaminergic pathway innervating cortex, striatum, hippocampus, and amygdala of the forebrain with cell bodies originating in the posterior hypothalamus and midbrain regions.[52,53] In the rat, a circadian rhythm of HA concentration has its peak in the light phase. The enzyme that synthesizes HA, histidine decarboxylase, and the one that destroys it, histamine-N-methyl-transferase, also show a circadian pattern such that their activity is highest during the dark phase.[54] This seems to indicate that the peak turnover rate occurs during darkness. This is further supported by the observation in rats that 2-thiazolylethlamine, a H_1-receptor agonist, increases wakefulness, whereas pretreatment with pyralimine, a selective H_1-receptor blocker, prevents this effect. In addition, inhibition of HA synthesis decreases waking and increases NREM sleep.[55]

It would appear that HA antagonism has a more obvious effect during wakefulness than during sleep, so it is suggested that the histaminergic system may be more concerned with vigilance than with the underlying state of sleep and wakefulness. The tendency to decrease wakefulness and increase NREM sleep suggests complementary roles for the H_1 and H_2 systems in the control of sleep, and it is tentatively suggested that they may modulate the balance between wakefulness and NREM sleep.[56] In summary, experiments in humans support the role of histaminergic mechanisms in the control of the sleep-wakefulness continuum, though their limited effect during nocturnal sleep, and their more obvious effect during wakefulness, suggest that the histaminergic system may be more concerned with maintaining vigilance during the wakeful state than with sustaining the underlying state of wakefulness itself. Histaminergic mechanisms may also have a subtle part to play in the balance between wakefulness and slow-wave activity during nocturnal sleep.

Acetylcholine

Cholinergic mechanisms clearly play a role in maintaining arousal at both cortical[57,58] and subcortical sites.[59,60] For example, ACh is released from cerebral cortex during activation,[61] including REM sleep.[62] In addition, intravenous administration of physostigmine to humans during NREM sleep in small doses induces REM sleep and in large doses wakefulness.[63] On the other hand, diminished cortical cholinergic activity is associated with a synchronized EEG (delta waves or high-amplitude, slow-frequency waves), whether it is achieved by lesions of the nucleus basalis (the origin of cholinergic projections to the cortex) or the administration of muscarinic antagonists.[58]

Slow-Wave Sleep

Lesion and recording studies have identified cells located within the lower brain stem[2] as well as the anterior hypothalamus–preoptic area and basal forebrain area that are most active during slow-wave sleep and that may be necessary for it.[64–66] These "sleep-on" cells located in the anterior hypothalamus–preoptic area are intermingled with cells involved in heat loss, so many anatomic and chemical substrates that produce increases in temperature and result in heat loss may also induce slow-wave sleep. This suggests that sleep-generating and temperature-regulating mechanisms are closely linked, anatomically, chemically, or in both ways. However, the causal and functional relationship of this link is speculative at this time.

The initiation of slow-wave sleep involves damping of the activity of the systems involved in wakefulness. The process, by nature of the anatomic connections of the neurons, involves an antagonistic, inhibitory action by other neuronal populations, which are discussed later.

Serotonin

A role for 5-HT in sleep has been suggested by the observation that L-tryptophan, a precursor of 5-HT, is a "natural hypnotic" that increases slow-wave sleep time and decreases sleep latency.[67,68] It should be noted, however, that tryptophan is not currently used clinically because it was implicated in the eosinophilic myalgia syndrome.

The mechanism responsible for the role of 5-HT in sleep is not clear. Jouvet's original monoamine theory of sleep[25,69] first recognized the importance of 5-HT in initiating and maintaining sleep. Briefly, lesions of the dorsal raphe nucleus, as well as pharmacologic depletion of brain 5-HT by p-chlorophenylalanine (PCPA), a tryptophan hydroxylase inhibitor, produced insomnia lasting 3 to 4 days in cats.[70,71] This insomnia could be reversed by treatment with 5-hydroxytryptophan, the 5-HT precursor, which bypassed synthesis inhibition. Later studies have refuted the original hypothesis that 5-HT was the sleep neurotransmitter. In cats given daily PCPA treatment, non-REM sleep returned to 70% of normal in 1 week while brain 5-HT levels were still depleted by 90% to 95%.[72] Other methods of depleting brain 5-HT, such as the neurotoxin 5,7-dihydroxytryptamine, did not affect sleep in spite of 78% forebrain depletion of 5-HT.[73] Furthermore, in vivo voltametric studies demonstrated that the intracerebral release of serotonin did not increase with sleep onset.[74]

The profound but temporary insomnia induced by serotonin depletion, by either PCPA or lesions of the dorsal raphe nucleus, may have resulted from the rapidity with which brain serotonin levels fell rather than the absolute levels of serotonin. This interpretation is consistent with the hyperexcitable state in schizophrenic patients,[75] including convulsions, associated with abrupt discontinuation of large 5-hydroxytryptophan doses.

Not only the level of 5-HT but also the number of specific 5-HT–binding sites exhibits a 24-hour rhythm,[76] but, unlike the 5-HT levels, which are increased in the forebrain during recovery following sleep deprivation,[77] the receptor levels are unchanged by sleep deprivation.[78] Numerous distinct binding sites for 5-HT have been identified.[79-81] The role of the 5-HT$_2$ receptor in sleep has been implicated by studies using ritanserin, a specific antagonist at this receptor. Administration of ritanserin (5 or 10 mg), increased stage 3 and 4 sleep in humans and tended to decrease waking and REM sleep.[82-84]

More recently, Jouvet and his colleagues have formulated a new conception of 5-HT in sleep mechanisms: 5-HT, released by axonal nerve endings in the basal hypothalamus as a neurotransmitter during waking, might act as a neurohormone and induce synthesis or liberation of hypnogenic factor(s), which would be secondarily responsible for slow-wave and REM sleep.[85]

Circulating factors

Pieron and coworkers as well as Ishimori introduced the idea of a sleep-inducing factor, "hypnotoxin." Sleep was induced in a naive recipient following intracerebroventricular (ICV) injection of a cerebrospinal fluid sample obtained from a sleep-deprived dog.[86-88] Pieron's hypnotoxin theory was confirmed with the use of better quantitative measurements and properly controlled experiments by Schnedorf and Ivy.[89]

Delta sleep–inducing peptide. The ICV infusion of extracorporeal dialysates from blood of donor rabbits that were in a state of electrically induced sleep, has been reported to induce delta (slow-wave) sleep in recipient rabbits.[90] A nonapeptide, delta sleep–inducing peptide (DSIP), isolated from these dialysates appears to be responsible for this effect.[91,92] Further experiments have shown that this effect is repeatable in rats and cats, even when the drug is administered intravenously or subcutaneously, instead of ICV (for review see reference 93). In humans, intravenous infusions of DSIP in the morning or at night increased total sleep time.[94-98] In rats and humans, plasma DSIP exhibited a circadian rhythm—a peak in the late afternoon and a trough in the early morning[99-101]—but there was no correlation between levels and sleep stage.[99] Constant exposure to light abolishes this circadian rhythm.[101]

In addition to its effects on sleep, DSIP has many "extrasleep" effects. It increased body temperature[102] but had no apparent effect on brain temperature.[103] Decreases in blood pressure,[104] anxiousness,[105] and locomotor activity[106-108] have also been reported.

In humans, beneficial applications of DSIP have been reported for insomniacs,[95,98,109,110] a narcoleptic,[111] opiate addicts and alcoholics,[105] and patients with chronic, pronounced pain episodes.[112] Recent reports in chronic psychophysiologic insomniacs have claimed complete elimination of insomnia plus improvement in sleep, daytime mood state, circadian rhythmicity of sleep, and cognitive and psychomotor performance following 6 days' DSIP treatment.[113-118] Monti and coworkers[119] have not been able to replicate these findings, so the clinical usefulness of DSIP still needs to be determined.

It has been observed that DSIP not only affects sleep but also modulates a variety of physiologic activities in humans and animals.[114-117] Graf and coworkers[120] have proposed that DSIP, in addition to facilitating sleep, may exert a chronopharmacologic action as a natural programming substance. According to them, DSIP-induced changes in cerebral neurotransmitters and plasma proteins may underlie the programming effects.[121] Tobler and Borebely[107] noted a delayed effect of DSIP on rat locomotor activity. Inoue[122,123] observed circadian rest-activity, rhythm-dependent, sleep-modulating effects of DSIP in rats. From these observations, it has been formulated that DSIP might be the first peptide representative of a possibly large group of "psychophysiologic programming substances" within a yet-unknown hierarchical, multidimensional network of priming molecular mechanisms.[118]

Sleep-promoting substances: Uridine and SPS-B. Sleep-promoting substance (SPS) extracted from the water dialysates of brain stems of 24 hour sleep–

deprived rats contains a number of active components. In addition to uridine, which was first identified in 1983,[124,125] there are at least four other partially purified fractions.[126] Of these, SPS-B has been shown to cause an excess of sleep. ICV infusion of the most recently purified form of SPS-B has been shown to elicit a profound sleep-enhancing effect in freely moving rats at the beginning of their nocturnal period.[93] This effect was caused by the more frequent occurrence of NREM and REM sleep episodes with normal sleep-waking behavior. Further purification, as well as identification, of this substance is necessary before its definitive role in sleep modulation can be assessed.

Nocturnal ICV infusion of uridine caused more frequent episodes of NREM and REM sleep without affecting the duration of the episodes; diurnal infusion had no effect on sleep patterns. Extra-sleep effects of uridine include a reduction of spontaneous locomotor activity[127,128] with no change in temperature.[126,129,130] These data support the conclusion that uridine may be involved in the feedback mechanisms that keep the sleep pressure at a dependent normal level, which is preprogrammed in accordance with the phase of the circadian rest-activity rhythm.[126,129,131]

Muramyl peptides. In 1984, Martin[132] and Krueger and their coworkers[133,134] reported that factor S, which was obtained from the cerebrospinal fluid of sleep-deprived goats, from bovine and rabbit cerebral tissue, and human urine, was identified as a muramyl tetrapeptide. In addition, a muramyl tripeptide from humans was identified as an active somnogen. It was recently proposed that muramyl peptides (MPs) can induce sleep, which in turn enhances immunoreactivity, and that it thus has a recuperative function in the mammalian body.[135-138] Evidence for this includes the following fact: MPs are known as components of peptidoglycans, which form the backbone of bacterial cell walls and exert profound pyrogenic and immunostimulatory activities in the mammalian body.[139-141] The pyrogenic effects can be dissociated from the sleep-inducing effects.[134,142-144] Although MPs cannot be biosynthesized in the mammalian body,[140] during the digestion of bacteria by macrophages a chemically unidentified sleep-enhancing substance was produced.[145] This suggests that mammals can process bacterial cell walls to produce biologically active MPs. It appears that the somnogenic activity of MPs, which are concerned mainly with the induction of excess slow-wave sleep, is mediated through the monokine interleukin 1 (IL-1), since the effect can be elicited sooner in rabbits by IL-1 than by MPs.[135,140,142-144]

Interleukin 1. Kreuger and coworkers[136] have proposed that sleep has a reciprocal relationship with the immune system. That is, sleep itself may enhance certain aspects of immune regulation and may, in turn be enhanced by certain immune modulators. Moldofsky and colleagues[146] supported this view with their finding that serum IL-1 and other immune modulators were elevated during sleep in humans. IL-1 belongs to a family of polypeptides that mediate a variety of host defense functions and possesses pyrogenic activity. IL-1 is liberated by macrophages to activate T lymphocytes and induce fever by acting on hypothalamic cells.

IL-1 purified from human or rabbit mononuclear cells enhanced NREM sleep in a dose-dependent fashion immediately following ICV or intravenous infusion into rabbits or rats.[147-150] Additionally, IL-1 elicited hyperthermia. In rabbits, this hyperthermic response, but not the typical temperature changes that occur at transition time, could be prevented by simultaneous ICV infusion of anisomycin without abolishing the somnogenic effect.[147,151] Additionally, in rats the increase of slow-wave activity was not correlated with the elevated body temperature.[148] These results indicate that the effect of IL-1 on sleep is not secondary to hyperthermia. In humans, a peak is the plasma IL-1 level occurs during slow-wave sleep shortly after sleep onset.[146]

The central nervous system and the immune system play a role in host defense mechanisms. Many regulatory substances, such as IL-1, MPs, and vasoactive intestinal peptide/growth-hormone releasing factor (VIP/GRF)–like peptides, are shared by both systems and have profound effects on both sleep and specific aspects of the immune response. Krueger and coworkers[136] have found close relationships between immune reactions and slow-wave sleep. Furthermore, mammalian macrophages process bacterial cell walls, which contain polymers of MPs and release somnogenic substances. Both glia and macrophages possess binding sites for MPs and both produce several somnogenic immunoactive substances, such as IL-1, PGs, and interferon-α. Recent studies suggest that the gene responsible for canine narcolepsy is homologous to the human immunoglobulin μ-switch gene, thereby supporting a possible relationship between immune function and control of sleep.[152] Together, these findings strongly suggest an interaction between sleep and the immune response, and suggest a role for sleep in recuperative processes.

Recently, Irwin and coworkers[153] reported that natural killer cell activity was positively and significantly correlated with various aspects of NREM sleep in both normal controls and depressed patients.

Arginine vasotocin. Arginine vasotocin (AVT), a naturally occurring peptide isolated from the pineal gland, inhibits gonadotropin release, modifies conditioned behavior, and may enhance slow-wave sleep. ICV administration of AVT in cats and rabbits induces NREM and decreases REM sleep.[154,155] In rats, only a decrease in REM latency was observed.[107,156] Additionally, in humans, subcutaneous administration of AVT increased REM sleep. The conclusion from these ambiguous results is that the somnogenic properties of AVT appear to be mediated through indirect effects and await further confirmation.

Adenosine.   Adenosine is a naturally occurring purine nucleoside that causes sedation and inhibits neuronal firing activity. Caffeine, on the other hand, decreases sleep, particularly NREM sleep, and shortens REM latency, presumably because it blocks the adenosine receptors.[157]

Many studies indicate that adenosine enhances deep NREM and REM sleep. Briefly put, in rats and dogs intraventricular or intraperitoneal administration of adenosine or an adenosine A_1–receptor agonist increases NREM sleep.[158-160] Additionally, deoxycoformycin, an adenosine deaminase inhibitor, enhanced REM sleep, and in larger doses, NREM sleep.[160,161] Last, the adenosine precursor S-adenosylhomocysteine enhanced NREM and REM sleep in rats, cats, and rabbits.[162]

Adenosine A_1 receptors, which are more responsive to the doses of adenosine used in the previously mentioned study,[159] have been studied following REM sleep deprivation. Following 48 of 96 hours' deprivation, the adenosine receptor number was elevated; however, following the 48-hour deprivation adenosine levels were unchanged.[163] Consequently, the exact role of adenosine on alertness remains to be determined.

Prostaglandins.   Hayaishi and coworkers[164-166] have developed the prostaglandin (PG)-dependent humoral theory of sleep regulation. Two different PGs, PGD_2 and PGE_2, have been shown to interact reciprocally to affect sleep. Whereas PGD_2 increases sleep time, PGE_2 decreases it in a dose-dependent manner. PGD_2 injected into the preoptic area or infused intracerebroventricularly in femtomolar quantities induces both slow-wave and REM sleep in rats and monkeys.[167-170] Additionally, the PGD synthetase activity exhibits a circadian fluctuation that parallels the sleep-wake cycle, so there is more activity during the quiescent phases of the animal's activity cycle. Last, when diclofenac sodium, an inhibitor of PG synthesis, was infused into rats, a dose-dependent decrease in sleep occurred.[171] After termination of the infusion, a rebound in sleep was reported. These results are consistent with the notion that PGD_2 is involved in physiologic induction of sleep in rats.

It was further shown that PGE_2 increases wakefulness. When AH6809, a PGE_2 antagonist, was infused centrally into both monkeys and rats, a dose-dependent increase in sleep was reported.[166,172] Therefore, reciprocal activity of PGD_2 and PGE_2 may regulate the state of vigilance.

Melatonin.   Melatonin is a major hormone of the mammalian pineal gland. Its synthesis and release into the general circulation are timed by one or more biologic clocks but in humans they occur only in darkness. When subjects are studied under near-dark conditions, the onset and shutoff of melatonin secretion has been used to determine the phase position of the circadian oscillator or oscillators. The general physiologic function of melatonin in humans remains unknown, although in some other mammals it appears to regulate seasonal breeding behavior.

Abnormalities of melatonin secretion have been described in three psychiatric syndromes: (1) seasonal affective disorder (SAD) with winter depression, (2) major depressive disorders, and (3) premenstrual disorder. SAD is associated with hypersomniac, hyperphagic depressions during winter in northerly climates.[173] It can be treated by extending the daily photoperiod with bright lights. It has been suggested that SAD in humans is closely associated with a phase delay of the circadian rhythm of melatonin secretion. In contrast, in most but not all studies of patients with major depression, the total amount of nocturnal melatonin (the area under the curve) tends to be low.[174] Finally, in women with premenstrual depression, total melatonin secretion is low at all phases of the menstrual cycle, possibly because of early shutoff of melatonin secretion.[175]

Melatonin has been reported to enhance sleep in cats, rats, young chickens, and humans.[176-180] In humans, for example, an intravenous bedtime dose of 50 mg reduced sleep latency,[179,181] whereas three oral daytime doses of 80 mg enhanced sleepiness.[182] On the other hand, no effect (except prolongation of REM sleep latency after the large dose) was reported following a 1-mg or a 5-mg oral dose administered at bedtime.[183] Daily administration of 2 mg melatonin in the late afternoon induced unusual tiredness in the early evening after 4 to 5 days and an increase in plasma level that exceeded endogenous nighttime levels by a factor of 10 to 100.[184,185]

While it appears unlikely that melatonin is directly involved in sleep regulation, owing to the extremely large doses needed to alter sleep, it does appear that it may affect sleep indirectly by altering the phase of the circadian pacemaker (A. Lewy, personal communication). If this preliminary finding is confirmed by further studies, it will be important from both clinical and preclinical points of view.

Clinically, it might provide the first pharmacologic means of shifting the phase position of the circadian rhythm. Preclinically, it will be the first demonstration that a pharmacologic agent affects the human circadian rhythm in a manner that is consistent with a traditional phase-response curve.

γ-aminobutyric acid

Early evidence for a role of γ-aminobutyric acid (GABA) in the induction of sleep was supplied by the benzodiazepine hypnotics, which enhance GABA-ergic inhibitory transmission.[186] The benzodiazepines also have nonspecific effects, such as anxiolysis and muscle relaxation. Nevertheless, lowering of the level of behavioral vigilance and induction, as well as maintenance of sleep, are among the more prominent effects. Following administration of L-clcyloserine, an inhibitor of the GABA-degrading enzyme GABA transaminase, to rats, rabbits, and cats, similar results to that obtained with benzodiazepines (except no increased agitation with large doses) was noticed.[187] For example, with small doses, augmentation of REM sleep with no change in NREM sleep was reported, whereas with large doses REM sleep was inhibited. Additionally, a prolonged transition phase between NREM and REM sleep was noticed.[187] As proposed by Koella,[17] the SORA may constitute a coordinating center with two programs, one to sustain wakefulness and the other to sustain sleep. The output of these different channels is controlled by the various neurotransmitters; however, GABA, which is an inhibitory neurotransmitter, may play a local transmission-modulation role in coordination of the excitatory and inhibitory flow as processed through the SORA.

REM Sleep

REM sleep has been called paradoxical sleep because the brain is metabolically, physiologically, and psychologically active, as it is not during NREM sleep. During REM sleep the brain neither depends on external stimuli for its increased activity nor expresses a motor output in response to activation of the central motor systems. Because of this cyclic central activation, some have suggested that REM sleep is important to brain metabolic processes.

In any species the amount of REM sleep increases as body and brain size increase. The time between any two REM sleep episodes decreases as the basal metabolic rate of a given homeothermic species increases,[2] a finding consistent with the hypothesis that REM sleep is important to some brain metabolic process.

The anatomic substrates responsible for the generation of REM sleep are apparently located within the pons. By using complete transections of the brain at specific points, Jouvet[25] demonstrated in the pontine cat preparation the cyclic appearance of REM sleep–like phenomena such as REMs and atonia. More specific intrapontine lesions indicated that different pathways were involved in tonic and phasic events. Lesions of the dorsolateral pontomesencephalic tegmentum, which sends projections to the thalamus, caused phasic events such as PGO spikes to disappear, but not tonic events (muscle atonia and cortical activation).[188] Anatomic studies in the rat suggest that cortical activation depends on projections from the pons to the thalamus, hypothalamus, and basal forebrain[59,189,190] and thus offer a possible explanation of why these lesions which disrupted the connections to the thalamus but may not have altered those connections to either the hypothalamus or the basal forebrain, did not affect cortical activation during REM sleep in cats. The tonic atonia that accompanies REM sleep is generated at the level of the pons but involves a critical relay at the medulla. As early as 1946 it was shown that electrical stimulation of the ventromedial medulla induced muscle atonia not unlike that seen in REM sleep.[191]

The prime candidates for the cholinergic cells that facilitate REM sleep are located in the dorsolateral tegmentum, the lateral dorsal tegmental (LDT) nuclei, and the pedunculopontine tegmental (PPT) group.[192-195] These cells display increased firing rates before and during REM sleep, especially in association with PGO spikes. Nonselective lesions of the dorsolateral tegmentum with kainic acid as well as electricity markedly attenuate REM sleep. The LDT and PPT send projections to the thalamus that may inhibit the mechanisms responsible for sleep spindles and delta EEG waves, to the medial pontine reticular formation, where application of cholinomimetic agents triggers REM sleep, and to the medulla, where they facilitate the atonia of REM sleep. The NE and 5-HT neurons in the LC and dorsal raphe, respectively, lie close to the cholinergic neurons in LDT and PPT and apparently can inhibit them, either directly or indirectly via GABA interneurons.

The ability of several types of pharmacologic agents to affect REM sleep can be understood within the conceptual framework provided by the reciprocal interaction model. Thus, some cholinomimetic agents and some aminergic antagonists augment REM sleep, whereas anticholinergic agents and aminergic agonists often attenuate or block it. Although this model is of heuristic value, it is undoubtably simplistic, as other endogenous substances affect REM sleep and not all pharmacologic predictions of the model have been confirmed in actual experiments. For example, lesions of LC and dorsal raphe do not increase total REM sleep.[2]

Cholinergic agents

The importance of cholinergic mechanisms is now firmly established in the control of REM sleep, and an interesting historical footnote recalls that a dream inspired Otto Loewe to conduct the experiment that established ACh as a neurotransmitter.[196] Thus, we may surmise that ACh triggered the dream that led to the discovery of this role in the brain.

By placing ACh crystals directly on the pons of the cat, Hernandez-Peon was the first to observe that cholinergic agonists induce REM sleep.[197-199] Although this technique was crude and fraught with interpretational problems, the observation of REM sleep induction by cholinomimetic agents has been repeatedly confirmed using a variety of cholinergic agonists, such as carbachol (a nonhydrolyzable analog of ACh), bethanechol (a muscarinic agonist), and neostigmine (a cholinesterase inhibitor). The effects of physostigmine, also an anticholinesterase inhibitor, on REM sleep were variable in animals, sometimes increasing REM sleep and at other times having no effect. Injections of cholinergic agonists into the medial pontine reticular formation effectively induce REM sleep or its components but may exhibit longer latency than those in the dorsal or medial pontine tegmentum. In contrast, injections of carbachol into the rostral midbrain or the medullary reticular formation induced waking and decreased REM sleep.[200-203] Similar results have also been observed in the rat.[204] A particularly striking recent observation notes that a single injection of carbachol into the parabrachial region of cats increases REM sleep threefold, following a latency of about 1 day, and that increased REM sleep lasts at least 2 weeks. Since this region of the brain stem is involved in the generation of PGO spikes, this finding suggests that prolonged periods of PGO spikes prime REM sleep.[205]

Other pharmacologic evidence that favors a role for ACh in the generation of REM sleep was that hemicholinium-3, an inhibitor of the high-affinity choline uptake system and thus of ACh synthesis, given to cats ICV completely blocked the appearance of REM sleep and decreased the animals' waking time.[206] A recent report has indeed demonstrated increased release of ACh from the feline pons during REM sleep as compared with either slow-wave sleep or waking,[207] further strengthening the evidence for a role for endogenous ACh in REM sleep.

Acetylcholine receptor subtypes.   Administration of scopolamine, a muscarinic antagonist, has been shown to inhibit REM sleep in both rats and humans; tolerance to the REM sleep suppression develops over a period of several days.[208] REM sleep rebound occurred when scopolamine was abruptly discontinued and was accompanied, in rats, by a significant increase in the density of muscarinic receptors in caudate but not in brain stem.[209]

Administration of cholinomimetic agonists to humans also induces REM sleep, depending upon the timing and dose of drug. For example, physostigmine can induce either REM sleep in small doses or wakefulness in large doses when infused during the first or second NREM period; the latency to REM sleep induction was longer when physostigmine was infused just after sleep onset than when it was infused 35 minutes after sleep onset. Furthermore, the dose of physostigmine (0.5 mg) that induced REM sleep when infused 35 minutes into the first NREM period induced wakefulness when infused midway through the second NREM period.[63] These differential effects of physostigmine may reflect the dynamic relationships between REM inhibitory and facilitatory processes that evolve with the sleep cycle and have been partially modeled according to the mathematical implications of the reciprocal interaction model.[210] Furthermore, pretreatment with scopolamine (but not methylscopolamine, which fails to cross the blood-brain barrier) blocked the REM-inducing effects of arecoline in humans, further suggesting that arecoline-induced REM sleep is mediated by muscarinic receptors. Other cholinergic agonists reported to facilitate REM sleep in humans include RS 86 and pilocarpine.[211,212] Of clinical interest, both arecoline and RS 86 shorten REM sleep latency more in patients with depression than in control volunteers.[211,213] This finding has now been replicated in seven separate studies, including one group of patients who had never received antidepressants before or who had been off antidepressants at least 4 months. In some but not all studies, the arecoline-induced REM sleep was significantly correlated with REM sleep latency. Since REM sleep latency is typically short in patients who meet formal diagnostic criteria for depression, it suggests that short REM sleep latency might be related to upregulated muscarinic neurotransmission or diminished aminergic neurotransmission. These observations are consistent with the cholinergic-aminergic imbalance hypothesis of depression, which suggests that depression results from an increased ratio of cholinergic to aminergic neurotransmission.[214] More recently, however, Riemann and colleagues[215] have reported faster REM sleep induction with RS 86 in schizophrenic patients than in normal controls. Although they did not specifically assess their patients with this hypothesis in mind, this observation may be consistent with the suggestion that the so-called negative symptoms of schizophrenia (anhedonia, apathy, dysphoria) reflect muscarinic, cholinergic receptor supersensitivity.[216]

ACh interacts with several types of cholinergic receptors that are generally classified as either nicotinic or muscarinic. The muscarinic receptors are further subdivided on the basis of molecular biologic methods into M_1, M_2, M_3, M_4, and M_5. In order to determine the cholinergic receptor specificity in the generation of REM sleep, Velazquez-Moctezuma and coworkers administered equimolar amounts of the M_2 receptor agonists, cisdioxolane and oxotremorine-M, into the medial pontine reticular formation (mPRF) and reported rapid induction of REM sleep and an increased percentage of REM sleep seen over a 5-hour recording period.[217–219] The same molar dose of the M_1 agonist, McN-A-343, had no effect on REM sleep compared with saline. Though these results suggest that in the cat an M_2 receptor in mPRF mediates REM sleep, the study does not exclude the possible role of other muscarinic receptor subtypes. After all, M_2 receptor subtypes are located predominately in the mPRF, whereas M_1 receptor subtypes are located in forebrain areas. Consistent with the hypothesis that M_1 receptor subtypes may be involved, systemic administration of biperiden and other relatively selective antagonists of M_1 receptors have been reported to reduce REM sleep when administered systemically. In humans and cats, acute administration of biperiden (2 to 8 mg in humans, 0.1 mg/kg in cats) increased the latency to REM sleep and decreased REM sleep time.[220–223] Furthermore, Salin-Pascual and colleagues found that biperiden blocked the increase in REM sleep induced by auditory stimulation during REM sleep in humans.[222] In addition, Zoltoski and colleagues[224] have reported that systemic administration of scopolamine, trihexyphenidyl (a relatively selective M_1 antagonist), and biperiden exerted a dose-dependent inhibition of REM sleep in rats.

Of possible interest are the observations that the REM sleep rebound is different following repeated administration of biperiden (4 nights)[221] and scopolamine (3 nights)[220] to humans: while REM sleep latency is shortened in both instances, REM sleep time was increased compared to baseline following abrupt discontinuation of scopolamine but not of biperiden. This observation suggests that both receptor subtypes may mediate induction of REM sleep but that only M_2 receptors increase total REM sleep time.

The role of muscarinic receptors was further suggested by a study of the Flinders Sensitive Line (FSL) of rats. These rats have been selectively bred by Overstreet and coworkers[225] for more than 20 generations for their sensitivity to the hypothermic effects of cholinergic agonists. They display an increased density of muscarinic cholinergic receptors as assessed by binding of 3-quinuclidinyl benzilate (QNB). Of interest to sleep researchers, they showed a short REM latency and significantly increased REM sleep percentage which resulted from shorter REM sleep cycle length, not a longer duration of each REM sleep period.[226] Also of interest, the FSL strain has been proposed as a rodent model of depression.[227] The exact mechanisms of the sleep and behavior changes in the FSL remain to be determined.

In human narcolepsy, a well as the canine model of narcolepsy, REM sleep latency is very short. Although the neural mechanisms responsible are unknown, an increased density of muscarinic receptors, assessed by QNB binding, has been described in the brain stem of narcoleptic dogs, as compared with nonnarcoleptic ones.[228] In addition, other data suggest decreased turnover of dopamine.[22]

The role of nicotinic receptors in the control of sleep has been relatively neglected. Hu and colleagues have reported that both mecamylamine and hexamethonium, antagonists of neuronal nicotinic receptors, blocked the generation of PGO spikes in reserpinized cats.[229] Velazquez-Moctezuma and colleagues reached similar conclusions.[230] These authors concluded that PGO spike generation is partially mediated by a nicotinic mechanism, that cortical activation, measured a desynchronized EEG, contains an M_1 component, and that the muscle atonia seen during REM sleep is mediated by an M_2 receptor. Furthermore, Velazquez-Moctezuma's group reported that administration of nicotine into the mPRF induced REM sleep in cats.[231]

To our knowledge, the effects of nicotine on human sleep have not been investigated at this time. In a study of smokers, Soldatos and associates[232] reported that smokers had significantly longer sleep latency than nonsmokers and that their sleep improved immediately upon discontinuing smoking. Interestingly, anecdotal reports suggest that smokers who use the nicotine patch to help stop smoking report increased amounts of dreaming, which may be consistent with the report of Velazquez-Moctezuma's group[231] that nicotine injected into the medial pontine reticular formation induces REM sleep.

Noradrenergic compounds

Many cells of the LC cease firing during the transition from NREM sleep to REM sleep (or during REM sleep) and regain their activity once the state is terminated. This, along with evidence provided below, suggests not only that REM sleep needs cholinergic action to be generated but that the effects of NE are directly inhibitory. In fact, a recent hypothesis by Siegel and Rogawski proposes that REM sleep resensitizes or upregulates noradrenergic receptors.[233] In general, compounds that decrease the norepinephrine (NE) content or release increase the amount of REM sleep and compounds that increase NE activity decrease REM sleep.

Amphetamine releases NE (as well as other amines) from nerve terminals, inhibits its reuptake, and can have other adrenergic effects. As reviewed earlier, D-amphetamine decreases both the percentage of REM sleep and total sleep. Long-term (but not short-term) treatment with this stimulant leads to a large REM sleep rebound.[234] In addition, stimulant addicts shown hypersomnia, short REM sleep latency, and increased amounts and percentage of REM sleep during the first several weeks after withdrawal from cocaine or amphetamine.[20] Although the amphetamine and other stimulants do release NE, they have numerous other neuropharmacologic effects that complicate interpretation. For example, pretreatment with a dopamine antagonist, pimozide, blocked the REM-inhibiting and alerting effects of amphetamine in humans.[21]

The compound α-methyl-*p*-tyrosine (AMPT) is an inhibitor of the catecholamine-synthesizing enzyme tyrosine hydroxylase and depletes the neurotransmitter stores of NE and DA at the nerve terminal. Cats treated with this compound show an increase in the amount of REM sleep, while little happens to NREM sleep.[235] The same basic observation was made when healthy volunteers were given AMPT, except that there was an increase in NREM sleep as well[236,237] Furthermore, profound insomnia for a day or two followed the discontinuation of AMPT which had been administered for 3 days previously. Reserpine, a drug that depletes tissue of NE, DA, and 5-HT by preventing its entry into the vesicles whence it is released, can also increase the amount of REM sleep and shorten the latency to REM sleep in both cats and humans.[238] These findings are consistent with the view that aminergic neurotransmitters are inhibitory to REM sleep. Work with more selective adrenergic agonists and antagonists further supports the idea of an inhibitory role for NE in REM sleep.

As part of the reciprocal interaction hypothesis, it has been postulated that NE systems are inhibitory to the generation of PGO spike.[239] Clonidine reduced PGO spike activity while idazoxan antagonized this effect.[240] As stated earlier, many noradrenergic cells in the LC cease firing in association with PGO spikes.

The narcolepsy syndrome is characterized by excessive daytime sleepiness, cataplexy, sleep paralysis, and hypnagogic hallucinations. The noradrenergic and serotonergic systems appear to be involved because antidepressants, which mainly potentiate both systems by reuptake blockade, are effective in treating the various symptoms of narcolepsy, both human and canine.[241,242] Moreover, in both narcoleptic patients and dogs, prazosin, an α1-adrenergic blocker, precipitates cataplexy, whereas clonidine, an α2-adrenergic agonist, decreases cataplectic attacks.[242] In general, it appears that NE acts to suppress cataplexy,[243] though its exact mechanism and role in the narcoleptic tetrad still need to be determined.

Adrenergic receptor subtypes. Adrenergic receptors are subdivided into two major types, α- and β- adrenergic receptors, based on their ability to interact differentially with a family of adrenergic pharmacologic agents. Like cholinergic receptors, these major classifications of receptors are further subdivided into the α_1, α_2, β_1, and β_2 receptors, based on similar pharmacologic criteria of differential compound effects.

An interesting topology of the α-adrenergic receptors in the synaptic connection is that α_1 receptors are mainly found postsynaptically to the noradrenergic terminal whereas α_2 receptors are preferentially found on the terminal itself and usually function to decrease release of NE. Thus, one would expect that activation of α_1 receptors should lead to positive NE effects while activation of α_2 receptors normally decreases the amount of NE released into the synaptic cleft and acts as an antagonist of NE action. As predicted by the reciprocal interaction hypothesis, the compound methoxamine an α_1 agonist, decreases REM sleep in rats whereas the α_1 antagonist prazosin increases it.[244] In addition, intravenous administration of thymoxamine, an α_1-receptor antagonist, increases REM sleep in humans.[245] Furthermore, activation of α_1 receptors leads to increased wakefulness and a decrease in both NREM and REM sleep. Interestingly, studies conducted using the α_2-receptor agonist clonidine reported modest decreases in REM sleep in both humans and cats.[246,247] Yohimbine, an α_2 antagonist, does decrease REM sleep in rats, supposedly by increasing release of NE.[244] The use of β-selective drugs such as propranolol, has produced inconsistent effects, or none, on REM sleep. The role played by the β receptors in mediating NE's action in the pons is therefore unclear.[244]

Serotonergic compounds

The second major group of cells that are relatively quiescent during REM sleep are located within the raphe nucleus. For this reason, 5-HT has also been proposed to be inhibitory to the state of REM sleep. However, pharmacologic manipulations of 5-HT in humans and animals has had mixed effects which are not readily interpretable (for reviews and general discussion see references 25, 248, and 249). Other attempts to investigate the importance of 5-HT have used the 5-HT–depleting drug PCPA. Of interest is the fact that this drug can initially abolish sleep when given in large enough doses to animals, but even with continued treatment, sleep returns to normal with time though the 5-HT level remains low.[72] Nonetheless, PGO spikes continued to appear during wakefulness and NREM sleep, suggesting that serotoninergic cells inhibit PGO spikes. Smaller doses of the drug (about one-tenth that used in animals), when given to humans, decreased REM sleep but had little effect on NREM sleep. Furthermore, the decrease in REM sleep could be sustained several weeks. When some of these patients were given the 5-HT precursor, 5-hydroxytryptophan, which can circumvent the PCPA block, REM sleep returned to normal with no rebound.[236] Likewise, when PCPA treatment was discontinued, normal REM sleep returned within a few days in both humans and animals.

Lysergic acid diethylamide (LSD) tends to increase REM sleep in humans,[250,251] possibly because it shuts down serotonergic neurons, at least in the dorsal raphe of the rat.[252] Furthermore, 5-HT agonists such as fenfluramine, which releases 5-HT, and fluoxetine, which is a potent reuptake blocker, decreased both total sleep and REM sleep.[249] Though these results appear to indicate a fundamental difference between sleep in animal models and in humans, with regard to 5-HT such a conclusion is at best premature. A much larger set of studies using more selective agents with large ranges of doses will be needed to better understand the possible role of 5-HT in REM sleep.

Neuropeptides and other possible modulators

Knowledge of the biology of central nervous system neuropeptides and neuromodulators is growing quickly but is not yet as detailed as knowledge of the classical neurotransmitters. Thus, the location and function of many of these compounds is not clearly understood, and this precludes their integration into any present model of REM sleep. Furthermore, since many of these substances may not cross the blood-brain barrier, studies carried out in humans may point to systemic effects and not to a central function. Whether some of the effects noted in animals represent pharmacologic rather than physiologic effects also remains to be determined.

AVT can totally block REM sleep and much increase NREM sleep, for at least 5 hours, in cats that receive as little as 10^{-18} into a cerebral ventrical (ICV). The same effect can be obtained by a 100-fold larger dose of the peptide given intraperitoneally.[154] When anti-AVT antiserum is given ICV to cats, not only is there an increase in the amount of REM sleep but there is also the intrusion of REM sleep episodes occurring at sleep onset, a condition not seen in normal animals.[155] If the dorsal raphe nucleus is lesioned no effect of ICV AVT is observed in cats 5 days following the lesion.[253] This suggests that the inhibition of REM sleep by AVT in the cat is dependent on the actions of 5-HT, an area of investigation that requires more work as we discussed above. However, because antiserum raised against AVT can augment REM sleep, this supports the notion of an endogenous role for AVT in regulating REM sleep.

A large body of literature suggests that vasoactive intestinal polypeptide (VIP) increases REM sleep in animals. ICV administration of 30 pmol of VIP to rats at the beginning of the light or rest phase enhanced REM sleep within 1 hour after injection. A tenfold larger dose produced the same effect but with a 24-hour delay, suggesting a complicated modulatory role of REM sleep by VIP.[254] Cats treated with 30 picomoles ICV gave similar results to those obtained in the rats but with a 5-hour delay to the effects.[255] To better estimate whether VIP normally plays a role in modulating REM sleep, a VIP antiserum was administered to rats ICV, resulting in an increase in waking and a decrease in REM sleep that was not associated with a decrease in NREM sleep.[254] Thus, there is reasonable support for the theory that both VIP and AVT may play a normal role in modulating the REM sleep–generating or –sustaining system of the brain, or both.

A third peptide with interesting effects on REM sleep is somatostatin (SS). When rats were infused ICV with SS over 2 days, REM sleep increased and no effect on NREM sleep was observed. When SS administration was discontinued, animals sleep state percentages returned to pretreatment levels.[256,257] Furthermore, if cysteamine, a drug that depletes SS stores, is given ICV (40 or 90 µg/per day) there is a dose-dependent decrease in the amount of REM sleep, again with no statistically significant change in NREM sleep.[256,257] Analogues of SS have similar effects on REM sleep. Furthermore, SS has been reported to overcome the REM sleep–suppressing effect of scopolamine.[258,259] In addition, increased REM sleep induced by carbachol treatment may be dependent on SS, since pretreatment with an anti-SS antiserum was reported to block the carbachol stimulatory effect.[260]

CONCLUSIONS

Sleep researchers have made significant progress in recent years in identifying the neurochemical and neurophysiologic mechanisms responsible for sleep, and especially REM sleep. Indeed, we now probably know as much about the physiologic control of REM sleep as we know about any higher basic behavioral state such as eating, sexual behavior, or memory. Clearly, the current widely accepted paradigm is that REM sleep is promoted by cholinergic neurons that originate in the brain stem, most probably the LDT nucleus and PPT group, and that it is inhibited by noradrenergic and serotoninergic neurons located in the LC and dorsal raphe, respectively. Cholinergic neurons exert a widespread and crucial role in the orchestration of REM sleep, through their projections to mPRF, medulla, and forebrain areas in the thalamus and basal forebrain.

Though many interesting "leads" now exist as to the neurochemical and neurophysiologic mechanisms involved in the control of NREM sleep, we must still be humble and admit that much remains to be firmly established. Clearly, the role of the thalamus and basal forebrain has been established in specific EEG manifestations of NREM sleep. Still, the specific mechanisms involved in the induction and maintenance of NREM sleep appear to be varied and complicated, not yet readily put into a simple framework.

Considerable interest is currently directed toward hypothetical endogenous "sleep hormones," immunomodulating factors that might promote sleep, and thermoregulatory processes involved in the induction (and, possibly, functions) of sleep.

What also is emerging is a broader view of sleep, which must include wakefulness and a relationship to underlying circadian processes. Moreover, as we learn more about the manipulation of underlying circadian processes and thermoregulation we can anticipate new approaches to the management of sleep-wake disorders.

REFERENCES

1. Rechtschaffen A, Kales AA. A manual of standardized terminology, techniques, and scoring system for sleep stages of human subjects. Los Angeles: Brain Research Institute, UCLA, 1968.
2. Jones BE. Paradoxical sleep and its chemical/structural substrates in the brain. Neuroscience 1991;40:637–656.
3. Daan S, Beersma DGM, Borbely AA. Timing of human sleep: Recovery process gated by a circadian pacemaker. Am J Physiol 1984;246:R161–R183.
4. Buchsbaum M, Gillin JC, Wu J, et al. Regional cerebral glucose metabolic rate in human sleep assessed by positron emission tomography. Life Sci 1989;45:1349–1356.
5. Kennedy C, Gillin JC, Mendelson WB, et al. Local cerebral glucose utilization in non-REM sleep. Nature 1982;17:275–280.
6. Nakamura R, Kennedy C, Gillin JC, et al. Hypnogenic center theory of sleep: No support from metabolic mapping in monkeys. Brain Res 1983;268:372–376.
7. Moore RY, Eichler VB. Loss of a circadian adrenal coricosterone rhythm following suprachiasmatic lesions in the rat. Brain Res 1972;42:201–206.
8. Moore RY, Lenn NJ. A retinohypothalamic projection in the rat. J Comp Neurol 1972;142:1–14.
9. Smale L, Blanchard J, Moore RY, et al. Immunocytochemical characterization of the suprachiasmatic nucleus and the intergeniculate leaflet in the diurnal ground squirrel *Spermophilus lateralis*. Brain Res 1991;563:77–86.
10. Moore RY, Card JP. Visual pathways and the entrainment of circadian rhythms. Ann NY Acad Sci 1985;453:123–133.
11. Eastman CI, Mistlberger RE, Rechtschaffen A. Suprachiasmatic nuclei lesions eliminate circadian temperature and sleep rhythms in the rat. Physiol Behav 1983;32:357–368.
12. Mistlberger RE, Bergmann BM, Waldenar W, et al. Recovery sleep following sleep deprivation in intact and suprachiasmatic nuclei–lesioned rats. Sleep 1983;6:217–233.
13. Zwyghuizen-Doorenbos A, Roehrs T, Lamphere J, et al. Increased daytime sleepiness enhances ethanol's sedative effects. Neuropsychopharmacology 1988;1:279–286.
14. Edgar DM, Seidel WF, Martin CE, et al. Triazolam fails to induce sleep in suprachiasmatic nucleus-lesioned rats. Neurosci Lett 1991;125:125–128.
15. McCarley RW, Hobson JA. Neuronal excitability modulation over the sleep cycle: A structural and mathematical mode. Science 1975;189:58—60.
16. Hobson JA, McCarley RW, Wyzinski PW. Sleep cycle oscillation: Reciprocal discharge by two brainstem neuronal groups. Science 1975;189:55—58.
17. Koella WP. The organization and regulation of sleep. A review of the experimental evidence and a novel integrated model of the organizing and regulating apparatus. Experientia 1984;40:309–338.
18. Gillin JC, van Kammen DP, Graves J, et al. Differential effects of D- and L-amphetamine on the sleep of depressed patients. Life Sci 1975;17:1233–1240.
19. Post RM, Gillin JC, Goodwin FK, et al. The effect of orally administered cocaine on sleep of depressed patients. Psychopharmacology 1974;37:59–66.
20. Watson R, Hartmann E, Schildkraut JJ. Amphetamine withdrawal: Affective state sleep patterns, and MHPG excretion. Am J Psychiatry 1972;129:39–45.
21. Gillin JC, van Kammen D, Bunney WE Jr. Pimozide attenuates effects of *d*-amphetamine in EEG sleep patterns in psychiatric patients. Life Sci 1978;22:1805–1810.
22. Faull KF, Zeller-DeAmicis LC, Radde L, et al. Biogenic amine concentrations in the brains of normal and narcoleptic canines: Current status. Sleep 1986;9:107–110.
23. Benkert O, Kohler B. Intrahypothalamic and intrastriatal dopamine and norepinephrine injection in relation to motor hyperactivity in the rat. Psychopharmacology 1972;24:318–325.
24. Fog R. Stereotyped and non-stereotyped behavior in rats induced by various stimulant drugs. Psychopharmacology 1969;14:299–304.
25. Jouvet M. The role of monoamines and acetylcholine-containing neurons in the regulation of the sleep-waking cycle. Ergeb Physiol 1972;64:166–308.
26. Jones BE, Bobillier P, Jouvet M. Effets de la destruction des neurones contenant des catecholamines du mesencephale sur le cycle veille sommeils du chat. C R Soc Biol 1969;163:176–180.

27. Jones BE, Bobillier P, Pin C, et al. The effects of lesions of catecholamine containing neurons upon monoamine content of the brain and EEG and behavioral waking in the cat. Brain Res 1973;58:157–177.

28. Scheving LE, Harrison WH, Gordon P, et al. Daily fluctuation (circadian and ultradian) in biogenic amines of the rat brain. Am J Physiol 1968;214:166–173.

29. Kovacevic R, Radulovacki M. Monoamine changes in the brain of cats during slow wave sleep. Science 1976;193:1025–1027.

30. Kafi S, Gaillard JM. Brain dopamine receptors and sleep in the rat: Effects of stimulant blockade. Eur J Pharmacol 1976;38:357–364.

31. Wauquier A, Van den Broeck WAE, Niemegeers CJE. On the antagonistic effects of pimozide and clompenidine on apomorphine-disturbed sleep-wakefulness in dogs. In: Koella WP, ed. Sleep 1980. Basel: S Karger, 1981;279–282.

32. Wauquier A, Van den Broeck WAE, Janssen PAJ. Biphasic effects of pimozide on sleep-wakefulness in dogs. Life Sci 1980;27:1469–1475.

33. Cianchetti C, Masala C, Corsini GU, et al. Effect of apomorphine on human sleep. Life Sci 1978;23:403–408.

34. Cianchetti C. Dopamine agonists and sleep in man. In: Wauquier A, Gaillard JM, Monti JM, et al., eds. Sleep: Neurotransmitters and Neuromodulators. New York: Raven Press, 1985;121–134.

35. Miller JD, Farber J, Gatz P, et al. Activity of mesencephalic dopamine and non-dopamine neurons across stages of sleep and walking in the rat. Brain Res 1983;273:133–141.

36. Aston-Jones G, Bloom FE. Norepinephrine-containing locus coeruleus neurons in behaving rats exhibit pronounced responses to non-noxious environmental stimuli. J Neurosci 1981;1:887–900.

37. Kleinlogel H, Scholtysik G, Sayers AC. Effects of clonidine and BS 100–141 on the EEG sleep pattern in rats. Eur J Pharmacol 1975;33:159–163.

38. Autret A, Beillevaire T, Cathala H-P, et al. The effect of clonidine on sleep patterns in man. Eur J Clin Pharmacol 1977;12:319–322.

39. Gaillard JM, Kafi S. Involvement of pre- and postsynaptic receptors in catecholaminergic control of paradoxical sleep in man. Eur J Clin Pharmacol 1979;15:83–89.

40. Putkonen PTS, Leppavuori A, Stenberg D. Pardoxical sleep inhibition by central alpha-adrenoceptor stimulant clonidine antagonized by alpha-receptor blocker yohimbine. Life Sci 1977;21:1059–1066.

41. Depoortere H. EEG study of drug interactions with the sedative effect of clonidine in the rat. In: Koella WP, ed. Sleep 1982. Basel: S Karger, 1983;273–275.

42. Autret A, Minz M, Beillevaire T, et al. The REM sleep-suppressing effect of clonidine and its antagonism by yohimbine. In: Koella WP, Levin P, eds. Sleep 1976. Basel: S. Karger, 1977;366–369.

43. Skarby T, Andersson K-E, Edvinsson L. Characterization of the postsynaptic alpha-adrenoceptor in isolated feline cerebral arteries. Acta Physiol Scand 1981;112:105–107.

44. Tononi G, Pompeiano M, Pompeiano O. Modulation of desynchronized sleep through microinjection of β-adrenergic agonists and antagonists in the dorsal pontine tegmentum of the cat. Eur J Physiol 1989;415:142–149.

45. Monnier M, Sauer R, Hatt AM. The activating effects of histamine on the central nervous system. Int Rev Neurobiol 1970;12:265–305.

46. Wolf P, Monnier M. Electroencephalographic, behavioural, and visceral effects of intraventricular infusion of histamine in the rabbit. Agents Actions 1973;3:196.

47. Bye C, Dewsbury D, Peck AW. Effects on the human central nervous system of two isomers of ephedrine and triprolidine, and their interaction. Br J Clin Pharmacol 1974;1:71–78.

48. Bye CE, Claridge R, Peck AW, et al. Evidence for tolerance to the central nervous system effects of the histamine antagonist, triprolidine, in man. Eur J Clin Pharmacol 1984;12:181–186.

49. Peck AW, Fowle ASE, Bye C. A comparison of triprolidine and clemastine on histamine antagonism and performance tests in man: Implications for the mechanism of drug induced drowsiness. Eur J Clin Pharmacol 1975;8:455–463.

50. Nicholson AN, Pascoe PA, Stone BM. Histaminergic systems and sleep: Studies in man with histamine H1 and H2 receptor antagonists. Neuropharmacology 1985;24:245–250.

51. Nicholson AN, Stone BM. The H2 antagonists cimetidine and ranitidine: Studies on performance. Eur J Clin Pharmacol 1984;26:579–582.

52. Garbarg M, Barbin G, Bischoff S, et al. Dual localization of histamine in an ascending neuronal pathway and in non-neuronal cells evidenced by lesions in the lateral hypothalamic area. Brain Res 1976;106:333–348.

53. Schwartz JC, Barbin G, Duchemin AM, et al. Histamine receptors in the brain and their possible functions. In: Ganellin CR, Parsons ME, eds. Pharmacology of Histamine Receptors. Bristol: John Wright and Sons, 1982;351–391.

54. Orr E, Quay WB. Hypothalamic 24-hour rhythms in histamine, histidine decarboxylase, and histamine-*N*-methyltransferase. Endocrinology 1975;96:941–945.

55. Monti JM, Pellejero T, Jantos H, et al. Role of histamine in the control of sleep and waking. In: Wauquier A, Gaillard JM, Monti JM, et al. eds. Sleep: Neurotransmitters and Neuromodulators. New York: Raven Press, 1985;197–209.

56. Nicholson AN. Histaminergic systems: Daytime alertness and nocturnal sleep. In: Wauquier A, Gaillard JM, Monti JM, et al. eds. Sleep: Neurotransmitters and Neuromodulators. New York: Raven Press, 1985;211–220.

57. Vanderwolf CH, Robinson TE. Reticulo-cortical activity and behavior: A critique of the arousal theory and new synthesis. Behav Brain Sci 1981;4:459–476.

58. Buzsaki G, Bickford R, Ponomareff G, et al. Nucleus basalis and thalamic control of neocortical activity in the freely moving rat. J Neurosci 1988;8:4007–4026.

59. Steriade M, Datla S, Pare D, et al. Neuronal activities in brainstem cholinergic nuclei related to tonic activation patterns in thalamocortical systems. J Neurosci 1990;10:2541–2559.

60. Steriade M, Dossi RC, Nunez A. Network modulation of a slow intrinisic oscillation of cat thalamocortical neurons implicated in sleep delta waves: Cortically induced synchronization and brainstem cholinergic suppression. J Neurosci 1991;11:3200–3217.

61. Celesia GG, Jasper HH. Acetylcholine released from cerebral cortex in relation to state of activation. Neurology 1966;16:1053–1064.

62. Jasper H, Tessier J. Acetylcholine liberation from cerebral cortex during paradoxical (REM) sleep. Science 1971;172:601–602.

63. Sitaram N, Gillin JC. Development and use of pharmacological probes of the CNS in man: Evidence of cholinergic abnormality in primary affective illness. Biol Psychiatry 1980;15:925–955.

64. McGinty DJ, Sterman MB. Sleep suppression after basal forebrain lesions in the cat. Science 1968; 160:1253–1255.

65. Szymusiak R, McGinty DJ. Sleep-suppression after kainic acid–induced lesions of the basal forebrain in cats. [Abstr]. Sleep Res 1985;14:2.

66. McGinty D. Hypothalamic thermoregulatory control of slow wave sleep. In: Mancia M, Marini G, eds. The Diencephalon and Sleep. New York: Raven Press, 1990;97–110.

67. Wyatt RJ, Kupfer DJ, Sjoersma A, et al. Effects of L-tryptophan (a natural sedative) on human sleep. Lancet 1970;2:842–845.

68. Hartmann E. L-Tryptophan as an hypnotic agent: A review. Waking Sleeping 1977;1:155–161.

69. Jouvet M. Neuropharmacology of the sleep-waking cycle. Handb Psychopharmacol 1977;8:233–293.

70. Koella WP, Feldstein A, Czicman JS. The effect of para-chlorophenylalanine on the sleep of cats. Electroencephalogr Clin Neurophysiol 1968;25:481–490.

71. Weitzman E, Rapport MM, McGregor P, et al. Sleep patterns of the monkey and brain serotonin concentration: Effect of p-chlorophenylalanine. Science 1968;160:1361–1363.

72. Dement W, Mitler M, Henriksen S. Sleep changes during chronic administration of parachlorophenylalanine. Rev Can Biol (Suppl) 1972;31:239–246.

73. Ross CA, Trulson ME, Jacobs BL. Depletion of brain serotonin following intraventricular 5,7-dihydroxytryptamine fails to disrupt sleep in the rat. Brain Res 1976;114:517–523.

74. Cespuglio R, Saika N. Gharib A, et al. Voltammetric detection of the release of 5-hydroxyindole compounds through the sleep-waking cycle of the rat. Exp Brian Res 1990;80:121–128.

75. Wyatt RJ, Gillin JC. Development of tolerance to and dependence of endogenous neurotransmitters. In: Mandell AJ, ed. Neurobiological Mechanisms of Adaptation and Behavior. New York: Raven Press, 1975; 47–59.

76. Wesemann W, Rotsch M, Schulz E, et al. Circadian rhythm of serotonin binding in rat brain. I. Effect of the light-dark cycle. Chronobiol Int 1986;3:135–139.

77. Borbely AA, Steigrad P, Tobler I. Effect of sleep deprivation on brain serotonin in the rat. Behav Brain Res 1980;1:205–210.

78. Weseman W, Rotsch M, Schulz E, et al. Circadian rhythm of serotonin binding in rat brain. II. Influence of sleep deprivation and imipramine. Chronobiol Int 1986;3:141–146.

79. Conn PJ, Sanders-Bush E. Central serotonin receptors: Effector systems, physiological roles and regulation. Psychopharmacology 1987;92:267–277.

80. Martin GR. Current problems and future requirements for 5-hyroxytryptamine receptor classification. Neuropsychopharmacology 1990;3:321–333.

81. Hartig P, Kao H-T, Macchi M, et al. The molecular biology of serotonin receptors: An overview. Neuropsychopharmacology 1990;3:335–347.

82. Declerck AC, Wauquier A, Van der Ham-Veltman PHM, et al., Increase in slow wave sleep in humans with serotonin-S2 antagonist ritanserin. Curr Ther Res Clin Exp 1987;41:427–432.

83. Idzikowski C, Cowen PJ, Nutt D, et al. The effects of chronic ritanserin treatment on sleep and the neuroendocrine response to L-tryptophan. Psychopharmacology 1987;93:416–420.

84. Idzikowski C, Mills FJ, Glennard R. 5-Hydroxytryptamine-2 antagonist increases human slow wave sleep. Brain Res 1986;378:164–168.

85. Jouvet M, Buda C, Cespuglio R, et al. Hypnogenic effects of some hypothalamo-pituitary peptides. In: Bunney WE Jr, Costa E, Potkin SG, eds. Clinical Neuropharmacology, vol 9, suppl 4. New York: Raven Press, 1986;465–467.

86. Legendre R, Pieron H. Le probleme des facteurs du sommeil. Resultats d'injections vasculaires et intracerebrales de liquides insomniques. C R Soc Biol 1910;62:1077–1079.

87. Legendre R, Pieron H. Recherches sur le besoin de sommeil consecutif a une veille prolongee. Z Allg Physiol 1913;14:235–262.

88. Ishimori K. True cause of sleep—A hypnogenic substance as evidenced in the brain of sleep-deprived animals. Igakkai Zasshi (Tokyo) 1909;23:429–457.

89. Schnedorf JG, Ivy AC. An examination of the hypnotoxin theory of sleep. Am J Physiol 1939;125:491–505.

90. Monnier M, Hosli L. Dialysis of sleep and waking factors in blood of rabbit. Science 1964;146:796–798.

91. Schoenenberger GA, Monnier M. Characterization of a delta-electroencephalogram (sleep)–inducing peptide. Proc Natl Acad Sci USA 1977;74:1282–1286.

92. Schoenenberger GA, Maier PF, Tober HJ, et al. The delta EEG (sleep)–inducing peptide (DSIP). XI. Amino-acid analysis, sequence, synthesis and activity of the nonapeptide. Pflugers Arch 1978;376:119–129.

93. Inoue S. Biology of Sleep Substances. Boca Raton, Fla: CRC Press, 1989.

94. Schneider-Helmert D, Gnirss F, Monnier M, et al. Acute and delayed effects of DSIP (delta sleep-inducing peptide) on human sleep behavior. Int J Clin Pharmacol Ther Toxicol 1981;19:341–345.

95. Schneider-Helmert D, Schoenenberger GA.Effects of DSIP in man. Multifunctional psychophysiological

properties besides induction of natural sleep. Neuropsychobiology 1983;9:197–206.

96. Blois R, Monnier M, Tissot R, et al. Effect of DSIP on diurnal and nocturnal sleep in man. In: Koella WP, ed. Sleep 1980. Basel: S. Karger, 1981;301–303.

97. Schneider-Helmert D, Gnirss F, Schoenenberger GA. Effect of DSIP applications in healthy and insomniac adults. In: Koella WP, ed. Sleep 1980. Basel: S Karger, 1981;417–420.

98. Schneider-Helmert D. Influences of DSIP on sleep and waking behavior in man. In: Koella WP, ed. Sleep 1982. Basel: S Karger, 1983;117–125.

99. Kato N, Nagaki S, Takahashi Y, et al. DSIP-like material in rat brain, human cerebrospinal fluid, and plasma as determined by enzyme immunoassay. In: Inoue S. Borbely AA, eds. Endogenous Sleep Substances and Sleep Regulation. Tokyo: Japan Science Solciety Press, 1985;141–153.

100. Kastin AJ, Nissen C, Coy DH. DSIP-like immunoreactivity in the developing rat brain. Brain Res Bull 1981;7:687–690.

101. Fischman AJ, Kastin AJ, Graf M. Circadian variation of DSIP-like material in rat plasma. Life Sci 1984;35:2079–2084.

102. Kovalzon VM, Kalikhevich VN, Churkina SI. The active analogue of the inactive "sleep peptide". Bull Eksp Biol Med 1986;101:707–709.

103. Obal F Jr, Torok A, Alfoldi P, et al. Effects of intracerebroventricular injection of delta sleep–inducing peptide (DSIP) and an analogue on sleep and brain temperature in rats at night. Pharmacol Biochem Behav 1985;23:953–957.

104. Graf MV, Kastin AJ, Schoenenberger GA. Delta sleep–inducing peptide in spontaneously hyperactive rats. Pharmacol Biochem Behav 1986;24:1797–1799.

105. Dick P, Costa C, Foyolle K, et al. DSIP in the treatment of withdrawal syndromes from alcohol and opiates. Eur Neurol 1984;23:364–371.

106. Monnier M, Hatt AM, Cueni LB, et al. Humoral transmission of sleep. VI. Purification and assessment of a hypnogenic fraction of "sleep dialysate" (factor delta). Pflugers Arch 1972;331:257–265.

107. Tobler I, Borbely AA. Effect of delta sleep inducing peptide (DSIP) and arginine vasotocin (AVT) on sleep and locmotor activity in the rat. Waking Sleeping 1980;4:139–153.

108. Schoenenberger GA, Graf M. Effects of DSIP and DSIP-P on different biorhythmic parameters. In: Wauquier A, Gaillard JM, Monti JM, Radulovacki M, eds. Sleep: Neurotransmitters and Neuromodulators. New York: Raven Press, 1985;265–277.

109. Schneider-Helmert D. DSIP in insomnia. Eur Neurol 1984;23:358:363.

110. Kaeser HE. A clinical trial with DSIP. Eur Neurol 1984;23:386–388.

111. Schneider-Helmert D. Effects of DSIP on narcolepsy. Eur Neurol 1984;23:353–357.

112. Larbig W, Gerber WD, Kluck M, et al. Therapeutic effects of delta sleep–inducing peptide (DSIP) in patients with chronic, pronounced pain episodes. A clinical pilot study. Eur Neurol 1984;23:372–385.

113. Schneider-Helmert D. Efficacy of DSIP to normalize sleep in middle-aged and elderly chronic insomniacs. Eur Neurol 1986;5:448–453.

114. Hermann E, Ernst A, Schneider-Helmert D. Effects of DSIP on daytime mood states of insomniacs [Abstr]. Sleep Res 1987;16:222.

115. Hofman WF, Schneider-Helmert D. The influence of DSIP on the rhythm of spontaneous sleep tendency in insomniacs and normal subjects [Abstr]. Sleep Res 1987;16:615.

116. Schneider-Helmert D, Hermann E, Schoenenberger GA. Efficacy of DSIP for withdrawal treatment of low-dose benzodiazepine dependent insomniacs [Abstr]. Sleep Res 1987;16:133.

117. Schneider-Helmert D, Schoenenberger GA, Hermann E. Advancing delayed sleep phase by treatment with DSIP [Abstr]. Sleep Res 1987;16:222.

118. Schneider-Helmert D. DSIP: Clinical application of the programming effect. In: Inoue S, Schneider-Helmert D, eds. Sleep Peptides: Basic and Clinical Approaches. Berlin: Springer-Verlag, 1988;175–198.

119. Monti JM, Debellis J, Alterwain P, et al. Study of delta sleep–inducing peptide efficacy in improving sleep on short-term administration of chronic insomniacs. Int J Clin Pharmacol Res 1987;7:105–110.

120. Graf MV, Christen H, Tobler HJ, et al. Effects of repeated DSIP and DSIP-P administration on the circadian locomotor activity of rats. Pharmacol Biochem Behav 1981;15:717–721.

121. Graf MV, Christen H, Schoenenberger GA. DSIP/DSIP-P and circadian motor activity of rats under continuous light. Peptides 1982;3:623–626.

122. Inoue S, Honda K, Komoda Y, et al. Little sleep-promoting effects of three sleep substances diurnally infused in unrestrained rats. Neurosci Lett 1984;49:207–211.

123. Inoue S, Honda K, Komoda Y, et al. Differential sleep-promoting effects of five sleep substances nocturnally infused in unrestrained rats. Proc Natl Acad Sci USA 1984;81:6240–6244.

124. Komoda Y, Ishikawa M, Nagasaki H, et al. Uridine, a sleep-promoting substance from brainstems of sleep-deprived rats. Biomed Res 1983;4(Suppl):223–227.

125. Komoda Y, Ishikawa M, Nagasaki H, et al. Purification, isolation, and identification of sleep-promoting substances (SPS) from brainstems of sleep-deprived rats. Folia Psychiatr Neurol Jpn 1985;39:210–211.

126. Inoue S, Honda K, Komoda Y. Sleep-promoting substances. In: Wauquier A, Gaillard JM, Monti JM, et al. eds. Sleep: Neurotransmitters and Neuromodulators. New York: Raven Press, 1985;305–318.

127. Krooth RS, Hsaio WL, Lam GFM. Effects of natural pyrimidines and of certain related compounds on the spontaneous activity in the mouse. J Pharmacol Exp Ther 1978;207:504–514.

128. Yamamoto I, Kimura T, Tateoka Y, et al. Central depressant activities of N3-allyluridine and N3-allylthymidine. Res Commun Chem Pathol Pharmacol 1986;52:321–332.

129. Honda K, Komoda Y, Inoue S. Effects of sleep-promoting substances on the rat circadian sleep-waking cycles. In: Inoue S, Borbely AA, eds. Endogenous Sleep

Substances and Sleep Regulation. Tokyo: Japan Scientific Society Press, 1985;203–214.

130. Honda K, Komoda Y, Nishida S, et al. Uridine as an active component of sleep-promoting substance: Its effects on the nocturnal sleep in rats. Neurosci Res 1984;1:243–252.

131. Inoue S. Sleep substances: Their roles and evolution. In: Inoue S, Borbely AA, eds. Endogenous Sleep Substances and Sleep Regulation. Tokyo: Japan Scientific Society Press, 1985;3–12.

132. Martin SA, Karnovsky ML, Krueger JM, et al. Peptidoglycans as promoters of slow-wave sleep. I. Structure of the sleep-promoting factor isolated from human urine. J Biol Chem 1984;259:12652–12658.

133. Krueger JM, Karnovsky ML, Martin SA, et al. Peptidoglycans as promotors of slow wave sleep. II. Somnogenic and pyrogenic activities of some naturally occurring muramyl peptides; correlations with mass spectrometric structure determination. J Biol Chem 1984;259:12659–12662.

134. Krueger JM. Muramyl peptides and interleukin-1 as promoters of slow-wave sleep. In: Inoue S, Borbely AA, eds. Endogenous Sleep Substances and Sleep Regulation. Tokyo: Japan Scientific Society Press, 1985;181–192.

135. Krueger JM. Muramyl peptide enhancement of slow-wave sleep. Methods Find Exp Clin Pharmacol 1986;8:105–110.

136. Krueger JM, Walter J, Levin C. Factor S and related somnogens: An immune theory for slow wave sleep. In: McGinty DJ, Drucker-Colin R, Morrison A, et al., eds. Brain Mechanisms of Sleep. New York: Raven Press, 1987;253–275.

137. Krueger JM, Toth LA, Cady AB, et al. Immunomodulation and sleep. In: Inoue S, Schneider-Helmert D, eds. Sleep Peptides: Basic and Clinical Approaches. Berlin: Springer-Verlag, 1988;95–129.

138. Krueger JM, Karnovsky ML. Sleep and immune response. Ann NY Acad Sci 1987;496:510–516.

139. Adam A, Lederer E. Muramyl peptides: Immunomodulators, sleep factors, and vitamins. Med Res Rev 1984;4:111–152.

140. Karnovsky ML. Muramyl peptides in mammalian tissues and their effects at the cellular level. Fed Proc 1986;45:2556–2560.

141. Werner GH, Floc'h F, Migliore-Samour D, Jolles P. Immunomodulating peptides. Experientia 1986;42:521–531.

142. Krueger JM. Pappenheimer JR, Karnovsky ML. Sleep-promoting effects of muramyl peptides. Proc Natl Acad Sci USA 1982;79:6102–6106.

143. Krueger JM, Walter J, Karnovsky ML, et al. Muramyl peptides. Variation of somnogenic activity with structure. J Exp Med 1984;159:68–76.

144. Krueger JM. Endogenous sleep factors. In: Wauquier A, Gaillard JM, Monti JM, et al., eds. Sleep: Neurotransmitters and Neuromodulators. New York: Raven Press, 1985;319–331.

145. Johanssen L, Wecke J, Krueger JM. Macrophase processing of bacteria; CNS-active substances are produced [Abstr]. Soc Neurosci 1987;13:260.

146. Moldofsky H, Lue FA, Eisen J, et al. The relationship of interleukin-1 and immune functions to sleep in humans. Psychosom Med 1986;48:309–318.

147. Walter J, Davenne D, Shoham S, et al. Brain temperature changes coupled to sleep states persist during interleukin-1–enhanced sleep. Am J Physiol 1986;250:R96–R103.

148. Tobler I, Borbely AA, Schwyzser M, et al. Interleukin-1 derived from astrocytes enhances slow wave activity in sleep EEG of the rat. Eur J Pharmacol 1984;104:191–192.

149. Shoham S, Davenne D, Cady AB, et al. Recombinant tumor necrosis factor and interleukin-1 enhance slow-wave sleep in rabbits. Am J Physiol 1987;253:R142–R149.

150. Krueger JM, Walter J, Dinarello CA. Sleep-promoting effects of endogenous pyrogen (interleukin-1). Am J Physiol 1984;246:R994–R999.

151. Krueger JM, Karaszewski JH, Davenne D, et al. Somnogenic muramyl peptides. Fed Proc 1986;45:2552–2555.

152. Mignot E, Wang C, Rattazzi C, et al. Genetic linkage of autosomal recessive canine narcolepsy with a μ-immunoglobulin heavy chain switch-like segment. Proc Natl Acad Sci USA 1991;88:3475–3478.

153. Irwin M, Smith TL, Gillin JC. Electroencephalographic sleep and natural killer cell activity in depressed patients and controls. Psychosom Med 1992;54:10–21.

154. Pavel S, Psatta D, Goldstein R. Slow wave sleep induced in cats by extremely small amounts of synthetic and pineal vasotocin injected into the third ventricle of the brian. Brain Res Bull 1977;2:251–254.

155. Goldstein R, Psatta D. Sleep in the cat: Raphe dorsalis and vasotocin. Sleep 1984;7:373–379.

156. Mendelson WB, Gillin JC, Pisner G, et al. Arginine vasotocin and sleep in the rat. Brain Res 1980;182:246–249.

157. Karacan I, Thornby JI, Anch AM. Dose-related sleep disturbances induced by coffee and caffeine. Clin Pharmacol Ther 1976;20:682–689.

158. Radulovacki M, Miletich RS, Green RD. N-6 (L-phenylisopropyl) adenosine (L-PIA) increases slow wave sleep (S2) and decreases wakefulness in rats. Brain Res 1982;246:178–180.

159. Radulovacki M, Virus RM, Djuricic-Nedelson M, et al. Adenosine analogs and sleep in rats. J Pharmacol Exp Ther 1984;228:268–274.

160. Radulovacki M, Virus RM, Rapoza D, et al. A comparison of the dose response effects of pyrimidine ribonucleosides and adenosine on sleep in rats. Psychopharmacology 1985;87:136–140.

161. Radulovacki M, Virus RM, Djuricic-Nedelson M, et al. Hypnotic effects of deoxycoformycin in rats. Brain Res 1983;271:392–395.

162. Sarda N, Dubois M, Gharib A, et al. Increase of paradoxical sleep induced by S-adenosyl-L-homocysteine. Neurosci Lett 1982;30:69–72.

163. Yanik G, Radulovacki M. REM sleep deprivation upregulates adenosine A1 receptors. Brain Res 1987;402:362–364.

164. Ueno R, Hayaishi O, Osama H, et al. Prostaglandin D_2 regulated physiological sleep. In: Inoue S, Borbely AA, eds. Endogenous Sleep Substances and Sleep Regulation. Tokyo: Japan Scientific Society Press, 1985;193–201.

165. Ueno R, Honda K, Inoue S, et al. Prostaglandin D_2, a cerebral sleep-inducing substance in rats. Proc Natl Acad Sci USA 1983;80:1735–1737.

166. Matsumura H, Honda K, Goh Y, et al. Awaking effect of prostaglandin E_2 in freely moving rats. Brain Res 1989;481:242–249.

167. Ueno R, Ishikawa Y, Nakayama T, et al. Prostaglandin D_2 induces sleep when microinjected into the preoptic area of conscious rats. Biochem Biophys Res Commun 1982;109:576–582.

168. Hayaishi O, Ueno R, Onoe H, et al. Prostaglandin D_2 induces sleep when infused into the cerebral ventrical of conscious monkeys. Adv Prostaglandin Thromboxane Leukot Res 1987;17B:946–948.

169. Hayaishi O. Prostaglandin D_2 and sleep. Adv Prostaglandin Thromboxane Leukot Res 1989;19:26–33.

170. Onoe H, Ueno R, Fujita I, et al. Prostaglandin D_2, a cerebral sleep-inducing substance in monkeys. Proc Natl Acad Sci USA 1988;85:4082–4086.

171. Naito K, Osama H, Ueno R, et al. Suppression of sleep by prostaglandin synthesis inhibitors in unrestrained rats. Brain Res 1988;71(3A):A298.

172. Matsumura H, Goh Y, Ueno R, et al. Awaking effect of Pg E_2 microinjected into the preoptic area of rats. Brain Res 1988;444:265–272.

173. Rosenthal NE, Sack DA, Gillin JC, et al. Seasonal affective disorder. Arch Gen Psychiatry 1984;41:72–80.

174. Wetterberg L, Beck-Frus J, Kjellman BF. Melatonin as a marker for a subgroup of depression in adults. In: Shafii M, Shafii SL, eds. Biological Rhythms, Mood Disorder, Light Therapy, and the Pineal Gland. Washington, DC: American Psychiatric Press, 1990;69–95.

175. Parry BL, Berga S, Kripke D, et al. Altered waveform of plasma nocturnal melatonin secretion in premenstrual depression. Arch Gen Psychiatry 1990;47:1139–1145.

176. Marczynski TJ, Yamaguchi N, Ling GM, et al. Sleep induced by the administration of melatonin (5-methoxy-N-acetyltryptamine) to the hypothalamus in unrestrained cats. Experientia 1964;20:435–437.

177. Hishikawa Y, Cramer H, Kuhlo W. Natural and melatonin-induced sleep in young chickens—a behavioral and electrographic study. Exp Brain Res 1969;7:84–94.

178. Anton-Tay F, Diaz JL, Fernandez-Guardiola A. On the effect of melatonin upon human brain. Its possible therapeutic implications. Life Sci 1971;10:841–850.

179. Cramer H, Rudolph J, Consbruch U, et al. On the effects of melatonin on sleep and behavior in man. Adv Biochem Psychopharmacol 1974;11:187–191.

180. Holmes SW, Sugden D. Effects of melatonin on sleep and neurochemistry in the rat. Br J Pharmacol 1982;76:95–101.

181. Cramer H, Bohme W, Kendel K, et al. Freisetzung von Wachstumshormon und von Melanozyten stimulierendem Hormon im durch Melatonin gebahnten

Schlaf beim Menschen. Arzneimittelforschung 1976;26:1076–1078.

182. Lieberman HR, Waldhauser F, Garfield G, et al. Effects of melatonin on human mood and performance. Brain Res 1984;323:201–207.

183. James SP, Mendelson WB, Sack DA, et al. The effect of melatonin on normal sleep. Neuropsychopharmacology 1987;1:41–44.

184. Arendt J, Borbely AA, Franey C, et al. Effects of chronic, small doses of melatonin given in the late afternoon on fatigue in man: A preliminary study. Neurosci Lett 1984;45:317–321.

185. Arendt J, Bojkowski C, Folkard S, et al. Some effects of melatonin and the control of its secretion in man. In: Evered D, Clark S, eds. Photoperiodism, the Pineal Gland, and Melatonin. Ciba Symposium 1985;266–279.

186. Mendelson WB, Canin M, Cook JM, et al. A benzodiazepine receptor antagonist decreases sleep and reverses the hypnotic actions of flurazepam. Science 1983;219:414–416.

187. Scherschlicht R. Role for GABA in the control of the sleep-wakefulness cycle. In: Wauquier A, Gaillard J, Monti JM, et al eds. Sleep: Neurotransmitters and Neuromodulators. New York: Raven Press,1985;237–249.

188. Henley K, Morrison AD. A re-evaluation of the effects of lesions of the pontine tegmentum and locus coeruleus on phenomena of paradoxical sleep in the cat. Acta Neurobiol Exp 1974;34:215–232.

189. Jones BE, Tian-Zhu Y. The efferent projections from the reticular formation and the locus coeruleus by anterograde and retrograde axonal transport in the rat. J Comp Neurol 1985;242:56–92.

190. Steriade M, McCarley RW. Brainstem Control of Wakefulness and Sleep. New York: Plenum Press, 1990.

191. Magoun HW, Rhines R. An inhibitory mechanism in the bulbar reticular formation. J Neurophysiol 1946;9:165–171.

192. Friedman L, Jones BE. Computer graphic analysis of sleep-wakefulness state changes after pontine lesions. Brain Res Bull 1984;13:53–68.

193. Friedman L, Jones BE. Study of sleep-wakefulness states by computer graphics and cluster anlaysis before and after lesions of pontine tegmentum in the cat. Electroencephalogr Clin Neurophysiol 1984;57:43–56.

194. Mitani A, Ito K, Hallanger AE, et al. Cholinergic projections from the laterodorsal and pedunculopontine tegmental nuclei to the pontine giganticellular tegmental field in the cat. Brain Res 1988;451:397–402.

195. Shiromani PJ. Armstrong DM, Gillin JC. Cholinergic neurons from the dorsolateral pons project to the medial pons: A WGA-HRP and choline acetyltransferase immunohistochemical study. Neurosci Lett 1988;95:19–23.

196. Friedman AK. Circumstances influencing Otto Loewi's discovery of chemical transmission in the nervous system. Pflugers Arch 1971;325:85–86.

197. Mazzuchelli-O'Flaherty AL, O'Flaherty JJ, Hernandez-Peon R. Sleep and other behavioral responses induced by acetylcholinergic stimulation of frontal and mesial cortex. Brain Res 1967;4:268–283.

198. Hernandez-Peon R, Chavez-Ibarra G, Morgane PJ, et al. Limbic cholinergic pathways involved in sleep and emotional behavior. Exp Neurol 1963;8:93–111.

199. Hernandez-Peon R, O'Flaherty JJ, Mazzuchelli-O'Flaherty AL. Sleep and other behavioral effects induced by acetylcholinergic stimulation of basal temporal cortex and striate structures. Brain Res 1967;4:243–267.

200. Baghdoyan HA, Rodrigo-Angula ML, McCarley RW, et al. Site-specific enhancement and suppression of desynchronized sleep signs following cholinergic stimulation of three brainstem sites. Brain Res 1984;306:39–52.

201. Baghdoyan HA, Lydic R, Clifton CW, et al. The carbachol-induced enhancement of desynchronized sleep signs is dose dependent and antagonized by centrally administered atropine. Neuropsychopharmacology 1989;2:67–79.

202. Vanni-Mercier G, Sakai K, Lin DS, et al. Mapping of cholinoreceptive brainstem structures responsible for the generation of paradoxical sleep in the cat. Arch Ital Biol 1989;127:133–164.

203. Baghdoyan HA, Rodrigo-Angulo ML, McCarley RW, et al. A neuroanatomical gradient in the pontine tegmentum for the cholinoceptive induction of desynchronized sleep signs. Brain Res 1987;414:245–261.

204. Gnadt JW, Pegram GV. Cholinergic brainstem mechanisms of REM sleep in the rat. Brain Res 1986;384:29–41.

205. Datta S, Calvo JM, Quattrochi JJ, et al. Long-term enhancement of REM sleep following cholinergic stimulation. Neuroreport 1991;2:619–622.

206. Hazra J. Effect of hemicholinium-3 on slow wave and paradoxical sleep of cat. Eur J Pharmacol 1970;11:395–397.

207. Kodama T, Takahashi Y, Honda Y. Enhancement of ACh release during paradoxical sleep in the dorsal tegmental field of the cat brain stem. Neurosci Lett 1990;114:277–282.

208. Gillin JC, Sutton L, Ruiz C, et al. The effects of scopolamine on sleep and mood in depressed patients with a history of alcoholism and a normal comparison group. Biol Psychiatry 1991;30:157–169.

209. Sutin EL, Shiromani PJ, Kelsoe JR, et al. Rapid eye movement sleep and muscarinic receptor binding in rats are augmented during withdrawal from chronic scopolamine treatment. Life Sci 1986;39:2419–2427.

210. McCarley RW, Massaquoi SG. A limit cycle mathematical model of the REM sleep oscillatory system. Am J Physiol 1986;251:R1011–R1029.

211. Berger M, Reimann D, Hoechli D, et al. The cholinergergic REM sleep induction test with RS86: State or trait-marker of depression? Arch Gen Psychiatry 1989;46:421–428.

212. Berkowitz A, Janowsky D, Gillin JC. Pilocarpine, an orally active, muscarinic, cholinergic agonist, induces REM sleep and reduces Delta sleep in normal volunteers. Psychiatry Res 1990;33:113–119.

213. Gillin JC, Sutton L, Ruiz C, et al. The cholinergic REM induction test with arecoline in depression. Arch Gen Psychiatry 1991;48:264–270.

214. Janowsky DS, El-Yousef MK, Davis JM. A cholinergic-adrenergic hypothesis of mania and depression. Lancet 1972;2:632–635.

215. Riemann D, Gann H, Fleckenstein P, et al. Effect of RS 86 on REM latency in schizophrenia. Psychiatry Res 1991;38:89–92.

216. Tandon R, Greden JF. Cholinergic hyperactivity and negative schizophrenic symptoms. Arch Gen Psychiatry 1989;46:747–758.

217. Velazquez-Moctezuma J, Shalauta MD, Gillin JC, Shiromani PJ. Cholinergic antagonists and REM sleep generation. Brain Res 1991;543:175–179.

218. Velazquez-Moctezuma J, Gillin JC, Shiromani PJ. Effect of specific M1, M2 muscarinic receptor agonists on REM sleep generation. Brain Res 1989;503:128–131.

219. Velazquez-Moctezuma J, Shiromani PJ, Gillin JC. Acetylcholine and acetylcholine receptor subtypes in REM sleep generation. In: Aquilonius SM, Gillberg PG, eds. Progress in Brain Research. Amsterdam: Elsevier Science Publications, 1990:407–413.

220. Gillin JC, Sutton L, Ruiz C, et al. Dose dependent inhibition of REM sleep in normal volunteers by biperiden, a muscarinic antagonist. Biol Psychiatry 1991;30:151–156.

221. Salin-Pascual RJ, Granados-Fuentes D, Galacia-Polo L, et al. Biperiden administration in normal sleep and after REM sleep deprivation in healthy volunteers. Neuropsychopharmacology 1991;5:97–102.

222. Salin-Pascual RJ, Granados-Fuentes D, Galicia-Polo L, et al. Rapid eye movement (REM) sleep increases by auditory stimulation reverted with biperiden administration in normal volunteers. Neuropsychopharmacology 1991;5:183–186.

223. Salin-Pascual RJ, Jimenez-Anguiano A, Granados-Fuentes D, et al. Effects of biperiden on sleep at baseline and after 72 h of REM sleep deprivation in the cat. Psychopharmacology (Berl) 1992;106:540–542.

224. Zoltoski RK, Velazquez-Moctezuma J, Shalauta M, et al. Effects of muscarinic antagonists on sleep [Abstr]. Soc Neurosci 1990;16:1254.

225. Overstreet DH, Russell RW, Helps SC, et al. Selective breeding for sensitivity to the anticholinesterase DFP. Psychopharmacology 1979;65:15–20.

226. Shiromani PJ, Overstreet D, Levy D, et al. Increased REM sleep in rats genetically bred for cholinergic hyperactivity. Neuropsychopharmacology 1988;1:127–133.

227. Overstreet DH. Selective breeding for increased cholinergic function: Development of a new animal model of depression. Biol Psychiatry 1986;21:49–58.

228. Kilduff TS, Bowersox S, Kaitin K, et al. Muscarinic cholinergic receptors and the canine model of narcolepsy. Sleep 1986;9:102–106.

229. Hu B, Bouhassira D, Steriade M, et al. The blockage of PGO waves in the cat LGN by nicotinic antagonists. Brain Res 1988;473:394–397.

230. Velazquez-Moctezuma J, Shalauta MD, Gillin JC, et al. Differential effects of cholinergic antagonists on REM sleep components. Psychopharmacol Bull 1990;26:349–353.

231. Velazquez-Moctezuma J, Shalauta MD, Gillin JC, et al. Microinjections of nicotine in the medial pontine reticular formation elicits REM sleep. Neurosci Lett 1990;115:265–268.

232. Soldatos CR, Kales JD, Scharf MB. Cigarette smoking associated with sleep difficulty. Science 1980;207: 551–553.

233. Siegel JM, Rogawski MA. A function for REM sleep: Regulation of noradrenergic receptor sensitivity. Brain Res Rev 1988;13:213–233.

234. Rechtschaffen A, Maron L. The effect of amphetamine on the sleep cycle. Electroencephalogr Clin Neurophysiol 1964;16:438–445.

235. Stern WC, Morgane PJ. Theoretical view of REM sleep function: Maintenance of catecholamine systems in the central nervous system. Behav Biol 1974;11:1–32.

236. Wyatt RJ. The serotonin-catecholamine dream bicycle: A clinical study. Biol Psychiatry 1972;5:33–63.

237. Sitaram N, Gillin JC, Bunney WE Jr. Cholinergic and catecholaminergic receptor sensitivity illness: Strategy and theory. In: Post RM, Ballenger JC, eds. Neurobiology of Mood Disorders. Baltimore: William & Wilkins, 1984;629–651.

238. Coulter JD, Lester BK. Reserpine and sleep. Psychopharmacology 1971;19:134–147.

239. Ruch-Monachon MA, Jalfre M, Haefely W. Drugs and PGO waves in the lateral geniculate body of the curarized cat. I. PGO wave activity induced by Ro4-1284 and by *p*-chloropheylalanine (PCPA) as a basis for neuropharmacological studies. Arch Int Pharmacodynam 1976;219:251–346.

240. Depoorte H. Adrenergic agonists and antagonists and sleep-wakefulness stages. In: Wauquier A, Gaillard JM, Monti JM, et al. eds. Sleep: Neurotransmitters and Neuromodulators. New York: Raven Press, 1985;79–92.

241. Guilleminault C. Narcolepsy syndrome. In: Kryger MH, Roth T, Dement WC, eds. Principles and Practices of Sleep Medicine. Philadelphia: WB Saunders, 1989;338–347.

242. Mignot E, Guilleminault C, Bowersox S, et al. Role of central alpha-1 adrenoceptors in canine narcolepsy. J Clin Invest 1988;82:885–894.

243. Aldrich MS, Rogers AE. Exacerbation of human cataplexy by prazosin. Sleep 1989;12:254–256.

244. Hilakivi I, Leppavouri A. Effects of methoxamine, an alpha-1 adrenoceptor agonist, and prazosin, an alpha-1 antagonist, on the stages of the sleep-wake cycle in the rat. Acta Physiol Scand 1984;120:363–372.

245. Oswald I, Adam K, Allen S, et al. Alpha-adrenergic blocker, thymoxamine and mesoridazine both increase human REM sleep duration [Abstr]. Sleep Res 1974;3:62.

246. Nicholson AN, Pascoe PA. Presynaptic alpha$_2$-adrenoceptor function and sleep in man: Studies with clonidine and idazoxan. Neuropharmacology 1991;30: 367–372.

247. Hilakivi I. The role of beta- and alpha-adrenoreceptors in the regulation of the stages of the sleep-waking cycle in the cat. Brain Res 1983;277:109–118.

248. Borbely AA, Tobler I. Endogenous sleep-promoting substances and sleep regulation. Physiol Rev 1989; 69:605–652.

249. Shiromani P, Gillin JC, Henriksen SJ. Acetylcholine and the regulation of REM sleep: Basic mechanisms and clinical implication for affective illness and narcolepsy. Annu Rev Pharmacol Toxicol 1987;27:137–156.

250. Muzio JN, Roffwarg HP, Kaufman E. Alterations in the nocturnal sleep cycle resulting from LSD. Electroencephalogr Clin Neurophysiol 1966;21:313–324.

251. Torda C. Contribution to the serotonin theory of dreaming (LSD infusion). NY State J Med 1968; 68:1135–1138.

252. Haigler HJ, Aghajanian GK. Lysergic acid diethylamide and serotonin: A comparison of effects on serotonergic neurons and neurons receiving a serotonergic input. J Pharmacol Exp Ther 1974;188:688–699.

253. Pavel S. Pineal vasotocin and sleep: Involvement of serotonin containing neurons. Brain Res Bull 1979; Nov–Dec 4:731–734.

254. Riou F, Cespuglio R, Jouvet M. Endogenous peptides and sleep in the rat. III. The hypnogenic properties of vasoactive intestinal peptide. Neuropeptides 1982; 2:265–277.

255. Prospero-Garcia O, Morales M, Arankowsky-Sandoval G, et al. Vasoactive intestinal polypeptide (VIP) and cerebrospinal fluid (CSF) of sleep-deprived cats restores REM sleep in insomniac recipients. Brain Res 1986;385:169–173.

256. Danguir J, De Saint-Hilaire Kafi S. Reversal of desipramine-induced suppression of paradoxial sleep by a long-acting somatostatin analogue (octreotide) in rats. Neurosci Lett 1989;98:154–158.

257. Danguir J. Intracerebroventricular infusion of somatostatin selectively increases paradoxical sleep in rats. Brain Res 1986;367:26–30.

258. Danguir J. The somatostatin analogue SMS 201–995 promotes paradoxical sleep in aged rats. Neurobiol Aging 1989;93:349–350.

259. Danguir J, De Saint-Hilaire-Kafi S. Scopolamine-induced suppression of paradoxical sleep is reversed by the somatostatin analogue SMS 201–995 in rats. Pharmacol Biochem Behav 1988;30:295–297.

260. Danguir J, De Saint-Hilaire-Kafi S. Somatostatin antiserum blocks carbachol-induced increase in paradoxical sleep in the rat. Brain Res Bull 1988;20:9–12.

5

Physiologic Changes
in Sleep

Sudhansu Chokroverty

Awareness is growing about the importance of sleep and its effect on the human organism. Adult human beings spend approximately one third of life sleeping, yet we do not have a clear idea of the functions of sleep. We do know that a vast number of physiologic changes take place during sleep in humans and other mammals. Almost every system in the body undergoes changes during sleep, most in the direction of reduced activity though certain ones indicate increased activity. The "physiology of wakefulness" has been studied intensively, but until recently very little was written about physiologic changes during sleep. It is important to know these changes in different body systems, to understand the physiology of several sleep disorders. A striking example is sleep apnea syndrome, which causes dramatic changes in respiratory control and the upper airway muscles during sleep that direct our attention to a very important pathophysiologic mechanism, and a therapeutic intervention, for this disorder. Similarly, physiologic changes in several other body systems are important to understanding the pathophysiology of many medical disorders, including disturbances of sleep.

Physiologic changes are known to occur in both the somatic and the autonomic nervous system during sleep. Important changes in the endocrine system and temperature regulation also are associated with sleep. All these factors have important effects, in terms of understanding the clinical disorders. In this chapter, I review the physiologic changes in the respiratory, cardiovascular and neuromuscular systems and gastrointestinal tract during sleep, as well as thermal and endocrine regulation. For details readers are referred to excellent reviews by Orem and Barnes[1] and Lydic and coworkers.[2]

RESPIRATION AND SLEEP

Functional Neuroanatomy of Respiration

Legallois[3] discovered in 1812 that breathing depends on a circumscribed region of the medulla. Following an intensive period of research on the respiratory centers in the nineteenth century, Lumsden,[4,5] and later Pitts and coworkers[6] in the twentieth century, laid down the foundation for the modern concepts of the central respiratory neuronal networks. Based on sectioning at different levels of the brain stem of cats, Lumsden[4,5] proposed pneumotaxic and apneustic centers in the pons and expiratory and gasping centers in the medulla. Later, Pitts' group,[6] concluded from experiments in cats that the inspiratory and expiratory centers were located in the medullary reticular formation.

There is a close interrelationship between the respiratory,[7-9] central autonomic,[10,11] and lower brain stem hypnogenic neurons[12-19] in the pontomedullary region. The hypothalamic and the lower brain stem hypnogenic neurons are also connected.[20] Reciprocal connections exist between hypothalamus, central nucleus of amgydala, parabrachial and Kolliker-Fuse nucleus, and nucleus tractus solitarius (NTS) of the medulla (Figures 5-1, 5-2).[11,21-24] In addition, the NTS connects with the nucleus ambiguus and retroambigualis (Figure 5-2).[21-24] Thus, the anatomic relationship suggests close functional interdependence between the central autonomic network and respiratory and hypnogenic neurons. In addition, peripheral respiratory receptors (arising from the pulmonary and tracheobronchial tree) and chemoreceptors (peripheral and central) interact with the central autonomic network in the region of the NTS.[7-9,25,26]

Breathing is controlled during wakefulness and sleep by two separate and independent systems[8,9,27-30]: the metabolic or automatic[8,9] and the voluntary or behavioral systems.[30] Both voluntary and metabolic systems operate during wakefulness, but breathing during sleep is entirely dependent upon the inherent rhythmicity of the autonomic (automatic) respiratory control system located in the medulla.[27-29] The voluntary control is mediated through the behavioral system that influences ventilation during wakefulness as well as nonrespiratory functions[31,32] such as phonation and speech. Additionally, the wakefulness stimulus, which is probably derived from the ascending reticular activating system,[33,34] represents a tonic stimulus to

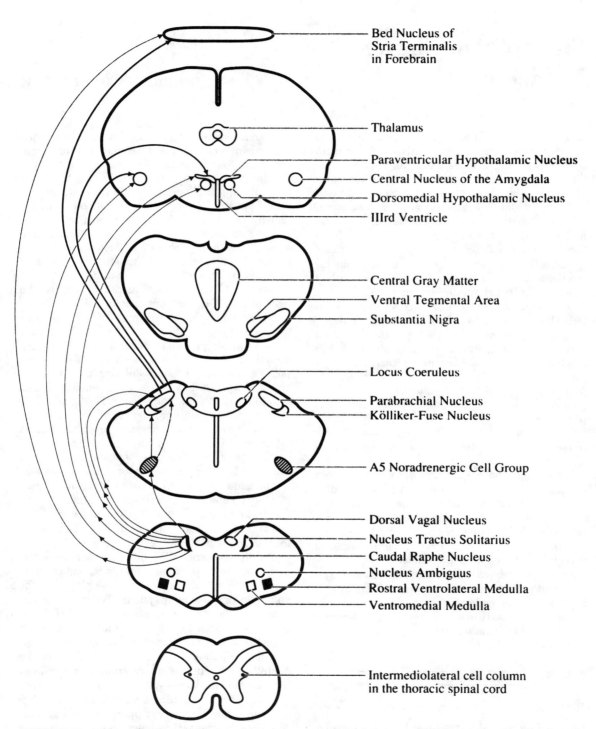

FIGURE 5-1.   *The ascending projections from the central autonomic network. (Reprinted with permission from Chokroverty S. Functional anatomy of the autonomic nervous system correlated with symptomatology of neurologic disease. In American Academy of Neurology Course No. 246, San Diego, CA, 1992;49–76.)*

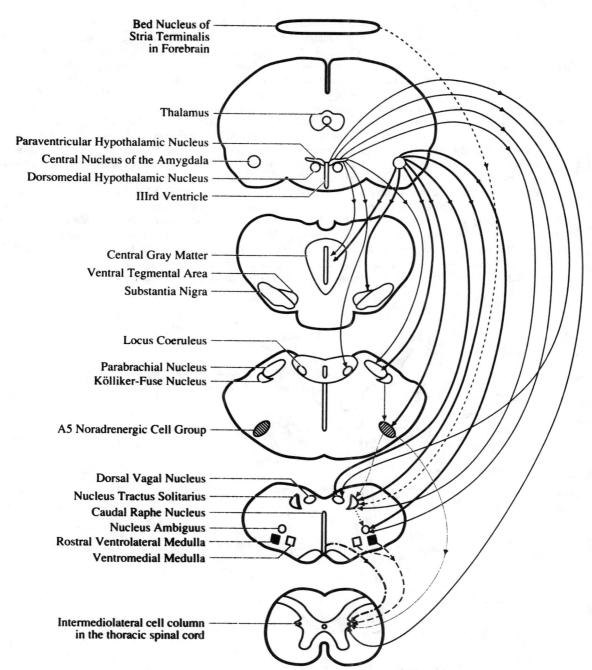

Bed Nucleus of
Stria Terminalis
in Forebrain

Thalamus

Paraventricular Hypothalamic Nucleus
Central Nucleus of the Amygdala
Dorsomedial Hypothalamic Nucleus
IIIrd Ventricle

Central Gray Matter
Ventral Tegmental Area
Substantia Nigra

Locus Coeruleus

Parabrachial Nucleus
Kölliker-Fuse Nucleus

A5 Noradrenergic Cell Group

Dorsal Vagal Nucleus
Nucleus Tractus Solitarius
Caudal Raphe Nucleus
Nucleus Ambiguus
Rostral Ventrolateral Medulla
Ventromedial Medulla

Intermediolateral cell column
in the thoracic spinal cord

FIGURE 5-2.   *The descending projections from the central autonomic network. (Reprinted with permission from Chokroverty S. Functional anatomy of the autonomic nervous system correlated with symptomatology of neurologic disease. In American Academy of Neurology Course No. 246, San Diego, CA, 1992;49–76.)*

ventilation during wakefulness. McNicholas and coworkers[35] mentioned the reticular arousal system, which is probably the same as the wakefulness stimulus,[33,34,36] exerting a tonic influence on the brain stem respiratory neurons.

Upper brain stem respiratory neurons are located in the rostral pons, in the region of the parabrachial and Kolliker-Fuse nuclei (pneumotaxic center), and in the dorsolateral region of the lower pons (apneustic center.[26] These two centers influence the automatic medullary respiratory neurons, which comprise two principal groups.[7-9,25-29,37,38] The dorsal respiratory group located in the NTS is responsible principally, but not exclusively, for inspiration, and the ventral respiratory group located in the region of the nucleus ambiguus and retroambigualis is responsible for both inspiration and expiration (Figure 5-3). These respiratory premotor neurons send axons that decussate below the obex and descend in the reticulospinal tracts in the ventrolateral cervical spinal cord to form synapses with the spinal respiratory motor neurons innervating the various respiratory muscles (Figures 5-3, 5-4). Respiratory rhythmogenesis depends on tonic inputs from the peripheral and central structures converging on the medullary neurons.[4,25,39,40] The parasympathetic vagal afferents from the peripheral respiratory tracts, the carotid and aortic body peripheral chemoreceptors, the central chemoreceptors located on the ventrolateral

surface of the medulla lateral to the pyramids, the supramedullary (forebrain, midbrain, and pontine regions) and the reticular activating systems all influence the medullary respiratory neurons to regulate the rate, rhythm, and amplitude of breathing and internal homeostasis.[10,25,26,40] Figure 5-5 schematically shows the effects of various brain stem and vagal transections on ventilatory patterns.

The voluntary control system for breathing originating in the cerebral cortex (forebrain and limbic system) controls respiration during wakefulness and has some nonrespiratory functions.[25,30,40] This system descends partly to the autonomic medullary controlling system and integrates in part there, but mostly it descends with the corticobulbar and the corticospinal tracts to the spinal respiratory motor neurons, where the fibers finally integrate with the reticulospinal fibers originating from the automatic medullary respiratory neurons.[8,9,22,29,41]

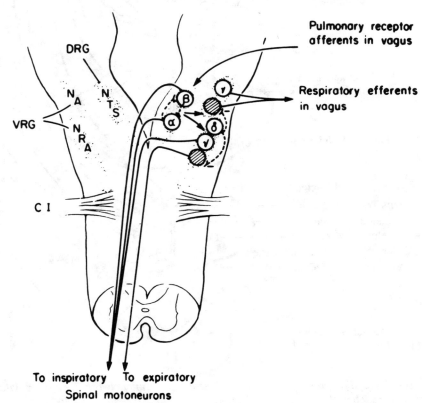

FIGURE 5-3.   *Schematic diagram shows medullary respiratory neurons, cell types, and their interconnections. Key: DRG, dorsal respiratory group; VRG, ventral respiratory group; NTS, nucleus tractus solitarius; NA, nucleus ambiguus; NRA, nucleus retroambigualis; CI, First cervical root; α, β, γ, δ, designations for inspiratory cell subtypes; open circles, inspiratory cells; hatched circles, expiratory cells. (Reproduced with permission from Berger AJ, Mitchell RA, Severinghaus JW. Regulation of respiration. N Engl J Med 1977;297:92–97,138–143,194–201.)*

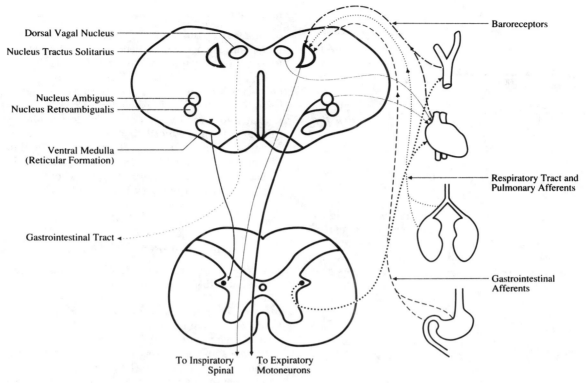

Dorsal Vagal Nucleus
Nucleus Tractus Solitarius
Nucleus Ambiguus
Nucleus Retroambigualis
Ventral Medulla
(Reticular Formation)
Gastrointestinal Tract
To Inspiratory Spinal
To Expiratory Motoneurons
Baroreceptors
Respiratory Tract and Pulmonary Afferents
Gastrointestinal Afferents

FIGURE 5-4. *The visceral afferents to and efferents from the nucleus tractus solitarius. (Reprinted with permission from Chokroverty S. Functional anatomy of the autonomic nervous system correlated with symptomatology of neurologic disease. In American Academy of Neurology Course No. 246, San Diego, CA, 1992;49–76.)*

Control of Ventilation During Wakefulness

The function of ventilation is to maintain arterial homeostasis (i.e., normal PO_2 and PCO_2.)[42] To maintain optimal PO_2 and PCO_2 levels, the metabolic or autonomic respiratory system utilizes mainly the peripheral and central chemoreceptors but also to some extent the body's metabolism and the intrapulmonary receptors.[42] It is well known that hypoxia and hypercapnia stimulate breathing.[43,44] Hypoxic ventilatory response is mediated through the carotid body chemoreceptors.[45,46] Normally, this response represents a hyperbolic curve[42,43] that shows a sudden increase in ventilation when PO_2 falls below 60 mm Hg (Figure 5-6). On the other hand, hypercapnic[42,44] ventilatory response is linear (Figure 5-6). This is mediated mainly through the medullary chemoreceptors[47] but also to some extent through the carotid body peripheral chemoreceptors.[45] When PCO_2 falls below a certain minimum level, resting ventilation is inhibited.[42] The metabolic rate (e.g., carbon dioxide production [VCO_2] or oxygen consumption [VO_2], particularly VCO_2, affects ventilation in part.[42] During sleep metabolism slows. The intrapulmonary receptors do not seem to play a major role in normal

human ventilation.[42] An important reflex, the Hering-Breuer reflex, depends on pulmonary stretch receptors. Vagal afferent stimulation by increasing lung inflation terminates inspiration.

In normal persons, during both rapid eye movement (REM) and non-REM (NREM) sleep, clear alterations are noted in tidal volume, alveolar ventilation, blood gases, and respiratory rate and rhythm.[27–29,40,48–52]

Changes in ventilation

During NREM sleep, minute ventilation falls by about 0.5 to 1.5 l per minute,[42,49,51,53–56] and this is secondary to reduction in the tidal volume. REM sleep shows a similar reduction of minute ventilation, up to about 1.6 l per minute.[42,51,54,56–58] Although there is a discrepancy in the literature regarding REM sleep–related ventilation in humans, it is generally accepted that most reduction occurs during phasic REM.

The following factors, in combination, may be responsible for alveolar hypoventilation during sleep[42]: reduction of VCO_2 and VO_2 during sleep;

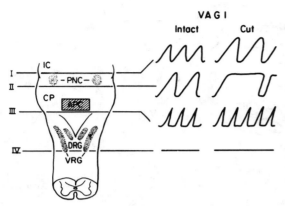

FIGURE 5-5.   *Effects of various brain stem and vagal transections on the ventilatory pattern of the anesthetized animal. On the left is a schematic representation of the dorsal surface of the lower brain stem, and on the right a representation of tidal volume with inspiration upward. Key: IC, inferior colliculus; PNC, pneumotaxic center; CP, cerebellar peduncle; APC, apneustic center; DRG, dorsal respiratory group; VRG, ventral respiratory group. Transection I, just rostral to PNC, causes slow, deep breathing in combination with vagotomy but does not affect normal breathing. Transection II, below PNC but above APC, causes slow, deep breathing with intact vagi but apneusis (sustained inspiration) or apneustic breathing (increase in inspiratory time) when the vagi are cut. Transection III, at the pontomedullary junction, generally causes regular gasping breathing which is not affected by vagotomy. Transection IV, at the medullospinal junction, causes respiratory arrest. (Reproduced with permission from Berger AJ, Mitchell RA, Severinghaus JW. Regulation of respiration. N Engl J Med 1977;297:92–97,138–143,194–201.)*

absence of the tonic influence of the brain stem reticular formation (i.e., absence of the wakefulness stimulus); reduced chemosensitivity (see later); increased upper airway resistance to airflow resulting from reduced activity of the pharyngeal dilator muscles during sleep.[54,59,60]

Changes in blood gases

As a result of the fall of alveolar ventilation, the P_{CO_2} rises by 2 to 8 mm Hg, P_{O_2} decreases by 3 to 10 mm Hg, and oxygen saturation (Sa_{O_2}) decreases by less than 2% during sleep.[49,51,52,61,62] These changes occur despite reductions of V_{O_2} and V_{CO_2} during sleep.[63]

Respiratory rate and rhythm

In NREM sleep the respiratory rate mostly shows an increment (sometimes a decrement), whereas in REM sleep the respiration becomes irregular, especially during phasic REM.[42] There is also waxing and waning of the tidal volume during sleep onset resembling Cheyne-Stokes breathing.[49,52,64–67] This is related to several factors[42]: sudden loss of wakefulness stimulus, reduced chemosensitivity at sleep onset (see later), and transient arousal. During the deepening stage of NREM sleep the respiration becomes stable and rhythmic and depends entirely on the metabolic controlling system.[27–29,40,42,51]

Control of Ventilation During Sleep

Chemosensitivity and sleep

Hypoxic ventilatory response in humans is decreased in NREM sleep and further decreases during REMs (Figure 5-7).[68–71] This reduction could result from two factors, increased upper airway resistance to airflow during all stages of sleep[54,59,60] and decreased chemosensitivity.

Hypercapnic ventilatory response also decreases by about 20% to 50% during NREM sleep[49,52,55,72,73] and further during REM sleep (Figure 5-8).[72,73] This results from a combination of two factors[10]: decreasing number of functional medullary respiratory neurons during sleep and increased upper airway resistance.[54,59,60] During sleep the carbon dioxide response curve shifts to the right so that increasing amounts of P_{CO_2} are needed to stimulate ventilation.[66,74] All these findings suggest decreased sensitivity of the central chemoreceptors subserving medullary respiratory neurons.[10]

Metabolism and ventilation during sleep

There is a definite decrease in V_{CO_2} and V_{O_2} during sleep.[63,75,76] Metabolism slows suddenly at sleep onset and accelerates slowly in the early morning, around 5 A.M.[63] During sleep, ventilation falls in parallel to metabolism. The rise of P_{CO_2} during sleep, however, is due to alveolar hypoventilation and is not related to reduced metabolism.[42] The role of the intrapulmonary receptors during normal sleep in humans is unknown.[42]

Changes in the upper airway and in intercostal muscle and diaphragm tone

The upper airway resistance increases during sleep as a result of hypotonia of the upper airway–dilating muscle[54,59,60,77,78] (see Physiologic Changes in the Neuromuscular System). There is also hypotonia of the intercostal muscles and atonia during REM

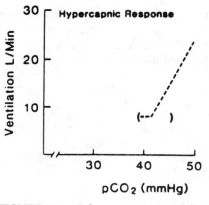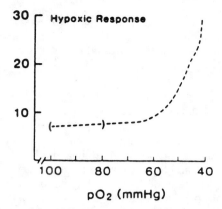

FIGURE 5-6. *Schematic representation of normal hypercapnic and hypoxic ventilatory response. Normal ranges are indicated by parentheses. (Reproduced with permission from White DP. Central Sleep Apnea. Clin Chest Med 1985;6:626.)*

sleep. The phasic activities in the diaphragm are maintained, but the tonic activity is reduced during REM sleep.[29] As a result of the supine position and hypotonia of intercostal muscles the functional residual capacity (FRC) decreases.[79,80]

Arousal responses during sleep

Hypercapnia is a stronger arousal stimulus than hypoxemia during sleep. An increase of P_{CO_2} of 6 to 15

mm Hg would cause consistent arousal during sleep,[81] whereas oxygen saturation (SaO_2) would have to decrease to 75% before a normal person is aroused.[68,82]

Laryngeal stimulation normally causes cough reflex response, but this is decreased during both states of sleep and is more markedly decreased during REM than NREM sleep.[83] Thus, clearance of aspirated gastric contents is impaired during

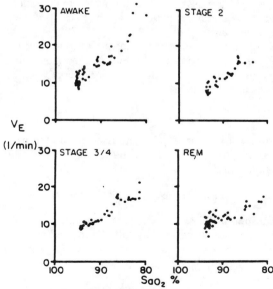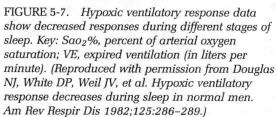

FIGURE 5-7. *Hypoxic ventilatory response data show decreased responses during different stages of sleep. Key: SaO_2%, percent of arterial oxygen saturation; VE, expired ventilation (in liters per minute). (Reproduced with permission from Douglas NJ, White DP, Weil JV, et al. Hypoxic ventilatory response decreases during sleep in normal men. Am Rev Respir Dis 1982;125:286–289.)*

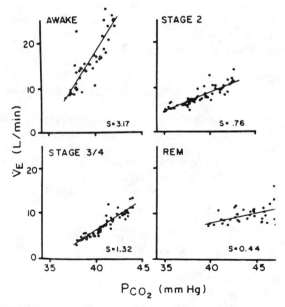

FIGURE 5-8. *Hypercapnic ventilatory response data show decreased responses in sleep, the most marked ones in REM sleep. (Reproduced with permission from Douglas NJ, White DP, Weil JV, et al. Hypercapnic ventilatory response in sleeping adults. Am Rev Respir Dis 1982;126:758–762.)*

sleep. It must be noted that in infants laryngeal stimulation causes obstructive apnea, and this has been postulated as one mechanism for sudden infant death syndrome.[84]

Summary and Conclusions

During wakefulness both metabolic and voluntary control systems are active. In NREM sleep the voluntary system is inactive and respiration is entirely dependent on the metabolic controller; the behavioral influences and the wakefulness stimuli are not controlling respiration. The ventilatory control during REM sleep is not definitely known, but most likely the behavioral mechanism is responsible for controlling breathing in REM sleep. Ventilation is unstable during sleep, and apneas may occur, particularly at sleep onset and during REM sleep. Respiratory homeostasis is thus relatively unprotected during sleep.

The major cause of hypoventilation and reduced ventilatory response to chemical stimuli during sleep is increased airway resistance.[54,59,60,85] The increased resistance results from reduced activity of the pharyngeal dilator muscles as well as decreased output of the sleep-related medullary respiratory neurons.[86] The reduction of the medullary respiratory neuronal activity in sleep causes a loss of the tonic and phasic motor output to the upper airway muscles resulting in an increase in airway resistance. Other factors that also contribute to sleep-related hypoventilation include these[27–29,40,42,87]: reduction of metabolic rate by about 10% to 15%; absence of the wakefulness stimuli; reduced chemosensitivity; increased blood flow to brain (maximal during REM sleep), which may depress central chemoreceptor activity; and functional alterations in the central nervous system (CNS) during sleep (e.g., cerebral cortical suppression due to reticular inhibition and physiologic cortical deafferentation [pre- and postsynaptic inhibition of the afferent neurons[88]] as well as postsynaptic inhibition of motor neurons during REM sleep [see later]).

PHYSIOLOGIC CHANGES IN THE HEART AND CIRCULATION DURING SLEEP

Physiologic changes during sleep in the heart include alterations in heart rate and cardiac output, and in the circulation include changes in blood pressure, peripheral vascular resistance, and blood flow in the various systems and regions.

Heart Rate

The heart rate decreases during NREM and shows frequent upward and downward swings during REM sleep.[89–93] Bradycardia during NREM sleep results from a tonic increase in parasympathetic activity (sympathectomy has little effect.)[89–93] Bradycardia persists during REM sleep and becomes intense owing to tonically reduced sympathetic discharge. Phasic heart rate changes (brady-tachycardia) during REM sleep are due to transient changes in both the cardiac sympathetic and parasympathetic activities.[89–93] Thus, parasympathetic activity predominates during sleep and an additional decrease of sympathetic activity is observed during REM sleep.

Cardiac Output

Cardiac output falls progressively during sleep, the greatest decrement occurring during the last sleep cycle, particularly during the last REM cycle early in the morning.[90,94] This may help explain why normal persons and patients with cardiopulmonary disease are most likely to die during the early morning hours.[95] Maximal oxygen desaturation and periodic breathing are also noted at this time.

Arterial Blood Pressure

During NREM sleep, blood pressure (BP) falls by about 5% to 14%; during REM sleep it fluctuates.[90,91,96] These changes are related to alterations in the autonomic nervous system.[89] Coote[97] concluded that the fall in BP during NREM sleep was secondary to a reduction in cardiac output while the BP changes during REM sleep resulted from alterations in cardiac output and peripheral vascular resistance (see later).

Pulmonary Arterial Pressure

Pulmonary arterial pressure rises slightly during sleep; during wakefulness the mean value is 18/8 mm Hg and during sleep 23/12 mm Hg.[98]

Peripheral Vascular Resistance

During NREM sleep peripheral resistance (PR) remains unchanged or may fall slightly, whereas in REM sleep there is a decrease in PR due to vasodilation.[90,99,100]

Blood Flow

Cutaneous, muscular, and mesenteric vascular blood flow show little change during NREM sleep, but blood flow increases, along with vasodilation, during REM sleep.[90,100,101] In muscle vascular bed there is vasoconstriction during REM sleep.[100] Mullen and coworkers[102] reported a decrease of plasma renin activity in humans during REM sleep, which indirectly suggests increased renal blood flow.

Cerebral blood flow increases during NREM but is maximal during REM sleep.[103,104] The largest increases are noted in the hypothalamus and the brain stem structures, and the smallest increases in cerebral cortex and white matter.

These hemodynamic changes in the cardiovascular system result from alterations in the autonomic nervous system.[89,93,97] In general, parasympathetic activity predominates during both NREM and REM sleep and is most predominant during REM sleep. In addition, there is sympathetic inhibition during REM sleep. The sympathetic activity during REM sleep is decreased in cardiac, renal, and splanchnic vessels but increased in skeletal muscles, owing to an alteration in the brain stem sympathetic controlling mechanism. Furthermore, during phasic REM sleep blood pressure and heart rate are unstable owing to phasic vagal inhibition and sympathetic activation resulting from changes in brain stem neural activity. Heart rate and blood pressure, therefore, fluctuate during REM sleep.

PHYSIOLOGIC CHANGES IN THE NEUROMUSCULAR SYSTEM

Physiologic changes have been noted during sleep in both the somatic and autonomic nervous system that in turn produce changes in the somatic and smooth muscles of the body. In this section I discuss the physiologic changes noted during sleep in the somatic muscles, including cranial and limb muscles and respiratory muscles.

Changes in Limb and Cranial Muscles

Alterations of limb and cranial muscle tone are noted during sleep. Muscle tone is maximal during wakefulness, and is slightly decreased in NREM sleep but markedly decreased or absent in REM sleep. Electromyography (EMG), particularly of the submental muscle, is necessary to identify REM sleep and is thus important for scoring technique. In addition, transient myoclonic bursts are noted during REM sleep. An important EMG characteristic is documentation of periodic limb movements of sleep (PLMS), which are noted in the majority of patients with restless legs syndrome but also noted in a variety of sleep disorders, and even in normal persons, particularly elderly ones.

Mechanism of Muscle Atonia or Hypotonia in REM Sleep

Dorsal pontine tegmentum appears to be an important central region responsible for limb muscle atonia in REM.[105] Axonal projections from this pontine area via a medial[106] and a lateral tract[107] terminate

on the medullary reticular formation (gigantocellular and magnocellular regions). Long descending axons from this area terminating in the spinal cord[108,109] are responsible for REM-specific inhibitory postsynaptic potentials (IPSPs) to produce muscle atonia.[110] Lesions of the dorsal pontine tegmentum abolish muscle atonia of REM sleep.[111-113] Similar lesions have also been found to cause increased diaphragm activity in REM sleep.[105]

Postsynaptic inhibition of the motor neurons is responsible for the atonia of the somatic muscles, as evidenced by intracellular recordings of spinal motor neurons in chronic spinal preparation of cats.[114] There is lumbar motor neuron hyperpolarization of 2 to 10 mV during REM sleep. Intracellular recordings revealed increased number and appearance of REM-specific IPSPs in the lumbar motor neurons of cats.[115,116] These potentials are derived from inhibitory interneurons, which may be located either in the spinal cord or in the brain stem, from which long axons project to the spinal motor neurons.[115,117] These REM-specific IPSPs are responsible for muscle atonia in REM sleep.[118] The neurotransmitter for mediation of such IPSPs appears to be glycine, not γ-aminobutyric acid (GABA).[118] Strychnine, a glycine antagonist, administered by microiontophoresis near the motor neurons antagonizes the IPSP, though picrotoxin and bicuculline, GABA antagonists, do not. The identity of the individual interneurons in the spinal cord remains unknown; they could be Ia inhibitory neurons but they are not Renshaw cells.

The IPSPs in the cranial motor neurons are also most likely strychnine sensitive, and a neurotransmitter could be GABA-B neurotransmitter.[118]

Upper Airway Muscles and Sleep

Changes occur in the function of the upper airway muscles during sleep that have important clinical implications, particularly for patients with sleep apnea syndrome. Upper respiratory tract subserves both respiratory and nonrespiratory functions.[119] In experimental studies in cats, pharyngeal motor neurons in the vagus and glossopharyngeal nerves are located in the medulla, overlapping the medullary respiratory neurons.[120] The experimental study of Bianchi and colleagues[121] demonstrated that after changes induced by chemical stimuli (normocapnic hypoxia and normoxic hypercapnia) pharyngeal motor activities are more sensitive than phrenic nerve activation.

The genioglossus muscle[122]

Genioglossal EMG activities consist of phasic inspiratory bursts and variable tonic discharges, and these are decreased during sleep, particularly REM sleep.[123-125] Selective reduction of genioglossal or hypoglossal nerve activity (i.e., disproportionately more reduction than the diaphragmatic or phrenic activities) has been noted with alcohol, diazepam, and many anesthetic agents. On the other hand, protriptyline and strychnine each selectively increase such activity.

The masseter muscle[126]

Masseter contraction closes the jaw and elevates the mandible. In sleep apnea patients, masseter activation is present during eupneic episodes but decreased during apneic ones. Masseter EMG activity decreases immediately before the apnea, is absent during the early part of the episode, and increases at the end of the apneic period. Based on the experiments using chemical stimuli, Suratt and Hollowell[126] concluded that masseter activity can be increased by hyperoxic hypercapnia and inspiratory resistance loading. It appears that phasic EMG bursts start in the masseter at the same time as in the genioglossus and the diaphragm. Suratt and Hollowell[126] did not find phasic activity in masseter muscle in normal subjects during regular breathing but noted such activity during inspiratory stimulation, such as inspiratory resistance loading or hypercapnia; however, in sleep apnea patients spontaneous phasic masseter activity was noted.

Intrinsic laryngeal muscle activity[127]

Intrinsic laryngeal muscles, controlled by the brain stem neuronal mechanism, play an important role in the regulation of breathing. In addition, the larynx participates in phonation, deglutition, and airway protection.[128] The posterior cricoarytenoid (PCA) muscle is the main vocal cord abductor. Laryngeal EMG can be performed by placing hooked wire electrodes percutaneously through the cricothyroid membrane.[129]

PCA demonstrates phasic inspiratory bursts in normal subjects during wakefulness and NREM sleep.[127] In addition, there is also tonic expiratory activity in wakefulness that disappears with NREM sleep. In REM sleep, PCA EMG shows fragmented inspiratory bursts and variable expiratory activity. During isocapnic hypoxia and hyperoxic hypercapnia normal subjects show increased phasic inspiratory PCA activity but minimal increase of tonic expiratory activity.[127]

Hyoid muscles[130]

Suprahyoid muscles (those inserted superiorly on hyoid bone) include geniohyoid, mylohyoid, hyoglossus, stylohyoid, and digastric. Infrahyoid muscles (those that insert inferiorly) include sternohyoid, omohyoid, and sternothyroid. It should be noted that the size and shape of the upper airways can be altered by movements of the hyoid bone. Motoneurons supplying these muscles are located in the pons, the medulla, and the upper cervical spinal cord. The hyoid muscles show inspiratory bursts during wakefulness and NREM sleep that are increased by hypercapnia. According to van Lunteren,[130] the relative contribution of hyoid, genioglossus, and other tongue muscles in the maintenance of pharyngeal patency needs to be clarified.

REM-related alterations in respiratory muscle acitivity

During REM sleep activity of upper airway muscle and diaphragm is reduced. Three types of REM-related alterations in the respiration muscles have been described.[105] One is *atonia* of EMG activity throughout the REM period. Somatic muscles characteristically show this response, which is related to glycine-mediated postsynaptic inhibition of motor neurons.[118] Rhythmic activity of the diaphragm persists in REM sleep, but certain diaphragmic motor units cease firing. Kline and coworkers[131] recently described *intermittent decrement of diaphragmatic activity* during single breaths. Upper airway muscles also show similar changes. A third alteration is *fractionations of diaphragmatic activity*. Pauses last 40 to 80 msec and occur in clusters correlated with PGO waves, which are phasic events of REM sleep.[132]

Recent experimental observations suggest that the brain stem neuronal circuitry responsible for limb muscle atonia in REM sleep can also produce phasic and tonic decrements of respiratory muscle activity by inhibiting brain stem respiratory motor neuron pools.[105] Thus, apneas in REM sleep may result from intermittent inhibition of the upper airway respiratory motor neurons.

GASTROINTESTINAL PHYSIOLOGY DURING SLEEP

A brief summary of the physiology of the gastrointestinal tract during sleep is given in this section; for details readers are referred to Orr.[133] Gastrointestinal changes include alterations in gastric acid secretion, changes in gastric volume and motility, swallowing, and alterations in esophageal peristalsis and intestinal motility.

Studying the physiology of the gastrointestinal system has been difficult because of lack of an adequate technique. Recently techniques, as well as facilities for making simultaneous polysomnographic (PSG) recordings, became available that allow study of the alterations in gastrointestinal physiology during different stages of sleep. Before the advent of these techniques scattered reports showed in general decreased motor and secretory functions during sleep. Modern methods have produced better and more consistent results, though, overall, findings are still somewhat contradictory. There is a dearth of adequate studies that utilized PSG and other modern techniques to understand the physiologic alterations of gastrointestinal motility and secretions during sleep.

Gastric Acid Secretion

During wakefulness gastric acid secretion depends on food ingestion, increased salivation, and the activity of the gastric vagus nerve. Moore and Englert[134] showed a clear circadian rhythm for gastric acid secretion in humans. These authors noted peak gastric acid secretion between 10:00 P.M. and 2:00 A.M. in patients with duodenal ulcer. Acid secretion increases considerably both during daytime and at night.[135,136] The importance of vagal stimulation for the control of circadian oscillation of gastric acid secretion has been provided by the absence of circadian rhythm for gastric acid secretion following vagotomy.[137]

Several studies have attempted to understand gastric acid secretion during different stages of sleep, but the results have not been consistent because of methodologic flaws and cumbersome techniques.[138–140] An important study was made by Orr and colleagues,[141] who studied five duodenal ulcer patients for 5 consecutive nights using PSG technique and continuous aspiration of gastric contents. They found no relationship between acid secretion and different stages of sleep or REM versus NREM sleep. The most striking finding was failure of inhibition of acid secretion during the first 2 hours of sleep, findings that agree with the previous report by Levin and associates.[135]

Gastric Motility[133]

Findings have been contradictory: both inhibition and enhancement of gastric motility have been noted during sleep.[142–144] In 1922 Wada[145]described cyclic gastric contractions in normal subjects during wakefulness and sleep. Finch and coworkers[146] later showed that gastroduodenal motility during sleep was related to sleep stage shifts and body movements. Orr[133] stated that, although no definite statement regarding gastric motility can be made, there seems to be overall inhibition of gastric motor function during sleep.

Esophageal Function

Swallowing is suppressed during sleep, particularly stage III and IV NREM sleep,[147–149] resulting in prolonged mucosal contact with refluxed acid.

Johnson and DeMeester[150] considered prolonged acid clearance an important factor in the pathogenesis of esophagitis caused by nocturnal gastroesophageal reflux (GER). Salivary flow, which is important for acid neutralization, also is decreased during sleep,[133] a phenomenon that contributes to prolonged acid clearance.[151] In normal subjects during wakefulness, reflux may occur in the upright position, mainly postprandially, and these episodes are terminated in less than 4 minutes.[150] Studies by Orr and colleagues[147,151] clearly show that the arousal response associated with swallowing during sleep prevents prolonged acid clearance and GER during sleep in normal subjects. In normal persons who experience episodes of GER there is generally a reduction in lower esophageal sphincter pressure.[152] The availability of the method to measure GER during sleep by esophageal pH monitoring[153] has advanced our understanding of swallowing and esophageal function during sleep.

Intestinal Motility

Although methods are now available to accurately measure intestinal motility, the results of motility studies during sleep are contradictory.[133]

THERMAL REGULATION IN SLEEP

Changes in Body Temperature and Circadian Rhythm

That body temperature follows a circadian rhythm independent of the sleep-wake rhythm[154] has been demonstrated in experiments involving desynchronization and resynchronization of human circadian rhythms. It has been shown that when all environmental cues (*Zeitgebers*) are removed the endogenous rhythms are freed from the influence of exogenous rhythms and a free-running rhythm ensues. During this time, it is clear that body temperature has a rhythm independent of the sleep-wake rhythm (Figure 5-9).[155] Nevertheless, body temperature has been linked intimately to the sleep-wake cycle.[156] Body temperature begins to fall with the onset of sleep, and the lowest temperature is noted during the third sleep cycle.[157,158]

Role of REM Sleep in Thermal Regulation

During REM sleep, the thermoregulating mechanism appears to be inoperative.[156,159,160] Body temperature increases during REM sleep, and there are cyclic changes in the temperature during this period. Thermoregulatory responses such as sweating and panting are noted in NREM sleep, but they are absent in REM sleep, and in fact the animals display a state of poikilothermia. Brain temperature rises during REM

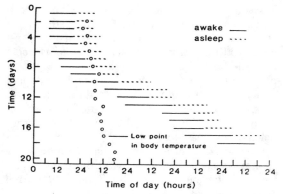

FIGURE 5-9.   *Synchronized (light-entrained) and desynchronized (free-running) rhythms in a person showing dissociation between body temperature and sleep-activity cycles. (Reproduced with permission from Aschoff J. Desynchronization and resynchronization of human circadian rhythms. Aerospace Med 1969;40:847.)*

sleep. Szymusiak and McGinty[161] speculated that REM sleep, by elevating brain temperature or by reversing the cooling trend in slow-wave sleep (SWS), prepares the body for behavioral activation. It should be noted that the loss of thermoregulation in REM sleep is not related to inhibition of motor control but is determined by central integration or thermoafferent pathways, or by both mechanisms.[156]

Mechanism of Thermoregulation in Sleep

The function of sleep appears to be energy conservation, as evidenced by a reduction in body temperature and metabolism during sleep, especially NREM sleep.[157,158,162] Sleep onset in humans is associated with a reduction of body temperature of 1° to 2°C accompanied by heat loss due to vasodilation and increased sweating. These changes appear to be related to reduced thermal sensitivity of the preoptic nucleus of the hypothalamus.[162] MacFadyen and colleagues[163] observed increased SWS after 2 to 3 days' starvation in humans, suggesting that the length of hypometabolism helps conserve energy. Increased body temperature[164] and hypothalamic heating[165] are associated with increased SWS. If the body temperature is elevated during the waking periods, SWS increases.[166,167] SWS is accompanied by a drop in body and brain temperature. According to Aschoff[154] the independent circadian rhythm of body temperature is unrelated to a reduction of motor activities at sleep onset. Based on experiments in cats, Szymusiak and McGinty[161,168] hypothesized that the neuronal mechanisms in the preoptic–anterior hypothalamic region are responsible for both thermal regulation and SWS generation and that SWS is essentially a thermoregulatory process. Jet lag and shift work may disrupt this linkage and change the rhythms of sleep and body temperature, which may cause disorganization of sleep architecture and of daytime function.[156]

ENDOCRINE REGULATION IN SLEEP

Neuroendocrine secretion appears to be under circadian control; that is, it shows circadian rhythm in the plasma concentrations of the hormones. The characteristic pattern of endocrine gland secretion is episodic or pulsatile secretion every 1 to 2 hours, which suggests ultradian rhythmicity. Hormone secretion thus depends on the stages of sleep and time of the day. In the following paragraphs changes in secretion of some major hormones during sleep are described. Figure 5-10 schematically shows the patterns of neuroendocrine secretion during sleep in an adult.

Growth Hormone

Takahashi and colleagues[169] observed that the plasma concentration of growth hormone (GH) peaks 90 minutes after sleep onset in seven of eight normal subjects and lasts some 1½ to 2½ hours. The peak is related to SWS (stages 3 and 4 NREM sleep). Several reports since then showed nocturnal peaks of GH in association with SWS.[170-173] The sleep-related release of GH is absent before age 3 months and is reduced in old age. The timing of the release of GH shifts if sleep is phase-advanced or -delayed, suggesting a close relationship between episodic GH secretion and sleep.[174] There is some evidence from a jet lag study by Goldstein and associates[175] of possible circadian influences on the regulation of GH secretion. Increased GH secretion has been noted after flights both eastward and westward.

The tightly linked normal relationship between GH and SWS is disrupted during sleep disturbances. For example, in narcolepsy[176] depression of GH secretion is associated with sleep disturbance, and in some cases of insomnia[177] there is a dissociation between SWS and GH secretion. Such dissociation also occurs in old age.[178,179] These findings suggest there are two independent mechanisms for controlling GH secretion and SWS. It is interesting to note that such a tight relationship is observed only in humans and baboons and not in rhesus monkeys and dogs,[180] a fact that may relate to the monophasic sleep patterns observed in the baboons and humans.[181]

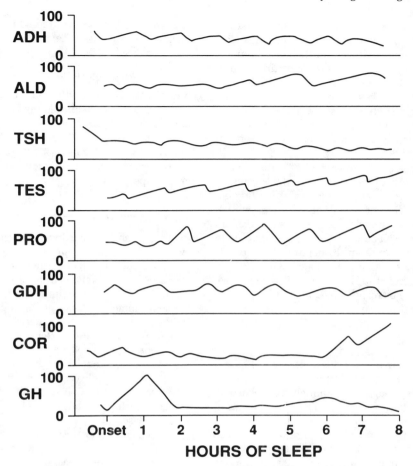

FIGURE 5-10.   *Schematic representation of the plasma levels of hormones in an adult during an 8-hour sleep. Key: ADH, antidiuretic hormone; ALD, aldosterone; TSH, thyroid-stimulating hormone; TES, testosterone; PRO, prolactin; GDH, gonadotropic hormone; COR, cortisol; GH, growth hormone. Zero indicates lowest secretary episode and 100 indicates peak. (Modified and adapted from Rubin R. Sleep endocrinology studies in man. Prog Brain Res 1975;42:73–80.)*

In acromegaly patients, GH secretion remains high throughout sleep and has no relationship to sleep onset or SWS.[182,183]

Diminished sleep-related secretion of GH is found in both sleep apnea and narcolepsy.[184] The pattern of GH secretion associated with clinical depression is contradictory: both impairment and normal sleep-related GH secretion have been noted.[177,185,186] GH secretion is somewhat disturbed in alcoholics.[187]

Schizophrenia, alcoholism, and depression in adults are associated with impaired sleep-related GH secretion.[186] Whether this is related to an associated decrease in SWS or abnormalities of biogenic amine

metabolism in these disorders cannot be stated with certainty. Cushing's syndrome is associated with decreased SWS and GH secretion. Nocturnal GH secretion was found to be higher than normal and SWS increased in two patients with thyrotoxicosis.[188] These abnormal findings normalized in response to antithyroid medication.

Adrenocortocotrophic Hormone and Cortisol Secretion

Adrenocorticotropic hormone (ACTH) stimulates cortisol secretion by the adrenal cortex. ACTH-cortisol secretion appears to be under circadian influence. Secretion is inhibited by sleep. The cortisol level is generally lowest in the early hours of sleep and highest in the early morning hours, around 4:00 to 8:00 A.M.[189,190] Alford and coworkers,[191,192] however, documented both a circadian and an ultradian episodic pattern of secretion for cortisol and ACTH. Cortisol secretion is suppressed during the first few hours of sleep but it rises later.[193,194]

Generally, the circadian rhythm of cortisol secretion remains undisturbed in disease states, such as Cushing's syndrome and narcolepsy.[186] With depression, the earlier occurrence of the lowest point of cortisol levels is thought to indicate a circadian phase advance.[195] The failure of dexamethasone to suppress cortisol secretion in depressed persons is not necessarily positively correlated with reduced REM latencies noted in depression.[196] Sleep deprivation itself may be responsible for such failure as is noted in normal persons.[197]

Prolactin Secretion

The plasma prolactin level does not seem to have a definite circadian rhythm, but it seems to be linked significantly to sleep,[198,199] though not related to specific sleep stages.[186] The prolactin level peaks in the early morning hours, around 5:00 to 7:00 A.M., but it begins to rise about 60 to 90 minutes after sleep onset.[200] Studies by Mendelson,[201] Rubin,[202] and Van Cauter and their coworkers[203] clearly show no relationship between prolactin secretion and NREM-REM cycles.

Prolactin secretion is suppressed by dopamine but stimulated by thyrotropin-releasing hormone.[186] Although prolactin secretion is related to sleep, the secretory pattern of prolactin does not decline with age[204] like that of GH.

Gonadotrophic Hormone (Gonadotropin)

There is no clear relationship between follicle-stimulating hormone (FSH) and leutinizing hormone (LH) levels and sleep-wake cycle or sleep stages in children or adults. However, in pubertal boys and girls gonadotropin levels increase in sleep.[205-208]

FSH and LH show pulsatile activities throughout the night without showing any relationship to testosterone secretion. However, early in puberty[205] during sleep there is a marked rise of plasma LH concentration, in contrast to testosterone or prolactin. LH and FSH secretion show no distinct circadian rhythms. Plasma testosterone levels rise at sleep onset and continue to rise during sleep at night.[209] Based on the observations that LH and prolactin secretion precede

testosterone secretion by 60 to 80 minutes, Rubin[181] suggested a relationship among these hormones

Thyroid-Stimulating Hormone

A distinct circadian rhythm has been established for secretion of thyroid-stimulating hormone (TSH) in normal humans.[191,210,211] Despite inconsistent results, there is general agreement that TSH levels increase before sleep onset and are inhibited by sleep,[186,211,212] but TSH secretion does not depend on any specific sleep stage.[213]

Miscellaneous Hormones

Aldosterone shows a maximal rise just before a sleeper awakes.[214] *Antidiuretic hormone* shows episodic secretion without any relationship to sleep or sleep stages.[214] *Plasma renin activity* shows a marked drop during REM sleep.[102] Renin is a hormone secreted by the juxtaglomerular cells of the kidneys under the influence of the sympathetic nervous system, circulation, blood volume, and systemic blood pressure.

In normal persons nocturnal urine volume decreases owing to decreased glomerular filtration, alteration of renin release, and increased reabsorption of water.[215,216] Brandenberger and coworkers[217] reported an ultradian, but not a circadian, rhythm for renin release.

Kripke and associates[218] studied *parathyroid hormone* (PTH) in seven normal subjects for 8 nights in the sleep laboratory. Plasma samples were obtained at 10- to 20-minute intervals for PTH and calcium determinations. PTH peaks tended to occur every 100 minutes, and PTH concentration was significantly related to cycles of stages 3 and 4 NREM sleep. Total plasma calcium, however, was significantly related to cycles of REM and stage 2 NREM sleep. *Melatonin* is synthesized and released by the pineal gland and is derived from serotonin.[214] Melatonin levels are highest at night but show a marked drop during REM sleep. The level peaks when the sleeper awakes.[219]

REFERENCES

1. Orem J, Barnes CD, Physiology in Sleep. New York: Academic Press, 1980.
2. Lydic R, Biebuyck. Clinical Physiology of Sleep. Bethesda, Md: American Physiological Society, 1988.
3. Legallois C. Experiences sur le Principe de la Vie. Paris: d'Hautel, 1812.
4. Lumsden T. Observations on the respiratory centres in the cat. J Physiol 1922–1923;57:153–160,354–367.
5. Lumsden T. The regulation of respiration., J Physiol 1923–1924;58:81–91,111–126.

6. Pitts RF, Magoun HW, Ranson SW. Localization of the medullary respiratory centers in the cat. Am J Physiol 1939;126:673–688.

7. Mitchell RA, Berger AJ. Neural regulation of respiration. Am Rev Respir Dis 1975;111:206–244.

8. Berger AJ, Mitchell RA, Severinghaus JW. Regulation of respiration. N Eng J Med 1977;297:92–97,138–143, 194–201.

9. Mitchell RA. Neural regulation of respiration. Clin Chest Med 1980;1:3–12.

10. Chokroverty S. Sleep apnea and autonomic failure. In: Low PA, ed. Clinical Autonomic Disorders. Boston: Little, Brown, 1993;589–603.

11. Loewy AD, Spyer KM. Central Regulation of Autonomic Functions. New York: Oxford University Press, 1990.

12. Steriade M, McCarley RW. Brainstem control of wakefulness and sleep. New York: Plenum, 1990.

13. Vertes RP. Brainstem control of the events of REM sleep. Progr Neurobiol 1984;22:241–288.

14. Moruzzi G. The sleep waking cycle. Ergeb Physiol 1972;64:1–165.

15. Hobson JA, Lydic R, Baghdoyan HA. Evolving concepts of sleep cycle generation: From brain centers to neuronal populations. Behav Brain Sci 1986;9:371–448.

16. Jouvet M. The role of monoamines and actylcholine containing neurons in the regulation of the sleep-waking cycle. Ergeb Physiol 1972;64:166–307.

17. Batini C, Magni F, Palestini M, et al. Neural mechanisms underlying the enduring EEG and behavioral activation in the mid-pontine pretrigeminal preparation. Arch Ital Biol 1959;97:1–12.

18. Batini C, Moruzzi G, Palestini M, et al. Effect of complete pontine transections on the sleep-wakefulness rhythm: The mid-pontine pretrigeminal preparation. Arch Ital Biol 1959;97:1–12.

19. Bremer F. Cerebral hypnogenic centers. Ann Neurol 1977;2:1–6.

20. Ricardo JA, Koh ET. Anatomical evidence of direct projections from the nucleus of the solitary tract to the hypothalamus, amygdala, and other forebrain structures in the rat. Brain Res 1978;153:1.

21. Loewy AD. Central autonomic pathways. In: Low PA, ed. Clinical Autonomic Disorders. Boston: Little, Brown, 1993; 88–103.

22. Loewy AD. Anatomy of the autonomic nervous system: An overview. In: Loewy AD, Spyer KM, eds. Central Regulation of Autonomic Functions. New York: Oxford University Press, 1990; 3–16.

23. Barron KD, Chokroverty S. Anatomy of the autonomic nervous system: Brain and brainstem. In: Low PA, ed. Clinical Autonomic Disorders, Boston: Little, Brown, 1993;3–15.

24. Chokroverty S. Functional anatomy of the autonomic nervous system correlated with symptomatology of neurologic disease. In: American Academy of Neurology Course No. 246. San Diego, Cal, 1992;49–76.

25. Chokroverty S. The spectrum of ventilatory disturbances in movement disorders. In: Chokroverty S, ed. Movement Disorders. Costa Mesa, Calif: PMA, 1990; 365–392.

26. Cherniack NS, Longobardo GA. Abnormalities in respiratory rhythm. In: Fishman AF, Cherniack NS, Widdicombe JG, eds. Handbook of Physiology, sec 3. The Respiratory System, vol II, part 2. Bethesda, Md: American Physiological Society, 1986;729–749.

27. Phillipson EA. Control of breathing during sleep. Am Rev Respir Dis 1978;18:909–939.

28. Phillipson EA. Respiratory adaptations in sleep. Annu Rev Physiol 1978;40:133–156.

29. Phillipson EA, Bowes G. Control of breathing during sleep. In: Fishman AF, Cherniack NS, Widdicombe JG, eds. Handbook of Physiology, sec 3. The Respiratory System, vol II, part 2. Bethesda Md: American Physiological Society, 1986;649–689.

30. Plum F. Breathlessness in neurological disease: The effects of neurological disease on the act of breathing. In: Howell JBL, Campbell EJM, eds. Breathlessness. Oxford: Blackwell Scientific, 1966;203–222.

31. Sears TA, Newsom Davis J. The control of respiratory muscles during voluntary breathing. Ann NY Acad Sci 1968;155:183.

32. Procter DF. Breathing mechanics during phonations and singing. In Wyke B, ed. Ventilatory and Phonatory Control Systems. London: Oxford University Press, 1974;39.

33. Cohen MI, Hugelin A. Suprapontine reticular control of intrinsic respiratory mechanisms. Arch Ital Biol 1965;103:317–334.

34. Hugelin A, Cohen MI. The reticular activating system and respiratory regulation in the cat. Ann NY Acad Sci 1963;109:586–603.

35. McNicholas WT, Rutherford R, Grossman R, et al. Abnormal respiratory pattern generation during sleep in patients with autonomic dysfunction. Am Rev Respir Dis 1983;128:429–433.

36. Fink BR. Influence of cerebral activity in wakefulness on regulation of breathing. J Appl Physiol 1961;16:15.

37. Merrill EG. The lateral respiratory neurons of the medulla: Their associations with nucleus ambiguus, nucleus retroambigualis, the spinal accessory nucleus and the spinal cord. Brain Res 1970;24:11.

38. Nathan PW. The descending respiratory pathway in man. J Neurol Neurosurg Psychiatry 1963;26:487–499.

39. Wang SC, Ngai SH, Frumin MJ. Organization of central respiratory mechanisms in the brainstem of the cat: Genesis of normal respiratory rhythmicity. Am J Physiol 1957;190:333–342.

40. Sullivan CE. Breathing in sleep. In: Orem J, Barnes CD, eds. Physiology in Sleep. New York: Academic Press, 1980;213–272.

41. Newsom Davis J. Control of muscles in breathing. In: Widdicombe JG, ed. Respiratory Physiology: MTP International Review of Science, vol 2. London: Butterworth, 1974;221–246.

42. White DP. Ventilation and the control of respiration during sleep: Normal mechanisms, pathologic nocturnal hypoventilation, and central sleep apnea. In: Martin RJ, ed. Cardiorespiratory Disorders During Sleep. Mount Kisco, NY: Futura, 1990;53–108.

43. Weil J, Byrne-Quinn E, Sodal I, et al. Hypoxic ventilatory drive in normal man. J Clin Invest 1970;49:1061–1072.

44. Read DJC. A clinical method for assessing the ventilatory response to carbon dioxide. Australas Ann Med 1967;16:20–32.

45. Whipp BJ, Wasserman K. Carotid bodies and ventilatory control dynamics in man. Fed Proc 1980;39:2668–2673.

46. Hornbein TF. The relationship between stimulus to chemoreceptors and their response. In: Torrance TW, ed. Arterial Chemoreceptors. Oxford: Blackwell, 1968;65–78.

47. Loeschcke HH. Review lecture: Central chemosensitivity and the reaction therapy. J Physiol (Lond) 1982;332:1–24.

48. Bulow K, Ingvar DH. Respiration and state of wakefulness in normals, studied by spirography, capnography and EEG. Acta Physiol Scand 1961;51:230–238.

49. Bulow K. Respiration and wakefulness in man. Acta Physiol Scand Suppl 1963;59:1–110.

50. Cherniack N. Respiratory dysrhythmias during sleep. N Engl J Med 1981;305:325–330.

51. Douglas J, White DP, Pickett CK, et al. Respiration during sleep in normal man. Thorax 1982;37:840–844.

52. Robin ED, Whaley RD, Crump CH, et al. Alveolar gas tensions, pulmonary ventilation, and blood pH during physiologic sleep in normal subjects. J Clin Invest 1958;37:981–989.

53. Skatrud J, Dempsey J. Interaction of sleep state and chemical stimuli in sustaining rhythmic ventilation. J Appl Physiol 1983;55:813–822.

54. Hudgel DW, Martin RJ, Johnson B, et al. Mechanics of the respiratory system and breathing during sleep in normal humans. J Appl Physiol 1984;56:133–137.

55. Goethe B, Altose MD, Gotham MD, et al. Effect of quiet sleep on resting and CO_2-stimulated breathing in humans. J Appl Physiol 1981;50:724–730.

56. Tabachnik E, Muller NL, Bryant AC, et al. Changes in ventilation and chest wall mechanics during sleep in normal adolescents. J Appl Physiol 1981;51:557–564.

57. Krieger J, Turlot JC, Mangin P, et al. Breathing during sleep in normal young and elderly subjects: Hypopneas, apneas, and correlated factors. Sleep 1983;6:108–120.

58. Lopes JM, Tabachnik E, Muller NL, et al. Total airway resistance and respiratory muscle activity during sleep. J Appl Physiol 1983;54:773–777.

59. Skatrud JB, Dempsey JA. Airway resistance and respiratory muscle function in snorers during NREM sleep. J Appl Physiol 1985;59:328–335.

60. Wiegand L, Zwillich CW, White DP. Collapsibility of the human upper airway during normal sleep. J Appl Physiol 1989;66:1800–1808.

61. Birchfield RI, Sieker HO, Heyman A. Alterations in respiratory function during natural sleep. J Lab Clin Med 1959;54:216–222.

62. Reed DJ, Kellogg RH. Changes in respiratory response to CO_2 during natural sleep at sea level and at altitude. J Appl Physiol 1958;13:325–330.

63. White DP, Weil JV, Zwillich CW. Metabolic rate and breathing during sleep. J Appl Physiol 1985;59:384–391.

64. Block AJ, Boysen PG, Wynne JW, et al. Sleep apnea, hypopnea, and oxygen desaturation in normal subjects. N Engl J Med 1979;300:513–517.

65. Webb P. Periodic breathing during sleep. J Appl Physiol 1974;37:899.

66. Bellville JW, Howland WS, Seed JC, et al. The effect of sleep on the respiratory response to carbon dioxide. Anesthesiology 1959;20:628–634.

67. Gillam PMS. Patterns of respiration in human beings at rest and during sleep. Bull Eur Physiopathol Respir 1972;8:1059–1070.

68. Berthon-Jones M, Sullivan CE. Ventilatory and arousal responses to hypoxia in sleeping humans. Am Rev Respir Dis 1982;125:632–639.

69. Douglas NJ, White DP, Weil JV, et al. Hypoxic ventilatory response decreases during sleep in normal men. Am Rev Respir Dis 1982;125:286–289.

70. Hedemark LL, Kronenberg RS. Ventilatory and heart rate responses to hypoxia and hypercapnia during sleep in adults. J Appl Physiol 1982;53:307–312.

71. White DP, Douglas NJ, Pickett CK, et al. Hypoxic ventilatory response during sleep in normal women. Am Rev Respir Dis 1982;126:530–533.

72. Douglas NJ, White DP, Weil JV, et al. Hypercapnic ventilatory response in sleeping adults. Am Rev Respir Dis 1982;126:758–762.

73. Berthon-Jones M, Sullivan CE. Ventilatory and arousal responses to hypercapnia in normal sleeping adults. J Appl Physiol 1984;57:59–57.

74. Reed DJ, Kellog RH. Changes in respiratory response to CO_2 during natural sleep at sea level and at altitude. J Appl Physiol 1958;17:325–330.

75. Brebbia DR, Altshuler KZ. Oxygen consumption rate and electroencephalographic stage of sleep. Science 1965;150:1621–1623.

76. Buskirk ER, Thompsonn RH, Moore R, et al. Human energy expenditure studies in the National Institute of Arthritis and Metabolic Diseases metabolic chamber. Am J Clin Nutr 1960;8:602–613.

77. Anch AM, Remmers JE, Bunce H III. Supraglottic airway resistance in normal subjects and patients with occlusive sleep apnea. J Appl Physiol 1982;53:1158–1163.

78. Skatrud JB, Dempsey JA, Badr S, et al. Effect of airway impedance on CO_2 retention and respiratory muscle activity during NREM sleep. J Appl Physiol 1988;65:1676–1685.

79. Hudgel DW, Devadatta P. Decrease in functional residual capacity during sleep in normal humans. J Appl Physiol 1984;57:1319–1322.

80. Tusiewicz K, Moldofsky H, Bryan AC, et al. Mechanics of the rib cage and diaphragm during sleep. J Appl Physiol 1977;43:600–602.

81. Hedemark LL, Kronenberg RS. Ventilatory and heart rate responses to hypoxia and hypercapnia during sleep in adults. J Appl Physiol 1982;53:307–312.

82. Gothe B, Goldman MD, Cherniack NS, et al. Effect of progressive hypoxia on breathing during sleep. Am Rev Respir Dis 1982;126:97–102.

83. Hara KS, Shepard JW Jr. Sleep and critical care medicine. In: Martin RJ, ed. Cardiorespiratory Disorders During Sleep. Mount Kisco, NY: Futura, 1990;323–363.

84. Thach BT, Davies AM, Koenig JS. Pathophysiology of sudden airway obstruction in sleeping infants and its relevance for SIDS. In: Schwartz PJ, Southall DP, Valdes-Dapena M, eds. The Sudden Infant Death Syndrome: Cardiac and Respiratory Mechanisms and Interventions. [Monogr]. Ann NY Acad Sci 1988;533:314–328.

85. Dempsey JA, Henke KG, Skatrud JB. Regulation of ventilation and respiratory muscle function in NREM sleep. In: Issa FG, Suratt PM, Remmers JE, eds. Sleep and Respiration. New York: Wiley-Liss, 1990;145–155.

86. Orem J. The nature of the wakefulness stimulus for breathing. In: Issa FG, Suratt PM, Remmers JE, eds. Sleep and Respiration. New York: Wiley-Liss, 1990;23–31.

87. Douglas NJ. Breathing during sleep in normal subjects. In: Peter JH, Podszus T, Von Wichert P, eds. Sleep-Related Disorders and Internal Diseases. Berlin: Springer-Verlag, 1987;254–260.

88. Pompeiano O. Mechanism of sensorimotor integration during sleep. Prog Physiol Psychol 1973;3:1–179.

89. Parmeggiani PL, Morrison AR. Alterations in autonomic functions during sleep. In: Loewy AD, Spyer KM, eds. Central Regulation of Autonomic Functions. New York: Oxford University Press, 1990; 367–386.

90. Khatri IM, Freis ED. Hemodynamic changes during sleep. J Appl Physiol 1967;22:867–873.

91. Snyder F, Hobson JA, Morrison DF, et al. Changes in respiration, heart rate, and systolic blood pressure in human sleep. J Appl Physiol 1964;19:417–422.

92. Burdick JA, Brinton G, Goldstein L, et al. Heart-rate variability in sleep and wakefulness. Cardiology 1970;55:79–83.

93. Baust W, Bohnert B. The regulation of heart rate during sleep. Exp Brain Res 1969;7:169–180.

94. Miller JC, Horvath SM. Cardiac output during human sleep. Aviat Space Environ Med 1976;47:1046–1051.

95. Smolensky M, Halberg F, Sargent F. II. Chronobiology of the life sequence. In: Itoh S, Ogata K, Yoshimura H, eds. Advances in Climatic Physiology. New York: Springer-Verlag, 1971.

96. Coccagna G, Mantovani M, Brignani F, et al. Arterial pressure changes during spontaneous sleep in man. Electroencephalogr Clin Neurophysiol 1971;31:277–281.

97. Coote JH. Respiratory and circulatory control during sleep. J Exp Biol 1982;100:223–244.

98. Lugaresi E, Coccagna G, Cirignotta F, et al. Breathing during sleep in man in normal and pathological conditions. Adv Exp Med Biol 1978;99:35–45.

99. Kumazawa T, Baccella G, Guazzi M, et al. Haemodynamic patterns during desynchronized sleep in intact cats and in cats with sino-aortic deafferentiation. Circulation Res 1969;24:923–937.

100. Mancia G, Baccella G, Adams DB, et al. Vasomotor regulation during sleep in the cat. Am J Physiol 1971;220:1086–1093.

101. Watson WE. Distensibility of the capacitance blood vessels of the human hand during sleep. J Physiol 1962;161:392–398.

102. Mullen PE, James VHT, Lightman SL, et al. A relationship between plasma renin activity and the rapid eye movement phase of sleep in man. J Clin Endocrinol Metab 1980;50:466–469.

103. Reivich M, Isaacs G, Evarts E, et al. The effect of slow wave sleep and REM sleep on regional cerebral blood flow in cats. J Neurochem 1968;15:301–306.

104. Greenberg JH. Sleep and the cerebral circulation. In: Orem J, Barnes CD, eds. Physiology in Sleep. New York: Academic Press, 1980;57–95.

105. Pack AI, Kline LR, Hendricks JC, et al. Neural mechanisms in the genesis of sleep apnea. In: Issa FG, Suratt PM, Remmers JE, eds. Sleep and Respiration. New York: Wiley-Liss, 1990;177–190.

106. Ohta Y, Mori S, Kimura H. Neuronal structures of the brainstem participating in postural suppression in cats. Neurosci Res 1988;5:181–202.

107. Sakai K, Sastre JP, Salvert D, et al. Tegmentoreticular projections with special reference to the muscular atonia during paradoxical sleep in the cat. An HRP study. Brain Res 1979;176:233–254.

108. Bowker RM, Westlund KN, Sullivan MC, et al. Descending serotonergic, peptidergic and cholinergic pathways from the raphe nuclei: A multiple transmitter complex. Brain Res 1983;288:33–48.

109. Jones BE, Pare M, Beaudet A. Retrograde labeling of neurons in the brain stem following injections of [³H] choline into the rat spinal cord. Neuroscience 1986;18:901–916.

110. Chase MH, Morales FR, Boxer PA, et al. Effect of stimulation of the nucleus reticularis gigantocellularis on the membrane potential of cat lumbar motoneurons during sleep and wakefulness. Brain Res 1986;386:237–244.

111. Jouvet M. Locus coeruleus et sommeil paradoxal. C R Soc Biol 1965;159:895–899.

112. Henley K, Morrison AR. A re-evaluation of the effect of lesions on the pontine tegmentum and locus coeruleus on phenomena of paradoxical sleep in the cat. Acta Neurobiol Exp 1974;34:215–232.

113. Hendricks JC, Morrison AR, Mann GL. Different behaviors during paradoxical sleep without atonia depend on pontine lesion site. Brain Res 1982;239:81–105.

114. Chase MH. Synaptic mechanisms and circuitry involved in motoneuron control during sleep. Int Rev Neurobiol 1983;24:213–258.

115. Morales FR, Boxer PA, Chase MH. Behavioral state-specific inhibitory postsynaptic potentials impinge on cat lumbar motoneurons during active sleep. Exp Neurol 1987;98:418–435.

116. Morales FR, Chase MH. Repetitive synaptic potentials responsible for inhibition of spinal cord motoneurons during active sleep. Exp Neurol 1982;78:471–476.

117. Takakusaki K, Ohta Y, Mori S. Single medullary reticulospinal neurons exert postsynaptic inhibitory effects via inhibitory interneurons upon alpha-motoneurons innervating cat hindlimb muscles. Exp Brain Res 1989; 74:11–23.

118. Soja PJ, Morales FR, Chase MH. Postsynaptic control of lumbar motoneurons during the atonia of active sleep. In: Issa FG, Suratt PM, Remmers JE, eds. Sleep and Respiration. New York: Wiley-Liss, 1990;9–22.

119. Iscoe S. Central control of the upper airway. In: Mathew OP, Sant'Ambrogio G, ed. Respiratory function of the upper airway. New York: Marcel Dekker, 1988;125–192.

120. Kalia M. Anatomical organization of the central respiratory neurons. Ann Rev Physiol 1981;43:105–120.

121. Bianchi AL, Grelot L, Barillot JC. Motor output to the pharyngeal muscles. In: Issa FG, Suratt PM, Remmers JE, eds. Sleep and Respiration. New York: Wiley-Liss, 1990;89–97.

122. Bartlett D Jr, Leiter JC, Knuth SL. Control and actions of the genioglossus muscle. In: Issa FG, Suratt PM, Remmers JE, eds. Sleep and Respiration. New York: Wiley-Liss, 1990; 99–108.

123. Sauerland EK, Harper RM. The human tongue during sleep: Electromyographic activity of the genioglossus muscle. Exp Neurol 1976;51:160–170.

124. Sauerland EK, Orr WC, Hairston LE. EMG patterns of oropharyngeal muscles during respiration in wakefulness and sleep. Electromyogr Clin Neurophysiol 1981;21:307–316.

125. Doble EA, Leiter JC, Knuth SL, et al. A noninvasive intraoral electromyographic electrode for genioglossus muscle. J Appl Physiol 1985;58:1378–1382.

126. Suratt PM, Hollowell DE. Inspiratory activation of the masseter. In: Issa FG, Suratt PM, Remmers JE, eds. Sleep and Respiration. New York: Wiley-Liss, 1990; 109–116.

127. Kuna SI, Insalaco G. Respiratory-related intrinsic laryngeal muscle activity in normal adults. In: Issa FG, Suratt PM, Remmers JE, eds. Sleep and Respiration. New York: Wiley-Liss, 1990;117–124.

128. Sant'Ambrogio G, Mathew OP. Laryngeal Function in Respiration. New York: Marcel Dekker, 1988.

129. Kuna ST, Smickley JS, Insalaco G. Posterior cricoarytenoid muscle activity during wakefulness and sleep in normal adults. Am Rev Respir Dis 1989; 139:A446.

130. van Lunteren E. Role of mammalian hyoid muscles in the maintenance of pharyngeal patency. In: Issa FG, Suratt PM, Remmers JE, eds. Sleep and Respiration. New York: Wiley-Liss, 1990;125–136.

131. Kline LR, Hendricks JC, Davies RO, et al. Control of activity of the diaphragm in rapid eye movement sleep. J Appl Physiol 1986;61:1293–1300.

132. Orem J. Neuronal mechanisms of respiration in REM sleep. Sleep 1980;3:251–267.

133. Orr WC. Gastrointestinal physiology. In: Kryger MH, Roth T, Dement WC. Principles and Practice of Sleep Medicine. Philadelphia: WB Saunders, 1989; 293–299.

134. Moore JG, Englert E. Circadian rhythm of gastric acid secretion in man. Nature 1970;226:1261–1262.

135. Levin E, Kirsner JB, Palmer WL, et al. A comparison of the nocturnal gastric secretion in patients with duodenal ulcer in normal individuals. Gastroenterology 1948;10:952–964.

136. Feldman M, Richardson CT. Total 24-hour gastric acid secretion in patients with duodenal ulcer: Comparison with normal subjects and effects of cimetidine and parietal cell vagotomy. Gastroenterology 1986;90:540–544.

137. McCloy RF, Girvan DP, Baron JH. Twenty-four–hour gastric acidity after vagotomy. Gut 1978;19:664–668.

138. Reichsman F, Cohen J, Colwill J, et al. Natural and histamine-induced gastric secretion during waking and sleeping states. Psychosomat Med 1960;1:14–24.

139. Armstrong RH, Burnap D, Jacobson A, et al. Dreams and acid secretions in duodenal ulcer patients. New Physician 1965;33:241–243.

140. Stacher G, Presslich B, Starker H. Gastric acid secretion and sleep stages during natural night sleep. Gastroenterology 1975;68:1449–1455.

141. Orr WC, Hall WH, Stahl ML, et al. Sleep patterns and gastric acid secretion in duodenal ulcer disease. Arch Intern Med 1976;136:655–660.

142. Orr WC, Dubois A, Stahl ML, et al. Gastric function during sleep. Sleep Res 1978;7:72.

143. Bloom PB, Ross DL, Stunkard AJ, et al. Gastric and duodenal motility, food intake and hunger measured in man during a 24-hour period. Dig Dis Sci 1970;15:719–725.

144. Yaryura-Tobias HA, Hutcheson JS, White L. Relationship between stages of sleep and gastric motility. Behav Neuropsychiatry 1970;2:22–24.

145. Wada T. An experimental study of slumber in its relation to activity. Arch Psychol (Frankf) 1922;8:1–65.

146. Finch P, Ingram D, Henstridge J, et al. Relationship of fasting gastroduodenal motility to the sleep cycle. Gastroenterology 1982;83:605–612.

147. Orr W, Robinson M, Johnson L. Acid clearance during sleep in the pathogenesis of reflux esophagitis. Dig Dis Sci 1981;26:423–427.

148. Lear C, Flanagan J, Moorees C. The frequency of deglutition in man. Arch Oral Biol 1965;10:83–96.

149. Litcher J, Muir RC. The pattern of swallowing during sleep. Electroencephalogr Clin Neurophysiol 1975;38:427–432.

150. Johnson LF, DeMeester TR. Twenty-four-hour pH monitoring of the distal esophagus: A quantitative measure of gastroesophageal reflux. Am J Gastroenterol 1974;62:325–332.

151. Orr WC, Johnson LF, Robinson MG. The effect of sleep on swallowing, esophageal peristalsis, and acid clearance. Gastroenterology 1984;86:814–819.

152. Dent J, Dodds WJ, Friedman RH, et al. Mechanisms of gastroesophageal reflux in recumbent asymptomatic human subjects. J Clin Invest 1980;65:256–257.

153. Orr WC, Bollinger C, Stahl M. Measurement of gastroesophageal reflux during sleep by esophageal pH monitoring. In: Guilleminault C, ed. Sleeping and Waking Disorders: Indications and Techniques. Menlo Park, Calif: Addison-Wesley Publishing Company, 1982;331–342.

154. Aschoff J. Circadian control of body temperature. J Therm Biol 1983;8:143–147.

155. Aschoff J. Desynchronization and resynchronization of human circadian rhythms. Aerospace Med 1969;40:847.

156. Heller HC, Glotzback S, Grahn D, et al. Sleep-dependent changes in the thermoregulatory system. In: Lydic R, Biebuyck JF. Clinical Physiology of Sleep. Bethesda, Md: American Physiological Society, 1988;145–158.

157. Aschoff J. Circadian rhythm of activity and body temperature. In: Hardy JD, Gagge AP, Stolwijk JAJ, eds. Physiological and Behavioral Temperature Regulation. Springfield, Ill: Charles C Thomas, 1970; 905–919.

158. Timbal J, Colin J, Boutelier C. Circadian variations in the sweating mechanism. J Appl Psychol 1975; 39:226–230.

159. Parmeggiani PL. Temperature regulation during sleep: A study in homeostasis. In: Orem J, Barnes CD, eds. Physiology in Sleep. New York: Academic Press, 1980; 97–143.

160. Henane R, Buguet A, Roussel B, et al. Variations in evaporation and body temperatures during sleep in man. J Appl Physiol 1977;42:50–55.

161. Szymusiak R, McGinty D. Control of slow wave sleep by thermoregulatory mechanisms. In: Issa FG, Suratt PM, Remmers JE, eds. Sleep and Respiration. New York: Wiley-Liss, 1990;53–66.

162. Berger RJ, Phillips NH. Comparative physiology of sleep, thermoregulation and metabolism from the perspective of energy metabolism. In: Issa FG, Suratt PM, Remmers JE, eds. Sleep and Respiration. New York: Wiley-Liss, 1990;41–52.

163. MacFadyen H, Oswald I, Lewis SA. Starvation and human slow wave sleep. J Appl Physiol 1973;35:391–394.

164. Horne JA, Shackell BS. Slow wave sleep elevations after body heating: Proximity to sleep and effects of aspirin. Sleep 1987;10:383–392.

165. Benedek GF, Obal F Jr, Lelkes Z, et al. Thermal and chemical stimulation of the hypothalamic heat detectors. The effects on the EEG. Acta Physiol Acad Sci Hungar 1982;60:27–35.

166. Bunnell DE, Agnew JA, Horvath SM, et al. Passive body heating and sleep: Influence of proximity to sleep. Sleep 1988;11:210–219.

167. Horne JA, Reid AS. Night-time sleep EEG changes following body heating in a warm bath. Electroencephalogr Clin Neurophysiol 1985;60:154–157.

168. McGinty D, Szymusiak R. The basal forebrain and slow wave sleep: Mechanistic and functional aspects. In: Wauquier A, ed. Slow-Wave Sleep: Physiological, Pathophysiological and Functional Aspects. New York: Raven Press, 1989;61–73.

169. Takahashi Y, Kipnis D, Daughaday W. Growth hormone secretion during sleep. J Clin Invest 1968; 47:2079–2090.

170. Honda Y, Takahashi K, Takahashi S, et al. Growth hormone secretion during nocturnal sleep in normal subjects. J Clin Endocrinol Metab 1969;29:20–29.

171. Parker D, Sassin J, Mace J, et al. Human growth hormone release during sleep: Electroencephalographic correlation. J Clin Endocrinol Metab 1969;29:871–874.

172. Sassin J, Parker D, Mace J, et al. Human growth hormone release: Relation to slow-wave sleep and sleep-waking cycles. Science 1969;165:513–515.

173. Quabbe H. Chronobiology of growth hormone secretion. Chronobiologia 1977;4:217–246.

174. Weitzman E, Boyar R, Kapen S, et al. The relationship of sleep and sleep stages to neuroendocrine secretion and biological rhythms in man. Rec Prog Hormone Res 1975;31:401–406.

175. Goldstein J, Cauter EV, DeSir D, et al. Effects of "jet lag" on hormonal patterns. IV. Time shifts increase growth hormone release. J Clin Endocrinol Metab 1983;56:433–440.

176. Besset A, Bonardet A, Billiard M, et al. Circadian pattern of GH and cortisol in narcoleptic patients. Chronobiologia 1979;6:19–31.

177. Schilkrut R, Chandra O, Oswald N, et al. Growth hormone release during sleep and with thermal stimulation in depressed patients. Neuropsychobiology 1975;1:70–79.

178. Mendelson W. Studies of human growth hormone secretion in sleep and waking. Int Rev Neurobiol 1982;23:367–389.

179. Orr W, Vogel G, Stahl M, et al. Sleep patterns in growth hormone–deficient children and age-matched controls: Developmental considerations. Neuroendocrinology 1977;24:347–352.

180. Takahashi Y. Growth hormone secretion during sleep: A review. In: Kawakami M, ed. Biological Rhythms in Neuroendocrine Activity. Tokyo: Igaku-Shoin, 1974;316–325.

181. Rubin R. Sleep endocrinology studies in man. Prog Brain Res 1975;42:73–80.

182. Carlson HE, Gillin JC, Gorden P, et al. Absence of sleep related growth hormone peaks in aged normal subjects and in acromegaly. J Clin Endocrinol Metab 1972;34:1102–1105.

183. Sassin J, Hellman L, Weitzman E. A circadian pattern of growth hormone secretion in acromegalics. Sleep Res 1972;1:189.

184. Clark RW, Schmidt HS, Malarkey WB. Disordered growth hormone and prolactin secretion in primary disorders of sleep. Neurology 1979;29:855–861.

185. Amsterdam JD, Schweitzer E, Winoker A. Multiple hormonal responses to insulin-induced hypoglycemia in depressed patients and normal volunteers. Am J Psychiatry 1987;144:170–175.

186. Mendelson WB. Human Sleep. New York: Plenum, 1987;129–179.

187. Othmer E, Goodwin D, Levine W, et al. Sleep-related growth hormone secretion in alcoholics. Clin Res 1972;20:726.

188. Dunleavy DL, Oswald I, Brown E, et al. Hyperthyroidism, sleep and growth hormone. Electroencephalogr Clin Neurophysiol 1974;36:259–263.

189. Weitzman ED, Fukushima D, Nogeri C, et al. Twenty-four hour pattern of the episodic secretion of cortisol in normal subjects. J Clin Endocrinol Metab 1971; 33:14–22.

190. Hellman L, Nakada R, Curta J, et al. Cortisol is secreted episodically by normal man. J Clin Endocrinol Metab 1970;30:411–422.

191. Alford FP, Baker HW, Burger HG, et al. Temporal patterns of integrated plasma hormone levels during sleep and wakefulness. I. Thyroid-stimulating hormone, growth hormone and cortisol. J Clin Endocrinol Metab 1973;37:841–847.

192. Jacoby JH, Sassin JF, Greenstein M, et al. Patterns of spontaneous cortisol and growth hormone in rhesus monkeys during the sleep-wake cycle. Neuroendocrinology 1974;14:165.

193. Jarrett DB, Coble PA, Kupfer DJ. Reduced cortisol latency in depressive illness. Arch Gen Psychiatry 1983;40:506.

194. Kupfer D, Bulik C, Jarrett D. Nighttime plasma cortisol secretion and EEG sleep—are they associated? Psychiatr Res 1983;10:191–199.

195. Fullerton DT, Wenzel FJ, Lohrenz FN, et al. Circadian rhythm of adrenal cortical activity in depression. Arch Gen Psychiatry 1968;19:674–682,682–688.

196. Rush AJ, Giles DE, Roffwarg HP, et al. Sleep EEG and dexamethasone suppression test findings in outpatients with unipolar major depressive disorders. Biol Psychiatry 1982;17:327–341.

197. Klein HE, Seibold B. DST in healthy volunteers and after sleep deprivation. Acta Psychiatr Scand 1985; 72:16–19.

198. Sassin JF, Frantz AG, Kepen S, et al. The nocturnal rise of human prolactin is dependent on sleep. J Clin Endocrinol Metab 1973;37:436–440.

199. Parker D, Rossman L, Vanderhaan E. Sleep-related nyctohemeral and briefly episodic variation in human prolactin concentration. J Clin Endocrinol Metab 1973;36:1119–1124.

200. Sassin J, Frantz A, Weitzman E, et al. Human prolactin: 24 hour patterns with increased release during sleep. Science 1972;17:1205–1207.

201. Mendelson W, Jacobs L, Reichman J, et al. Methysergide suppression of sleep-related prolactin secretion and enhancement of sleep-related growth hormone secretion. J Clin Invest 1975;56:690.

202. Rubin RT, Poland RE, Gouin PR, et al. Secretion of hormones influencing water and electrolyte balance (antidiuretic hormone, aldosterone, prolactin) during sleep in normal adult men. Psychosomat Med 1978;40:44–59.

203. Van Cauter E, Desir D, Refetoff S, et al. The relationship between episodic variations of plasma prolactin and REM-non-REM cyclicity is an artifact. J Clin Endocrinol Metab 1982;54:70–75.

204. Parker DC, Rossman LG, Kripke TF, et al. Endocrine rhythms across sleep-wake cycles in normal young men under basal state conditions. In: Orem J, Barnes CD, ed. Physiology in Sleep. New York: Academic Press, 1980;145–179.

205. Boyar R, Finkelstein J, Roffwarg H, et al. Synchronization of augmented lutenizing hormone secretion with sleep during puberty. N Engl J Med 1972; 287:582–586.

206. Boyar RM, Rosenfeld RS, Kapen S, et al. Human puberty: Simultaneous augmented secretion of luteinizing hormone and testosterone during sleep. J Clin Invest 1974;54:609–618.

207. Kapen S, Boyar RM, Finkelstein J, et al. Effect of sleep-wake cycle reversal on LH secretory pattern in puberty. J Clin Endocrinol Metab 1974;39:283–289.

208. Fevre M, Segel T, Marks JF, et al. LH and melatonin secretion patterns in pubertal boys. J Clin Endocrinol Metab 1978;47:1383–1387.

209. Evans JI, MacLean AM, Ismail AAA, et al. Concentration of plasma testosterone in normal men during sleep. Nature 1971;229:261–262.

210. Weeke J, Gundersen HJG. Circadian and 30 minute variations in serum TSH and thyroid hormones in normal subjects. Acta Endocrinol 1978;89:659–672.

211. Lucke C, Hehrmann R, von Mayersbach K, et al. Studies in circadian variations of plasma TSH, thyroxine and triiodothyronine in man. Acta Endocrinol 1976;86:81.

212. Parker D, Pekary A, Hershman J. Effect of normal and reversed sleep-wake cycles upon nyctothemeral rhythmicity of plasma thyrotropin: Evidence suggestive of an inhibitory influence in sleep. J Clin Endocrinol Metab 1976;43:318.

213. Peters J, Santa-Cruz F, Tower B, et al. Differential endocrine responses to thyrotropin-releasing hormone during the rapid eye movement and slow-wave sleep in man. J Clin Endocrinol Metab 1981;52:975–981.

214. Anch AM, Browman CP, Mitler MM, et al. Sleep: A Scientific Perspective. Engelwood Cliffs, NJ: Prentice Hall, 1988.

215. Brod J. The Kidney. London: Butterworths, 1973.

216. Leaf A, Liddle GW. Summarization of the effects of hormones of water and electrolyde metabolism. In: Williams RH, ed. Textbook of Endocrinology. Philadelphia: WB Saunders, 1972;938–947.

217. Brandenberger G, Follenius M, Muzet A, et al. Ultradian oscillations in plasma renin activity: Their relationships to meals and sleep stages. J Clin Endocrinol Metab 1985;61:280–284.

218. Kripke DF, Lavie P, Parker D, et al. Plasma parathyroid hormone and calcium are related to sleep stage cycles. J Clin Endocrinol Metab 1978;47:1021–1027.

219. Birkeland AJ. Plasma melatonin levels and nocturnal transitions between sleep and wakefulness. Neuroendocrinology 1982;34:126–131.

II

Technical Considerations

6

Polysomnographic Technique: An Overview

Sharon A. Keenan

The term *polysomnography* (PSG) was proposed by Holland, Dement, and Raynal[1] in 1974 to describe the recording, analysis, and interpretation of multiple, simultaneous physiologic parameters. As a tool, PSG is essential in the formulation of diagnoses for sleep disorders patients and in the enhancement of our understanding of both normal sleep and its disorders.[2-14] It is a complex procedure that should be performed by a trained technologist. Today's sleep laboratory is undergoing rapid technologic evolution, particularly in terms of the increased use of computers and the collection of data outside the traditional sleep laboratory setting. This evolution requires sophisticated knowledge of equipment and procedures.

This chapter is a review of the technical aspects of PSG, providing a step-by-step approach to traditional, classical in-laboratory PSG recording techniques. Problems likely to be encountered during a recording are examined, as are ways to alleviate them. Figures and actual tracings augment the text and help identify artifacts. Elsewhere in this volume, specified protocols are discussed and physiologic recording techniques are reviewed.

PATIENT CONTACT

A number of factors need to be kept in mind when a PSG study is scheduled. Issues such as shift work, time zone change, or suspected advanced or delayed sleep phase syndrome should be taken into consideration. The study should be conducted during the patient's usual major sleep period, to avoid confounding circadian rhythm factors.

When PSG is scheduled, the patient is sent a questionnaire about his or her sleep-wake history and a sleep diary that solicits information about major sleep periods and naps for 2 weeks before the study (Appendix 6-1). This history-gathering instrument should also include basic information for the patient about the purpose and procedures of the sleep study. The goal — to make the patient's stay at the sleep laboratory as uncomplicated and comfort-

able as possible — might be facilitated if the patient brings along a favorite pillow, pajamas, or book.

The technologist should ensure that patients arriving at the laboratory are familiar with the surroundings and that they receive explicit information about the process. Patients should be shown to a bedroom and through the laboratory. They are made aware that someone will be monitoring their sleep throughout the entire study and told how to contact the technologist if necessary.

Before the study is undertaken, a full medical and psychiatric history should be completed and made available to the technologist performing the study. Without this information, the technologist is at a loss to understand how aspects of the medical or psychiatric history may affect the study or to anticipate difficulties. Obviously, technologists must also understand what questions the study seeks to answer. This enhances their ability to make protocol adjustments when necessary and ensures that the most pertinent information is recorded.

Pre-Study Questionnaire

It is not uncommon for patients, particularly those with excessive sleepiness, to have a diminished capacity to evaluate their level of alertness. In addition, many patients with difficulty initiating and maintaining sleep often report a subjective evaluation of their total sleep time and quality that is at odds with the objective data collected in the laboratory. For these reasons it is recommended that subjective data be collected systematically as part of the sleep laboratory evaluation.

The Stanford Sleepiness Scale (SSS, Appendix 6-2)[15,16] is an instrument used to assess a patient's subjective evaluation of sleepiness prior to the PSG. The SSS is presented to the patient immediately before the beginning of the study. It offers a series of phrases from which to choose the one that best describes their state of arousal or sleepiness. Patients respond by selecting the set of adjectives that most closely corresponds to their current state of sleepiness or alertness. The scale is used extensively in both clinical and research environments, but it has two noteworthy limitations. It is not suitable for children who have a limited vocabulary or for adults whose primary language is not English. In these situations a linear analog scale is recommended. One end of the scale represents extreme sleepiness and the other end alertness. Patients mark the scale to describe their state just prior to testing.,

Patients are also asked about their medication history, smoking history, any unusual events during the course of the day, their last meal prior to study, alcohol intake, and a sleep history for the last 24 hours, including naps. Involvement of the patient in providing this information usually translates into increased cooperation for the study. A technologist's complete awareness of specific patient idiosyncrasies, in the context of the questions to be addressed by the study, ensures a good foundation for the collection of high-quality data.

Nap Studies

A proposed alternative to nocturnal PSG has been the nap study (to be distinguished from the Multiple Sleep Latency Test [MSLT].[17] The rationale is that if a patient has a sleep disorder it will be expressed during an afternoon nap as well as during a more extensive PSG. The nap study approach has been used most frequently for the diagnosis of sleep-related breathing disorders and was proposed in an effort to reduce the cost of the sleep laboratory evaluation. The short study in the afternoon avoids the necessity of having a technologist present for an overnight study. There are serious limitations to the use of nap studies, however, including the possibility of false negative results or the misinterpretation of the severity of sleep-related breathing disorders if the patient is sedated or sleep deprived prior to the study. (When a nap study is performed, it should follow the guidelines published by the American-Thoracic Society:[18,19])

Although minimal systematic data exist on the value of nap recordings, nap studies of 2 to 4 hours' duration may be used to confirm the diagnosis of sleep apnea, provided that all routine polysomnographic variables are recorded, that both non-REM and REM sleep are sampled, and that the patient spends at least part of the time in the supine posture. Sleep deprivation or the use of drugs to induce a nap are contraindicated. Nap studies are inadequate to definitively exclude a diagnosis of sleep apnea.

PREPARATION OF THE EQUIPMENT

For the purpose of this chapter we refer to the polygraph, an instrument in which the main component is a series of amplifiers (see also Chapter 7). Usually there is a combination of alternating current (AC) channels, greater in number, and direct current (DC) channels, fewer in number. Typically, at least 12 to 16 channels are available for recording. The data from the amplifiers are typically written to a moving chart or to a computer, which converts the analog signal to a digital signal. The digital signal is then stored by the computer for subsequent manipulation or analysis.

Equipment for recording PSGs is produced by a number of manufacturers. Each may have a distinctive appearance and some idiosyncratic features, but there is a remarkable similarity when the basic functioning of the instrument is examined.

Equipment preparation includes an understanding of how the filters and sensitivity of the amplifiers affect the data collected. Inasmuch as the major difference between traditional clinical polysomnography and computer-based systems lies principally in data collection and storage, it is important that all technologists, regardless of the system used, have adequate knowledge of the operation of the equipment.

The amplifiers used to record physiologic data are very sensitive, so it is essential to eliminate unwanted signals from the recording. By using a combination of a high-frequency filter, and appropriate sensitivity settings, we maximize the likelihood of recording and displaying the signals of interest and decrease the possibility of recording extraneous signals. Care must be taken, when using the high- and low-frequency filters, however, to ensure that an appropriate window for recording specific frequencies is established and that the filters do not eliminate important data.

Alternating current amplifiers

Differential AC amplifiers are used to record physiologic parameters of high frequency, such as the electroencephalogram (EEG), the electrooculogram (EOG), the electromyogram (EMG), and the electrocardiogram (ECG). The AC amplifier has both high- and low-frequency filters. The presence of the low-frequency filter makes it possible to attenuate slow potentials not associated with the physiology of interest; these include galvanic skin response, DC electrode imbalance, and breathing reflected in an EMG, EEG, or EOG channel. Combinations of specific settings of the high- and low-frequency filters make it possible to focus on specific band widths associated with the signal of interest. For example, respiration is a very slow signal (roughly 12 to 18 breaths per minute) in comparison with the signal of an EMG, which has a much higher frequency (approximately 30 to 120 Hz).

Direct current amplifiers

In contrast to the AC amplifier, the DC amplifier does not have a low-frequency filter. DC amplifiers are typically used to record slower-moving potentials, such as output from oximeters or pH meters, changes in pressure in continuous positive airway pressure (CPAP) equipment, or output from transducers that record endoesophageal pressure changes or body temperature. Airflow and effort of breathing can be successfully recorded with either AC or DC amplifiers.

An understanding of the appropriate use of filters in clinical PSG is essential to proper recording technique.[20] Table 6-1 provides recommendations for filter settings for a number of physiologic parameters.

Calibration of the Equipment

The PSG recording instrument must be calibrated to ensure adequate functioning of amplifiers and appropriate settings for the specific protocol. The first calibration is an all-channel calibration (Figure 6-1). During this calibration all amplifiers are set to the same sensitivity, high-frequency filter, and low-frequency filter settings. The proper functioning of all amplifiers is thus demonstrated, ensuring that all are functioning in identical fashion.

A second calibration is performed for the specific study protocol. During this calibration amplifiers are set with the high-frequency filter, low-frequency filter, and sensitivity settings appropriate for each channel; the settings are dictated by the requirements of the specific physiologic parameter recorded on each channel (see Table 6-1, Figure 6-2). The protocol calibration ensures that all amplifiers are set to ideal conditions for recording the parameter of interest. All filter and sensitivity settings, as well as paper speed and time, should be clearly documented on each channel.

Paper Speed

The paper speed of the instrument establishes the epoch length or the amount of time that appears on each page of the recording. The process of sleep stage scoring and analysis of abnormalities is accomplished by an epoch-by-epoch review of the data.

A common paper speed for traditional polysomnography is 10 mm/sec, providing a 30-sec epoch. Another widely accepted paper speed is 15 mm/sec, which gives a 20-sec epoch length. Significant portions of tracings at a paper speed of 30 mm/sec should be used when recording patients with suspected sleep-related seizure activity. This enhances the ability to visualize EEG data, specifically the spike activity associated with epileptic discharges. In general, paper speeds slower than 10 mm/sec should be avoided because they compromise an adequate display of EEG data. Data such as oxygen saturation, respiratory signals, or changes in penile circumference, however, can sometimes be more easily visualized with slower paper speeds. If compressed data are required it is possible to output the signal from the polysomnograph to a slower-moving strip chart recorder. Simultaneous display of the signal on both the polysomnogram and the slower-moving chart is advantageous.

THE STUDY

Electrode/Monitor Application Process

The quality of the tracing generated in the sleep laboratory depends a great deal on the quality of the electrode application.[21] Before any electrode or monitor is applied the patient should be instructed about the procedure and given an opportunity to ask questions. The first step in the electrode application procedure involves measurement of the patient's head. The International 10-20 System[22] of electrode placement is used to localize specific electrode placements (Figure 6-3). The following sections address the application process for EEG, EOG, EMG, and ECG channels.

TABLE 6-1. Amplifier Conditions for a Routine PSG

Channel*	Low-Frequency Filter (Hz)	Time Constant(s)	High-Frequency Filter (Hz)	Sensitivity (μV/cm)
EEG	0.3	0.4	35	50
EOG	0.3	0.4	35	50
EMG	5[†]	0.03	90 to 120	50
ECG[‡]	1.0	0.12	15	1 MV/cm to start, adjust as necessary
Airflow (AC-amp)	0.15	1 to 2	15	50 to start, adjust as necessary
Effort (AC-amp)	0.15	1 to 2	15	50 to start, adjust as necessary

*EEG includes C3/A2,C4/A1,O1/A2,O2/A1, etc. EOG include right outer canthus and left outer canthus.
†If shorter time constant or higher low-frequency filter is available, it should be used. This includes settings for all EMG channels, including mentalis, submentalis, masseter, anterior tibialis, intercostal.
‡The sensitivity for ECG is set at 1 MV/cm to start and adjusted as necessary.
(From Keenan SA. Polysomnography: Technical aspects in adolescents and adults. J Clin Neurophysiol 1992;9(1):21–31.)

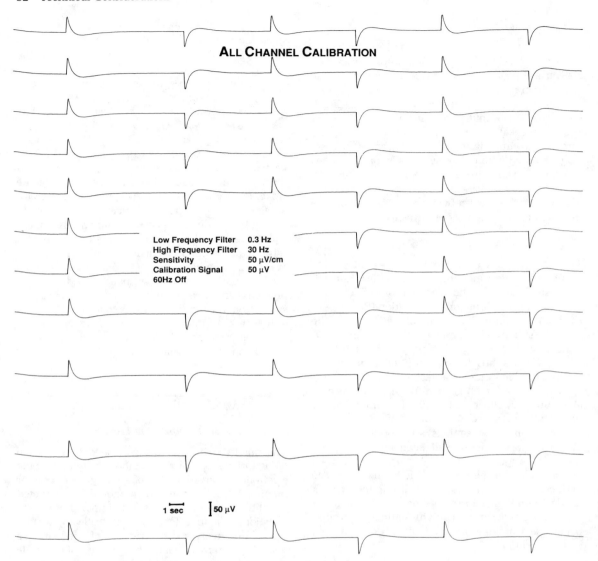

ALL CHANNEL CALIBRATION

Low Frequency Filter	0.3 Hz
High Frequency Filter	30 Hz
Sensitivity	50 μV/cm
Calibration Signal	50 μV
60Hz Off	

1 sec   50 μV

FIGURE 6-1.   *All channel calibration is shown. All amplifiers have the same sensitivity and high- and low-frequency filter settings.*

Electroencephalography

Standard electrode derivations for monitoring EEG activity during sleep are C_3-A_1 or C_4-A_2, and O_1-A_2 or O_2-A_1, but in many situations there may be a need for additional electrodes. For example, to rule out the possibility of epileptic seizures during sleep, or the presence of any other sleep-related EEG abnormality, it may be necessary to apply the full complement of EEG electrodes according to the International 10–20 System (Appendix 6-3).

For recording EEG, a gold cup electrode with a hole in the center is commonly used. Silver–silver chloride electrodes are also useful to record EEG, though they may have limitations such as increased maintenance (evidenced by the need for repeated chloriding) and the inability to attach these electrodes to the scalp.

The placement of C_3, C_4, O_1, and O_2 are determined by the International 10-20 System of electrode placement. Reference electrodes are placed on the bony surface of the mastoid process. A description of the measurement procedure appears in Appendix 6-4.

The preferred method of application for EEG scalp and reference electrodes is the collodion technique.[23,24] This technique ensures long-term placement and allows for correction of high impedances, those over 5000 Ω, after application.

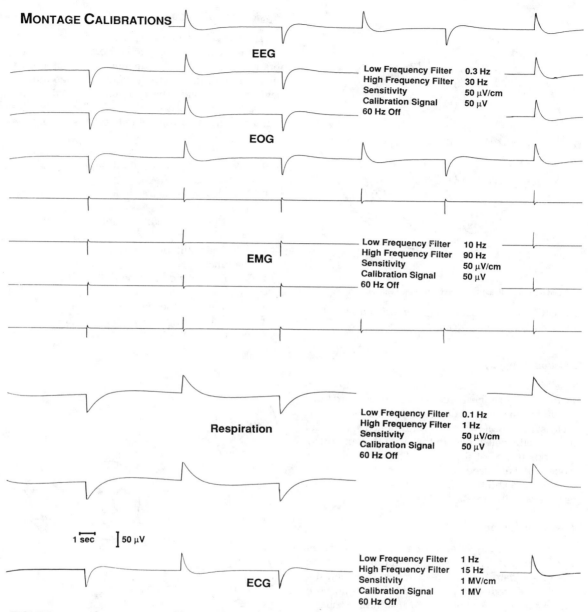

FIGURE 6-2. *The Montage Calibration shows changes in high and low filter settings from the all-channel calibration to accommodate the display of a variety of physiologic signals for the PSG.*

Electrooculography (see also Chapter 7)

The EOG is a recording of the movement of the cornea-retinal potential difference that exists in the eye. It is important to recognize that it is the movement of this dipole, not muscle activity of the eyes, that is recorded. Gold cup electrodes, or silver–silver chloride electrodes can be used to monitor the EOG.

An electrode is typically applied at the outer canthus of the right eye (ROC) and is offset 1 cm above the horizontal. Another electrode is applied to the

outer canthus of the left eye (LOC) and is offset by 1 cm below the horizontal. The reference electrodes are connected to the contralateral ears. Additional electrodes can be applied infraorbitally and supraorbitally for either eye. The infraorbital and supraorbital electrodes enhance the ability to detect eye movements that occur in the vertical plane and can be particularly useful in the MSLT (Figure 6-4).[17] EOG electrodes are typically applied to the surface of the skin with an adhesive collar; this method avoids the risk of collodion contacting the patient's eyes.

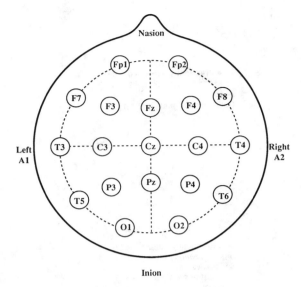

Standard international 10-20 electrode placement (superior view)

FIGURE 6-3.   *The complete International 10–20 System of electrode placement.*

Electromyography

A gold cup or a silver–silver chloride electrode attached with an adhesive collar is used to record EMG activity from the mentalis and submentalis muscles. At least three EMG electrodes are applied to allow for an alternative electrode, in the event that an artifact develops in one of the others. The additional electrode can be placed over the masseter muscle to enhance the ability to detect bursts of EMG activity associated with bruxism (Figure 6-5).

Electrocardiography

There are a variety of approaches for recording the ECG during PSG. The simplest approach involves use of standard gold cup electrodes. However, disposable electrodes are also available for this purpose. ECG electrodes are applied with an adhesive collar to the surface of the skin, just beneath the right clavicle and on the left side at the level of the seventh rib. A stress loop is incorporated into the lead wire to ensure long-term placement.

Impedances

Before recording, electrodes should be visually inspected to check the security of their placement and an impedance check should be obtained and documented. This requires the use of an impedance meter, which is either built in to the polygraph or separate from it. Any EEG, EOG, ECG, or EMG electrode with an impedance greater than 5000 Ω should be adjusted.

Physiologic Calibrations

Physiologic calibrations are performed after the electrode and monitor application is complete. This calibration both allows for documentation of proper functioning of the electrodes and other monitoring devices and provides baseline data for review and comparison when scoring the PSG. The specific instructions given to the patient for this calibration include these:

- Eyes open, look straight ahead for 30 seconds.
- Eyes closed, look straight ahead for 30 seconds.
- Look to left and right, up and down. Repeat.
- Hold head still, blink eyes slowly, five times.
- Grit teeth, clench jaw, or smile.
- Inhale and exhale.
- Hold breath 10 seconds.
- Flex right foot, flex left foot.
- Flex right hand, flex left hand

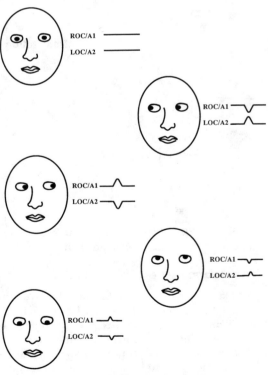

FIGURE 6-4.   *The recording montage for a two-channel EOG demonstrates out-of-phase pen deflection in association with conjugate eye movements.*

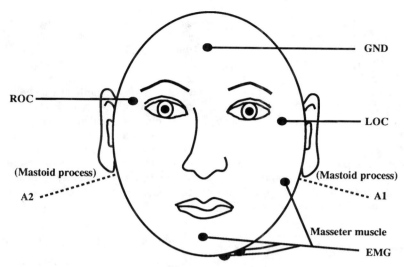

FIGURE 6-5. *Schematic diagram shows placement of the EMG electrodes to record activities from the mental, submental, and masseter muscles. Key: ROC, LOC, outer canthus of the right and left eyes, respectively.*

As these instructions are given to the patient, the technologist examines the tracing and documents the patient's responses. When the patient stares straight ahead for 30 seconds with eyes open, the background EEG activity is examined. As the patient looks right and left the tracing is examined for out-of-phase deflections of the pens associated with recording the EOG. Out-of-phase deflection occurs if the inputs to consecutive channels of the polygraph are ROC/A1 for the first EOG channel and LOC/A2 for the second. It is also important, when the patient closes the eyes, to observe the reactivity of the alpha rhythm in the EEG. The patient is also asked to blink five times.

The EMG signal is checked by asking the patient to grit the teeth, smile, or yawn. The patient is asked to flex the right big toe and the left big toe; then the right foot and the left foot in turn. The technologist documents proper functioning of the electrodes and amplifiers used to monitor anterior tibilialis EMG activity. If the patient is in the laboratory to rule out suspected REM sleep behavior disorder additional electrodes should be applied on the extensor digitorum muscles of each arm. Should this condition exist, physiologic calibrations for those electrodes are performed as well. Specifically, patients are asked to extend their wrists while the technologist examines the recording for the corresponding increase in amplitude on the extensor digitorum EMG channel.

Inhalation and exhalation allow for examination of channels monitoring airflow and breathing.[25,26] A suggested convention is that inhalation causes an upward deflection of the pens and exhalation a downward deflection. It is most important that the signals on all the channels monitoring breathing are in phase with each other, to avoid misinterpreting paradoxical breathing. The technologist should also observe a flattening of the trace for the duration of a voluntary apnea.

If the 60- or 50-Hz notch filter is in use, a brief examination (2 to 4 seconds) of portions of the tracing with the filter in the *out* position is essential. Identification of any 60- or 50-Hz interference that may be masked by the filter is thus possible. Care should be taken to eliminate any source of this interference and to ensure that the notch filter is used only as a last resort. This is most important when recording patients suspected of having seizure activity, because the notch filter attenuates the amplitude of spike activity. If other monitors are used, the technologist should incorporate the necessary calibrations.

After physiologic calibrations are completed, the technologist determines if any adjustment to electrodes or other monitoring devices is needed before the PSG begins. If artifact is noted during the physiologic calibrations, it is imperative that every effort be made to correct the problem; the condition is likely to get worse through the remaining portions of the recording. The functioning of alternative (spare) electrodes should also be examined during this calibration.

When a satisfactory calibration procedure is completed and all other aspects of patient and equipment preparation are completed, lights are turned out in the patient's room and the patient is told to assume a comfortable sleeping position and attempt to fall asleep. The lights-out time should be clearly noted on the tracing.

Monitoring Recording

Documentation

Complete documentation for the PSG is essential. This includes patient identification (patient's full name and medical record number), date of recording, and a full description of the study. The names of the technologist performing the recording should be noted and any other technologists involved in preparation of patient and equipment. In laboratories that use multiple pieces of equipment, the specific instrument used to generate the recording should be identified. This is particularly useful in the event that artifact is noted during the analysis portion (scoring) of the sleep study.

Specific parameters recorded on each channel should be clearly noted, as should a full description of sensitivity, filter, and calibration settings for each channel. Paper speed must also be documented to provide information on epoch length. The time of the beginning and end of the recording must be noted, as well as specific events that occur during the night. For instruments that lack a time code generator or other device that would automatically note clock time it is important that the technologist make manual notes of clock time at hourly intervals. Any changes made to filter and sensitivity settings or paper speed should be clearly noted on the tracing.

The technologist is also responsible for providing a clinical description of unusual events. For example, if a patient experiences an epileptic seizure during the study, the clinical manifestations of the seizure must be detailed: deviation of eyes or head to one side or the other, movement of extremities, presence of vomiting or incontinence, duration of seizure, and postictal status. Similar information should be reported on any clinical event observed in the laboratory, such as somnambulism. Physical complaints reported by the patient are also noted.

Troubleshooting and artifact recognition

In general, when difficulties arise during recording, the troubleshooting inquiry begins at the patient and follows the path of the signal to the recording device. More often than not the problem can be identified as a difficulty with an electrode or other monitoring device. It is less likely that an artifact is the result of a problem with an amplifier. If the artifact is generalized (i.e., on most channels), then the integrity of the ground electrode and the instrument cable

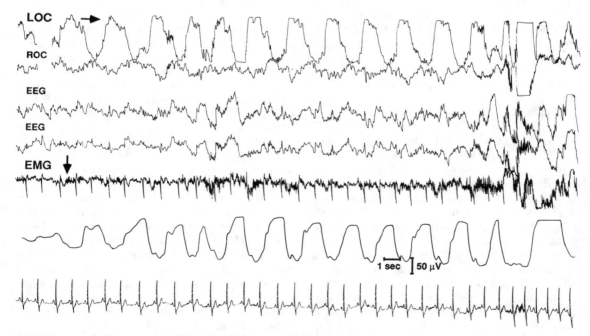

FIGURE 6-6.   *Artifact in LOC channel (LOC/A₁) can be localized to the LOC electrode. The EEG channels in the trace are C₃/A₂ and O₂/A₁. Because the artifact does not appear in the O₂/A₁ channel it is localized to the LOC electrode. The electrode placement may be insecure or the patient may be lying on the electrode, which could move as the patient breathes. Additional artifact is noted in the EMG channel. This signal is contaminated with ECG artifact, and the intermittent slower activity and the wandering baseline are most likely due to a loose lead. The ECG channel also shows a pattern consistent with a loose electrode wire.*

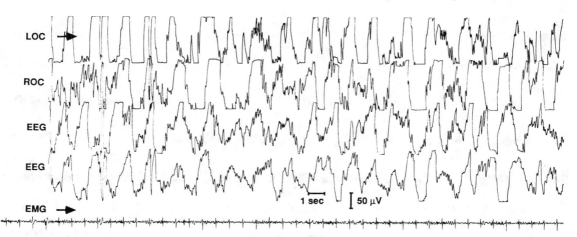

FIGURE 6-7. *This figure illustrates the blocking artifact seen with inappropriate sensitivity settings, which can be abolished by decreasing sensitivity. If adjustments to sensitivity are made, they should be clearly noted and should be made on all channels that display EEG data. It is common procedure to calibrate the equipment with decreased sensitivities (i.e., 100 μv/cm) for children's studies and with increased sensitivity (i.e., 30 μv/cm) for older patients. Typically, sensitivity settings are not changed frequently during the recording (as they may be in routine EEG). As a result, it is not uncommon to see this artifact when the patient enters slow-wave sleep.*

should be checked. If the artifact is localized (i.e., on a limited number of channels), then the question should be, which channels have this artifact in common and what is common to the channels involved? The artifact is probably the result of a problem located in an electrode or monitoring device that is common to both channels. If the artifact is isolated to a single channel, the source of artifact is limited to the inputs to the specific amplifier, the amplifier itself, or the ink-writing system for the channel. Figures 6-6 through 6-14 depict some frequently encountered artifacts seen during PSG.

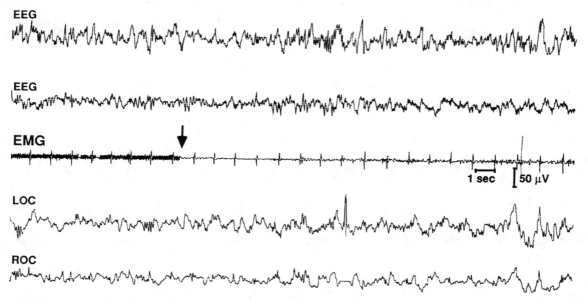

FIGURE 6-8. *A 60-Hz artifact exists in the EMG channel in this tracing. At the arrow, the 60-Hz filter is turned on, but there is continued evidence of difficulty with electrodes on this channel, as evidenced by the ECG artifact and occasional spikelike activity. Turning on the 60-Hz filter is not the correct response to eliminate the artifact. If possible, the technologist should switch to an alternative electrode or fix the one involved.*

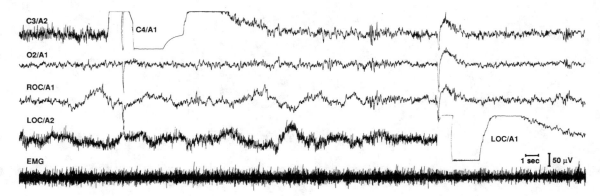

FIGURE 6-9.   *The high-frequency (probably EMG) artifact noted in the C_3/A_2 and LOC/A_2 channels can be localized to the A_2 electrode. This problem can be solved by switching to the alternative reference (A_1) electrode. A high-amplitude discharge is noted during the switch from C_3/A_2 to C_4/A_1 and LOC/A_2 to LOC/A_1. This can be avoided by placing the amplifier in standby mode while making the change.*

ENDING THE STUDY

Clinical circumstances and laboratory protocol dictate whether the patient is awakened at a specific time or is allowed to awaken spontaneously. After awakening, to end the study the patient should be asked to perform the physiologic calibration movements, to ensure that the electrodes and other monitoring devices are still functioning properly. The equipment should be calibrated at the settings used for the study, and, finally, the amplifiers should be set to identical settings for high- and low-frequency filters and sensitivity and an all-channel calibration should be performed. This is essentially the reverse of the calibration procedures mentioned at the beginning of the study.

A subjective evaluation by the patient is made. The patient is asked to estimate how long it took to fall asleep, the amount of time spent asleep, and if there were any disruptions during the sleep period. Patients should report on quality of sleep and the level of alertness they experience on arousal.

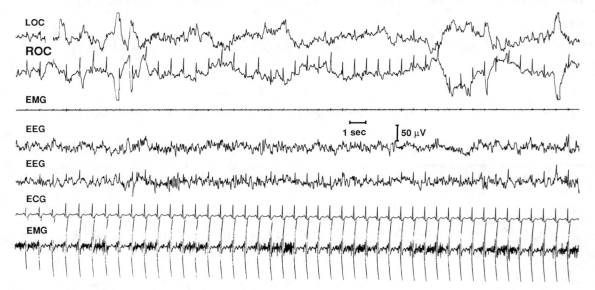

FIGURE 6-10.   *The ROC channel (ROC/A_1) and the second EEG (O_2/A_1) channels are contaminated with ECG artifact. The artifact can be identified by aligning the spikelike activity noted in channels with the R wave on the ECG channel. It is localized to the A1 electrode because it is seen in both ROC/A_1 and O_2/A_1 channels and A1 is common to both. It should be noted that the high-amplitude ECG artifact seen in the EMG channel below the ECG channel is unavoidable. This artifact is due to the proximity of EMG electrodes to the heart, which superimposes a robust signal on the intercostal EMG signal.*

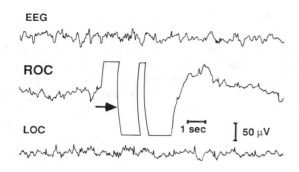

FIGURE 6-11. *The high-amplitude deflection in the ROC (ROC/A₁) channel is associated with an electrode artifact commonly referred to as an electrode pop. This can be the result of compromised electrode placement or insufficient electroconductive gel under the electrode. When it is observed, the involved electrode should not be trusted to give reliable data.*

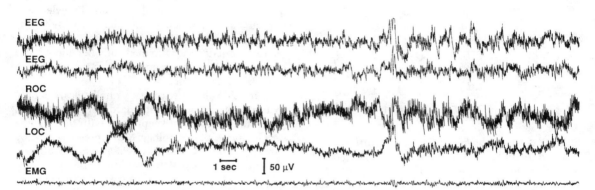

FIGURE 6-12. *The generalized, high-frequency activity superimposed on the EEG and EOG channels is most likely secondary to muscle activity. The EMG channel shows only artifact. In addition, it appears there is a slant to the left, particularly in channels 1 through 4, which is probably secondary to difficulty with mechanical baseline of the pens.*

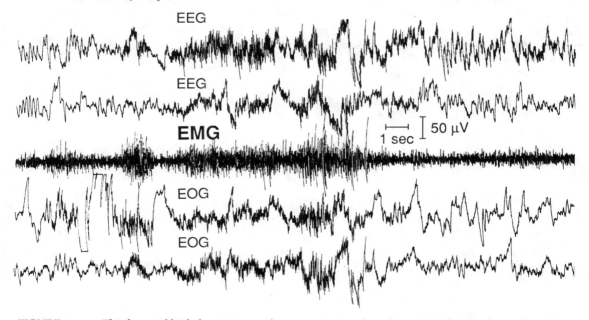

FIGURE 6-13. *This burst of high-frequency artifact, superimposed on the EEG and EOG channels, is due to a brief movement by the subject. As in Figure 6-12, this is a superimposition of EMG activity on the EEG and EOG channels. It should also be noted that in the first EOG channel there is an electrode pop. The EMG channel in this tracing is of good quality and should be compared to that in Figure 6-12.*

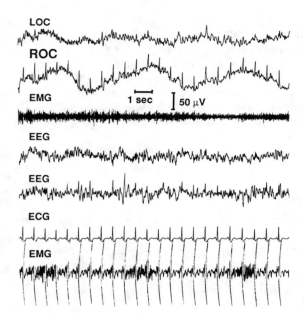

LOC

ROC

EMG

1 sec   50 µV

EEG

EEG

ECG

EMG

FIGURE 6-14.   *A high-amplitude, slow artifact is noted in the ROC (ROC/A₁) channel. This is most likely asociated with the patient's breathing and is secondary to a loose electrode or the patient is lying on the right side and disturbing the electrode in synchrony with breathing. A relatively high-amplitude ECG artifact is also seen. The artifact can be localized to the ROC electrode. The EMG tracing noted at the bottom of this example is an intercostal EMG. The high-amplitude ECG spike in this channel is impossible to eliminate, but the brief bursts of EMG activity can be noted in association with the artifact seen in the ROC/A₁ channel. This is further evidence that the artifact noted in the ROC electrode is probably associated with breathing, as the bursts of intercostal EMG activity are asociated with the effort of breathing.*

It is also worthwhile for the sleep laboratory staff to know how patients intend to leave the laboratory. A patient who has a severe sleep disorder should avoid driving. An arranged ride or public transportation should be used, particularly if the patient has withdrawn from stimulant medications in anticipation of the study.

CONCLUSION

PSG is a complex, labor-intensive procedure. It requires specialized technical skills and knowledge of normal sleep and sleep disorders. Technologists need to be experts with sleep laboratory equipment, competent in dealing with medically ill patients, and capable of dealing with emergencies that may arise in the sleep laboratory.

Our field is faced with many challenges, not only in terms of developing standards of practice and procedures but also of keeping up with the ongoing developments of technology. Much pressure is being exerted to make PSG readily available to the millions of sleep disorders patients waiting to be diagnosed. This needs to be achieved in a cost-effective manner that does not compromise high-quality data and detailed analysis necessary for the formulation of accurate and complete diagnoses.

Throughout its evolution PSG has proven a robust tool for enhancing our understanding of sleep and its disorders. It is an essential diagnostic procedure. The next few years will prove interesting, particularly in terms of advances in technology and its consequent enhancement of our ability to understand normal sleep and sleep disorders.

APPENDIX 6-1.   Template for 24 Hour Sleep-Wake Log. This log should be completed by the patient for a period of 2 weeks prior to the study.

Date			Date			Date		
Time	**Awake**	**Asleep**	**Time**	**Awake**	**Asleep**	**Time**	**Awake**	**Asleep**
12:00			12:00			12:00		
13:00			13:00			13:00		
14:00			14:00			14:00		
15:00			15:00			15:00		
16:00			16:00			16:00		
17:00			17:00			17:00		
18:00			18:00			18:00		
19:00			19:00			19:00		
20:00			20:00			20:00		
21:00			21:00			21:00		
22:00			22:00			22:00		
23:00			23:00			23:00		
24:00			24:00			24:00		
01:00			01:00			01:00		
02:00			02:00			02:00		
03:00			03:00			03:00		
04:00			04:00			04:00		
05:00			05:00			05:00		
06:00			06:00			06:00		
07:00			07:00			07:00		
08:00			08:00			08:00		
09:00			09:00			09:00		
10:00			10:00			10:00		
11:00			11:00			11:00		
Exercise			Exercise			Exercise		
Treatment			Treatment			Treatment		
Sleep quality			Sleep quality			Sleep quality		
Medications			Medications			Medications		
Comments			Comments			Comments		

For each hour of the day,
- Indicate sleep or wake time with an *X* in the appropriate box(es).
- Indicate naps with an *N* in the appropriate box(es).
- Indicate periods of extreme sleepiness with an *S* in the appropriate box(es).

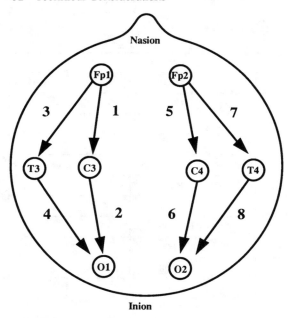

FIGURE 6-15.   *Suggested montage to be used to screen for possible seizure activity during sleep. Use of wide interelectrode distance affords a global view of EEG activity and conserves channels. To more adequately localize epileptogenic activity, a full complement of electrodes should be used. For a more comprehensive review of montages the reader is referred to* Standard EEG Montages *as proposed by American EEG Society Guidelines 1980 No. 7, Grass Instruments.*

APPENDIX 6-2.

Subjective Evaluation of Sleepiness

Stanford Sleepiness Scale[16]

1. Feeling active and vital; alert; wide awake.
2. Functioning at a high level, but not at peak; able to concentrate.
3. Relaxed; awake; not at full alertness; responsive.
4. A little foggy; not at peak; let down.
5. Fogginess; beginning to lose interest in remaining awake; slowed down.
6. Sleepiness; prefer to be lying down; fighting sleep; woozy.
7. Almost in reverie; sleep onset soon; lost struggle to remain awake.

Linear Analog Scale

Ask patient to make a mark on the scale that corresponds to his/her state prior to testing.

Alert   Sleepy

|————————————————————————————————|

APPENDIX 6-3.   Suggested EEG montages for recording sleep-related seizure activity

Suggested Montage for Recording Sleep-Related Seizure Activity for a 12-Channel Study.

1. $Fp_1 = C_3$
2. $C_3 = O_1$
3. $Fp_1 = T_3$
4. $T_3 = O_1$
5. $Fp_2 = C_4$
6. $C_4 = O_2$
7. $Fp_2 = T_4$
8. $T_4 = O_2$
9. EMG – submentalis-mentalis
10. Right outer canthus – left outer canthus
11. Nasal/oral airflow
12. ECG

Suggested Montage for Recording Sleep-Related Seizure Activity for a 21-Channel Study.

1. $Fp_1 = F_3$ 9. $Fp_1 = F_7$
2. $F_3 = C_3$ 10. $F_7 = T_3$
3. $C_3 = P_3$ 11. $T_3 = T_5$
4. $P_3 = O_1$ 12. $T_5 = O_1$
5. $Fp_2 = F_4$ 13. $Fp_2 = F_8$
6. $F_4 = C_4$ 14. $F_8 = T_4$
7. $C_4 = P_4$ 15. $T_4 = T_6$
8. $P_4 = O_2$ 16. $T_6 = O_2$
17. EMG – mentalis - submentalis
18. Right outer canthus / A_1
19. Left outer canthus / A_2
20. Nasal/oral airflow
21. ECG

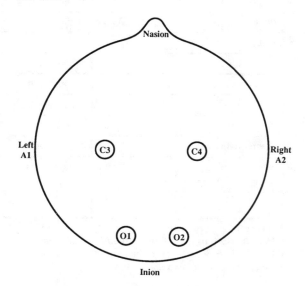

EEG electrode placement for sleep (superior view)

FIGURE 6-16.   *The International 10–20 EEG electrode placement for sleep recordings are shown.*

APPENDIX 6-4.   Measuring the Head for C_3, C_4, O_1, and O_2

Before measuring the head, it is helpful to make an initial mark at the inion, the nasion, and the two preauricular points.

1. Measure the distance from the nasion to inion along the midline through the vertex. Make a preliminary mark at the midpoint (C_z). An electrode will not be placed on this spot, but it will be used as a landmark.
2. Center this point in the transverse plane by marking the halfway point between the left and right preauricular points. The intersection of marks from steps 1 and 2 give the precise location of C_z.
3. Reposition the measuring tape at the midline through C_z and mark the points 10% up from the inion (O_z) and nasion (Fp_z).
4. Reposition the measuring tape in the transverse plane through C_z and mark 10% (T_3) and 30% (C_3) up from the left preauricular point and 10% (T_4) and 30% (C_4) up from the right preauricular point.
5. Position the tape around the head through Fp_z, T_3, O_z, and T_4. Ten percent of this circumference distance is the distance between Fp_1 and Fp_2 and between O_1 and O_2. Mark these four locations on either side of the midline.
6. The second marks for O_1 and O_2 are made by continuing the horizontal mark for O_z. Do this by holding the tape at T_3 and T_4 through O_z, and extend the horizontal mark to intersect the previous O_1 and O_2 marks.
7. To establish the final mark for C_3 place the tape from O_1 to Fp_1 and make a mark at the midpoint of this line. When extended, this mark will intersect the previous C_3 mark. Repeat on the right side for C_4.

REFERENCES

1. Holland JV, Dement WC, Raynall DM. "Polysomnography": A response to a need for improved communication. Presented at the 14th Annual Meeting of the Association for the Psychophysiological Study of Sleep, Jackson Hole, Wyoming, June, 1974.
2. Broughton RJ. Polysomnography: Principles and applications in sleep and arousal disorders. In: Niedermeyer E, Lopes da Silva F, eds. Electroencephalography: Basic Principles, Clinical Applications, and Related Fields. ed 2. Baltimore: Urban & Schwarzenberg, 1987; 687–724.
3. Coleman RM, Pollack C. Weitzman ED. Periodic movements in sleep (nocturnal myoclonus): Relation to sleep-wake disorders. Ann Neurol 1980; 8:416–421.
4. Dement WC, Kleitman N. Cyclic variations of EEG during sleep and their relation to eye movements, body motility and dreaming. Electroencephalogr Clin Neurophysiol 1957;9:673–690.
5. Dement WC, Rechtschaffen A. Narcolepsy: Polygraphic aspects, experimental and theoretical considerations. In: Gastaut H, Lugaresi E, Berti Ceroni G, eds. The Abnormalities of Sleep in Man. Bologna: Aulo Gaggi Editore, 1968; 147–164.
6. Dement WC, Zarcone V, Guilleminault C, et al. Diagnostic sleep recording in narcoleptics and hypesomniacs. Electroencephalogr Clin Nuerophysiol 1973; 35:220.
7. Dement WC. Sleep Apnea Syndromes. New York: Alan R Liss, 1978:357–363.
8. Karacan I. Evaluation of nocturnal penile tumescence and impotence. In: Guilleminault C, ed. Sleeping and Waking Disorders: Indications and Techniques. Menlo Park, Calif: Addison-Wesley, 1982:343–372.
9. Keenan SA. Polysomnography: Technical aspects in adolescents and adults. J Clin Neurophysiol 1992; 9:21–31.
10. McGregor, P, Weitzman ED, Pollack CP. Polysomnographic recording techniques used for diagnosis of sleep disorders in a sleep disorders center. Am J EEG Technol 1978; 18:107–132.
11. Orr WC, Bollinger C, Stahl M. Measurement of gastroesophageal reflux during sleep by esophageal pH monitoring. In: Guilleminault C, ed. Sleeping and Waking Disorders: Indications and Techniques. Menlo Park, Calif: Addison-Wesley, 1982:331–343.
12. Raynal DM. Polygraphic aspects of narcolepsy. In: Guilleminault C, ed. Narcolepsy. New York: Spectrum, 1976: 669–684.
13. Schenk CH, Bundlie SR, Ettinger MG, et al. Chronic behavioral disorders of human REM sleep: A new category of parasomnia. Sleep 1986; 9:293–308.
14. Weitzman ED, Pollack CP, McGregor P. The polysomnographic evaluation of sleep disorders in man. In: Aminoff MJ, ed. Electrodiagnosis in Clinical Neurology. New York: Churchill Livingstone, 1980: 496–524.
15. Hoddes E, Dement WC, Zarcone V. The development and use of the Stanford Sleepiness Scale (SSS). Psychophysiology 1972; 9:150.
16. Hoddes E, Zarcone V, Smythe H, et al. Quantification of sleepiness: A new approach. Psychophysiology 1973; 10:431–436.
17. Carskadon MA. Measuring daytime sleepiness. In: Kryger MH, Roth T, Dement WC, eds. Principles and Practice of Sleep Medicine. Philadelphia: WB Saunders, 1989:684–689.
18. American Thoracic Society. Indications and standards for cardiopulmonary sleep studies. Am Rev Respir Dis 1989; 139: 562.
19. Martin RJ, Block AJ, Cohn MA, et al. Indications and standards for cardiopulmonary sleep studies. Sleep 1985; 8(4):371–379.

20. Cooper R, Osselton JW, Shaw JC. EEG technology, ed 2. London: Butterworths, 1974.

21. Carskadon MA. Basics for polygraphic monitoring of sleep. In: Guilleminault C, ed. Sleeping and Waking Disorders: Indications and Techniques. Menlo Park, Calif: Addison-Wesley, 1982: 1–16.

22. Jasper HH. The ten-twenty electrode system of the International Federation. Electroencephalogr Clin Neurophysiol 1958; 10:371–375.

23. Cross C. Technical tips: Patient specific electrode application techniques. Am J EEG Technol 1992; 32:86–92.

24. Tyner FS, Knott JR, Mayer WB Jr. Fundamentals of EEG Technology. New York: Raven Press, 1983.

25. Keenan Bornstein S. Respiratory monitoring during sleep: Polysomnography. In: Guilleminault C, ed. Sleeping and Waking Disorders: Indications and Techniques. Menlo Park, Calif: Addison-Wesley, 1982: 183–212.

26. Kryger MH. Monitoring respiratory and cardiac function. In: Kryger MH, Roth T, Dement WC, eds. Principles and Practice of Sleep Medicine. Philadelphia: WB Saunders, 1989: 702–716.

7

Electroencephalography, Electromyography and Electrooculography: General Principles and Basic Technology

Thaddeus Walczak
Sudhansu Chokroverty

Traditional sleep studies typically include two channels to monitor eye movement and one channel each for electromyography (EMG) and electroencephalography (EEG). Though two channels probably remain sufficient for monitoring eye movements, we feel that multiple EEG and EMG channels should be recorded during routine nighttime studies. Various central nervous system and metabolic disorders may result in a syndrome that mimics excessive daytime somnolence. Unusual nocturnal spells may be seizures. EEG findings during polysomnography (PSG) may be the first indication of these medical disorders. Furthermore, EEG findings associated with epilepsy may occur only during sleep. Thus, a fairly thorough evaluation of electrocerebral activity is possible during routine PSG, and it may be very useful. It follows that polysomnographers should possess a thorough knowledge of both normal and abnormal EEG patterns. Similarly, variability in a single channel of EMG is often difficult to interpret. Multiple EMG channels help confirm that a decrease in tonic EMG is in fact physiologic. Multiple EMG studies are, of course, essential in suspected cases of restless legs syndrome or REM behavior disorder and in patients who have abnormal movements during sleep.

A complete description of the technical and interpretive issues in EEG, EMG, and electrooculography (EOG) is not possible in a single chapter. The reader is referred to several excellent monographs[1-5] on these subjects. Our discussion starts with basic technical and safety issues and then reviews measurement and interpretation of EOG and EMG. The bulk of the chapter is devoted to normal EEG findings in wakefulness and sleep and to frequently encountered abnormalities. Various artifacts in the PSG that may interfere with the interpretation are mentioned. Our discussion is limited to patients aged 2 months and older. Neonatal waking and sleep EEGs are not discussed. Several useful sources are available for the interested reader.[1,2,4,6]

ELEMENTARY CONCEPTS OF ELECTRICITY

At this point, a review of some elementary concepts of electricity may be useful. Electricity is largely the study of the concentration and flow of charged particles. A fundamental principle of electricity states that like charges repel and unlike charges attract. Thus, if particles of like charge are allowed to move freely, they quickly reach a relatively uniform distribution. The flow of charged particles is called *current* and is usually denoted by I. Various features of biologic systems, such as equilibrium constants of reactions or membrane permeability, often result in a concentration of particles of like charge. This concentration is a store of potential energy that is released when the charged particles are allowed to move and achieve more uniform distribution. *Voltage* (V) measures how much energy is released when a given amount of charge is allowed to move as current flow. Voltage, also known as potential difference, is always measured between two points. Because the concentration of charge may differ at any two points, the potential energy contained in a given concentration of charge can be measured only by relating it to the concentration of charge elsewhere. In the real world, movement of charge experiences *resistance* (R) as it passes through a conducting medium. The resistance is measured in ohms (Ω). Current, voltage, and resistance are related by Ohm's law, I = V/R. The law makes intuitive sense: The higher the voltage between two points, the greater the flow of charge one would expect. The greater the resistance to the movement of charge, the less flow of charge one would expect.

Concentrations of charges of different polarity often are separated by a poorly conducting medium. This situation can be modeled by an electrical device known as a capacitor. Capacitors can be thought of as two conducting plates separated by insulation. The ability of the capacitor to store charge is measured by the capacitance, which is the amount of charge the device can store for a given voltage. When a capacitor is attached to a source of constant voltage, such as a battery, positive charges flow from the positive pole of the battery to one plate and negative charges flow from the negative pole of the battery to the other plate. Charges continue flowing until the mutual repulsion of the accumulated charges on each plate equals the potential difference of the battery. At this point, current flow ceases.

The situation is different when the source of voltage varies with a predictable frequency. Voltages generated by the brain and recorded by the EEG do not stay constant but vary continuously within certain limits. In a circuit with such a voltage source and a capacitor it can be shown that at any time the current flow equals the capacitance multiplied by the change in voltage with respect to time.* Thus, the capacitor influences and resists the flow of current in a circuit with a varying voltage. The resistance to current flow exerted by the capacitor is measured by the capacitative reactance (X_c). It is clear that the concept of resistance must be expanded to include capacitative reactance in circuits with a voltage source that varies. Impedance (Z) is a measure of resistance that includes reactive capacitance and is, therefore, appropriate in circuits with varying voltages. In these situations, Ohm's law takes the form $I = V/Z$. Because intracerebral voltages vary over time, impedance is the proper measure of how well electrodes and gel transmit brain activity.

PHYSIOLOGIC BASIS OF ELECTROENCEPHALOGRAPHY

An EEG record is essentially a measure of the changes of electrocerebral voltages over a period of time. In order to interpret an EEG, it is important to understand the source of the voltages recorded at the scalp and how these voltages are organized into normal cerebral rhythms.

---

*Capacitance (c) is defined as the amount of charge (Q) the capacitor can store for a given voltage (V), or Q/V. Assuming that C is constant, and differentiating with respect to time (t), we find that $dC/dT = 0 = -(Q/V^2)(dV/dT) + (1/V)(dQ/dT)$. Rearranging, $dQ/dT = (Q/V)(dV/dT)$. Current flow or $I = dQ/dt$. Hence $I = C(dV/dt)$.

Electrocerebral activity measured by EEG does not appear to be caused by individual or summed action potentials. Action potentials are too short (usually less than 1 msec) and synchronized bursts of action potentials have too limited a distribution to account for the rhythms seen in normal EEG. Excitatory and inhibitory postsynaptic potentials, on the other hand, last much longer (15 to 200 msec or more). These synaptic potentials induce more extensive voltage changes in extracellular space. Scalp recorded EEG activity results from extracellular current flow induced by summated excitatory or inhibitory postsynaptic potentials.

Figure 7-1 illustrates, in simplified fashion, how synaptic potentials induce voltage changes recorded at the scalp. An excitatory input on a deep dendrite causes (positively charged) ions to flow into the pyramidal neuron, resulting in a lack of positive charges, or negative charge, outside the neuron. Everywhere else, including the superficial dendrite, positive ions flow out of the cell into the extracellular space to complete the current loop. This results in relative "positivity" in the superficial extracellular space. Because the superficial dendrite and surrounding extracellular space are closer to the scalp electrode, a positive deflection is recorded. The separation of superficial positive and deep negative charges allows one to view the pyramidal neuron as a dipole. This permits a more complete analysis of how synaptic potentials result in scalp EEG changes.[7,8]

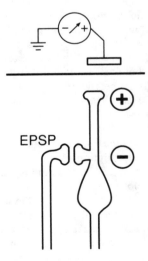

FIGURE 7-1.   *Scalp EEG voltage recordings resulting from an excitatory input on a deep synapse (see text). (Modified from Kandel ER, Schwartz JH, eds. Principles of Neural Science, ed 2. Amsterdam: Elsevier, 1985;642.)*

EEG voltage recordings are rhythmic (i.e. they are regularly recurring waveforms of similar shape and duration). It is important to understand how voltage changes induced by individual neurons are organized into the widely distributed rhythms recorded with EEG. The dominant theory of EEG rhythmicity advanced by Anderson and Andersson[9] is based on studies of barbiturate-induced spindle activity. These investigators recorded synchronous rhythmic spindles from the cerebral cortex and thalamus. Neither removal of cerebral cortex nor transection of the brain stem below the thalamus eliminated thalamic spindles, but ablation of the entire thalamus abolished spindle activity. These findings led to the proposal that rhythmic oscillations of thalamic neurons induce synchronous synaptic excitatory or inhibitory potentials over broad areas of cortex, and thus the rhythmic voltage changes recorded with scalp EEG. Diffuse thalamocortical neuronal projections were known to exist and could mediate this thalamic influence. This model was expanded to explain most EEG rhythmic activity.

Recent authors have emphasized that barbiturate-induced spindles differ significantly from other cerebral rhythms.[10] The role of the thalamus in synchronizing barbiturate spindle activity over broad areas of cortex may not be relevant to other EEG rhythms. Neurons in other brain structures, including inferior olive, hippocampus, and temporal neocortex, exhibit oscillatory behavior and may play a role in generating EEG rhythms.[11] Though widespread subcortical influences probably play an important role in organizing EEG rhythms it is premature to conclude that all EEG rhythms are induced by oscillations of thalamic neurons.

Cerebral activity recorded at the scalp has approximately one-tenth the voltage of activity simultaneously recorded at the cortical surface. This attenuation is due in large part to the cerebrospinal fluid, dura, and skull overlying the cortical surface. The area and location of the cortex generating the activity also play a role.

COMPONENTS OF THE POLYGRAPHIC CIRCUIT

Voltages and current flows generated by cortex, eyes, and heart during polysomnographic studies are exceedingly small. The function of the polygraph is to transform these tiny voltages into an interpretable record. The major components necessary to accomplish this are illustrated in Figure 7-2. Each component is briefly considered.

Electrodes and conducting gel transmit biologic voltages from skin or muscle to the polygraphic

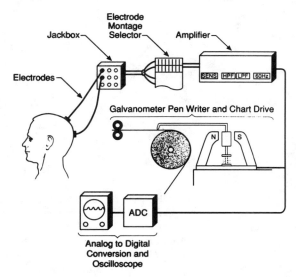

FIGURE 7-2. *Components of the polygraphic circuit.*

circuit. Various types of electrodes have been designed.[3,12] Disk electrodes are preferred for recording EEG, EOG, ECG, and EMG. These are typically made of chlorided silver or noble metals such as gold or platinum. Needle electrodes generally are not recommended.

The critical component of the conducting gel is an electrolyte, usually sodium chloride, that easily dissociates into its ionic components. The anions and cations establish a layer of negative and positive charges between the scalp and recording electrode. This charged double layer allows transmission of scalp voltage changes to the electrode and the rest of the polygraphic circuit.

The electrode-electrolyte interface is the most critical link in the polygraphic circuit. Most artifact originates here; consequently, careful technique in electrode application largely determines the quality of the recording. The impedance in any electrode pair should not exceed 10 kΩ. High impedance can decrease the amount of signal the electrode presents to the amplifier. Methods to achieve low impedance are described in Chapter 6. Additionally, the impedance in the two electrode inputs into the amplifier should not differ by more than 10 kΩ. Higher values degrade the ability of a differential amplifier to eliminate environmental noise and increase artifact (see later). Impedance varies with the composition and surface area of the electrode and with the surface area of the conducting jelly beneath the electrode. Thus, these factors should be kept constant in an electrode pair attached to the same amplifier. For example, a disk electrode and needle electrode have different surface

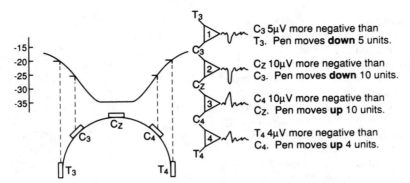

FIGURE 7-3.   *Scalp voltage distribution of a vertex wave. A plot of hypothetical absolute voltages at various electrode positions is shown on the left. Resulting EEG tracing is shown on the right with explanation. A transverse bipolar chain is utilized with amplifiers connected from left to right. The same electrode is connected to input 2 of an amplifier and input 1 of the next amplifier in the chain (see text for details).*

areas and conducting gel is not used with needle electrodes. Therefore, impedances of the two electrodes will be significantly different. If the two electrodes are attached to the same amplifier, environmental artifact is likely to contaminate the recording.

Electrodes are attached to electrode wires, which conduct the EEG signal to the electrode box or jackbox. The electrode wires terminate in a pin, which is then plugged into a receptacle in the electrode box known as a jack. The jacks are usually numbered or identified according to the 10-20 electrode system. Wires from each of the jacks run together in a shielded conductor cable to the polygraph. There, wires from each of the jacks are connected to a specific point on a multiple contact switch known as the *electrode selector*. The selector contains rows of switches, arranged in pairs corresponding to the two inputs of an amplifier. Depressing or otherwise activating the switches allows the technician to select which two electrodes contribute signal to each amplifier.

The amplifiers used in polygraphic recording have several important features. Differential amplifiers are usually used. These amplify the difference in voltage between the two amplifier inputs. Figure 7-3 provides an illustration. Let us assume that T_3 is connected to input 1 of an amplifier and C_3 is connected to input 2 of the same amplifier. The amplifier determines the difference between the two inputs ($5\mu V$) and the galvanometer pen registers a deflection of 5 units. The actual amount of the deflection in millimeters depends on the sensitivity used (see later). The fact that the differential amplifier amplifies the difference between electrode inputs, rather than the absolute voltage at any electrode, is a useful feature, because environmental noise, which is likely to be the same at the two electrodes is "sub-

tracted out" and so does not contaminate the recording. The common mode rejection ratio (CMRR) expresses the ability of the amplifier to suppress a signal, such as noise, that is present simultaneously at both electrodes. This ratio should exceed 1000:1; most contemporary polygraphic amplifiers have values exceeding 10,000:1.

A differential amplifier multiplies the small difference in cerebral voltages by a constant, referred to as *gain*. This multiplication is necessary because the recording galvanometer pen requires voltages much higher than those generated by the brain to generate an EEG record. Amplifiers can faithfully amplify input voltages only within a certain range, known as the *dynamic range*. Input voltages below the lower limit of the dynamic range are lost in noise; voltages above the upper limit result in distorted EEG output. Flexible control of amplification within the dynamic range is achieved by manipulating the sensitivity switch. The sensitivity switch is connected to a series of voltage dividers that attenuate the amplified cerebral voltages enough for the EEG record to be interpretable. Sensitivity is defined as the amount of voltage needed to produce a set deflection of the pen. The usual units are microvolts per millimeter or millivolts per centimeter. One of the technologist's most important tasks is to maintain sensitivity settings low enough for the input voltage to result in a pen deflection of sufficient amplitude to be detectable. However, the sensitivity cannot be so low that the amplitude of pen deflection interferes with or "blocks" pen movements in adjacent channels. Because the voltage of electrocerebral activity varies during the study, sensitivity settings may need to be adjusted to maintain an appropriate amplitude of recorded EEG activity. Because amplitude of various waveforms is an important consideration in scoring sleep stages, these adjustments must be carefully documented. Initial recommended sensitivity settings for the biologic signals routinely encountered in PSG are summarized in the preceding chapter.

Whereas the sensitivity settings determine the amplitude of pen deflection, the polarity of the cerebral activity determines its direction. The differential amplifier compares polarity at the two electrodes. The resulting pen deflection is determined according to the polarity convention. If input 1 is negative relative to input 2, the pen moves up. If input 1 is positive relative to input 2, the pen moves down. If input 2 is negative relative to input 1 the pen moves down. If input 2 is positive relative to input 1 the pen moves up. It follows that *phase reversals* of EEG waveforms can be used to roughly localize the scalp distribution of those waveforms. The scalp voltage distribution of a typical vertex wave serves to illustrate (see Figure 7-3). Here we see hypothetical absolute voltages at several electrode positions. The electrodes are linked in serial pairs from left to right. When C_3 is connected to input 1 and C_z is connected to input 2 in amplifier 2, the amplifier determines that the difference between the two electrodes is 10 μV. Input 2 is more negative than input 1. Thus the galvanometer pen recording from this amplifier registers a downward deflection of 10 units. In amplifier 3, C_z is connected to input 1 and C_4 to input 2. The amplifier determines that the difference in voltages is also 10 μV, but input 1 is now more negative than input 2. Consequently, the galvanometer pen recording from this amplifier registers an upward deflection of 10 units. The phase reversal in the adjacent channels marks the electrode where the vertex wave is most negative. This is the electrode shared by both amplifiers, namely C_z. Because most cerebral activ-

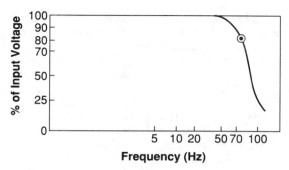

FIGURE 7-5. *Frequency-response curve of a hypothetical low-pass filter with a cutoff frequency of 70 Hz and a roll-off of − 6 dB per octave. (Modified from Tyner F, Knott J, Mayer W Jr. Fundamentals of EEG Technology, vol 1. New York: Raven Press, 1983.)*

ity is negative at the scalp, phase reversals with the pen deflections pointing toward each other, as in Figure 7-3, are most common. Positive cerebral activity would result in a phase reversal with the pen deflections pointing away from each other at the electrode that was most positive. Note that localization by phase reversal is accurate only when electrodes spaced at relatively short distances are serially linked in adjacent amplifiers. This is known as a bipolar montage.

After voltages at the two inputs are subtracted and amplified, the result is passed through a series of filters. The goal of filtering is to attenuate voltages occurring at undesirable frequencies (e.g., environmental noise) without disturbing frequencies found in the biologic signal of interest. A frequency-response curve measures the ability of a filter to attenuate various frequencies. Frequency-response curves for 2 types of filter included in most polygraphs are presented in Figures 7-4 and 7-5. A high-pass filter (also known as a low-frequency filter), allows higher-frequency activity to pass unchanged while it progressively attenuates lower frequencies (Figure 7-4). A low-pass filter (also known as a high-frequency filter), allows lower frequencies to pass unchanged while it progressively attenuates higher frequencies (Figure 7-5). Both filters are defined by cutoff frequency and roll-off. The filter with a given cutoff frequency will attenuate voltage of that frequency by 20%* (e.g., the high-pass filter in Figure 7-4 has a cutoff frequency of 1 Hz, so a 100-μV 1-Hz wave passed through this filter will have an amplitude of 80-μV). Attenuation of frequencies above the

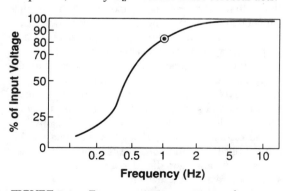

FIGURE 7-4. *Frequency-response curve of a hypothetical high-pass filter with a cutoff frequency of 71 Hz and a roll-off of − 6 dB per octave. (Modified with permission from Tyner F, Kott J, Mayer W Jr. Fundamentals of EEG Technology, vol 1. New York: Raven Press, 1983.)*

---

*In electrophysiology, a widely used convention dictates that voltage at the cutoff frequency is attenuated at 20%. In electrical engineering, voltage at the cutoff frequency is attenuated by approximately 30%.

cutoff frequency is more or less linear for the high-pass filter. Attenuation of frequencies below the cut-off frequency is progressively more severe as lower frequencies are encountered. This progressively more severe attenuation is defined by the filter's roll-off. Roll-off for most EEG filters is -6 dB per octave. For the high-pass filter this means that the voltage of activity is decreased by half for every halving of the frequency.

The 60-Hz, or notch, filter is also a feature of most polygraphic amplifiers.* This filter is designed to attenuate mains frequency very harshly while attenuating activity of surrounding frequencies less.[3] Because electrical mains are ubiquitous, 60-Hz artifact may easily contaminate an EEG recording. The notch filter should be used sparingly, for at least two reasons. First, some biologic signals of interest to the polysomnographer have waveforms with important components in the range of 40 to 80 Hz. Examples include myogenic activity and epileptiform spikes, both of which may be significantly attenuated by the notch filter. For example, use of the notch filter in the chin EMG channel may create a false impression that tonic EMG has significantly decreased. Second, the capability of the differential amplifier to reject common signals (see earlier) should be sufficient to suppress 60-Hz artifact in most cases. Thus, the appearance of 60 Hz usually signals a problem somewhere in the polygraphic circuit that needs to be resolved. Most often the culprit is high impedance at the electrode-scalp interface. Less frequently defects in the amplifier or grounding of the polygraph are responsible. In these cases addressing the cause of the 60 Hz, rather than using the notch filter, is the appropriate course. There are circumstances in which a nearby source of 60 Hz (e.g., a critical piece of medical equipment that cannot be disconnected) renders the EEG uninterpretable. Use of the 60-Hz filter may be justified in these circumstances but must be clearly documented.

A writer unit transforms the amplified and filtered signal into a written record. The writer unit consists of an oscillograph and chart drive. A galvanometer pen unit is a widely used oscillograph (Figure 7-6). A specially designed coil of wire and a pen stylus are mounted on a rod. The coil of wire is placed between the two poles of a permanent magnet. Current flow from the amplifier enters the coil and induces a magnetic field. The induced magnetic field interacts with the field of the permanent magnet, resulting in a deflection of the pen stylus on the paper. The amount of deflection is proportional to the magnetic field, which is proportional to the current from the amplifier, which in turn is proportional

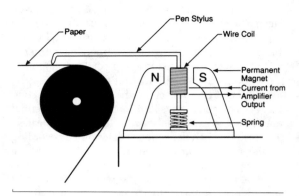

FIGURE 7-6. *Hypothetical galvanometer pen writer unit (not to scale). (Modified from Tyner F, Knott J, Mayer W Jr. Fundamentals of EEG Technology, vol 1. New York: Raven Press, 1983.*

to the biologic signal. A spring attached to the rod returns the pen stylus to baseline after the current responsible for the deflection has ceased. This spring, together with the friction of the pen stylus against the paper and the inertia of the galvanometer, are collectively known as *damping* and resist the pen movement. Very rapid signal changes (high-frequency signal) require very rapid galvanometer movement which disproportionately increases the amount of energy necessary to overcome damping. Because more energy is required to write out high-frequency signals, the galvanometer pen unit, in effect, acts as a high-frequency filter. Galvanometer pen writer units usually do not faithfully reproduce signals with frequencies higher than 80 to 90 Hz.

The chart drive pulls the paper below the pens at a constant speed to provide a continuous record of pen deflections (voltage changes) over time. Paper speeds slower than 10 mm/sec save paper but cannot be recommended because resolution of faster waveforms necessary for scoring sleep stages is impossible. When suspicious waveforms, such as epileptiform spikes, are noted, increasing paper speed to 30 mm/sec can aid interpretation. Many currently available polygraphic systems avoid the paper writeout by digitizing amplifier output and storing it on various nonpaper media. These signals can be processed and subsequently displayed on an oscilloscope. Selected portions can be printed out using traditional writer units. The issues that arise in analog-to-digital conversion of biologic signals are reviewed elsewhere.[13]

ELECTRICAL SAFETY

Contemporary polygraphic and EEG studies are very safe procedures. Nonetheless, the possibility of electrical injury exists whenever a patient is connected

---

*In Europe, mains frequency is 50 Hz, so a 50-Hz notch filter is widely available.

to an electrical apparatus. Thus, technicians performing studies and physicians supervising sleep laboratories must understand the basic principles of electrical safety.

Electrical injury is caused by excessive current flow through biologic tissue. Electrical injury may cause burns, seizures, and irreversible damage to the CNS. When excessive current flows through the heart, ventricular arrythmias, including ventricular fibrillation, may occur. The amount of current necessary to induce ventricular fibrillation depends on skin impedance, the mass of tissue the current must traverse before reaching the heart, the health of the heart, and the general health of the patient, among other factors. In a healthy adult with dry, intact skin, 100 to 300 mA delivered at 60 Hz induces fibrillation (so-called macroshock).[3] Smaller amounts of current (microshock) induce fibrillation in electrically susceptible patients. These include patients with wet skin or wounds as well as patients with pacemaker electrodes inserted in the ventricular myocardium. Dry, intact skin offers high impedance to current flow, as technicians well appreciate. Moisture on or extensive interruption of the skin significantly reduces this impedance, allowing current to flow toward the heart more readily. Pacemaker wires allow the current to flow directly into the vulnerable myocardium rather than through the high impedance offered by the chest wall and pleural cavities. When 60-Hz current is applied directly to the heart, intensities as low as 100 μA result in fibrillation, though higher values are necessary in most cases.[14–16]

Current flow requires a source of current and the formation of a complete circuit. Thus, electrical safety has two goals: (1) the polygraph must not become a source of excessive current and (2) the polygraph and patient (or technician) must not form a complete circuit through which excessive current may flow and cause electrical injury. Proper maintenance, proper grounding, and use of isolation devices accomplish these goals.

The power unit of the polygraph is a potential source of excessive current. A fault in the power unit may result in a short circuit, which would allow current (a *fault current*) to flow to the polygraph chassis (Figure 7-7A). If the machine ground was disabled and the patient was touching a pipe or some other conducting substance, current would flow through the electrodes and the patient to the pipe, possibly causing electrical injury. Current would also flow through a technician touching the polygraph and a conducting substance. To guard against this possibility, the chassis of the polygraph is connected to the building ground through a three-pronged outlet (Figure 7-7B). Should a current-bearing element contact the chassis, the current

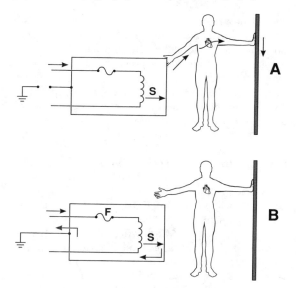

FIGURE 7-7. (A) *Technician touches polygraph chassis and water pipe. Polygraph chassis is ungrounded because of interruption in ground wire. A short circuit (S) in the power supply unit allows current to flow to chassis, through technician's heart, to water pipe. Arrows trace path of current flow. (B) Short circuit in polygraph with an intact chassis ground. A short circuit (S) in the power supply allows current to flow to chassis. The low-resistance chassis ground allows unimpeded flow of current to building ground. The current surge blows a fuse (F), quickly stopping further current flow. Bystanders are safe unless they touch the chassis at the moment of the short circuit.*

would be shunted through machine ground to the building ground because this path has the least resistance. The sudden high current flow would blow a fuse in the power unit or open a circuit breaker, stopping further current flow. A brief period is necessary for the excessive current to blow the fuse, and if the patient were touching a conducting substance during this period current would still flow through the patient, though the duration of the current flow would be briefer and the danger to the patient less.

It follows that the connection between the polygraph and building ground must not be compromised. Electrical outlets powering appliances connected to patients must have documented secure connections to building ground. Technicians should ensure good contact between the ground pin of the power cord and the outlet. Three-prong–to–two-prong adapters do not provide secure contact with building ground and must not be used. Resistance of the ground circuit in the polygraph should be checked periodically to detect interruptions. Fuses should never be defeated (i.e. short-circuited). Repeatedly blown fuses may indicate fault currents and potential danger to technician and patient. Finally, regular maintenance may prevent potentially dangerous fault currents.

Even in the absence of a fault, the complicated circuitry of the polygraph generates lower-intensity currents known as *leakage currents. Stray capacitance* is a major source of leakage current. Any circuit whose current flow is insulated from other conducting substances can be viewed as a capacitor: the current-carrying circuit can be considered one plate of a capacitor, the insulation and surrounding space can be considered the dielectric and the other conducting substances the other plate of the capacitor. Alternating current (AC) flowing through any insulated circuit, therefore, generates currents in other conducting substances in the area. One pertinent example is the power cord of the polygraph. AC current flow in the insulated "hot" wire of the power cord induces a smaller amount of current flow in the neutral and ground wires. Even though leakage currents are much smaller than fault currents, they can cause injury in electrically susceptible patients. Acceptable limits for leakage currents have been defined.[3,17] Adequate grounding protects both patient and technician in this circumstance as well. The leakage current is shunted to the low-resistance machine ground and then to building ground. Extension cords increase stray capacitance and thus leakage currents and should never be used during PSG. Isolation jackboxes, which limit the amount of possible current flow through electrodes, offer additional protection for electrically susceptible patients.

Current flow can also occur when machinery attached to the patient draws power from different outlets or when multiple grounds are attached to the patient. The voltage of the ground contact at different outlets may be quite different, causing current flow. Multiple grounds can result in a *ground loop*, which can act as a secondary coil of a transformer and generate current flow. A ground loop also acts as an antenna that can pick up environmental electromagnetic "noise" and increase artifact. These potentially dangerous situations can be avoided by plugging in all machinery attached to the patient to the same outlet cluster and using only one patient ground.

ELECTROOCULOGRAPHY
(See also Chapter 6)

The electrical field generated by the eye approximates a simple dipole (Figure 7-8A) with a posterior negativity centered at the retina and a relative positivity probably centered at the cornea. Eye movements change the orientation of this dipole relative to the skull. Polygraphic recording from strategically placed electrodes can detect these changes and can, therefore, be used to monitor eye movements. The standard sleep scoring manual[18] recommends that an electrooculogram utilize at least two channels (Figure 7-8B). One electrode is placed 1 cm superior and lateral to the outer canthus of one eye. This electrode is input 1 to an amplifier; input 2 to this amplifier is an electrode attached to one ear or mastoid. Another electrode is placed 1 cm inferior and lateral to the outer canthus of the other eye. This electrode forms input 1 to a second amplifier; input 2 to this amplifier is attached to the same ear as input 2 of the first amplifier. This placement scheme

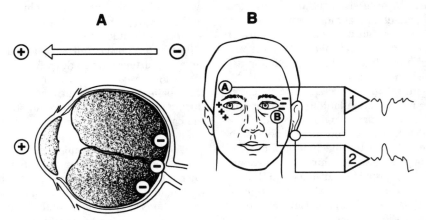

A   **B**

FIGURE 7-8.   (A) *The voltage field generated by the eye can be represented by a simple dipole, the cornea being positive and the retina negative.* (B) *Use of two polygraphic channels to detect conjugate eye movements according to the scheme suggested in the sleep scoring manual.*[18] *Eye movements result in out-of-phase potentials in the two channels.*

detects conjugate horizontal and vertical eye movements. For example, when the eyes look to the right (see Figure 7-8B), the cornea of the right eye approaches electrode A and electrode A becomes positive relative to the inactive ear. According to the polarity convention, amplifier 1 registers a downward deflection. Simultaneously, the retina of the left eye approaches electrode B. Consequently, electrode B becomes negative relative to the inactive ear and amplifier 2 registers an upward deflection. The out-of-phase deflections in the two adjacent channels indicate that a conjugate eye movement has occurred. Similarly, an upward eye movement results in a downward deflection in amplifier 1 and an upward deflection in amplifier 2. Eye blinks produce an identical pattern, because eye closure results in upward rotation of the eyeball (Bell's phenomenon).

Some laboratories attach electrodes to both ears and refer the periocular electrodes to the contralateral ear (e.g., right upper canthus to left ear and left lower canthus to right ear). This minor change has several advantages. The longer interelectrode distances increase the amplitude of the deflections. The amplitude of the deflections generated by movement of each eye is more likely to be equal because the interelectrode distances are equal. Finally, if one of the ear electrodes comes off during the study, the technician can refer both periocular electrodes to the remaining ear electrode and avoid waking the patient. Though these montages detect both horizontal and vertical eye movements, they cannot distinguish between them, but that can be easily accomplished by recording inputs from supraorbital and infraorbital electrodes with a third amplifier.[3,12]

Several varieties of eye movements are recorded during routine PSG. While the patient is awake, saccadic eye movements, as well as eye blinks, are noted. Eye blinks produce the same EOG pattern as vertical eye movement. One of the first signs of drowsiness is cessation of any eye movements. Somewhat "deeper" in drowsiness, slow eye movements are seen. These usually have a frequency of less than 0.5 Hz,[19] are most consistently recorded in the horizontal axis, gradually increase in amplitude as background alpha activity drops out, and usually disappear in stage 2 sleep. Rapid eye movements (REMs), occur during REM sleep. Movements along the horizontal axis are the most common, though oblique and vertical movements occur as well. REMs typically occur in bursts and may be preceded on the EEG by characteristic "sawtooth" waves. There is no widely accepted definition of REMs that would serve to distinguish them from slow eye movements. Parameters useful for computerized quantification of REMs have been reported,[20] but these are not directly applicable to visual scoring. Radtke[21] has suggested a reasonable clinically applicable definition for REMs, namely that the duration of the initial pen deflection is less than 200 msec and the duration of the entire waveform less than 1 second.

In a recent study of drowsiness in normal subjects, Santamaria and Chiappa[19] recorded eye movements with a sensitive motion transducer attached over the globe as well as with the traditional EOG. They found two types of eye movements not previously reported. What were named *small, fast, irregular eye movements* were observed in 60% of normal subjects in the early stage of drowsiness, before slow eye movements. They did not appear in the routine EOG channels. What were called *small, fast, rhythmic eye movements* were found in 30% of normal subjects, usually associated with the traditional slow eye movements. These occasionally appeared in the routine EOG channels, though usually with very low amplitude. If confirmed, these findings could be useful for determining early stages of drowsiness.

ELECTROMYOGRAPHIC RECORDINGS IN SLEEP DISORDERS

EMG activities are important physiologic characteristics that need to be recorded for diagnosis and classification of a variety of sleep disorders. EMG represents electrical activities of muscle fibers resulting from depolarization of the muscles following transmission of nerve impulses along the nerves and neuromuscular junctions.[5] EMG could represent tonic, phasic, and rhythmic activity. Physiologically, there is a fundamental tone in the muscles, at least throughout the period of wakefulness and non-REM (NREM) sleep, but it is markedly diminished or absent in antigravity muscles during REM sleep. Maintenance of muscle tone is a complex physiologic phenomenon that depends on suprasegmental, segmental, and peripheral afferent mechanisms.[22] Tone, therefore, may be influenced by a variety of extrinsic and intrinsic stimuli. Following a nerve impulse, the resting muscle membrane potential is altered, and when it reaches a threshold level, depolarization of the muscle results from a change in the external and internal ionic balance and muscle calcium channel alterations.[5] The threshold depolarization causes an action potential to develop in the muscle. A compound muscle action potential represents summation of the action currents in many muscle fibers. Surface EMG recordings record many muscle fibers, bundles, and groups; needle EMGs record about 15 to 20 muscle fibers near the needle tip.[5] Phasic EMG represents activities related to some physiologic alterations, either spontaneous or induced. Examples of phasic EMGs are EMG activities phasically related to inspiratory bursts and myoclonic muscle bursts that occur spontaneously or in response to some stimuli. If there are rhythmic activities, for example tremor, EMG bursts have a rhythm. In sleep disorders medicine the tonic and phasic EMG bursts are usually the most important ones, unless, as sometimes happens, rhythmic EMG bursts are noted in certain sleep disorders, such as patients with restless legs syndrome (see Chapter 19).

Method of Recording

EMG recordings from submental muscles using surface electrodes are routinely performed in PSG and multiple sleep latency tests. Electrodes placed in this area record mostly the activities of the mylohyoid and the anterior belly of the digastric muscles. The electrodes also record some activities from the genioglossus and hyoglossus muscles by volume conduction. This recording is important for identifying the presence or absence of muscle tone for sleep stage scoring.

In a patient suspected of restless legs syndrome, tibialis anterior muscles must be recorded, preferably bilaterally, because sometimes the periodic movements of legs alternate between the two legs. Ideally, the recording should also include 1 or 2 EMG channels from the upper limb muscles, as occasionally movements are noted in the upper limbs.

For understanding the pathophysiology of sleep apnea it is important to record the respiratory muscle activities (see also Chapter 9). These should include not only the intercostal muscles but also the diaphragmatic muscle, a variety of upper airway muscles, and the facial muscles. The true diaphragmatic activities characteristically are recorded by intraesophageal bipolar electrodes, which can also quantitate the diaphragmatic EMG activity.[23-25] This technique as well as esophageal pressure recording by inserting an esophageal balloon transnasally (which provides respiratory muscle mechanical activity) are invasive, uncomfortable, and not generally used at present. Noninvasive technique—placing surface electrodes to the right or left of the umbilicus or over the anterior costal margin—may also pick up diaphragmatic activity, though admixture of intercostal muscle activity makes this noninvasive technique unreliable for quantitative assessment of diaphragmatic EMG.[26] The intercostal EMG recorded from the seventh to the ninth intercostal space[27] with active electrodes on the anterior axillary line and the reference electrodes on the midaxillary line may record some diaphragmatic muscle activity in addition to the intercostal activity. An important muscle for recording respiratory activity is the alae nasi muscle.[27] It has been shown that this picks up

not only inspiratory activity but also some expiratory activity. Many upper airway muscles are accessory muscles of respiration. All the facial muscles, including the masseter muscles, show inspiratory bursts during the recordings.[27] To show the decrease of tone in the genioglossus and other oropharyngeal and laryngeal muscles it is important to record EMGs from them. For many of these muscles recordings can be made in a noninvasive manner by means of surface electrodes,[27] but for some, for example laryngeal muscle, an invasive technique that uses fine wire electrodes is required. To record the muscle activity from an individual muscle only, wire electrodes must be inserted into that particular muscle only.

Clinical Significance of EMG Recording

EMG shows decreasing tone from wakefulness through stages I to IV of NREM sleep. In REM sleep the EMG tone is markedly diminished or absent. It is important to use the appropriate filters and very high gain at the beginning of the recording, to appreciate the decreasing muscle tone during REM sleep. In certain pathologic conditions (e.g., REM behavior disorder) the EMG tone may persist or phasic muscle bursts may be seen repeatedly during REM sleep. This may also happen in patients being treated for narcolepsy, and may represent a medication side effect.

For the diagnosis of periodic limb movements of sleep, which are seen in most of the cases of restless legs syndrome, in a variety of other sleep disorders, and even in normal persons, particularly older ones, EMG recordings of the tibialis anterior muscles are essential. Characteristics of the EMG bursts in periodic limb movements of sleep are described in Chapter 19. In upper airway obstructive apnea, the EMG of the upper airway muscles shows marked decrease of tone during the apneic episodes while the diaphragmatic and intercostal muscle activity persists.[27] During REM sleep, however, intercostal and even diaphragmatic EMGs show marked diminution of the tonic activity.[28]

In certain neurodegenerative diseases such as the Shy-Drager syndrome laryngeal EMG recording may be important to detect vocal cord paralysis causing upper airway obstructive apnea.[29]

For certain movement disorders (for example, paroxysmal nocturnal dystonia), it is important to record multiple muscle EMGs during polysomnographic recordings at night, to document dystonic muscle activities.

Multiple muscle EMG recordings are also important in patients with restless legs syndrome because of the presence of a variety of EMG activity in these patients (e.g., periodic limb movements of sleep, myoclonic bursts both during wakefulness and sleep, a mixture of myoclonic and dystonic EMG bursts during wakefulness, and occasionally during sleep (see Chapter 19).

THE ELECTROENCEPHALOGRAPH

EEG is recorded in sleep studies mostly to assist scoring of sleep stages. Obviously, EEG can provide other useful information as well. Routine diagnostic EEGs usually sample at most one hour of electrocerebral activity. The polysomnograph records EEG activity for much longer periods, thus increasing the likelihood that abnormalities will be recorded. Consequently, the polysomnographer must be familiar with the broad range of normal EEG findings and the abnormalities encountered in various age groups. The following discussion is, at best, an incomplete review of some of the major patterns encountered in routine EEG.

Normal Waking Rhythms

Individual waves recorded on the EEG can be characterized by their frequency (i.e., how many of that wave would be required to occupy a given period of time, typically 1 sec). Frequency of EEG activity has been divided into four bands assigned the Greek letters beta, alpha, theta, and delta. Scoring of sleep is based largely on the amplitude and frequency of EEG waves. However, human electrocerebral activity is better characterized by the broader concept of EEG *rhythms*. EEG rhythms can be defined as sustained periods of electrocerebral activity of similar frequency that have stereotyped distribution, reactivity, symmetry, and synchrony and are associated with specific physiologic states. These rhythms have also been assigned Greek letters that correspond, in part, to letters assigned to frequency.

Several rhythms characterize the awake adult EEG. The most obvious is the *alpha rhythm* (see Figure 2-1). Alpha rhythm frequency varies between 8 and 13 Hz. This rhythm is distributed over the parietooccipital regions bilaterally. A normal alpha rhythm is synchronous and symmetric over the two hemispheres. Frequency of the rhythm should not vary by more than 1 Hz, and amplitude should not vary by more than 50% between the two hemispheres. The alpha rhythm is best seen during quiet alertness with eyes closed. Various maneuvers cause alpha to react or decrease in amplitude. The most effective is eye opening, but any sort of intense stimulation produces some degree of amplitude attenuation. As many as 10% of normal adults show no alpha rhythm during quiet wakefulness. The low-voltage EEG in these subjects is characterized by

poorly sustained beta and theta frequencies with amplitudes between 10 and 20 μV. Occasionally hyperventilation elicits a typical alpha rhythm in such patients. Low-voltage EEGs have not been recorded in normal subjects younger than 10 years.

Beta rhythms are present in virtually all adults, though they are usually less striking than alpha rhythms. Frequency of the beta rhythm is, by definition, above 13 Hz but typically is between 18 and 25 Hz. There are probably at least two beta rhythms, one distributed over the frontal and central regions and the other more diffusely distributed. Beta rhythms are present during wakefulness and drowsiness. They may appear more persistent during drowsiness, drop out during deeper sleep, and reappear during REM. Amplitude over the two hemispheres should not vary by more than 50%. Amplitude of beta activity is less than 20 μV in 98% of normal drug-free subjects. A persistent beta rhythm with higher amplitude suggests use of sedative-hypnotic medications, as most such medications increase the amplitude of beta activity.

Mu rhythms are most common in young adults. This rhythm consists of brief trains of 7 to 11-Hz waves over the central regions, often with phase reversals over C_3 or C_4. The waves have a wicket or arciform shape (Figure 7-9). Mu may occur synchronously or independently over the two hemispheres.

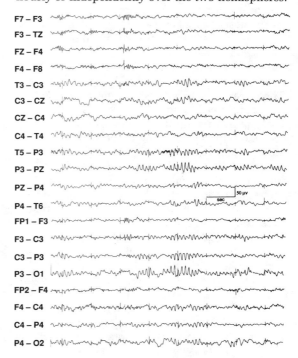

FIGURE 7-9. *Mu rhythm in the left parietal region (P_3). Note phase reversal of the 7 to 8-hz comblike rhythm at P_3 with spread of activity to C_3.*

This rhythm shows a characteristic reactivity: active or passive movement of the limbs, particularly contralaterally, or even an intention to move a limb attenuates mu activity. Mu is seen during wakefulness and may become more prominent during states I and II. It typically disappears in slow-wave sleep and may reappear during REM.[30] Direct EEG recordings from human motor cortex have demonstrated superharmonics of mu activity that react to limb movement.[31] This has led to the conclusion that mu is "a ubiquitous rhythm of the sensorimotor cortex at rest."[32]

Lambda rhythm is present in approximately 75% of young adults and becomes somewhat less common as they age. Lambda consists of a diphasic or triphasic waveform whose most prominent phase is a positivity at 01 or 02. The lambda rhythm is elicited by saccadic eye movements and appears to be an evoked response. It is present only during wakefulness when eyes are open.

EEG findings in infants and children undergo significant evolution with increasing age. In the following paragraph we emphasize a few major points; the reader is referred to other sources for details.[33-35] A sustained parietooccipital rhythm is not seen until approximately age 3 months. At that time, reactive 3-hz waves are recorded during wakefulness. Frequency of the parietooccipital rhythm increases rapidly over the next several years, reaching adult values in most children by age 3 years. Polyphasic slow waves (slow waves of youth) are found in the occipital regions bilaterally after 2 years in as many as 10% of normal subjects. Prevalence is highest around age 10 and gradually decreases afterward. These waveforms rarely occupy more than 25% of the record, and they do not significantly exceed other background rhythms in amplitude. Polyphasic slow waves react to eye opening in the same manner as alpha rhythm and in fact are considered to be a variant of the alpha rhythm. Greater amounts of random frontocentral theta waves are seen in children than in adults, but this decreases as the child ages. Brief runs of more sustained low-amplitude (less than 15 μV) frontal 6 to 7-Hz waves are seen in as many as 35% of adolescents. This rhythm is present during quiet wakefulness with eyes open and may be related to affective arousal.

In elderly persons frequency of the alpha rhythm slows somewhat, from a population mean of approximately 10.5 Hz to about 9 Hz, though alpha rhythm with a dominant frequency of less than 8 Hz remains abnormal in adults. Focal temporal theta is seen in as many as 35% of asymptomatic persons older than 50 years. Such activity is more commonly noted over the left temporal regions than the right and should probably occupy no more than 5% of the tracing. We feel that lower-frequency or more prevalent temporal slowing is abnormal. However, the exact point at which temporal slowing in elderly persons can be considered unequivocally abnormal remains controversial.[36-38]

Sleep EEG in Adults (see also Chapters 2 and 3)

The *Standard Scoring Manual*[18] divides sleep into four stages, and we discuss EEG findings in each of these four stages separately. (For scoring criteria see Chapter 12.) Drowsiness or stage I NREM sleep (see Figure 2-2) is used to designate transition between wakefulness and stage II and beyond. Stage I is also briefly seen after arousal from other sleep stages and often transiently precedes and follows periods of REM sleep. Because this is a transitional sleep stage it accounts for a relatively small percentage of a normal night's sleep, generally less than 5%.[39]

Recent studies have emphasized that EEG activity recorded during transition between wakefulness and stage 2 is variable and complex. EEG and physiologic changes that are inconsistent with wakefulness clearly occur before stage I as defined in the sleep scoring manual. Santamaria and Chiappa identified several phases of drowsiness and more than 20 distinct EEG patterns in a careful study of 55 normal adults.[19] The patterns of drowsiness varied in different subjects and varied in single subjects at different times. An early phase was characterized by changes in the alpha rhythm, which, however, persisted throughout this phase. Alpha may shift from its characteristic parietooccipital distribution to the frontocentral or temporal regions. Amplitude of alpha activity may either increase or decrease and frequency of the alpha rhythm may slow. Slower theta and delta frequencies may be superimposed in the central or temporal regions. These may have a paroxysmal or sharpish character and be confused with epileptiform potentials. Paroxysmal theta bursts may predominate in one temporal region and be misinterpreted as the temporal sharp waves often associated with complex partial seizures. Criteria for distinguishing these benign potentials from genuine focal epileptiform discharges have been outlined.[40]

As the alpha rhythm disappears, bursts of frontocentral beta and generalized delta slowing may appear. Frankly paroxysmal but nonetheless benign patterns are occasionally seen in normal adults at this time as well. *Benign epileptiform transients of sleep* (BETS) are seen in 5 to 24% of normal subjects.[19,41] These are spiky, often diphasic, transients (see Figure 27-8) with a broad field of distribution, usually involving both hemispheres. They typically shift from side to side and become less frequent during deeper sleep stags. Though BETS may superficially resemble epileptiform spikes, they are not associated with seizure disorders. White and coworkers[41] outlined useful criteria for distinguishing BETS from genuine epileptiform discharges. Less frequently, paroxysms of 6-Hz spike and wave (Figure 7-10) may be noted in either the frontal or occipital regions. The spike component usually has a relatively low amplitude whereas the following slow wave is more prominent. Paroxysms of such activity rarely last longer than 3 sec,[42] have an evanescent quality, and are less common during deeper sleep. In spite of their paroxysmal quality, they are not associated with seizures either.[42]

Eventually the alpha rhythm disappears altogether. *Vertex waves* are often recorded toward the end of stage I NREM sleep. These are high-voltage, sharp transients surface negative, followed by a lower-voltage surface-positive component. They have maximal voltage at the C_z electrode. Mild asymmetry between the two hemispheres and extension of the field to F_z, or less frequently P_z, is not uncommon. Vertex waves occur spontaneously or in response to stimuli that are insufficient to fully arouse the subject. *Positive occipital sharp transients of sleep* (POSTS) appear in posttransitional stage I, though these potentials are more common in deeper sleep stages (Figure 7-11). These are di- or triphasic sharp waves with a predominant positive phase at the occipital electrodes. They have a triangular appearance, similar to lambda waves. POSTS are noted synchronously over the two hemispheres and may occur singly or in runs. Occasional shifting amplitude asymmetry is noted in normal controls; however, persistent significant asymmetry should raise

suspicion of a posterior lesion. Because these potentials have a paroxysmal sharpish appearance, they may be confused with epileptiform discharges.

To summarize, drowsiness or stage I is a transitional state with many shifting and variable EEG patterns. Some of these resemble abnormal patterns, and determining whether an individual potential is normal may be difficult with the limited EEG montages typically used in PSG. It is important not to overinterpret. If there is uncertainty, routine EEG with a full complement of electrodes and multiple montages often clarifies the issue.

Stage II NREM sleep (see Figure 2-3) accounts for the bulk of a normal night's sleep (about 50% in normal adults).[39] *Sleep spindles* consist of a sequence of 12 to 16-Hz sinusoidal waves typically lasting a second or more. Voltage is usually maximal over the central regions. There is a high degree of symmetry and synchrony between the two hemispheres in normal subjects older than 1 year. Some investigators have proposed a classification of spindles based on topography and frequency,[32,43,44] but it is not clear that this has clinical utility at this time.

K complexes have been defined differently by sleep disorders specialists and electroencephalographers, which may confuse those trained in both disciplines. The sleep scoring manual[18] defines the K complex as a well-delineated negative sharp wave followed by a positive component. The K complex must be at least 0.5 seconds long and may or may not be accompanied by sleep spindles. Vertex waves are not specifically defined in the manual or the sleep disorders glossary of terms.[45] Most polysomnographers accept that vertex waves have a duration of

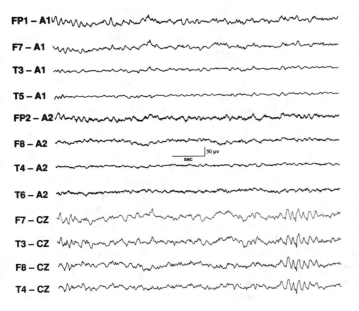

FIGURE 7-10. *Six-Hertz spike and wave (phantom spike and wave) seen in the last four channels.*

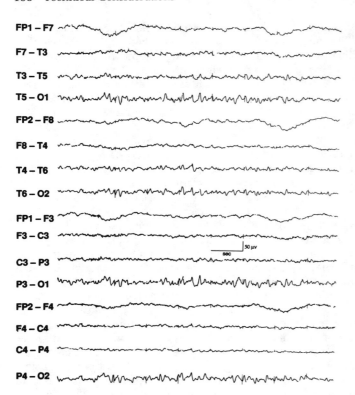

FP1 – F7

F7 – T3

T3 – T5

T5 – O1

FP2 – F8

F8 – T4

T4 – T6

T6 – O2

FP1 – F3

F3 – C3

C3 – P3

P3 – O1

FP2 – F4

F4 – C4

C4 – P4

P4 – O2

FIGURE 7-11.   *Positive occipital sharp transients (channels 4, 8, 12, 16 from the top) during stage I NREM sleep.*

less than 0.5 sec and distinguish vertex waves from K complexes on the basis of duration. This distinction is important when scoring sleep, because K complexes, even without spindles, are considered sufficient for scoring stage 2 sleep, whereas vertex waves alone do not allow scoring of stage 2 sleep. Glossaries of EEG terminology,[46] on the other hand, insist that K complexes always have associated sleep spindles and do not specify a duration.

EEG in NREM stages III and IV (see Figs. 2-4 and 2-5) is marked by high-amplitude slow waves. Computerized analyses indicate that sleep spindles, vertex waves, and POSTS[47,48] are abundant in stages III and IV, though they may be less noticeable to the interpreter's eye because of the abundant slow activity.

During REM sleep (see Figure 2-6) the background EEG is characterized by low-voltage mixed-frequency activity similar to that of early stage I. Alpha frequencies are often present and may be more persistent than in stage I. The alpha frequencies are usually 1 to 2 Hz less than the subject's waking rhythm.[49] Vertex waves, sleep spindles, and K complexes are absent. Characteristic sawtooth waves are frequently, though not inevitably, recorded. These are 2 to 6 Hz, sharply contoured triangular waves that usually occur serially for several seconds and are highest in amplitude over the C_z and F_z electrodes. A series of sawtooth waves typically precedes a burst of REMs.[50,51] REM sleep occupies 20% to 25% of the night's sleep of a normal subject.[39] Brief periods of state I sleep typically precede and follow a period of REM. Detailed rules for demarcating onset and termination of REM in these and other circumstances are outlined in the sleep scoring manual.[18]

Various atypical PSG patterns have been described. They usually are associated with some sleep disorder or with significant sleep disruption in normal persons. *Alpha-delta sleep* (see Figures 22-1 and 12-5) is characterized by persistence of alpha activity during stages 3 and 4. Excessive alpha "intrusion" may be seen in stage 2 as well, and the abundance of spindles appears to be decreased. This pattern appears to be associated with nonrestorative sleep and is seen in a variety of conditions.[52,53] It may be particularly characteristic of the fibromyositis syndrome. Moldovsky and colleagues[54] have elicited this EEG pattern in normal subjects by selectively depriving them of stage IV sleep. Deprivation of stage IV sleep also elicited complaints of diffuse arthralgias, myalgias, and fatiguability similar to the complaints of the fibromyositis syndrome. *REM-spindle sleep* (Figure 7-12) is characterized by the intrusion of sleep spindles into portions of the PSG that otherwise meet all criteria for REM sleep. This pattern may be seen in 1% to 7% of normal subjects[55] but is more common when sleep is disrupted and following the first night of continuous positive airway pressure (CPAP) treatment.

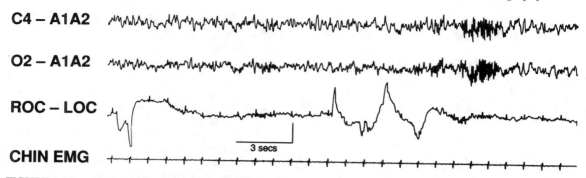

C4 – A1A2

O2 – A1A2

ROC – LOC

CHIN EMG

3 secs

FIGURE 7-12. *REM-spindle sleep. Note intrusion of sleep spindles in the EEG channels of a portion of a PSG that meet all criteria for REM sleep. There are REMs in the eye channel (ROC-LOC) and atonia in chin EM. Calibration (vertical bar) is 50 μV for the top three channels and 20 μV for the bottom channel.*

Broughton[56] recently reviewed other atypical patterns that occasionally occur during REM.

Normal Sleep EEG in Pediatrics
(see also Chapter 2)

The transition from neonatal to infantile EEG sleep patterns occurs between 1 and 3 months. Even after this period there is a great deal of change in the electrographic patterns until the adult patterns are reached. We emphasize the major points; the reader is referred elsewhere for details.[2,33-35,57]

Drowsiness in the pediatric age group differs from the adults' patterns in several ways. In children younger than 8 months drowsiness is marked by progressive slowing of EEG frequencies until delta waves predominate. After 8 months the onset of drowsiness is marked by long runs of continuous generalized high-voltage rhythmic theta or delta, which has been called *hypnagogic hypersynchrony.* Three types have been described in normal subjects.[34,35,57] In the most common type, the rhythmic slow waves have highest amplitude in the frontal and central regions. The continuous, rhythmic slowing may persist several minutes. Less commonly, amplitude is highest in the parietooccipital regions. Finally, a paroxysmal type occurs in approximately 10% of normal children. With this pattern, the alpha rhythm is gradually replaced by mixed frequencies. Diffuse bursts of 2 to 5-Hz slow waves, a few seconds in duration, then appear intermittently. Occasionally, random, poorly developed, sharpish waveforms are noted amidst the slow waves. These may be random superimposed alpha transients and should not be confused with epileptiform spike and wave. The first two types of hypnagogic hypersynchrony are rarely recorded after age 10 years. The paroxysmal type persists into the midteens, or rarely into adulthood.[34,35] In infancy and early childhood 20 to 25-Hz beta is also a prominent feature of drowsiness. The beta may have maximum voltage anteriorly or posteriorly or have a diffuse distribution. The amplitude may reach 60 μV. This pattern appears at 6 months and is seen most frequently from 12 to 18 months. Prevalence decreases subsequently, and prominent beta during drowsiness is rarely seen after 7 years.[57]

Vertex waves and K complexes appear at age 3 to 6 months. These potentials are rather blunt and may reach amplitudes exceeding 200 μV in infancy and early childhood. By age 5 years, both vertex waves and K complexes have an increasingly spiky configuration. Mild asymmetry is quite common. They may occur repetitively in brief bursts.

Sleep spindles appear at about 3 months of age. Between 3 and 9 months of age spindles occur in wicketlike trains, often more than several seconds long. These potentials are quite common at this age, occupying 15% of stage II sleep. Asynchrony between the hemispheres is the rule: only half the trains demonstrating interhemispheric synchrony at 6 months.[58,59] Interhemispheric synchrony increases to 70% by 12 months, and the duration and frequency of the spindle bursts gradually decrease. By 2 years of age virtually all spindle trains are synchronous; however, spindles are much less frequent, occupying only 0.5% of stage 2 sleep.[58,59] Spindles remain infrequent until approximately 5 years of age.[59]

Stage III and IV sleep is marked by high-amplitude slow activity, as in adults, though the amplitude of the slow activity is usually higher. An occipitofrontal gradient is often present: the very-high amplitude, slower frequencies predominate posteriorly and lower-amplitude, faster frequencies anteriorly.[60] This gradient becomes less striking with age, so that by 5 years the slow waves are distributed more diffusely.

EEG during REM sleep in infants and children is characterized by more slow activity than is seen in adults. The mature desynchronized EEG with scattered alpha emerges during the mid-teens.[61] The percentage of a normal night's sleep occupied by REM gradually decreases, from 40% at age 3 to 5 months to 30% at age 12 to 24 months and then gradually assumes adult values after puberty.[62] REM onset latency gradually lengthens over the first year of life as well.

THE ABNORMAL EEG

Many abnormal EEG patterns have been described. We discuss only the frequently encountered abnormalities. *Diffuse slowing of background activity* (Figure 7-13) is probably the most commonly recorded EEG abnormality. It can take several forms. One may see slowing of the parietooccipital alpha-type rhythm to a frequency below that allowable for the patient's age. Alternatively, frequency of the alpha-type rhythm may be normal but excessive diffuse theta and delta activity may be recorded. Finally, one may see both slowing of the alpha-type rhythm and excessive diffuse slower frequencies. Before concluding that an EEG has excessive slowing of background frequencies, the polysomnographer must

consider the patient's age and state of alertness. More diffuse theta is seen in normal children than is acceptable for adults. Frequency of background rhythms must be assessed while the patient is clearly awake (e.g., eyes blinking, talking). As noted above, both slowing of alpha-type rhythms and diffuse slower frequencies are commonly found in drowsiness in normal subjects. Consequently, the polysomnographer must be certain that the background frequencies are slow during wakefulness. Unfortunately, diffuse slowing of background frequencies is a very nonspecific pattern. It is commonly interpreted as being consistent with a variety of diffuse encephalopathies, including toxic, metabolic, and degenerative disorders.

Focal slowing (Figure 7-14) means that slow frequencies predominate over one region of the brain. Electrocerebral activity elsewhere is normal or the slowing is relatively mild. In experimental models, focal slowing is produced by focal white matter lesions, even when the cerebral cortex remains intact.[63] Focal cerebral lesions often involve both white matter and cortex, however, the usefulness of this distinction is blurred so in practice. A structural lesion must always be suspected when persistent focal slowing is recorded; however, not all patients

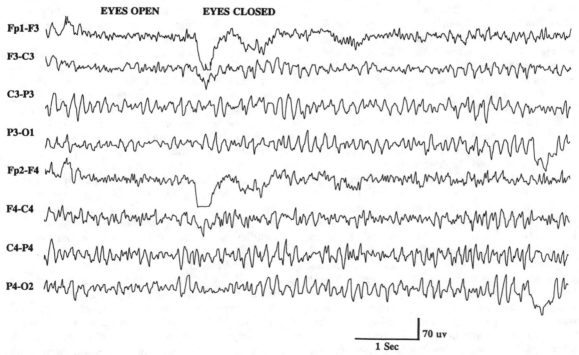

FIGURE 7-13.　*Diffuse slowing in a 67-year-old patient with dementia. Six- to seven-Hertz activity predominates over the parietooccipital regions. Although it is reactive to eye closure, the frequency of this rhythm is abnormally slow. (Reproduced with permission from Emerson RE, Walczak TS, Turner CA. EEG and evoked potentials. In Rowland, LP, ed. Merritt's Textbook of Neurology. Update 9, pp 3–20. Philadelphia, Lea and Febiger, 1992.*

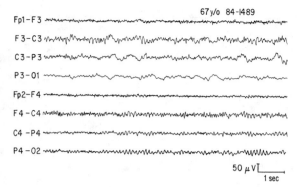

67y/o 84-1489

Fp1-F3

F3-C3

C3-P3

P3-O1

Fp2-F4

F4-C4

C4-P4

P4-O2

50 μV
1 sec

FIGURE 7-14. *Focal left hemispheric slowing in a 67-year-old patient with a large left hemispheric infarction. Left hemispheric alpha rhythm is also attenuated. (Courtesy of Dr. Timothy Pedly.)*

with focal slowing have neuroradiologically demonstrable lesions.[64] Patients with transient ischemic attacks or focal epilepsy often have focal EEG slowing, even though neuroradiologic investigations are normal. In epilepsy patients this slowing may be due to ongoing local inhibitory phenomena or may be a transient postictal finding.

Focal attenuation of background rhythms means that frequencies in one region of the brain have significantly lower amplitude than elsewhere. In experimental models, focal attenuation of background is produced when the gray matter is lesioned while underlying white matter remains intact.[63] Consequently, focal attenuation is often interpreted to indicate focal cortical dysfunction. In practice, attenuation of background frequencies is usually seen in combination with focal slowing (see Figure 7-14). Neuroradiologic investigations usually reveal large lesions involving both cortex and white matter.[65,66] Any fluid collection between the cortex and the recording electrode attenuates the recorded EEG activity. Thus, subdural fluid collections and subgaleal hematomas may result in focal attenuation of background rhythms even though the cortex may not be damaged.

The detection of *epileptiform discharges* is important because these potentials are highly associated with epilepsy. Pedley[67] has suggested that an epileptiform discharge should meet several criteria. It must be paroxysmal, which means that it must clearly stand out from the background. An epileptiform discharge must be "spiky" which means that the transition from ascending to descending phase is abrupt and the duration of the discharge is short (by convention less than 200 msec). It must have a clear field, that is it should not be confined to one electrode. It should have negative polarity because epileptiform discharges with positive polarity are un-

common.* Finally, a slow wave often follows an epileptiform discharge. Several different varieties of epileptiform discharges have been described, and these have been associated with different epilepsy syndromes.[67,68] A basic distinction is made between generalized and focal epileptiform discharges. Generalized epileptiform discharges indicate that the patient's seizure is likely to start simultaneously throughout the brain. An example is the generalized 3-Hz spike and wave (see Figure 27-2) that is characteristic of petit mal absence seizures. Focal epileptiform discharges indicate that the patient's seizure is likely to start in a restricted area of the brain, though subsequently it may spread. An example is the anterior temporal sharp wave that is characteristic of complex partial seizures of temporal lobe origin (Figure 7-15). This is an important distinction because the treatment and prognosis of these two epileptic syndromes is very different.[68] Approximately 90% of adults with epileptiform discharges have a history of seizures,[69,70] and incidental epileptiform discharges are very uncommon in normal adults.[71] The association of epileptiform discharges with seizures in the pediatric age group is not as strong and varies with patient age and type of epileptiform discharge.[72]

The polysomnographer must be able to recognize an *electrographic seizure* (see Figure 27-10). This may occur in patients with epilepsy or in patients with sleep apnea during severe hypoxia. The EEG patterns associated with seizures are extremely variable. In general, an electrographic seizure has abrupt onset and sustained and rhythmic evolution of frequencies, spreads to contiguous areas of the brain, terminates abruptly, and is often followed by irregular postictal slowing. Typically, faster frequencies are seen at seizure onset, and these gradually decrease in frequency as the seizure continues. Onset seizures associated with hypoxia usually are generalized. In practice, any sustained and evolving rhythm with abrupt onset raises concern about electrographic seizures; however, the polysomnographer must recall that drowsiness and arousal responses may begin abruptly and have rhythmic, sustained characteristics as well, especially in children.

Periodic lateralized epileptiform discharge (PLED) is another important pattern to be recognized. In this pattern, epileptiform discharges are recorded continuously over a given region (Figure 7-16). The epileptiform discharges occur at regular intervals, usually every 1 to 2 sec, and are thus labeled periodic.[73,74] Background activity is usually

---

*Positive rolandic sharp waves are occasionally recorded in premature infants with intraventricular hemorrhage or periventricular leukomalacia. Otherwise, positive sharp waves are very uncommon in older patients.

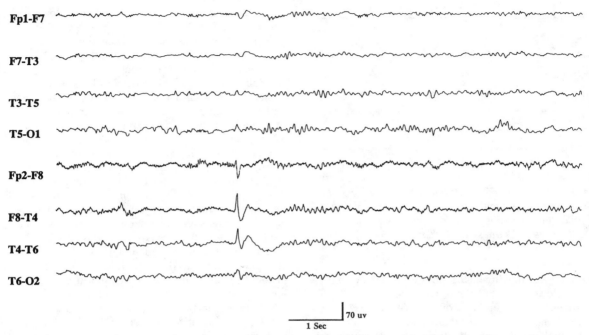

FIGURE 7-15.   *Right temporal interictal epileptiform discharge in a 32-year-old patient with complex partial seizures. (Reproduced with permission from Emerson RE, Walczak TS, Turner CA. EEG and evoked potentials. In Rowland, LP, ed. Merritt's Textbook of Neurology. Update 9, pp 3–20. Philadelphia, Lea and Febiger, 1992.*

significantly attenuated on the side with the discharges, and excessive slow frequencies are often seen bilaterally.[73,74] This pattern is usually associated with an acute focal cerebral insult. In a review of 586 cases reported in the literature,[75] 35% were related to an acute cerebral infarction, 26% to other sorts of mass lesions, and the remainder to infection, anoxia, or other causes. Clinically, PLEDs are associated with obtundation, seizures, and focal neurologic deficits. Some 70% to 90% of patients with PLEDs have seizures during the acute stage of their illness,[73-75] and 25% to 40% of patients with this pattern die in the hospital or shortly after discharge. Mortality may be especially high in patients with acute stroke and PLEDs.[73,74,76] PLEDS are almost always a transient phenomenon. The discharges become less frequent and lower in amplitude over the 2 weeks after the acute insult and are gradually replaced by focal delta slowing.[77]

Artifacts[1-4] (see also Chapter 6)

The polygraph is designed to record the relatively small voltages generated by the human brain, muscle, eye, and heart. Unfortunately, the remainder of the human body and the surrounding environment are not electrically silent. These generate abundant electrical activity that may obscure the biologic signals of interest. This extraneous electrical activity is called *artifact*. Making the distinction between the signal of interest and artifact is a central task for the polysomnographer, and the task is most difficult when interpreting EEG. Because high sensitivities are required to record the relatively low voltages generated by the brain, extraneous voltage sources are especially likely to contaminate the EEG recording.

There are four sources of artifact: (1) irrelevant physiologic signals, (2) environmental signals, (3) aberrant signals due to faulty or improperly applied electrodes, and (4) aberrant signals produced by the polygraph. More than one of these sources can contribute to a particular artifact. The following discussion summarizes frequently encountered artifacts and is by no means exhaustive. Indeed, artifacts are so diverse that it is probably not possible to construct a complete list. Each laboratory is encouraged to compile an atlas of artifacts commonly encountered in that particular location.

Irrelevant physiologic signals

Irrelevant signals may contaminate recording of the biologic signals of interest, especially EEG.

Myogenic potentials originating from scalp muscles may obscure EEG recording (see Figures 6-9 and 6-12). Myogenic activity may be difficult to distinguish from electrocerebral activity in the

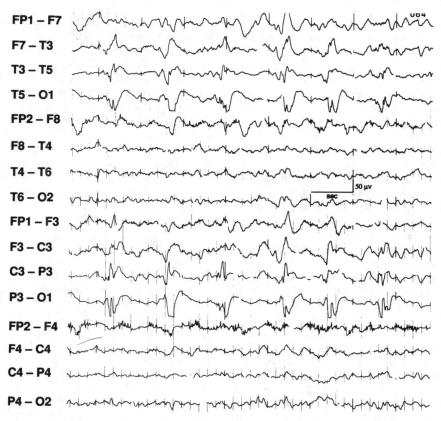

FIGURE 7-16. *Periodic lateralized epileptiform discharges (PLEDs) at a rate of 0.8 per second arising from the left parietal and posterior temporal regions (P_3, T_5) in a 72-year-old woman with a history of confusion and falling episodes.*

beta-frequency range, especially at slow paper speeds. It may obscure lower-amplitude electrocerebral activity.

Head movement also causes artifacts, frequencies of which are usually in the delta-range (see Figure 6-13). These artifacts are due to changes in electrode impedance, together with spurious static and capacitative potentials. Head movement artifacts are induced by slight movement of the electrodes on the scalp and the swaying of wires. The head movements associated with respiration often elicit movement artifact on the EEG, especially when the patient is lying on the recording electrodes. Correlating the spurious delta waves on the EEG with the respiratory monitor establishes their artifactual source. This may be important because these spurious potentials should not be used to score slow-wave sleep.

Sweating may result in very slow frequencies and changes in baseline, especially when direct current amplifiers are used in the polygraph. The salt content of sweat changes the ionic composition of the conducting gel, resulting in this particular artifact.

Potentials that arise from the sweat glands also play a role. Sweating may be asymmetric, and the resulting EEG asymmetry may mislead the interpreter.

Pulse artifact occurs when an electrode is placed on one of the scalp arteries. The electrode movement caused by the pulsations produces a delta wave. The regular relationship of the delta wave to ECG indicates the extracerebral origin of this activity.

The electrical fields generated by *ECG and eye movements* are commonly recorded from scalp electrodes (see Figure 6-10) and may be confused with electrocerebral activity. Again, referring to the channels recording ECG and eye movements demonstrates whether suspicious activity recorded at the scalp is caused by these extracerebral sources.

Environmental signals

The hospital environment contains many sources of electrical signals that may mimic electrocerebral or other physiologic activity. The *circulation of moistened air* through a respirator tube may induce bursts of alpha or theta frequencies at scalp electrodes. The electrostatic charges on drops entering an intravenous cannula—*intravenous drop artifacts*—may cause periodic spikelike artifacts. *Intravenous infusion pumps* can cause bursts of spiky transients followed by slower components. These artifacts are thought to be due to electromagnetic (rather than electrostatic) sources. *Telephones and pager systems* are among the many other potential sources of environmental artifacts. The interpreter relies on the technician to correlate unusual recorded potentials with specific events in the environment and, thus, to establish the artifactual nature of the potentials.

Sixty-Hertz electromagnetic radiation due to alternating current in power lines is ubiquitous in the hospital environment and may contaminate the recording (in Europe mains frequency is 50 Hz). The resulting 60-Hz artifact may be impossible to distinguish from myogenic activity at the slow paper speeds commonly used for PSG. The presence of this artifact in EMG leads may persuade the interpreter that a tonic EMG activity is high level when it is actually low. The 60-Hz artifact is verified when 60 cycles is counted in 1 sec of recording. Usually, paper speed must be increased to at least 60 mm/sec to distinguish adjacent potentials of this frequency and count them accurately. After the presence of 60 Hz is verified, the technician should proceed systematically to determine the source of the artifact. First, the technician must ensure that both of the involved electrodes are in fact attached to the patient, plugged into the jackbox, and connected to the relevant amplifier. The integrity of the patient ground must be similarly ensured. Next, the technician should check the impedances of the involved electrodes and the patient ground. Impedances in any electrode pair should not exceed 10 kΩ and the impedances of the two electrodes should be roughly equal. Only then can the technician conclude that the electrode-scalp interface is probably not the source of the artifact. At this point, the technician should search for 60-Hz sources in the environment. A "dummy patient," consisting of two leads shorted with a 10-kΩ resistor, may be carried around the room until the 60-Hz artifact reaches maximal amplitude and the source is identified. Finally, the technician should remember that faults with instrument ground may result in 60-Hz recording.

Aberrant signals from faulty electrodes

Improperly applied electrodes or electrode faults may result in other sorts of artifact.

Electrode "pops" are the most common electrode artifact. These are abrupt vertical transients (Figure 7-17), usually of positive polarity, that are confined to one electrode. They are superimposed upon but do not modify ongoing recording. Pops are due to abrupt changes in impedance and usually indicate either that the electrode is not securely attached or that electrolyte gel is insufficient. When confronted with a popping electrode, the technician should reset the electrode and apply more gel. If popping persists the electrode needs to be changed. Occasionally the electrode impedances change more gradually, mimicking slow activity. Again, the observation that the slow activity is confined to one electrode indicates that the electrode, rather than the body, is the source of the potential.

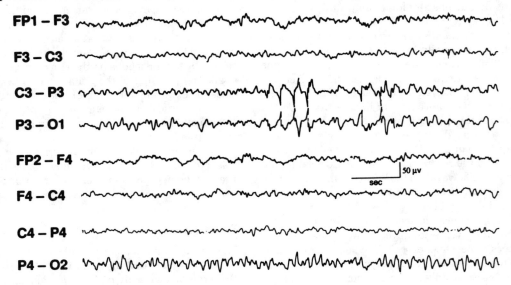

FIGURE 7-17.   *Electrode pops at P_3 electrode.*

Other electrode faults may result in artifact even if the electrode-scalp interface is intact. An interruption in the plating of the electrode may result in battery potentials, which can appear as bizarre, high-amplitude discharges confined to the faulty electrode. A similar artifact may occur when electrode gel connects the disk electrode and the wire lead, which are usually made of different metals.

Aberrant signals from the polygraph

Finally, the polygraph can be a source of artifact.

Random fluctuation of charges in any complicated recording instrument will result in some spurious output. In a well-built polygraph this *instrument noise* is infrequent and has low amplitude. It should not contaminate recording at standard sensitivities but may occasionally appear when sensitivities greater than 2 μV/mm are required.

Corrosion or loosening of contacts in switches or wires may cause abrupt changes in voltage or sudden loss of signal. The nonphysiologic nature of such potentials is usually readily apparent; though finding the source in the instrument may be difficult, especially if the artifact is intermittent.

A meticulous, alert, and experienced technician is the first and best defense against artifact. The critical importance of properly applied and gelled electrodes cannot be overemphasized for PSG, because adjusting or changing electrodes usually means waking the patient. The technician should be on the lookout for bizarre potentials and should seek to determine whether these are physiologic or artifactual. Observation of the patient and environment, correlations with the recorded activity, and careful documentation are critical. The technician must then decide whether the artifact significantly interferes with recording of the signal of interest. Deciding whether to change an electrode, and possibly wake the patient, or to allow a partially interpretable recording to continue requires experience and judgment. Ideally, the technician is aware of the major issues involved in interpreting a PSG and, so, is capable of making these important on-the-spot decisions wisely.

CONCLUSION

The interpretation of a PSG can be considered a pattern recognition task. The EEG is the most complicated and variable recording the polysomnographer interprets. Several issues continuously preoccupy the polysomnographer when interpreting the EEG. One question is whether the recorded signal is a true cerebral potential or whether it represents artifact. Another is whether the signal is present throughout the scalp or is confined to a single region of the scalp. The use of multiple channels for EEG recording allows the polysomnographer to answer these questions with greater certainty. Unfortunately, EEG recorded during routine PSG is often limited to a single channel. Limited montages and slow paper speeds often do not allow confident interpretation of unusual activity. This is especially unfortunate because EEG abnormalities important to the patient's care are more likely to occur during longer PSG recordings than during routine EEG. We feel that the cost of a few additional EEG channels is more than repaid by the greater certainty in interpretation and the greater likelihood that important abnormalities will be detected. Sometimes a confident decision on the nature of suspicious potentials cannot be made, even when several EEG channels are available. It is important not to overinterpret suspicious events. The polysomnographer should not be afraid to admit uncertainty when the collected data are insufficient. Referral for routine sleep EEG is usually appropriate in these circumstances. The full complement of scalp EEG channels often provides the necessary information. Similarly, information from additional EMG and EOG channels often clarifies ambiguities. Equivocal changes are often interpreted more confidently when more data is available.

REFERENCES

1. Daly DD, Pedley TA, eds. Current Practice of Clinical EEG, ed 2. New York: Raven Press, 1990.
2. Neidermeyer E, Lopes da Silva F, eds. Electroencephalography. Basic Principles, Clinical Applications and Related Fields, ed 2. Baltimore: Urban & Schwarzenberg, 1987.
3. Tyner F, Knott J, Mayer W Jr. Fundamentals of EEG technology, vol 1. New York: Raven Press, 1983.
4. Fisch BJ. Spehlman's EEG Primer, ed 2. Amsterdam, NY: Elsevier, 1991.
5. Kimura J. Electrodiagnosis in Diseases of Nerve and Muscle: Principles and Practice, ed 2. Philadelphia: FA Davis, 1989.
6. Werner SS, Stockard JE, Bickford RG. Atlas of Neonatal Electroencephalography. New York: Raven Press, 1977.
7. Creutzfeldt O, Houchin J. Neuronal basis of EEG waves. In: Creutzfeldt O, ed. Handbook of Electroencephalography and Clinical Neurophysiology, vol 2C. Amsterdam, Elsevier, 1974; 5–55.
8. Li CL, Cullen C, Jasper HH. Laminar microelectrode studies of specific somato-sensory cortical potentials. J Neurophysiol 1956;19:111–130.
9. Anderson P, Andersson SA. Physiological Basis of the Alpha Rhythm. New York: Appleton-Century-Crofts, 1968.

10. Steriade M, Gloor P, Llinas RR, et al. Basic mechanisms of cerebral rhythmic activities—report of IFCN committee on basic mechanisms. Electroencephalogr Clin Neurophysiol 1990;76:481–508.

11. Pedley TA, Traub RD. Physiological basis of the EEG. In: Daly DD, Pedley TA, eds. Current Practice of Clinical EEG, ed 2. New York: Raven Press, 1990; 107–137.

12. Geddes LA, Baker LE. Principles of Applied Biomedical Instrumentation. New York, John Wiley & Sons, 1968.

13. Gotman J. The use of computers in analysis and display of EEG and evoked potentials. In: Daly DD, Pedley TA, eds. Current Practice of Clinical EEG, ed 2. New York: Raven Press, 1990.

14. Whalen RE, Starmer CF, McIntosh HD. Electrical hazards associated with cardiac pacemaking. Ann NY Acad Sci 1964;3:922–931.

15. Starmer CF, McIntosh HD, Whalen RE. Electrical hazards and cardiovascular function. N Engl J Med 1971;284:181–186.

16. Geddes LA, Baker LE. Electrical safety in hospitals. J AAMI 1971;6(1).

17. Cooper R, Osselton JW, Shaw JC. EEG Technology. London: Butterworth's, 1980.

18. Rechtschaffen A, Kales A. A Manual of Standardized Terminology, Techniques and Scoring System for Sleep Stages of Human Subjects. Public Health Service GPO, Washington DC, 1968; (NIH Pub 204).

19. Santamaria J, Chiappa KH. The EEG of Drowsiness. New York: Demos, 1987.

20. McPartland RJ, Kupfer DJ. Computerized measures of EOG activity during sleep. Int J Biomed Comput 1978;9:409–419.

21. Radtke RA. Sleep disorders. In: Daly DD, Pedley TA, eds. Current Practice of Clinical EEG, ed 2. New York: Raven Press, 1990;561–592.

22. Lance JW. The control of the muscle tone, reflexes and movement. The Robert Wartenberg lecture. Neurology 1980;30:1303–1313.

23. Lourenco RV, Mueller EP. Quantification of electrical activity in the human diaphragm. J Appl Physiol 1967;22:598–600.

24. Lopata M, Evanich MJ, Lourenco RV. Quantification of diaphragmatic EM response to CO_2 rebreathing in humans. J Appl Physiol 1977;43:262–270.

25. Lopata M, Zubillaga G, Evanich MJ, et al. Diaphragmatic EMG response to isocapnic hypoxia and hyperoxic hypercapnia in humans. J Lab Clin Med 1978;91:698–709.

26. Lopata M, Lourenco RV. Evaluation of respiratory control. Clin Chest Med 1980;1:33–45.

27. Chokroverty S, Sharp JT. Primary sleep apnoea syndrome. J Neurol Neurosurg Psychiatry 1981;44:970–982.

28. Phillipson EA, Bowes G. Control of breathing during sleep. In: Fishman AF, Cherniack AS, Widdicombe JG, eds. Handbook of Physiology, sect 3, The Respiratory System, vol II, part 2. Bethesda, Md: American Physiological Society, 1986;649–689.

29. Guindi GM, Bannister R, Gibson W, et al. Laryngeal electromyography in multiple system atrophy with autonomic failure. J Neurol Neurosurg Psychiatry 1981;44:49–53.

30. Yamada T, Kooi KA. Level of consciousness and the mu rhythm. Clin Electroencephalogr 1975;6:80–88.

31. Jasper HH, Penfield W. Electrocorticograms in man: Effect of voluntary movement upon the electrical activity of the precentral gyrus. Arch Psychiat Nervenkr 1949;183:163–174.

32. Kellaway P. An orderly approach to visual analysis: Characteristics of the normal EEG of adults and children. In: Daley DD, Pedley TA, eds. Current Practice of Clinical EEG, ed 2. New York: Raven Press, 1990; 139–200.

33. Blume WT. Atlas of Pediatric Electroencephalography. New York: Raven Press, 1982.

34. Eeg-Olofsson O, Petersen I, Sellden U. The development of the EEG in normal children from the age of 1 to 15 years: Paroxysmal activity. Neuropaediatrie 1971;4:405–427.

35. Eeg-Olofsson O. The development of the electroencephalogram in normal adolescents from the age of 16 through 21 years. Neuropaediatrie 1971;3:11–45.

36. Obrist WD. The electroencephalogram of normal aged adults. Electroencephalogr Clin Neurophysiol 1954;6:235–244.

37. Katz RI, Horowitz GR. Electroencephalogram in the septuagenarian: Studies in a normal geriatric population. J Am Geriatr Soc 1982;30:273–275.

38. Torres F, Faoro A, Loewenson R, et al. The electroencephalogram of elderly subjects revisited. Electroencephalogr Clin Neurophysiol 1983;56:391–398.

39. Williams RL, Karacan I, Hursch CJ. Electroencephalography of human sleep: Clinical applications. New York: John Wiley and Sons, 1974.

40. Reiher J, Lebel M. Wicket spikes: Clinical correlates of a previously undescribed EEG pattern. Can J Neurol Sci 1977;4:39–47.

41. White JC, Langston JW, Pedley TA. Benign epileptiform transients of sleep: Clarification of the small sharp spike controversy. Neurology 1977;27:1061–1068.

42. Thomas JE, Klass DW. Six per second spike and wave pattern in the electroencephalogram. A reappraisal of its clinical significance. Neurology 1968;18:587–593.

43. Gibbs F, Gibbs E. Atlas of Electroencephalography, vol 1. Cambridge, Mass: Addison-Wesley, 1951.

44. Deebenham P. Sleep spindle symposium—introduction. Sleep 1981;4:384–386.

45. Association of sleep disorders centers and association for the psychophysiological study of sleep. Glossary of terms used in the sleep disorders classification. Sleep 1979;2:123–129.

46. Dutertre F. Catalogue of the main EEG patterns. In: Remond A, ed. Handbook of Electroencephalography and Clinical Neurophysiology, vol 11A. Amsterdam: Elsevier, 1977; 40–79.

47. Vignaendra V, Matthews RL, Chatrian GE. Positive occipital sharp transients of sleep: Relationships to nocturnal sleep cycle in man. Electroencephalogr Clin Neurophysiol 1974;37:239–246.

48. Gaillard J, Blois R. Spindle density in sleep of normal subjects. Sleep 1981;4:385–391.

49. Johnson LC, Nute C, Austin MT, et al. Spectral analysis of the EEG during waking and sleeping. Electroencephalogr Clin Neurophysiol 1967;23:80.

50. Schwartz RA. EEG et mouvements oculaires dans le sommeil de nuit. Electroencephalogr Clin Neurophysiol 1962;14:126–128.

51. Berger RJ, Olley P, Oswald I. The EEG, eye movements and dreams of the blind. Q J Exp Psychol 1962;14:183–186.

52. Hauri P, Hawkins DR. Alpha-delta sleep. Electroencephalogr Clin Neurophysiol 1973;34:233–237.

53. Moldofsky H, Lue FA. The relationship of alpha and delta EEG frequencies to pain and mood in fibrositis patients treated with chlorpromazine and L-tryptophan. Electroencephalogr Clin Neurophysiol 1980;50:71–80.

54. Moldofsky H, Scarisbrick P. Induction of neuroasthenic musculoskeletal pain syndrome by selective sleep stage deprivation. Psychosomat Med 1976;38:35–44.

55. Snyder F. Toward an evolutionary theory of dreaming. Am J Psychiatry 1966;123:121–136.

56. Broughton RJ. Polysomnography: Principles and applications in sleep and arousal disorders. In: Neidermeyer E, Lopes da Silva F, eds. Electroencephalography. Basic Principles, Clinical Applications and Related Fields, ed 2. Baltimore: Urban & Schwarzenberg, 1987;687–724.

57. Kellaway P, Fox BJ. Electroencephalographic diagnosis of cerebral pathology in infants during sleep. Its rationale, technique, and the characteristics of normal sleep in infants. J Pediatr 1952;41:262–287.

58. Lenard HG. The development of sleep spindles during the first two years of life. Neuropaediatre 1970;1:264–276.

59. Tanguay PE, Ornitz EM, Kaplan A, et al. Evolution of sleep spindles in childhood. Electroencephalogr Clin Neurophysiol 1975;38:175–181.

60. Slater GE, Torres F. Frequency-amplitude gradient. A new parameter for interpreting pediatric sleep EEGs. Arch Neurol 1979;36:465–470.

61. Niedermeyer E. Maturation of the EEG: Development of waking and sleep patterns. In: Neidermeyer E, Lopes da Silva F, eds. Electroencephalography. Basic Principles, Clinical Applications and Related Fields, ed 2. Baltimore: Urban & Schwarzenberg, 1987;133–157.

62. Roffwarg H, Muzio J, Dement W. Ontogenic development of the human sleep-dream cycle. Science 1966;152:604–619.

63. Gloor P, Ball G, Schaual N. Brain lesions that produce delta waves in the EEG. Neurology 1977;27:326–333.

64. Marshall DW, Brey RL, Morse MW. Focal and/or lateralized plymorphic delta activity. Association with either 'normal' or 'nonfocal' computed tomographic scans. Arch Neurol 1988;45:33–35.

65. Schaul N, Green L, Peyster R, et al. Structural determinants of electroencephalographic findings in acute hemispheric lesions. Ann Neurol 1986;20:703–711.

66. Ottonello GA, Regestga G, Tanganelli P. Correlation between computerized tomography and EEG findings in acute cerebrovascular disorders. In: Lechner H, Aranibar A, eds. EEG and Clinical Neurophysiology. Amsterdam: Excerpta Medica, 1980;148–161.

67. Pedley TA. Interictal epileptiform discharges: Discriminating characteristics and clinical correlations. Am J Electroencephalogr Technol 1980;20:101–119.

68. Roger J, Dravet C, Bureau M, et al. Epileptic Syndromes in Infancy, Childhood, and Adolescence. London: John Libbey Eurotext, 1985.

69. Ajmone-Marsan C, Zivin LS. Factors related to the occurrence of typical paroxysmal abnormalities in the EEG records of epileptic patients. Epilepsia 1970;11:361–381.

70. Salinsky M, Kanter R, Dasheiff RM. Effectiveness of multiple EEGs in supporting the diagnosis of epilepsy: An operational curve. Epilepsia 1987;28:331–334.

71. Zivin L, Ajmone Marsan C: Incidence and prognostic significance of 'epileptiform activity' in the EEG of nonepileptic subjects. Brain 1968;91:751–778.

72. Kellaway P. The incidence, significance and natural history of spike foci in children. In: Henry CE, ed. Current Clinical Neurophysiology. Update on EEG and Evoked Potentials. North-Holland: Elsevier, 1980;150–175.

73. Chatrian GE, Shaw C, Leffman H. The significance of periodic lateralized epileptiform discharges in EEG: An electrographic, clinical and pathological study. Electroencephalogr Clin Neurophysiol 1964;17:177–193.

74. Markand ON, Daly DD. Pseudoperiodic lateralized paroxysmal discharges in electroencephalogram. Neurology 1971;21:975–981.

75. Snodgrass SM, Tsuburaya K, Ajmone-Marsan C. Clinical significance of periodic lateralized epileptiform discharges, relationship to status epilepticus. J Clin Neurophysiol 1989;6:159–172.

76. Walsh JM, Brenner RP. Periodic lateralized epileptiform discharges—long term outcome in adults. Epilepsia 1987;28:533–536.

77. Schwartz MS, Prior PF, Scott DF. The occurrence and evolution in the EEG of a lateralized periodic phenomenon. Brain 1973;96:613–622.

8

Electrocardiographic Recognition of Cardiac Arrhythmias

Daniel M. Shindler
John B. Kostis

A wealth of information is available about cardiac rate and rhythm disturbances during sleep. Twenty-four–hour ambulatory electrocardiography (ECG) has made it possible to study cardiac rhythm in both awake and sleeping subjects. For most practical purposes, it is possible to think about cardiac rhythm during sleep in the same way as during wakefulness, though the heart rate is slower during sleep. As a result, escape-type arrhythmias may appear or become more frequent. One should first be familiar with the normal behavior of the heart and subsequently become familiar with a simple classification of cardiac arrhythmias.

NORMAL CARDIAC RHYTHM

The normal cardiac rhythm is defined as a normal sinus rhythm, that is, the cardiac rate is between 60 and 100 and the cardiac impulse originates in the sinus node. This is best confirmed by identifying a normal-looking P wave that is followed by a normal and constant PR interval and is always succeeded by a single QRS complex. It is quite normal for cardiac cycle length (RR interval) in a given patient to be somewhat variable. This is referred to as *sinus arrhythmia* (Figure 8-1).[1-3]

CARDIAC ARRHYTHMIAS

Arrhythmias are due to disturbances of impulse formation, impulse conduction, or a combination of the two. Arrhythmias can be separated into two large groups. Those that originate in the sinus node, atria, or atrioventricular (AV) node are referred to as *supraventricular arrhythmias;* those that originate in the ventricles are classified as *ventricular arrhythmias.* Figures 8-2 through 8-16 illustrate a variety of cardiac arrhythmias.

Supraventricular Arrhythmias

When the QRS complex is narrow, the arrhythmia is, with few exceptions, supraventricular. Unfortunately, when the QRS complex is wide, it is often impossible to determine conclusively whether an arrhythmia is supraventricular or ventricular. Inspection of the ECG is the first step in evaluating an arrhythmia. If the arrhythmia is considered potentially life threatening a specialized electrophysiologic study may be required to further assess its significance.[4]

Sinus Tachycardia

The most common rhythm disturbance (which may not be abnormal), sinus tachycardia, is an acceleration of the sinus heart rate above 100. In most cases sinus tachycardia does not exceed 180 beats per minute. Sinus tachycardia is best diagnosed by identifying P waves, determining that they are of normal morphology, subsequently establishing that the PR interval is normal and constant, and finally determining that (1) each QRS complex is preceded by the P wave and (2) each P wave is followed by a normal QRS. In the course of normal daily activity the heart rate rises in a gradual fashion and subsides in a gradual fashion.[5]

Sinus Bradycardia

The opposite boundary of normal heart rate is sinus bradycardia. Sinus bradycardia is defined as a rate slower than 60 beats per minute.[6] Again, it is manifested by a normal P wave appearance, normal and constant PR interval, and normal relationship of the P wave to the QRS complex, with a one-to-one sequence similar to that of sinus tachycardia. One observational pitfall in the patient with sinus bradycardia is the fact that at times U waves become very prominent and can easily be confused with P waves. As a result, blocked premature atrial contractions can be misdiagnosed.

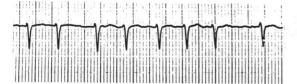

FIGURE 8-1.   *Normal sinus rhythm with sinus arrhythmia.*

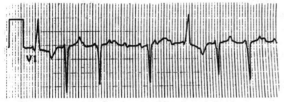

FIGURE 8-2.   *Atrial fibrillation.*

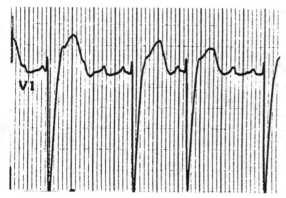

FIGURE 8-3.   *Atrial flutter with variable ventricular response.*

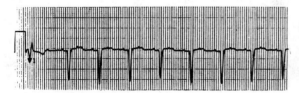

FIGURE 8-4.   *Atrial flutter.The first and fifth QRS complexes are aberrantly conducted.*

FIGURE 8-5.   *Atrial tachycardia with 2:1 block.*

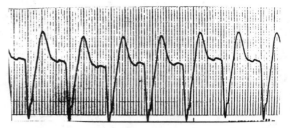

FIGURE 8-6.   *Undetermined wide complex rhythm, rate 100 beats per minute.*

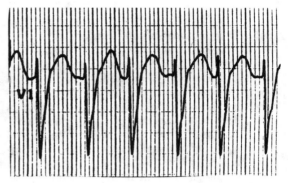

FIGURE 8-7.   *Undetermined wide complex tachycardia, rate 145 beats per minute.*

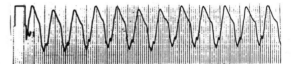

FIGURE 8-8.   *Ventricular tachycardia.*

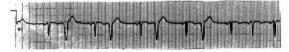

FIGURE 8-9.   *Normal sinus rhythm. Premature ventricular contractions in bigeminy.*

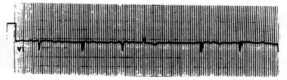

FIGURE 8-10.   *Atrial fibrillation. Premature ventricular contraction.*

Premature Atrial Contractions

Premature atrial contractions are observed frequently in normal subjects and patients with a variety of diseases. They are manifested as an interruption in the heart rhythm with a premature beat having a narrow QRS complex. Because the origin of the atrial impulse is ectopic, the appearance of the P wave is abnormal, denoting its abnormal early ori-

gin. There is quite a wide spectrum in the incidence and frequency of premature atrial contractions. There is a classification that describes their nature. If the premature atrial contractions occur singly, they are classified according to their incidence per period of time. Therefore, an ambulatory ECG report commonly describes how many premature atrial contractions were observed in a period of time, such as an

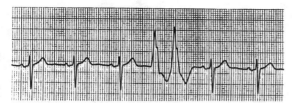

FIGURE 8-11. *Normal sinus rhythm. Premature ventricular couplet.*

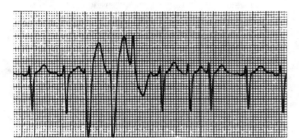

FIGURE 8-12. *Normal sinus rhythm. Three-beat multifocal ventricular tachycardia salvo. The eighth QRS complex is a premature atrial contraction.*

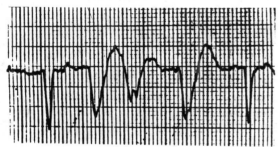

FIGURE 8-13. *Three-beat ventricular salvo resembling baseline artifact. Artifacts do not have T waves.*

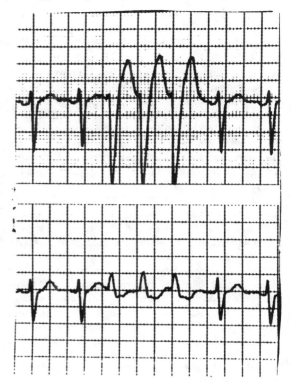

FIGURE 8-14. *Three-beat ventricular salvo demonstrated in two simultaneous leads.*

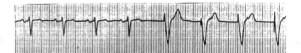

FIGURE 8-15. *Sinus rhythm with a demand pacemaker taking over in the last four beats. Note the disappearance of P waves.*

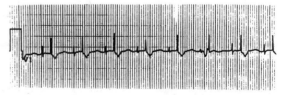

FIGURE 8-16. *AV sequential pacemaker. The sixth QRS complex is a native nonpaced premature beat. The pacemaker is programmed to deliver a ventricular pacing spike anyway.*

hour, a minute, or 24 hours, according to how common they are.

When premature atrial contractions are frequent, it is customary to further describe their nature (cyclic or noncyclic) and rate. For example, when premature atrial contractions occur cyclically they may show a bigeminal pattern.

Multifocal Atrial Tachycardia

A variant of frequent premature atrial contractions is tachycardia, which is called multiform atrial tachycardia or chaotic atrial tachycardia.[7] This is a rhythm disturbance that has definite clinical significance. It is identified by an irregular heart rhythm with narrow QRS complexes and rates in excess of 100 beats per minute. As the name implies, it is multifocal: the atrial beats originate in multiple sites in the atria. Consequently, the appearance of the P waves varies with the point of origin. There is variability in both the P-wave morphology and the PR interval. Multifocal atrial tachycardia is an arrhythmia that may have significant consequences and should not be confused electrocardiographically with another common arrhythmia, atrial fibrillation.

Atrial Fibrillation

Atrial fibrillation is a very common rhythm disturbance that is important to diagnose, as the initial heart rate can be quite fast and drug therapy (usually digitalis) may be required to slow it down. Patients with chronic atrial fibrillation are at increased risk for thromboembolic phenomena and are therefore often admitted to the hospital for further management when this rhythm is diagnosed.[8] The ECG hallmark of atrial fibrillation is a completely random and irregular heart rhythm with no reproducible RR interval. Because the atria are fibrillating at a rate of 500 beats per minute, there are no P waves. The electrocardiographic baseline may appear irregular and erratic. This should not be confused with the variable P waves of chaotic atrial tachycardia or with U waves, as mentioned above. The ventricular rate in patients with atrial fibrillation tends to be fast when it first occurs. The rate may range around 150 beats per minute. A clue to underlying conduction system disease is the fact that a patient with atrial fibrillation initially presents with a slow ventricular rate. At this point, caution needs to be exercised with therapeutic modalities, because therapy with an agent such as digitalis may produce undesirable AV conduction problems.[9,10]

Atrial Flutter

A variant of atrial fibrillation is a rhythm disturbance known as *atrial flutter*.[11] Atrial flutter differs in that atrial activity can be diagnosed as occurring 300 times per minute. At this rate, the ECG hallmark is a characteristic sawtooth pattern at a rate of 300 beats per minute. The usual presentation of atrial flutter is an atrial rate of 300 beats per minute with some degree of block between the atria and ventricles (the usual block being 2:1). Therefore, it is quite typical to recognize atrial flutter by the presence of sawtooth baseline with a ventricular response of 150 beats per minute. The therapeutic goal in atrial flutter (similar to atrial fibrillation) is to slow down the ventricular response when it is fast. Again, caution is exercised when the initial ventricular response (with no medications) is an unduly slow rate with a conduction block of 4:1 or greater.

Automatic versus Reentrant Tachycardia

The rhythm disturbances referred to above are classified as automatic rhythm disturbances. If properly diagnosed, they can be classified as disorders of cardiac automaticity. The warm-up phenomenon (gradual, nonabrupt increase in heart rate) is a hallmark of automatic tachycardia. Usually an automatic tachycardia dictates a search for its cause, which is then treated. For example, multifocal atrial tachycardia is typically seen in patients with lung disease, and improvement of hypoxemia often results in return of the cardiac rhythm to normal. Sinus tachycardia frequently indicates a metabolic disturbance such as fever, thyrotoxicosis, or hypovolemia. Again, therapy of the cause is the proper approach rather than addressing the mechanism of the rhythm disturbance itself.[12,13]

Conversely, a group of tachycardias referred to as reentrant ones are treated by addressing the mechanism of reentry. When this is corrected, the rhythm is restored to normal.

Paroxysmal Atrial Tachycardia

Paroxysmal atrial tachycardia is the classical reentrant tachycardia that is treated with medications that interrupt the mechanism of reentry.[14] As the name denotes, a paroxysmal atrial tachycardia begins abruptly. There is no warm-up phenomenon, and the heart rate instantly increases to between 140 and 180 beats per minute. It may cease spontaneously and just as abruptly, to return to sinus rhythm. It is quite common to observe these salvos of atrial tachycardia in patients, whether they are awake or asleep.

When paroxysmal atrial tachycardia is persistent it warrants treatment because of the unduly fast heart rate. Several maneuvers that increase vagal tone, such as Valsalva maneuver or carotid sinus massage, can break the arrhythmia.[15] When these are ineffective, it becomes necessary to employ medications. The calcium channel blocker, verapamil, is quite useful for this purpose. More recently, an agent that causes complete but very transient AV block, called adenosine, has emerged as the modality of choice.[16]

Sick Sinus Syndrome

Various combinations of tachycardia with bradycardia may suggest the diagnosis of sick sinus syndrome. Ambulatory ECG monitoring may be required to demonstrate the presence of sinus node dysfunction.[17-20]

Aberrant Supraventricular Conduction

A transient delay in intraventricular (IV) conduction can be seen in patients with supraventricular tachycardias. If the P waves are not clearly identifiable, the rhythm may be misdiagnosed as ventricular tachycardia (see later). QRS complex morphology may be useful in making the correct diagnosis. The initial aberrant conduction occurs in the QRS, which terminates a short cardiac cycle that was immediately preceded by a long cardiac cycle.[21,22]

VENTRICULAR ARRHYTHMIAS

The next group of rhythm disturbances, the ventricular arrhythmias, may be more hemodynamically significant and can be associated with clinically important heart disease. They can also be seen in normal patients.

Premature Ventricular Contractions

A very common rhythm disturbance often felt by patients (but many times not) is the premature ventricular contraction. It is most commonly an early beat that is easily recognized on the ECG as a wide QRS complex with abnormal repolarization.[23] The incidence on 24-hour ECG monitoring can be reported according to how often this finding is present; therefore, premature ventricular contractions are reported as occurring a certain number of times per hour. If rare they are classified by how many times they occur in 24 hours; if very common they may be classified in terms of occurrence per minute.[24]

Ventricular Bigeminy

A very common rhythm disturbance is a sustained rhythm, especially at night, consisting of an alternating normally conducted QRS complex with a premature ventricular contraction followed by a pause and a resumption of the sequence. This is referred to as ventricular bigeminy. It is, for most practical purposes, benign, but it has some clinical implications. For one, a patient taking a pulse may notice only the normally conducted beats. The pulse deficit then would result in a mistaken diagnosis of bradycardia.

Ventricular Tachycardia

The finding of three or more premature ventricular contractions in a row (at a heart rate faster than 100) is referred to as *ventricular tachycardia*.[25] It may be brief or sustained.[26] The most important distinction that needs to be made when ventricular tachycardia is suspected is the alternate diagnosis of supraventricular tachycardia with aberrant ventricular conduction. The diagnostic approach to this critical differential diagnosis is multifaceted. The diagnosis begins at the bedside. If the patient is hemodynamically decompensated, it is necessary to act rapidly.[27,28]

Multiple ECG leads should be employed to identify P waves that mark atrial activity. Atrial P waves that are unrelated to ventricular QRS complexes make ventricular tachycardia more likely than aberrant conduction. The appearance of the QRS complex was recently shown to be extremely useful in the recognition of a ventricular origin for tachycardia. Sustained ventricular tachycardia often degenerates into ventricular fibrillation, resulting in death.

Ventricular Fibrillation

Ventricular fibrillation is a lethal terminal dysrhythmia that requires immediate electrical defibrillation.[29] There are no identifiable QRS complexes. It may begin on a T wave (this is referred to as R on T). It may also be seen in association with a unique ventricular tachyarrhythmia called torsades de pointes.

Torsades de Pointes

The morphology of this ventricular tachyarrhythmia is unique. The points of the ventricular complexes vary in their height, appearing to turn around a central axis, the baseline of the ECG tracing. It is important to measure the QT interval. QT prolongation can be caused by electrolyte disturbances, antiarrhythmic drugs, or central nervous system or congenital disease.[30-34]

Accelerated Idioventricular Rhythm

The law of the heart states that the fastest pacemaker is the one that governs the heart. Accelerated idioventricular rhythm (AIVR) is a slow ventricular rhythm that captures the heart because the sinus rate is even slower. The rate of AIVR is less than 100 beats per minute. It is usually faster than the typical 40–beats per minute ventricular escape rate, thus the term *accelerated*. This is typically an escape rhythm that should not be suppressed with antiarrhythmic agents such as lidocaine. AIVR is often short lived and has no hemodynamic consequences. In this setting it does not require treatment. When AIVR is sustained and hypotension is observed, an agent such as atropine may be useful in overdriving the AIVR by accelerating the sinus node. The ECG diagnosis of AIVR consists of establishing the ventricular origin of the rhythm.

PACEMAKER RHYTHM

Pacemaker rhythms are identified by the pacemaker spike preceding the wide QRS complex. It is necessary to determine proper capture as well as proper sensing. Dual-chamber pacemakers are designed to restore the normal sequence of AV contraction. They are also associated with pacemaker-induced arrhythmias.[35] Some patients may have a pacemaker or defibrillator implanted to treat life-threatening ventricular arrhythmias.[36,37]

INTRACARDIAC RECORDINGS

Certain patients may be referred for electrophysiologic study to further evaluate their arrhythmia. The tracings obtained during those studies may demonstrate ECG information about the heart that is unobtainable from surface ECG studies. It is possible to record the electrical activity of the bundle of His. This may help decide which patients require a permanent pacemaker. The sinus node recovery time can be measured in patients with sick sinus syndrome. Ventricular arrhythmias can be induced to assess efficacy of antiarrhythmic therapy.[38]

SIGNAL-AVERAGED ECG

It is possible to amplify the electrocardiographic complex by as much as 1000 times with the use of signal averaging. The signal-averaged ECG can demonstrate the presence of late potentials (high-frequency, low-amplitude signals). Their absence is associated with a more favorable prognosis following myocardial infarction.

MANAGEMENT OF ARRHYTHMIAS DETECTED DURING SLEEP

The sophisticated monitoring equipment available today permits detection of cardiac arrhythmias and conduction disturbances as they occur during sleep. Sustained ventricular arrhythmias require immediate attention. The patient needs to be awakened, and blood pressure and mental status must be ascertained. If the ventricular arrhythmia causes hypotension or the patient is unarousable, emergency measures may be required. Fortunately, this event is extremely rare. Nonsustained ventricular arrhythmias are a more common finding. By the time the patient is aroused, blood pressure is usually normal, but the patient needs to be monitored for recurrence of the arrhythmia.

Conduction disturbances can also be detected. Sinus arrest is manifested by the disappearance of P waves and an area other than the sinus node taking over the cardiac rhythm. This can be a junctional rhythm, an ectopic atrial rhythm, or a ventricular rhythm. Now it is important to ascertain by ECG whether arrhythmias are, as mentioned, sustained or nonsustained. It is also worthwhile to determine whether a newly detected rhythm disturbance is a consequence of a conduction abnormality followed by an escape mechanism rather than a premature mechanism for arrhythmia initiation such as a premature ventricular contraction.

The hemodynamics, as measured by blood pressure, are the most important indicators of the significance of an arrhythmia as it is occurring. It is also important to take into account the underlying cardiac status of the particular patient in whom the arrhythmia is observed.

REFERENCES

1. Rawles JM, Pai GR, Reid SR. A method of quantifying sinus arrhythmia: Parallel effect of respiration on PP and PR intervals. Clin Sci 1989;12:954.
2. de Marneffe M, Jacobs P, Haardt R, et al. Variations of normal sinus node function in relation to age: Role of autonomic influence. Eur Heart J 1986;7:662.
3. Gomes JA, Winters SL. The origins of the sinus node pacemaker complex in man: Demonstration of dominant and subsidiary foci. J Am Coll Cardiol 1987;9:45.
4. Coelho A, Palileo E, Ashley W, et al. Tachyarrhythmias in young athletes. J Am Coll Cardiol 1986;7:237.
5. Yeh SJ, Lin FC, Wu DL. The mechanisms of exercise provocation of supraventricular tachycardia. Am Heart J 1989;117:1041.
6. Northcote RJ, Canning GP, Ballantyne D. Electrocardiographic findings in male veteran endurance athletes. Br Heart J 1989;61:155.
7. Scher DL, Arsura EL. Multifocal atrial tachycardia: Mechanisms, clinical correlates and treatment. Am Heart J 1989;118:574.
8. Wolf PA, Abbott RD, Kannel WB. Atrial fibrillation: A major contributor to stroke in the elderly. The Framingham Study. Arch Intern Med 1987;147:1561.
9. Fananapazir L, German LD, Gallagher JJ, et al. Importance of pre-excited QRS morphology during induced atrial fibrillation to the diagnosis and location of multiple accessory pathways. Circulation 1990;81:578.
10. Kopecky SL, Gersh BJ, McGoon MD, et al. The natural history of lone atrial fibrillation. A population-based study over 3 decades. N Engl J Med 1987;317:669.
11. Waldo AL, Carlson MD, Henthorn RW. Atrial flutter: Transient entrainment and related phenomena. In: Zipes DP, Jalife J, eds. Cardiac Electrophysiology: From Cell to Bedside. Philadelphia: WB Saunders, 1990;530.
12. Simpson RJ Jr, Amara I, Foster JR, et al. Thresholds, refractory periods, and conduction times of the normal and diseased human atrium. Am Heart J 1988; 116:1080.
13. Villain E, Vetter VL, Garcia JM, et al. Evolving concepts in the management of congenital junctional ectopic tachycardia. Circulation 1990;81:1544.
14. Pritchett EL, McCarthy EA, Lee KL. Clinical behavior of paroxysmal atrial tachycardia. Am J Cardiol 1988;62:30.
15. Morady F, Krol RB, Nostrant TT, et al. Supraventricular tachycardia induced by swallowing: A case report and review of the literature. PACE Pacing Clin Electrophysiol 1987;10:133.
16. Rankin AC, Oldroyd KG, Chong E, et al. Value and limitations of adenosine in the diagnosis and treatment of narrow and broad complex tachycardias. Br Heart J 1989;62:195.

17. Bharati S, Lev M. Cardiac Conduction System in Unexplained Sudden Death. Mt. Kisco, NY: Futura, 1990.
18. Choi YS, Kim JJ, Oh BH, et al. Cough syncope caused by sinus arrest in a patient with sick sinus syndrome. PACE Pacing Clin Electrophysiol 1989;12:883.
19. Sasaki Y, Shimotori M, Akahane K, et al. Long-term follow-up of patients with sick sinus syndrome: A comparison of clinical aspects among unpaced, ventricular inhibited paced, and physiologically paced groups. PACE Pacing Clin Electrophysiol 1988, 11:1575.
20. Schuger CD, Tzivoni D, Gottlieb S, et al. Sinus node and atrioventricular nodal function in 220 patients recovering from acute myocardial infarction. Cardiology 1988;75:274.
21. Akhtar M, Shenasa M, Jazayeri M, et al. Wide QRS complex tachycardia. Reappraisal of a common clinical problem. Ann Intern Med 1988;109:905.
22. Miles WM, Zipes DP. Electrophysiology of wide QRS tachycardia. Prog Cardiol 1988;1/2:77.
23. Moulton KP, Medcalf T, Lazzara R. Premature ventricular complex morphology. Circulation 1990;81:1245.
24. Funck-Brentano C, Coumel P, Lorente P, et al. Rate dependence of ventricular extrasystoles: Computer identification and quantitative analysis. Cardiovasc Res 1988;22:101.
25. Akhtar M. Clinical spectrum of ventricular tachycardia. Circulation 1990;82:1561.
26. Wilber DJ, Olshansky B, Moran JF, et al. Electrophysiological testing and nonsustained ventricular tachycardia. Circulation 1990;82:350.
27. Lucente M. Rebuzzi AG, Lanza GA, et al. Circadian variation of ventricular tachycardia in acute myocardial infarction. Am J Cardiol 1988;62–670.
28. Steinman RT, Herrera C, Schuger CD. Wide QRS tachycardia in the conscious adult. Ventricular tachycardia is the most frequent cause. JAMA 1989; 261:1013.
29. Trappe HJ, Brugada P, Talajic M, et al. Prognosis of patients with ventricular tachycardia and ventricular fibrillation: Role of the underlying etiology. J Am Coll Cardiol 1988;12:166.
30. Jackman WM, Friday KJ, Clark M, et al. The long QT syndromes: A critical review, new clinical observations and unifying hypothesis. Prog Cardiovasc Dis 1988;31:115.
31. Laks MM. Long QT interval syndrome. A new look at an old electrophysiologic measurement—the power of the computer. Circulation 1990;82:1539.
32. Nguyen PT, Scheinman MM, Seger J. Polymorphous ventricular tachycardia: Clinical characterization, therapy, and the QT interval. Circulation 1986;74:340.
33. Opie LH. Forum on torsades de pointes: Introduction. Cardiovasc Drugs Ther 1990;4:1167.
34. Rosen MR, Danilo P Jr, Robinson RB, et al. Sympathetic neural and alpha-adrenergic modulation of arrhythmias. Ann NY Acad Sci 1988;533:200.
35. Levander-Lindgren M, Lantz B. Bradyarrhythmia profile and associated diseases in 1,265 patients with cardiac pacing. PACE Pacing Clin Electrophysiol 1988;11:2207.
36. Rosenthal ME, Josephson ME. Current status of antitachycardia devices. Circulation 1990;82:1889.
37. Winkle RA, Mead RH, Ruder MA, et al. Long-term outcome with the automatic implantable cardioverter-defibrillator. J Am Coll Cardiol 1989;13:1353.
38. Zipes DP, Akhtar M, Denes P, et al. ACC/AHA guidelines for clinical intracardiac electrophysiologic studies. J Am Coll Cardiol 1989;14:1827 and Circulation 1989;80:1925.

9

Respiration and Respiratory Function: Technique of Recording and Evaluation

Richard A. Parisi
Teodoro V. Santiago

EVALUATION OF RESPIRATORY FUNCTION IN PATIENTS WITH SLEEP DISORDERS

A critical part of the initial medical evaluation of all patients with sleep disorders is the assessment of respiratory function. The reason for the importance of this assessment is relatively straightforward: Many of the most common and potentially serious sleep disorders (e.g., sleep apnea syndrome, nocturnal asthma, and sleep-related hypoventilation) are respiratory in nature and may be associated with respiratory abnormalities also evident in the awake state. Although a detailed discussion of the diagnostic evaluation of respiratory disease is beyond the scope of this volume, a general approach is presented here, in which a systematic assessment of key components of respiratory function is emphasized.

Clinical Evaluation

Patients with previously diagnosed lung disease are often referred for evaluation of sleep complaints. Patients with chronic obstructive pulmonary disease (COPD) present with symptoms of insomnia related to frequent awakenings.[1] Hypersomnia may also occur, particularly in persons who exhibit sleep-related hypoventilation. Many patients with asthma experience exacerbations of this disorder during sleep. Like patients with COPD, asthmatics often describe episodic arousal associated with dyspnea, cough, or wheezing.[2] Another important group of patients are those with respiratory neuromuscular disease. In many such cases symptoms of respiratory insufficiency at night, including frequent nocturnal arousals often associated with dyspnea, cough, choking, or morning headache, are frequently among the earliest signs of impending respiratory failure.[3] A related but distinct group of patients in whom sleep-disordered breathing is common are those with altered central neural respiratory drive. Such patients may exhibit hypoventilation syndromes while awake that are exacerbated by sleep.

Physiologic Testing

Formal testing of pulmonary mechanics, respiratory muscle strength, gas exchange, and central respiratory drive may be indicated for selected patients with clinical sleep disorders though none of these tests should be a routine part of a sleep evaluation.

Pulmonary mechanics

Spirometry is a dynamic analysis of maximal forced expiratory airflow. This basic test of pulmonary function, readily available at most centers and in many physicians' offices and relatively inexpensive and simple to perform, provides quantitative assessment of intrathoracic airway obstructive disease and is a moderately sensitive screening test for restrictive mechanical processes such as interstitial lung disease and respiratory muscle weakness. Although respiratory muscle weakness usually results in reduction of the forced vital capacity by spirometry, the most sensitive clinical test for muscle strength is measurement of maximal inspiratory and expiratory pressure at the mouth against an occluded airway. When restriction of vital capacity is evident on spirometry, more complete measurement of lung volumes is indicated to evaluate the pattern of restriction. For example, interstitial lung diseases generally decrease all lung volumes symmetrically, whereas extrapulmonary processes such as respiratory muscle weakness primarily reduce vital capacity without affecting functional residual capacity.

Arterial blood gases

Although arterial blood gases of most patients referred to a sleep disorders center need not be measured, this test provides valuable information in some patients with sleep-disordered breathing, particularly those found by pulse oximetry (during polysomnography) to be hypoxemic while awake. Most patients with obstructive sleep apnea syndrome have normal blood gases while awake. In contrast, patients with various hypoventilation syndromes are characteristically hypercapnic while awake, as are patients with advanced COPD or chronic neuromuscular diseases.

Respiratory control

The obstructive sleep apnea syndrome typically is not associated with overt abnormalities of respiratory drive,[4] and when chronic hypercapnia is present in awake patients, a primary impairment of respiratory drive should be considered. In the absence of significant ventilatory mechanical impairment due to chronic lung disease or neuromuscular weakness, chronic hypercapnia may be attributed to reduced respiratory carbon dioxide sensitivity, as in the obesity-hypoventilation syndrome. In patients with moderate ventilatory impairment whose respiratory carbon dioxide drive is suspected to be abnormal, the change in $PaCO_2$ during maximal voluntary ventilation may be measured.[5] Normalization of the $PaCO_2$ during a 2-minute maximal ventilation maneuver suggests that sufficient mechanical reserve is present to maintain normocapnia but that respiratory carbon dioxide chemosensitivity is diminished. A blunted ventilatory response to carbon dioxide and hypoxia, measured by standard techniques[6,7] can confirm this clinical impression; however, the value of these tests in an individual patient is limited by the variability of normal responses and by the confounding effect of mechanical ventilatory impairment, which may also decrease the measured responses.

RESPIRATORY MONITORING DURING SLEEP

General Principles

It should be evident from the following discussion that a wide array of methods are available to monitor respiratory output during sleep in the clinical setting. Clearly, the number and type of monitoring device employed are highly dependent on the purpose of the study to be performed. For some purposes, a single measure that ensures sufficient gas exchange, such as pulse oximetry, is sufficient. Detection of subtle changes in airflow due to increased upper air resistance requires more sensitive techniques. In discussing various modalities, an effort will be made to convey which ones are generally considered part of "standard" polysomnography.

Monitoring Respiratory Mechanical Output

Airflow and snoring

Clinically applicable airflow sensors can be classified as direct or indirect and as quantitative or semi-quantitative (Table 9-1). For most clinical purposes,

TABLE 9-1.   Methods for Monitoring Airflow During Sleep

	Principle	Signal Characteristics	Comments
Pneumotachygraph	Direct	Excellent; quantitative and easily integrated to yield tidal volume	Requires sealed facemask Can be incorporated into nasal CPAP systems
Thermistor/thermocouple	Indirect. Detects increased temperature of expired air.	Semiquantitative; only directional changes are reliable	Inexpensive, easy to use Signal quality reduced during nasal CPAP treatment
Capnograph	Indirect. Detects increased CO_2 in expired air.	Semiquantitative for airflow; significant time delay because air is sampled continuously for remote analysis	Easy to use Signal quality reduced during nasal CPAP treatment
Respiratory inductance plethysmograph	Indirect. Senses change in thoracic and abdominal cross-sectional areas. Sum of these compartments is proportional to airflow.	Good when properly calibrated	Least intrusive (no sensor near face) Calibration errors due to slippage or position changes a common problem
Tracheal sound	Indirect. Airflow through trachea produces sound audible via microphone.	Good; sound amplitude increases during snoring/partial upper airway obstruction	Inexpensive Can be used to quantitate snoring

semiquantitative indirect methods, such as an oro-nasal thermistor, are sufficient to identify apneas and hypopneas.

Quantitative measurement of airflow or tidal volume usually requires a sealed mask placed over the nose or the nose and mouth connected to a calibrated pneumotachygraph. Although this technique provides the accuracy necessary for some research applications, the method can be cumbersome and intrusive, thus limiting its value for clinical monitoring. One setting in which direct quantitative airflow monitoring is not only possible but preferable is during application of nasal continuous positive airway pressure (CPAP). Some commercially available CPAP units provide flow and volume outputs directly from the remote CPAP control. These devices are particularly useful because the more commonly used semiquantitative sensors, such as thermistors or carbon dioxide meters, must be placed under the nasal mask seal, potentially causing discomfort or pressure leakage, and because respiration-related temperature and PCO_2 changes at the nose may be damped considerably by the bias flow of room air required to maintain positive pressure in the nasal airway.

Snoring is an airflow-related phenomenon, though most measures of flow are not very sensitive to it. Many sleep laboratories document snoring with notes detailing the observations of a PSG technician. Quantitative assessment of snoring can be obtained with relative ease by a sound level meter connected to a microphone placed near the patient. Several studies have documented that sound detected by a microphone placed over the cervical trachea can also be used as a semiquantitative indicator of airflow and snoring.[8,9]

Respiratory muscle activity

The principal purpose of monitoring respiratory muscle activity, commonly described as *respiratory effort*, is to detect disparities between these measures and airflow. Both direct and indirect methods are employed to monitor respiratory muscle activity (Table 9-2). The most commonly employed methods are indirect, semiquantitative, or nonquantitative techniques that detect changes in circumference of the thorax and abdomen, including inductive plethysmography, magnetometers, and strain gauges. Figure 9-1 illustrates the manner in which these devices, employed in tandem, respond to normal tidal breathing and to respiratory muscle contractions against an obstructed upper airway. Although paradoxical expansion of the thorax and abdomen may occur under other circumstances, such as with fatigue or paralysis of the diaphragm, periodic reversal of this pattern is quite useful for detecting intermittent upper airway obstruction during sleep. Also, calibration of the relative thoracic and abdominal compartmental volume changes allows summation of the two impedance signals to obtain an indirect, and potentially quantitative, measure of lung volume changes (and thus, airflow).[10] These indirect techniques are noninvasive and simple to use, but one disadvantage is that volume changes do not reflect muscle activity when upper airway impedance changes. For example, respiratory motion of the chest wall invariably decreases during obstructive apnea despite increasing muscle activity.

Direct monitoring of respiratory muscle activity, either electrical or mechanical, has some advantages over the more commonly used indirect methods, in that such a method continues to accurately reflect

TABLE 9-2. Methods for Monitoring Respiratory Muscle Activity During Sleep

	Principle	*Signal Characteristics*	*Comments*
Esophageal pressure	Direct; esophageal pressure equivalent to intrathoracic pressure generated by respiratory muscles	Excellent; reliable; quantitative	Invasive; requires transnasal insertion Uncomfortable for patient/subject
Diaphragmatic EMG	Direct; measures neural activation rather than mechanical output	Quantitative; poor signal-noise ratio with surface electrodes	ECG artifact; nonrespiratory muscle EMG difficult to eliminate
Inductance plethysmography/strain gauge/magnetometer	Indirect; senses changes in thoracic and abdominal cross-sectional areas due to respiratory muscle contraction	Semiquantitative	Easy to use Amplitude decreases during obstructive apnea or hypopnea (despite increased effort) Paradoxical motion of thorax and abdomen during obstructive apnea or hypopnea

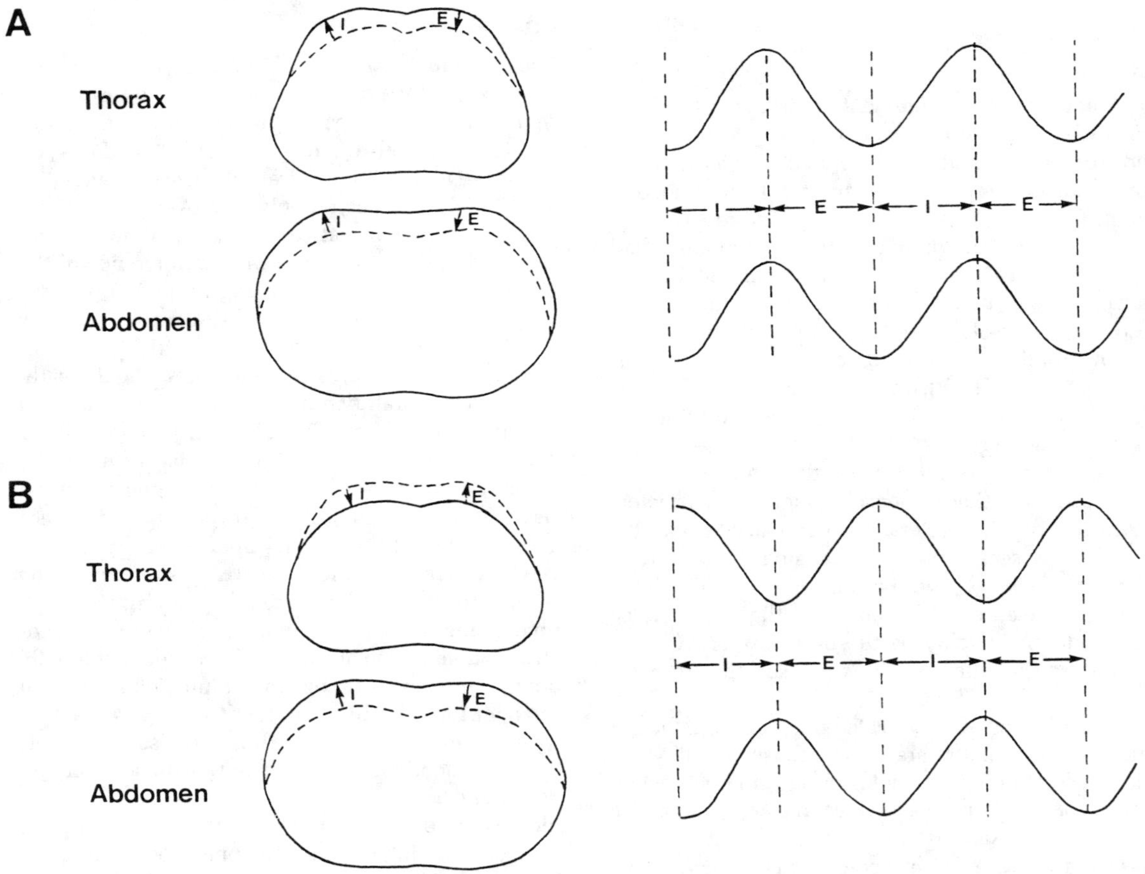

A

Thorax

Abdomen

B

Thorax

Abdomen

FIGURE 9-1.   *The diagrams illustrate changes in cross-sectional area of the thoracic and abdominal compartments during inspiration (I) and expiration (E), and the resultant appearance of polygraph recordings from a respiratory inductive plethysmograph placed around each compartment. (A) Normal synchronous inflation. (B) Paradoxical respiratory motion in the presence of upper airway obstruction.*

activity in the presence of partial or complete upper airway obstruction. Diaphragm or parasternal electromyography (EMG) is limited because reliable recordings are often difficult to obtain from the diaphragm using surface electrodes, and intercostal EMG typically is inhibited during rapid eye movement (REM) sleep. Esophageal pressure provides a reliable, quantitative, and sensitive measure of respiratory muscle mechanical activity, and this has been widely employed for PSG in the past. The requirement for transnasal insertion of a pressure catheter is quite uncomfortable and invasive, however, so this technique has been largely replaced by the indirect methods described earlier.

Monitoring Gas Exchange

Pulse oximetry

It is well known that oxyhemoglobin and deoxyhemoglobin differ in their absorption spectra for visible light. This principle underlies the technique of oximetry by which the degree of hemoglobin saturation by oxygen can be measured by transillumination of an accessible structure such as the earlobe or fingertip. Pulse oximetry is the simplest and most reliable noninvasive method for assessing adequacy of pulmonary gas exchange and has become an essential part of PSG assessment of respiratory disorders of sleep.

Carbon dioxide monitoring

By sampling expired air at the nose, carbon dioxide concentration can be monitored. Under optimal circumstances, end-tidal PCO_2 reflects alveolar PCO_2, and thus arterial PCO_2. End-tidal PCO_2 measurements should be interpreted with caution, however, since dilution of the sampled expired gas with room air (gas is typically sampled at flow rates of 50 to 150 ml per minute) systematically reduces the measured PCO_2. Transcutaneous monitoring of PCO_2 has been utilized in some studies of adults with sleep-disordered breathing, but its use is better established in neonatal monitoring.[11] Because transcutaneous PCO_2 may vary unpredictably from $PaCO_2$, and because of the long response times of the measurements, it is useful principally as a semiquantitative index of trends in alveolar ventilation.

CLASSIFICATION OF DISORDERED BREATHING EVENTS DURING SLEEP

Although respiratory events are identified and classified in various ways by different sleep disorders centers, the most common method requires concurrent measurement of respiratory airflow, respiratory muscle activity, and (in some cases) arterial oxygen saturation. More limited monitoring may be performed in some instances, as during unattended home monitoring, though identification of subtypes of respiratory dysrhythmias with these methods may be less reliable and is not yet considered "standard."

Apneas

In adults, apnea is defined as the absence of airflow for 10 seconds or more.[12-14] Apneas are classified as central, obstructive, or mixed by the concurrent pattern of respiratory muscle activity (Figure 9-2). Central apneas are due to absence of respiratory effort; thus, any measure of respiratory muscle activity is absent. During obstructive apnea, respiratory efforts continue (and indeed increase) while airflow is prevented by upper airway obstruction. Mixed apneas are a variant of obstructive apneas during which respiratory effort is absent for several seconds following the onset of upper airway occlusion. Obstructive apneas are by far the most common type in patients with a clinically significant sleep apnea syndrome. Arterial oxygen saturation characteristically declines during apneas, though the degree of desaturation varies considerably among patients.

Hypopneas

Hypopnea is generally defined as a transient decrease in respiratory airflow. Precise criteria defining such events have provoked disagreement, and several methods have been in common use.[14] One requires only a reduction in airflow of one half or two thirds, though such precision is difficult to apply when a semiquantitative, nonlinear method is used to monitor flow. Others have utilized decreased respiratory excursions measured by an inductive plethysmograph, a decrease in arterial oxygen saturation of 4%, or some combination of these criteria.

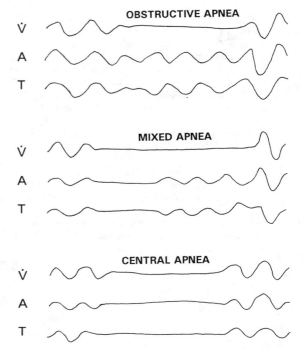

FIGURE 9-2.   *Simultaneous recordings of airflow (V) monitored with a thermistor, and motion of the abdomen (A) and thorax (T) recorded with a pair of circumferential inductive plethysmographic sensors, during an obstructive apnea, a mixed apnea, and a central apnea. Note the paradoxical abdominal and thoracic motion during the obstructive apnea and obstructive portion of the mixed apnea.*

More uncertainty surrounds the question of how to differentiate hypopneas that are predominantly central or obstructive. The most reliable way to achieve this is direct measurement of respiratory muscle activity, such as by esophageal pressure, which decreases during central hypopnea and increases during an obstructive event. Paradoxical motion of the thorax and abdomen is also more common during obstructive hypopneas than during central ones.

REFERENCES

1. Fleetham J, West P, Mezon B, et al. Sleep, arousals, and oxygen desaturation in chronic obstructive pulmonary disease. Am Rev Respir Dis 1982;126:429–433.
2. Cattarall JR, Douglas NJ, Calverley PM, et al. Irregular breathing and hypoxaemia during sleep in chronic stable asthma. Lancet 1982;1:301–304.
3. Smith PEM, Calverley PMA, Edward RHT, et al. Practical problems in the respiratory care of patients with muscular dystrophy. N Engl J Med 1987;316:1197–1204.

4. Garay SM, Rapoport D, Sorkin B, et al. Regulation of ventilation in the obstructive sleep apnea syndrome. Am Rev Respir Dis 1981;124:451–457.

5. Skatrud JB, Dempsey JA, Bhansali P, et al. Determinants of carbon dioxide retention and its correction in humans. J Clin Invest 1980;65:813–821.

6. Hirshman CA, McCullogh RE, Weil JV. Normal values for hypoxic and hypercapnic ventilatory drives in man. J Appl Physiol 1975;38:1095–1098.

7. Rajagopal KR, Abbrecht PH, Tellis CJ. Control of breathing in obstructive sleep apnea. Chest 1984;85:174–180.

8. Cummiskey JM, Williams TC, Krumpe PE, et al. The detection and quantification of sleep apnea by tracheal sound recordings. Am Rev Respir Dis 1982;126:221–224.

9. Peirick J, Shepard JW Jr. Automated apnea detection by computer: Analysis of tracheal breath sounds. Med Biol Eng Comput 1983;21:632–635.

10. Sackner MA. Monitoring of ventilation without a physical connection to the airway. In: Sackner MA, ed. Diagnostic Techniques in Pulmonary Disease. New York: Marcel Dekker, 1980;503–537.

11. McLellan PA, Goldstein RS, Ramcharan V, et al. Transcutaneous carbon dioxide monitoring. Am Rev Respir Dis 1981;124:199–201.

12. Martin RJ, Block AJ, Cohn MA, et al. Indications and standards for cardiopulmonary sleep studies. Sleep 1985;8:371–379.

13. Kurtz D, Krieger J. Analysis of apnea in sleep apnea. In: Guilleminault C, Dement WC, eds. Sleep Apnea Syndromes. New York: Alan R Liss, 1978;145–159.

14. American Thoracic Society Consensus Conference. Indications and standards for cardiopulmonary sleep studies. Am Rev Respir Dis 1989;139:559–568.

10

Measurement of Sleepiness/Alertness: Multiple Sleep Latency Test

Thomas Roth
Timothy Roehrs
Leon Rosenthal

Daytime sleepiness, a common experience for most adults, is the inevitable consequence of inadequate sleep the previous night. Given the universality of the acute experience of daytime sleepiness, it is typically minimized as a serious health problem, but increasingly chronic excessive daytime sleepiness is recognized as an important and significant symptom in medicine. Furthermore, excessive daytime sleepiness can and should be distinguished from fatigue, tiredness, and lassitude, though many patients may not make such distinctions themselves, unless they are carefully queried.

Surveys of the general population have found that between 0.5% and 5% of persons surveyed complain of excessive daytime sleepiness.[1-5] This symptom is associated with a number of different medical, behavioral, and pharmacologic causes, but, regardless of its cause, excessive daytime sleepiness per se has serious social and medical consequences. Nearly half of the patients with excessive sleepiness seen at sleep disorders centers report automobile accidents; more than half report occupational accidents, some life threatening; many have lost jobs because of their sleepiness; and the impact of sleepiness on family life is quite disruptive.[6] Information on traffic and industrial accidents in the general population suggests a link between sleepiness and life-threatening events. For example, the highest rate of automobile accidents occurs in the early morning hours, which is remarkable because fewer automobiles are on the road during these hours.[7] Shift workers, a particularly sleepy subpopulation, have the poorest job performance and the highest rate of industrial accidents of all workers.[8]

Problems in assessing sleepiness became evident during early research on the daytime consequences of sleep loss, before the clinical significance of sleepiness was recognized. Sleep loss compromises daytime functions. Virtually everyone experiences dysphoria and reduced performance efficiency when they do not sleep adequately. The majority of the performance tasks are insensitive to the effects of sleep loss.[9] Only long and monotonous tasks are reliably sensitive to changes in the quantity and quality of nocturnal sleep. Using various measures of mood, including factor analytic scales, the most consistent and systematic response to sleep loss is increased sleepiness. Among the various subjective measures of sleepiness, the Stanford Sleepiness Scale (SSS) is best validated.[10] Yet clinicians have found that patients may rate themselves alert on the SSS even as they are falling asleep.[11]

Normal and pathologic variations in daytime sleepiness and alertness (used as antonyms) can now be directly assessed and quantified by the Multiple Sleep Latency Test (MSLT), a test of the rapidity with which a subject falls asleep in a standardized, sleep-conducive setting, is repeated at 2-hour intervals throughout the day. The MSLT uses standard sleep recording methods to document both the rate of sleep onset and the appearance of rapid eye movement (REM) episodes at sleep onset. Other procedures that have been used to quantify sleepiness/alertness, including pupillometry, subjective rating scales, and tests of vigilance or reaction time, are all correlated to some extent with the MSLT, but because of a variety of shortcomings these are not widely used. The MSLT has become the standard method in clinical sleep disorders medicine for documenting complaints of excessive daytime sleepiness. It is also used to document sleep onset REM periods, a diagnostic sign of narcolepsy. Since the development of the MSLT by Carskadon and Dement in the late seventies[12] enormous progress has been made in the scientific investigation and understanding of both normal and pathologic variations in sleepiness and alertness.

MSLT METHODS

Recording Montage

General and specific technical guidelines for the administration of the MSLT have been previously published.[13] Briefly, the guidelines require that the standard Rechtschaffen and Kales recording montage be used to perform the MSLT.[14] The montage includes the referential electroencephalogram (EEG) from a central (C_3 or C_4) placement, two horizontal referential electrooculograms (EOGs) from right and left outer canthi, and a mental or submental electromyogram (EMG). Additionally helpful in the determination of sleep onset is a referential occipital EEG lead, which shows alpha activity in relaxed wakefulness with eyes closed and is followed by a characteristic change to mixed-frequency EEG activity at the onset of sleep. Also important for sleep onset determination is an EOG recording with filters set to allow visualization of slow rolling eye movements (e.g., 250 milliseconds), another sign of sleep onset.

Procedures

General

As indicated in the guidelines, to ensure a reliable and valid MSLT a number of general procedures are necessary.[13] A 1- or 2-week sleep diary recorded prior to the test and including information on usual bedtime, time of arising, napping, and drug use (i.e., caffeine, alcohol, illicit and licit drugs) is very helpful. Deviations from the subject's habitual sleep behavior should be noted, since sleep time accumulated or lost over the week prior to an MSLT can significantly affect the result. Central nervous system (CNS)–active drugs, as well as their discontinuation, can alter sleep and REM latencies and should be discontinued well in advance of the test, to avoid direct or residual effects. The sleep of the night preceding an MSLT should be documented with a standard nocturnal sleep recording. This nocturnal sleep recording should be scheduled to coincide with the timing and amount of the subject's usual sleep, as revealed in the diary.

The reliability of the MSLT is based on multiple determinations of sleep latency, as the studies discussed below have shown. Consequently, as indicated in the guidelines, four or five tests of sleep latency at 2-hour intervals throughout the day should be conducted.[13] Testing should be initiated 1½ to 3 hours after the nocturnal sleep period has been terminated, typically at 09:30 or 10:00 AM. The MSLT should be conducted in a sleep-conducive environment, quiet, dark, and at a comfortable temperature. Any potentially arousing stimuli should be removed from the test area.

Specific

The procedures specified by the guidelines for conducting the MSLT are these:[13] After arising from nocturnal sleep, the subject should toilet, dress in street clothes, and eat the usual breakfast (avoiding caffeinated beverages). Between the latency tests the subject should be kept out of the bed and monitored by technical staff to ensure that no napping occurs. Preparations for each latency test include smoking cessation 30 minutes before lights out, suspension of physical activity 15 minutes before lights out, bedtime preparation (removing shoes and restrictive clothes such as belt or necktie) at 10 minutes before lights out, all electrode connections and calibrations completed at 5 minutes before lights out, and the instructions to relax and fall asleep 5 seconds immediately before lights out, followed by lights out.

Ending a test

According to the guidelines, if sleep does not occur each test is concluded 20 minutes after lights out.[13] For the clinical version of the MSLT, in which the occurrence of REM sleep is at question, the test is concluded 15 minutes after the first 30-second epoch of sleep. In a research version of the MSLT, the test is concluded after three consecutive 30-second epochs of stage 1 sleep or one 30-second epoch of another sleep stage. When the recording is equivocal, it is safer to allow clearer signs of sleep (i.e., spindles and K complexes) to emerge rather than to terminate the test prematurely.

Scoring and Interpretation

Criteria for scoring sleep onset differ from those for test termination.[13] There has been some confusion in the MSLT literature in this regard; further, it should be noted that the MSLT sleep latency criteria differ from the typical definition of nocturnal sleep onset (stage 2 sleep or 10 continuous minutes of sleep) in much of the all-night sleep literature. MSLT sleep latency is the elapsed time in minutes from lights out to the first 30-second epoch scored as sleep. According to the scoring criteria of Rechtschaffen and Kales,[14] this implies that 16 seconds of sleep (i.e., more than 50% on a given epoch of the recording) is sufficient to score a sleep onset. REM sleep latency in a clinical test is scored as minutes from sleep onset (as defined above) to the first epoch of REM sleep.

Average sleep latency (minutes) for the four or five latency tests is the parameter typically used to express the level of sleepiness. In some of the clinical literature the MSLT result is expressed as a median sleep latency or a sleepiness index, which is merely the average latency subtracted from 100 and multiplied by 100% (corrected if fewer than five tests are conducted). The occurrence of REM sleep within 10 to 15 minutes of sleep onset is generally defined as a sleep-onset REM period (SOREMP), and the frequency of such SOREMPs is also tabulated.

Sources of Error

The level of sleepiness (defined as the average sleep latency) observed on the MSLT is affected by the sleep of the previous night and of the previous weeks. Any deviation from the subject's habitual sleep schedule (as revealed in the sleep diary) and sleep quality (as seen in the nocturnal sleep recording and the individual's estimate of its consistency with his usual sleep) is likely to overestimate or underestimate the usual level of daytime sleepiness. Similarly, the timing of the nocturnal sleep and daytime MSLT assessment relative to the subject's circadian phase is a potential source of error (an issue in studying shift and night workers). Out-of-phase sleep is likely to be disturbed and, so, associated with shorter MSLT latencies. Also, sleep latency itself varies as a function of circadian phase.

Sedating or alerting effects of drugs or discontinuation of long-term drugs can also be a source of error in documenting sleepiness. For some patients a urine drug screen may be necessary to confirm the absence of drugs. A noisy or stimulating test environment also invalidates an MSLT result. Instructions given to the subject at the initiation of the test are also important. Subjects should be aware that they are to close their eyes, lie still, and allow sleep to occur. Excessive tossing and turning are to be avoided. It should be recognized that the instruction *relax and fall asleep* may be emotionally loaded for patients with insomnia. This issue is discussed in the validity section.

Finally, while this has not yet been systematically studied, a possible "last-test" effect can be observed. In anticipation of going home for the day, subjects remain awake for the 20 minutes of the last latency test. The last-test effect could elevate the average sleep latency for the day. It can be avoided by scheduling other nonarousing activities after the last latency test. Scheduling a patient feedback session with the clinician, either before or after the last test, can be disruptive to that test and should be avoided.

REM sleep can also erroneously occur during the MSLT, and there are several important considerations. Many drugs suppress REM sleep, and discontinuing them increases the likelihood of SOREMPs on a MSLT. The circadian phase timing of the MSLT is also important with respect to the occurrence of REM sleep. REM sleep can occur on early morning latency tests in a person who is a late morning sleeper. Excessive disturbance of the sleep of the previous night also has the potential to result in REM sleep on early morning latency tests. For example, it has been suggested that apnea patients with highly fragmented sleep may have more SOREMPs than the general population. Thus, SOREMPs should be reevaluated in apnea patients if narcolepsy is suspected. However, it is unlikely that sleep restriction the week previous to an MSLT is likely to alter REM occurrence.

RELIABILITY AND VALIDITY

Reliability

Several studies of the reliability of the MSLT have been conducted. In healthy normal persons who maintained consistent sleep-waking schedules, the test-retest reliability of a four-test MSLT was .97 over a 4- to 14-month test-retest interval.[15] The test-retest interval (6 months or less versus more than 6 months) and the level of sleepiness (average latency 5 or less minutes versus 15 minutes or more) did not affect this MSLT reliability. The *number* of latency tests did alter MSLT reliability: the coefficient dropped to .85 for three tests and .65 for two tests. Another study of patients with insomnia over an interval of 3 to 90 weeks found a test-retest correlation of .65 on a five-test MSLT.[16]

There has also been interest in the test-retest reliability of SOREMPs in patients with narcolepsy. The current criteria require two or more SOREMPs out of five possible sleep onsets. In the only study done to date, 13 of 14 patients had two or more SOREMPs when retested ($\kappa = .62$, $P < .05$). Of interest, the REM latency on SOREMPS during the initial evaluation was also correlated to that during retesting ($r = .64$, $P < .02$).[17]

Validity

Determinants of daytime sleepiness

A number of different causes of pathologic sleepiness have been identified. The degree of daytime sleepiness is directly related to the amount of nocturnal sleep. Partial or total sleep deprivation in healthy normal subjects is followed by increased sleepiness the following day, which can reach pathologic levels.[18] Furthermore, modest sleep deprivation (as little as 1 hour per night) accumulates over time to progressively increase daytime sleepiness, again to pathologic levels.[19] On the other hand, in healthy normal young adults increased sleep time—

extending time in bed beyond the usual 7 or 8 hours per night—produces increased alertness (i.e., reduction in sleepiness).[20]

Daytime sleepiness also relates to the quality and continuity of the previous night's sleep. Sleep in patients with a number of sleep disorders is punctuated by frequent, brief arousals of 3 to 15 seconds duration. The arousals typically do not result in awakening, as judged by either Rechtschaffen and Kales sleep staging criteria or behavioral indicators, and the arousals recur in some conditions as often as one to four times per minute.[14] The arousing stimulus differs in the various disorders and can be identified in some cases (apneas, leg movements, pain) though not in others. The critical point is that the arousals generally do not result in shorter sleep, but rather in fragmented or discontinuous sleep, and this fragmentation produces daytime sleepiness.

Correlational evidence suggests a relation between sleep fragmentation and daytime sleepiness.[21] Fragmentation, as indexed by number of brief EEG arousals, number of shifts from other sleep stages to stage 1 sleep or wake, and the percentage of stage 1 sleep, correlate with excessive sleepiness in various patient groups.[22] Experimental fragmentation of the sleep of healthy normal persons has been produced by inducing arousal with an auditory stimulus. Studies have shown that subjects aroused at various intervals during the night demonstrate performance decrements and increased sleepiness on the following day.[23–26]

CNS depressant drugs, as might be expected, increase sleepiness. The benzodiazepine hypnotics hasten sleep onset at bedtime and shorten the latency to return to sleep after an awakening during the night, as demonstrated in a number of objective studies.[27,28] Long-acting benzodiazepines continue to shorten sleep latency on the MSLT the day after if taken at bedtime.[29] Ethanol administered at bedtime reduces latency to sleep and when administered during the daytime, ethanol also reduces sleep latency as measured by the MSLT.[30,31] One of the most commonly reported side effects associated with the use of H1 antihistamines is daytime sleepiness, and studies with objective measurement of sleepiness have confirmed the effect.[32,33]

Disorders of the CNS are assumed to be another determinant of daytime sleepiness. An unidentified CNS disturbance is thought to cause excessive sleepiness in patients with narcolepsy.[34] Another sleep disorder associated with excessive sleepiness and thought to be due to an unknown disorder of the CNS is idiopathic CNS hypersomnolence.[35] In both conditions, although the pathophysiology has not

been definitively established, the excessive sleepiness is well-documented.[36,37]

A number of case series have presented MSLT results in patients with complaints of excessive daytime sleepiness.[38] First, these series have clearly shown that patients with difficulties of excessive sleepiness can be differentiated from healthy normals based on the MSLT results. That is, these patients typically have average sleep latencies of 8 minutes or less, whereas normals usually have average latencies of 10 minutes or more. (Deviations from the norm in healthy adults is discussed later.) Also, SOREMPs are rarely seen in normal persons, while the occurrence of two or more is considered specific to narcolepsy. Second, the data have shown that differences in the severity of some sleep disorders are reflected in different levels of sleepiness on the MSLT. For example, patients with obstructive sleep apnea syndrome who have 40 or more apneas per hour of nocturnal sleep usually have average sleep latencies of 5 minutes or less, whereas those with fewer apneas per hour (20 to 40 per hour) have average latencies of 5 to 8 minutes, sometimes more. Finally, among different sleep disorders associated with excessive daytime sleepiness, a differentiation in levels of sleepiness and frequency of SOREMPs can be seen. Patients with chronic insufficient sleep usually have a more moderate level of sleepiness (5 to 8 minutes) than do patients with narcolepsy or severe obstructive sleep apnea syndrome (no more than 5 minutes). Among sleep disorders patients, only those with narcolepsy show two or more SOREMPs.

The relation of nocturnal sleep and daytime sleepiness (i.e., MSLT scores) in insomnia patients is not as clearly established. Insomnia patients do not necessarily complain of daytime sleepiness as the consequence of their perceived inadequate nocturnal sleep. Often the complaint is fatigue, tiredness, and dysphoria. In fact, some data suggest that insomnia patients may be hyperalert.[39] That is, while showing shortened nocturnal sleep compared to age-matched, healthy controls, this group of insomnia patients has an unusually long average sleep latency (i.e., more than 15 minutes).

Evaluation of therapeutic interventions

A number of studies have shown that MSLT levels in various sleep disorders are improved following appropriate therapeutic intervention. Two current treatments of obstructive sleep apnea syndrome are continuous positive airway pressure (CPAP) and uvulopalatopharyngoplasty (UPPP). CPAP provides a pneumatic splint of the airway, eliminating the upper airway obstructions and thus the brief arousals that fragment sleep. This improved sleep is associated with normalization of the MSLT.[40] UPPP, a surgical treatment aimed at removing excess upper airway tissue and thus establishing a patent airway, is less consistently successful. In patients who benefit from the surgery apneas are reduced, sleep is improved, and the MSLT level of sleepiness is normalized,[41] but in patients whose apnea does not improve, the MSLT result remains at presurgery levels, even though patients perceive a subjective improvement in alertness. This once again indicates the inaccuracy of subjective assessments of sleepiness/alertness.

MODIFICATIONS

The basic MSLT procedure has been modified in various ways, with no clear improvement. The first such modification was a change in the instructions to *try and stay awake*.[42] The instruction did produce longer sleep latencies, but the change did not increase sensitivity over that of the MSLT. A subsequent variation has been termed the Maintenance of Wakefulness Test (MWT), in which the instruction *Stay awake* is given to subjects while they are seated in a chair rather than lying in bed.[43] Again, longer latencies to stay awake are found, but improvement over the MSLT has not been documented. Finally, the Modified Assessment of Sleepiness Test (MAST) has been offered as an alternative to the MSLT.[44] It consists of three standard sleep latency tests (with a *Try to sleep* instruction) alternating with two tests of the ability to remain awake while seated in a chair reading a book. As indicated above, MSLT reliability begins to decline as the number of tests is reduced, as in the MAST. Improved sensitivity has not been established for the MAST.

The intent of all these MSLT modifications is to measure a subject's ability to remain awake. It is argued that, clinically, the patient's problem is remaining awake (which adds a certain face validity to the instruction to remain awake, but the ability to stay awake is a complex function of many factors, which can momentarily override the underlying physiologic state—motivation to remain awake, presence of competing motives, conduciveness of the environment, and time of day. Consequently, the ability to maintain wakefulness varies much between individuals and hour by hour within an individual. No single laboratory test is "generalizable" to the variety of circumstances under which wakefulness is to be maintained. The MSLT attempts to remove the confounding factors and measure the underlying physiologic state, thus defining the patient's maximal risk.

MSLT NORMS

Enough data on the MSLT have now been collected in normal and patient populations to describe the range of normal and abnormal values. In several reports of healthy, noncomplaining adults using a four-test MSLT, subjects aged 21 to 35 years had an average daily sleep latency of 10 minutes, adults aged 30 to 49 years had average latencies of 11 to 12 minutes, and subjects 50 to 59 years old averaged a latency of 9 minutes.[45,46] In the older subjects, nocturnal sleep efficiency was lower than that of the other age groups, and periodic leg movements during sleep were observed in 50% of the sample. In samples of healthy normal persons some have latencies in the pathologic range (no more than 5 minutes). However, they differ from sleep disorders patients in that the sleepiness is not persistent. With adequate sleep over a number of nights, the average daily sleep latency increases, reaching the population norm.[47]

Evidence for pathologic sleepiness is considered to be an average daily sleep latency of no more than 5 minutes. An average latency of 5 to 8 minutes is considered borderline pathologic. Latencies of 9 minutes and greater are considered normal.

REFERENCES

1. Karacan I, Thornby JI, Anch M, et al. Prevalence of sleep disturbance in a primarily urban Florida county. Soc Sci Med 1976;10:239–244.
2. Bixler ED, Kales JD, Scharf MB, et al. Incidence of sleep disorders in medical practice: A physician survey. Sleep Res 1976;5:160.
3. Lavie P. Sleep habits and sleep disturbances in industrial workers in Israel: Main findings and some characteristics of workers complaining of excessive daytime sleepiness. Sleep 1981;4:147–158.
4. Bixler ED, Kales A, Soldatos CR, et al. Prevalence of sleep disorders in the Los Angeles metropolitan area. Am J Psychiatry 1979;136:1257–1262.
5. Lugaresi E, Cirignotta F, Zucconi M, et al. Good and poor sleepers: An epidemiological survey of the San Marino population. In: Guilleminault C, Lugaresi E, eds. Sleep/Wake Disorders: Natural History, Epidemiology, and Long-Term Evolution. New York: Raven Press, 1983;2–12.
6. Navelet Y, Anders T, Guilleminault C. Narcolepsy in children. In: Guilleminault C, Dement WC, Passouant P, eds. Narcolepsy. New York: Spectrum, 1976;171–177.

7. Lavie P, Wollman M, Pollack I. Frequency of sleep-related traffic accidents and the hour of the day. Sleep Res 1986;15:275.

8. Folkard S. Shiftwork and performance. In: Johnson LC, Tepas DI, Colquhoun WJ, Colligan MJ, eds. The Twenty-Four Hour Workday: Proceedings of a Symposium on Variations in Work-Sleep Schedules. DHHS Publication No. (DIOSH) 81–127, Washington, DC: US Government Printing Office, 1981;347–373.

9. Webb WB. Sleep deprivation: Total, partial and selective. In: Chase MH, ed. The Sleeping Brain. Los Angeles: Brain Information Service/Brain Research Institute, University of California at Los Angeles, 1972;323–362.

10. Hoddes E, Zarcone VP, Smythe H, et al. Quantification of sleepiness: A new approach. Psychophysiology 1973;10:431–436.

11. Dement WC, Carskadon MA, Richardson GS. Excessive daytime sleepiness in the sleep apnea syndrome. In: Guilleminault C, Dement WC, eds. Sleep Apnea Syndromes. New York: Alan R Liss, 1978;23–46.

12. Carskadon MA, Dement W. The multiple sleep latency test: What does it measure? Sleep 1982;5:S67–S72.

13. Carskadon MA, Dement WC, Mitler M, et al. Guidelines for the Multiple Sleep Latency Test (MSLT): A standard measure of sleepiness. Sleep 1986;9:519–524.

14. Rechtschaffen A, Kales A: A Manual of Standardized Techniques and Scoring System for Sleep Stages of Human Sleep. Los Angeles: Brain Information Service/Brain Research Institute, University of California at Los Angeles, 1968.

15. Zwyghuizen-Doorenbos A, Roehrs T, Schaefer M, et al. Test-retest reliability of the MSLT. Sleep 1988;11:562–565.

16. Seidel WF, Dement WC. The Multiple Sleep Latency Test: Test-retest reliability. Sleep Res 1981;10:105.

17. Rosenthal LD, Krstevska S, Murlidmar A, et al. Reliability of sleep onset REM periods in narcolepsy. Sleep Res 1992;21:254.

18. Carskadon MA, Dement WC. Nocturnal determinants of daytime sleepiness. Sleep 1982;5:S73–S81.

19. Carskadon MA, Dement WC. Cumulative effects of sleep restriction on daytime sleepiness. Psychophysiology 1981;18:107–113.

20. Carskadon MA, Dement WC. Sleepiness during extension of nocturnal sleep. Sleep Res 1979;8:147.

21. Carskadon MA, Brown E, Dement WC. Sleep fragmentation in the elderly: Relationship to daytime sleep tendency. Neurobiol Aging 1982;3:321–327.

22. Stepanski E, Lamphere J, Badia P, et al. Sleep fragmentation and daytime sleepiness. Sleep 1984;7:18–26.

23. Bonnet MH. The effect of sleep disruption on performance, sleep, and mood. Sleep 1985;8:11–19.

24. Bonnet MH. Performance and sleepiness as a function of the frequency and placement of sleep disruption. Psychophysiology 1986;23:263–271.

25. Stepanski E, Salava W, Lamphere J, et al. Experimental sleep fragmentation and sleepiness in normal subjects: A preliminary report. Sleep Res 1984;13:193.

26. Levine B, Roehrs T, Stepanski E, et al. Fragmenting sleep diminishes its recuperative value. Sleep 1987;10:590–599.

27. Roth T, Zorick F, Wittig R, et al. Pharmacological and medical considerations in hypnotic use. Sleep 1982;5:S46–S52.

28. Nicholson AN. The use of short- and long-acting hypnotics in clinical medicine. Br J Clin Pharmacol 1981;11:615–695.

29. Roth T, Roehrs T. Determinants of residual effects of hypnotics. Accid Anal Prevent 1985;17:291–296.

30. MacLean A, Cairns J. Dose-response effects of ethanol on the sleep of young men. J Stud Alcohol 1982:43:433–444.

31. Zwyghuizen-Doorenbos A, Roehrs T, Lamphere J, et al. Increased daytime sleepiness exacerbates ethanol's sedative effects. Sleep Res 1987;16:160.

32. Roehrs T, Tietz E, Zorick F, et al. Daytime sleepiness and antihistamines. Sleep 1984;7:137–141.

33. Nicholson AN, Stone BM. Antihistamines: Impaired performance and the tendency to sleep. Eur J Clin Pharmacol 1986;30:27–32.

34. Kilduff TS, Bowersox SS, Kaitin KI, et al. Muscarinic cholinergic receptors and the canine model of narcolepsy. Sleep 1986;9:102–106.

35. Association of Sleep Disorders Centers. Diagnostic Classification of Sleep and Arousal Disorders, ed. 1. Sleep 1979;2:1–137.

36. Zorick F, Roehrs T, Koshorek G, et al. Patterns of sleepiness in various disorders of excessive daytime somnolence. Sleep 1982;5:S165–S174.

37. Coleman R, Roffwarg H, Kennedy S, et al. Sleep-wake disorders based upon a polysomnographic diagnosis—a national cooperative study. JAMA 1981;247:997–1103.

38. Roth T, Roehrs T, Carskadon M, et al. Daytime sleepiness and alertness. In: M Kryger, T Roth, WC Dement, eds. Principles and Practice of Sleep Medicine. Philadelphia: WB Saunders, 1989;14–23.

39. Stepanski E, Zorick F, Roehrs T, et al. Daytime alertness in patients with chronic insomnia compared with asymptomatic control subjects. Sleep 1986;11:54–60.

40. Lamphere J, Roehrs T, Wittig R, et al. Recovery of alertness after CPAP in apnea. Chest 1989;96:1364–1367.

41. Zorick F, Roehrs T, Conway W, et al. Effects of uvulo-palatopharyngoplasty on the daytime sleepiness associated with sleep apnea syndrome. Bull Eur Pathophysiol Res 1983;19:600–603.

42. Hartse KM, Roth T, Zorick FJ. Daytime sleepiness and daytime wakefulness: The effect of instruction. Sleep 1982;5:S107–S118.

43. Mitler MM, Gujavarty KS, Browman CP: Maintenance of wakefulness test: A polysomnographic technique for evaluating treatment efficacy in patients with excessive somnolence. Electroencephalogr Clin Neurophysiol 1982;53:658–661.

44. Erman MK, Beckham B, Gardner DA, et al. The Modified Assessment of Sleepiness Test (MAST). Sleep Res 1987;16:550.

45. Levine B, Roehrs T, Zorick F, et al. Daytime sleepiness in young adults. Sleep 1988;11:39–46.

46. Roehrs T, Zorick F, McLeaghan A, et al. Sleep and MSLT norms for middle adults. Sleep Res 1984;13:87.

47. Roehrs T, Timms V, Zwyghuizen-Doorenbos A, et al. Sleep extension in sleepy and alert normals. Sleep 1989;12:449–457.

11

Ambulatory Cassette Polysomnography

W. Vaughn McCall
Gail R. Marsh
C. William Erwin

A multichannel cassette recorder suitable for polysomnography (PSG) became available in 1971, and the first report of successful ambulatory PSG came 2 years later, when Wilkinson and Mullaney described recording a PSG on a train.[1] Since then, the growth and acceptance of ambulatory PSG has progressed as techniques, indications, and limitations have been clarified.

Ambulatory PSG implies freedom of movement for the patient. Nevertheless, the sleep literature continues to lump ambulatory PSG with telemetry and home-bound recording units that require the patient to stay within a few feet of the bed, either because of limited radio frequency broadcast range or the need for telephone transmission. In comparison, ambulatory cassette PSG can be recorded in the home, in an inpatient setting, or ad lib in the community. *Home recording* and *ambulatory recording* can coincide but are not synonymous. This chapter focuses on ambulatory cassette PSG and covers other noncassette ambulatory technology and cassette home recordings only indirectly.

THEORETICAL BASIS

In 1983, Oxford Medical, Ltd. introduced the eight-channel Medilog 9000 series cassette ambulatory recording and playback units (PBU) as an advance over existing four-channel systems. Our clinical experience has been with these systems, so they will be described in detail. Although the instrument was designed primarily as an electroencephalographic (EEG) recording device because of its continuous 24-hour recording capability, it was easily adaptable to PSG studies. The direct current 40-Hz system passband allowed for standard PSG parameters of chin electromyography (EMG), EEG, electrooculography (EOG), as well as electrocardiography (ECG), leg EMG, and impedance and thermistor respirometry. The 9200 series was introduced in 1989 and is fundamentally the same as the 9000. The newer model is based on a personal computer with software, providing a "windows"-like environment. The redesigned recorders are lighter, smaller, (1 pound and 5 by 4 by 1.5 inches) and quieter but continue the blocked analog recording of eight channels of physiology on audio (C-120) tape cassettes. Twenty-four hours' recording is achieved by a very slow tape transport speed (2 mm/sec). When played back at multiples of real time, the subauditory biologic signals are accelerated into the human auditory range. New software releases are more easily distributed via floppy disk, as compared to replacing a ROM, as required in the 9000 series. Automated sleep scoring became available on the 9000 series via a separate dedicated microprocessor using parallel processing. The same scoring system is available on the 9200 series using a 286 or 386 processor with the same algorithm. A separate analysis package is available for the multiparameter recorder that has built-in oximetry.

The PBU is the size of a personal computer and simultaneously displays all 8 channels of data and the corresponding time. The PBU replays the data at 20, 40, or 60 times real time. A minimum playback speed of 20 times is required to retrieve activity from analog tape. The PBU displays 16-second "pages" of data from the continuously moving tape transport onto the screen. The 20-, 40-, or 60-times display can be frozen at any time to inspect details of waveforms. Similarly, the PBU can present one page at a time, though this is a time-consuming strategy for reading an entire record because of the excessive time required to start and stop the tape transport at each page. The PBU also allows printing of portions or the entire record on paper in real time to a polygraph or a laser printer. This is rarely required in clinical PSG situations (though it is for clinical epilepsy).

The PBU provides stereo audio output (to headphones, external speakers, or a monaural internal speaker). Most frequencies of the waking and sleeping EEG fall well below the 20-Hz threshold of human hearing. By increasing tape transport speed in the PBU to at least 20 times real time, these EEG frequencies are accelerated into the audible range. A 10-Hz alpha wave becomes 200, 400, or 600 Hz, corresponding to 20-, 40-, or 60-times transport speed. The audible EEG (and other) signals are of great value in scoring PSG, as we detail later.

Independent of clinical considerations, ambulatory cassette PSG offers several logistic advantages over standard paper PSG. First is the sheer volume of space saved in storing clinical PSG. Second, cassettes are more easily transported or mailed than paper PSG. Third, a single technician can connect three patients in an afternoon, and no staff is required during night hours. Finally, the analog data on tape can be redigitized to allow on-line analysis of sleep events by computer that are otherwise laborious to quantify (counting spindles, slow waves, and eye movements). There are, of course, mixed blessings as well. It may be tempting to use computer analysis of basic sleep stages from the cassette, but the current position of the American Sleep Disorders Association (ASDA) requires human scoring.[2] Our experience with the Medilog automated scoring indicates it is generally accurate in scoring stage 2 and slow-wave sleep but makes frequent and clinically unacceptable errors in discriminating wakefulness, stage 1, and rapid eye movement (REM) sleep from each other. Apparently, the computer algorithms have difficulty when the data departs in minor ways from the programmers' concepts. Fortunately, the 9200 series allows for editing of the computer-scored data or direct entry of human-scored data. We do the latter by combination auditory-visual analysis (described later). Number keys when depressed enter a desired epoch of a sleep stage until a different key is pressed. The different stages are registered on the screen at the rate of tape playback in the form of a hypnogram.

TECHNIQUES OF RECORDINGS

The application of the ambulatory recorder to the patient deserves detailed attention because of the prolonged time of attended recording and the consequent risk of technical failures. The comments and suggestions that follow are based on our experience with more than 1450 ambulatory cassette PSGs during the last 6 years in clinical, research, and normative subject data collection.

Although they are capable of a full 25 hours' of monitoring, we usually apply the cassette recorders in the afternoon and remove them between 8:00 and 9:00 A.M. the following day. The technologist uses the remaining hours to clean electrodes, check returned recorders for proper operation, and put 20 minutes of 100-μV sine wave calibration on each tape (25 μV in the case of chin EMG). Patients are instructed to come to the laboratory with a freshly shampooed head to which no hair spray or tonic has been applied. The head is measured according to the 10-20 international system and is marked at C_3, C_z, and O_z.

The montage employed necessarily depends in large measure on what clinical suspicions are being investigated through PSG and is adapted to the limited number of channels available. We use a standard EEG recorder with two channels of EEG, two channels of EOG, and one chin EMG for the staging of sleep architecture. When PSG is used in the assessment of insomnia, we screen for periodic leg movements of sleep (PLMS) and apnea; thus, our three remaining channels are committed to left and right anterior tibialis EMG and a nasal-oral thermistor. Our montage order is as follows: nasal-oral thermistor, left leg EMG, right leg EMG, chin EMG, C_3-M_2, O_z-C_z, left EOG, right EOG. The EOG channels are superior oblique, referenced to the ipsilateral mastoid (M). This montage brings the polysomnographer's visual focus to the middle of the screen and avoids placing channels that often saturate in channel 7 or 8, where interference with the timing channel (9) can occur with saturation in either 7 or 8. Alternative montages (e.g., ECG) are deployed if clinical considerations merit it.

A 15-inch electrode lead is needed to reach C_3 and C_z, and an 8-inch lead is sufficient for O_z when the patient has short hair. Fifteen-inch electrode leads are preferable at all scalp sites if the patient has long hair. Six-foot electrode leads are required to reach the anterior tibialis at midcalf when screening for PLMS. Two reference electrodes (M_1 and M_2) and two grounds are used; this redundancy guards against losing the entire study if a single electrode lead is lost. We are now using disposable silver chloride electrodes for the EOG, chin EMG, and mastoid references (Hewlett Packard #40426A). The disposable electrodes are more quickly applied, more comfortable, and adhere better in these sites than metal cup electrodes.

The metal scalp electrodes are held in place with collodion. A lock of hair pulled over the top of the electrode and secured with additional collodion provides insurance against dislodgement. Electrode impedances are checked and must be less than 5000 Ω (preferably between 2000 and 3000 Ω).

The input cable from the recorder is run under the patient's shirt or blouse and undergarments to a collar that holds the input jacks. The leg electrodes are brought up from the legs, under the patient's undergarments and wrapped around the collar to provide strain relief against dislodgement. The functioning of each channel of the recorder is checked by having patients close their eyes, look up, look down, move the left leg, and so on. As patients prepare to leave, we instruct them not to chew gum, as this generates excessive artifact, not to immerse the device in liquid, and to complete a standard sleep diary on waking in the morning. If patients' urinary continence or cooperation is suspect, the recorder is placed in a zip-lock bag and sewn shut, to guard against moisture and patient curiosity. With practice, the attachment procedure can be completed in 60 to 90 minutes.

Upon patients' return to the laboratory the following morning, the collodion is removed with acetone. Some patients may be instructed in how to remove the electrodes at home. Upon its return, the PSG tape is briefly reviewed on the PBU for technical quality, against the possibility that a repeat study is required because of technical failure.

In the last 3 years we have experienced only 14 failures in 849 records (1.6%). The most frequent causes of failure include the patient removing the electrodes early (secondary to claustrophobia or dementia), immersion of the recorder in liquid (urine), or tape wrapping around the capstan of the tape transport. Patients tolerate the procedure well, and the most serious problem has been minor skin reactions to skin abrasion, collodion, or tape used to hold the electrodes in place. We have treated these with local application of hydrocortisone cream.

The ambulatory technique allows PSG to be recorded at a distant satellite laboratory without a clinical sleep specialist and sent later to an accredited sleep laboratory. The position of the ASDA, however, prohibits satellite recordings without on-site supervision of a clinical sleep specialist.[3]

SCORING AND DATA REDUCTION

In addition to evaluating nocturnal sleep, ambulatory PSG allows the sleep clinician to inspect daytime sleep propensity and sleep hygiene. To this end, the entire recording is scanned from the time patients leave the laboratory until they return. We have previously shown that sleep parameters generated from human rapid scanning (20 times) of the Medilog 9000 series cassette PSG correlate well with the standard sleep parameters derived from standard paper scoring.[4] In most instances, correlations greater than 0.95 were found, except in differentiating stage 2 from slow-wave sleep. Scoring in the rapid scanning mode is greatly facilitated by listening to the corresponding auditory output of the EEG channels. Each sleep stage has characteristic and readily identifiable sounds. The Medilog 9000 scanner stores data in a buffer before it is presented to a screen. The auditory signal is presented as the data enters the buffer and therefore precedes the visual record by several seconds. This scoring method, combining auditory and visual cues, is highly reproducible, with greater than 90% epoch-to-epoch agreement.[5]

At 60 times real time, the auditory signature of alpha rhythm is typified by nearly continuous droning of 480 to 660 Hz with little variation in pitch. As the patient drifts into stage 1, the tone becomes intermittent and interspersed with random sputtering, as the alpha attenuates and drops out. This quickly proceeds to include higher-pitched, intermittent 800- to 900-Hz chirping sounds, indicating the arrival of sleep spindles and stage 2. As slow-wave sleep approaches, a low, insistent 30- to 120-Hz rumbling (delta activity) mounts to an intensity suggesting a passing train, almost obliterating the gentle chirping of sleep spindles. The audible onset of REM sleep often precedes the earliest visual indications of this stage. This stage is quiet by comparison, reminiscent of the sound of wind blowing through pine trees. REM sleep's termination is usually announced by the reappearance of chirping spindles or the "crashing wave" white noise of a movement arousal (EMG).

Non-EEG channels also have characteristic aural qualities worth monitoring. The anterior tibialis EMG channels are usually quiet during sleep, but the rhythmic white noise discharge of PLMS immediately draws the attention of the polysomnographer. Occasionally a leg channel is sacrificed to allow a channel of ECG. The sharp peaks of the QRS complex present an irritating "buzzsaw" sound. The pitch of this noise rises and falls with accelerations and decelerations of the heart rate. This would be useful primarily for detecting the bradyarrhythmias or tachyarrhythmias that accompany obstructive sleep apnea, periods of asystole, or other irregularities of cardiac rate. The pitch of slow, undulating rhythms such as respiration and oximetry is too low to be heard without special equipment. For initial screening of a PSG, we prefer placing the output of C_3-M_2 and both anterior tibialis EMGs in our left ear and O_z-C_z in our right ear. Many artifacts also have characteristic aural qualities. Among the most common are the noisy, rhythmic white noise (EMG) discharges of chewing and the intermittent monotone 60-cycle interference of an electric blanket.

The trained polysomnographer can learn to use the rapid scanning combined visual-auditory method in a few hours. The efficiency of this method is underscored by the realization that at 60 times scanning, an 8-hour PSG can be initially reviewed in 8 minutes. This efficiency is compromised, however, if the polysomnographer interrupts the continuous flow of the rapid scanning to write down the various shifts in sleep stage and at what time they occur. We initially answered this problem by developing computer software to register the stage shifts as determined by a human scorer without distracting the scorer's attention. The PBU and computer are started at the same initial time, and the computer then maintains synchrony with the PBU. As the scorer identifies PSG stage shifts he depresses appropriate keys on the computer keyboard to register the corresponding stage changes. The computer, in effect, is functioning as an electronic secretary. At the end of the record, our computer software analyzes the raw human scored epoches to produce PSG parameters and a hypnogram. This approach combines the best of both worlds: hands-on human scoring and computer-assisted registry and calculation of sleep parameters. The Medilog 9200 has incorporated these functions, so an additional computer is not needed. The PBU can now simultaneously control tape transport functions and register human-entered stage changes.

CLINICAL APPLICATIONS

Ambulatory cassette PSG is tolerated well by the majority of patients and is preferred over standard in-house PSG by most patients who have had both. Only 18% of the first 339 patients in our laboratory complained that the apparatus significantly disturbed their usual sleep pattern, while 82% indicated their sleep was disturbed little or not at all.[6] While improving patient acceptance of PSG procedures, the ambulatory system may offer a more accurate picture of patients' sleep and eliminate the need for multiple recording nights, as practiced in some laboratories. Agnew and colleagues reported in 1966 that the first night of PSG sleep in a laboratory was not representative of subsequent nights.[7] This phenomenon was coined the *first-night effect* (FNE). The FNE includes lengthening of sleep onset latency and REM latency and an increase in the percentage of wakefulness and stage 1 sleep. These changes suggest that the first night's sleep in the laboratory is more restless, perhaps secondary to the sleeper's failure to immediately accommodate to the novel surroundings, the discomfort of the monitoring apparatus, and the presence of the technician.

To avoid the FNE, some laboratories conduct two or more consecutive nights of PSG to get a more representative appraisal of the patient. One advantage of the ambulatory cassette PSG is the marked reduction of FNE. Sharpley and colleagues examined the PSG of 12 normal subjects over three consecutive nights using the Medilog 9000.[8] No difference between the first and subsequent nights was noted for any parameters. The study suffered, however, from the use of computer scoring rather than hand scoring. Sharpley and coworkers repeated the study with PSGs scheduled once a week for 3 weeks and again found no difference between the first and subsequent nights.[9] This study, again, used only computer scoring.

We have recently examined the FNE in a group of 20 older insomniacs undergoing ambulatory PSG over three consecutive nights using the Medilog 9000.[10] All PSGs were completed after 2 weeks' or more abstinence from sleep-altering medications. We found no significant difference between the first and subsequent nights with regard to total sleep, wakefulness, sleep stage percentages, or latencies. These insomniacs did demonstrate large intraindividual variations from night to night. The lack of an FNE is postulated to be secondary to attaching the monitoring equipment hours in advance of bedtime allowing for acclimation, to the patient's familiarity with his own bed, and to the absence of an observing technician.

Despite these advantages for insomniacs, application of ambulatory PSG to a broader range of sleep clinic patients will depend on quality and ease of collection of respiratory data, as sleep apnea is the most common final diagnosis made in sleep centers. Standard PSG assessment of suspected sleep apnea requires one or more channels of EEG, two channels of EOG, chin EMG, a nasal airflow channel, an oral airflow channel, a thoracic effort channel, an abdominal effort channel, oximetry, ECG, two optional channels of anterior tibialis EMG, and recording of body position. This montage obviously exceeds the capacity of an eight-channel cassette recorder. Advocates of ambulatory assessment of sleep apnea have approached this problem either by expanding the number of recording channels or by sacrificing "unnecessary" channels. A new Medilog design will allow two eight-channel recorders to be linked together, to permit 16 channels of total capacity. Oxford Medilog also provides for synchronization of a standard eight-channel ambulatory recorder with a nonambulatory eight-channel "multiparameter" recorder continuing oximetry and respiratory effort channels. This later device is heavy (7 kg), because of the oximeter's requirement for the large current flow from nickel cadmium batteries. The display of 16 channels of EEG, EOG, ECG, EMGs, or thermistor monitoring may be viewed simultaneously on the 9200 PBU. Some specialized types of information, however, (e.g., oximetry, temperature) require special processing by the 9200 PBU and are not available for viewing in any raw data form.

Investigators who employ only one eight-channel cassette recorder often sacrifice standard PSG parameters (EEG, EOG, chin EMG,) to accommodate airflow, respiratory effort, ECG, and oximetry. Ancoli-Israel recently reviewed her experience with 1000 ambulatory cassette studies using a limited montage.[11] The limited montage appeared highly sensitive in uncovering apneic or PLMS episodes, and she thus concluded, "A diagnosis of sleep apnea and a determination of the severity of apnea can be accomplished without sleep stage information."[11] Peter and coworkers have also shown that ambulatory cassette recording omitting standard PSG parameters successfully captures apneic events.[12] Other commercial systems employ microprocessor recorders (instead of cassettes), omitting standard PSG measures in the study of sleep apnea. Comparison of simultaneous recordings using microprocessors and standard PSG have shown a high correlation in the two methods' ability to categorize apnea as absent, mild, or severe.[13,14] An example of an apneic event, as recorded by ambulatory cassette PSG, is shown in Figure 11-1.

Despite these successes, ambulatory assessment of apnea, omitting EEG, EOG, and chin EMG is compromised. Milder cases of sleep apnea may have apneic episodes confined to REM periods. This observation cannot be made in the absence of standard PSG data. Other variants of apnea may not be manifested unless the patient sleeps on his back. Such patients may respond to various behavioral position training techniques. If the patient does not spontaneously assume the supine position, it is desirable to have a technician present to roll the patient into position. The technician also is needed to reposition electrode leads dislodged by the apnea patient's body movements. Without a technician present, we have found that rarely more than 50% of the thermistor

tracing is interpretable for apnea patients. Finally, the technician's firsthand observation of disordered breathing is invaluable, and a technician is required later to titrate nasal continuous positive airway pressure (CPAP) if this treatment is elected. In summary, we agree with McDannold and colleagues[14] that ambulatory cassette assessment of sleep apnea is best reserved for use as an initial diagnostic test in patients with suspected severe sleep apnea, or for "follow-up of patients after initial CPAP titration or after surgical correction of obstructive sleep apnea."[14] As in adult sleep apnea, ambulatory cassette PSG may be useful for assessing apneic events in children with sudden infant death syndrome (SIDS), but this work is still preliminary.[15,16]

Broughton recently reviewed his investigations of ambulatory cassette PSG in the primary hypersomnias.[18] The foremost advantage of this method is using a full 24-hour recording to assess daytime sleep propensity and the total amount of sleep obtained in 24 hours. Broughton's[17] ambulatory studies have confirmed that narcolepsy patients have more disturbed and less nocturnal sleep, sleep more during the day, but get no greater total amount of sleep. Similar results are described by De Groen and associates.[18] Broughton's subjects followed ad lib

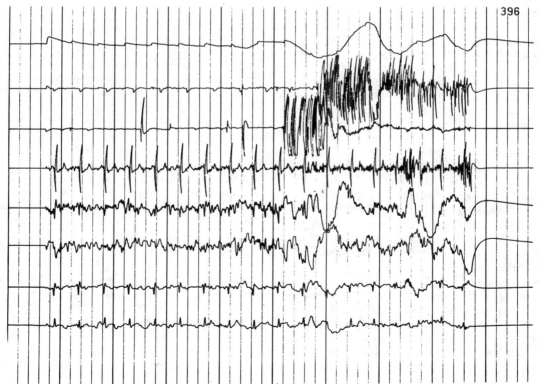

FIGURE 11-1. *Sleep apnea event terminated by an arousal as recorded by ambulatory cassette PSG. PSG montage: channel 1, nasal-oral thermistor; 2, left anterior tibialis EMG; 3, right anterior tibialis EMG; 4, chin EMG; 5, C_3-M_2; 6, O_z-C_z; 7, left EOG; 8, right EOG.*

behavior during these studies and demonstrated an average of 2.9 daytime naps. Surprisingly, the average duration of their longest daytime nap was 81 minutes, an observation that challenges the tenet that narcoleptics uniformly take brief naps. Fewer than half of the naps demonstrated a sleep-onset REM period, suggesting spontaneous naps monitored with ambulatory technique may be less robust than a standard multiple sleep latency test (MSLT) in identifying REM onsets.

Attempts to use ambulatory cassette recording for home MSLTs have been complicated by unanticipated disruptions at home that interfere with the MSLT protocol.[17] Other problems might include additional napping between scheduled MSLT naps. In summary, ambulatory cassette PSG may be useful in assessing narcolepsy but should not substitute for the standard MSLT. Reports of use of ambulatory cassette PSG for less common varieties of primary hypersomnia such as idiopathic hypersomnia or Kleine-Levin syndrome are few. Nevertheless, ambulatory PSG would be expected to provide valuable information on the 24-hour sleep-wake pattern in this group.

We are unaware of reports of ambulatory cassette recording to assess parasomnias, despite the possible advantages of ambulatory studies for following the progression of sleep-wake transitions during a parasomnia episode. In many instances the technician's firsthand observation or video recording is likely to be as useful as PSG data. Bennett and colleagues have shown that nocturnal penile tumescence may be registered on a Medilog ambulatory recorder,[19] but home studies would lack important measures of buckling force, and there would be no technician to reposition the easily dislodged mercury strain gauges.

Our laboratory's primary research interest has been evaluation of insomnia with ambulatory cassette PSG. Insomniacs tolerate the procedure well, and patients that have had both standard and ambulatory PSG prefer the latter.[6] As outlined above, interpretable records can be obtained 98% of the time with proper technique. Further, ambulatory PSG successfully separates groups of insomniacs and matched controls—revealing longer sleep latencies, more wakefulness, and more stage 1 in the insomniac group.[20] We have already noted some of the limitations of ambulatory PSG in the assessment of sleep apnea, parasomnias, and the MSLT. These limitations generally do not apply to the evaluation of insomnia. Sleep apnea infrequently contributes to complaints of insomnia, and the technician usually is not needed to document behavior in insomniac patients. On the contrary, ambulatory recording in the home environment may reveal the interplay of the patient and conditioned arousal stimuli. Some sleep clinicians believe that the vast majority of insomnia is secondary to psychological disorders and have questioned the necessity for PSG in the evaluation of insomnia.[21,22] Jacobs and colleagues, however, reviewed the preliminary diagnoses of 123 insomniacs undergoing standard PSG and found the PSG results "added to, refuted, or failed to support the clinical impression" in 49% of cases.[23] We have also pursued this issue using ambulatory cassette PSG.[24] We reported the results of evaluation of 100 outpatient insomniacs undergoing a thorough medical, psychiatric, behavioral, and ambulatory PSG evaluation. Eight-two percent of the PSGs were completed after a two-week drug-free interval. Two sleep clinicians formulated a consensual sleep diagnosis before the results of the PSG were known using only clinical data. The PSG results were subsequently found to yield important additional diagnostic information in 65% of the sample. The sleep diagnosis that most often went undetected by clinical examination alone was PLMS disorder associated with arousals and sleep fragmentation. The clinicians were able to predict PLMS disorder in only 14 of 25 cases revealed by PSG. In general, older insomniacs were more likely to have unsuspected PSG findings. Insomniacs with neurologic findings may also be more likely to have PLMS on their PSG.[25]

Because in insomniacs PSG may be most useful for clarifying PLMS disorder, we have focused on assessment of PLMS using ambulatory technique. Ambulatory Medilog recordings of PLMS were first described by Pollak and colleagues.[26] Ancoli-Israel and colleagues have simultaneously studied PLMS using both ambulatory cassette and standard PSG and demonstrated good correlation between the methods in detecting the leg movements.[27] We recently recruited twenty-three patients thought to have primary insomnia to complete three consecutive nights of ambulatory cassette PSG.[28] Eleven subjects showed no PLMS on any night, while the remaining twelve showed PLMS on all 3 nights. As a group, the 12 patients with PLMS disorder showed no FNE for either the number of movements per hour of sleep (movement index, MI) or the number of movement-related arousals per hour (AI). Individuals showed some intrasubject night to night variability in the MI ($r = 0.77$) and AI ($r = 0.8$), but not enough to affect the International Classification of Sleep Disorders (ICSD) PLMS severity rating between night 1 and night 2 in more than 80% of the cases.[29] Although standard PSG parameters, MI, and AI show considerable random night-to-night variability in insomnia, there are no FNEs with ambulatory technique, and a single night of recording is usually sufficient for clinical purposes. Research specifically addressing variability in insomnia may require multiple study nights.

An example of PLMS as recorded by ambulatory cassette PSG is shown in Figure 11-2.

We have concluded that ambulatory PSG provides useful clinical information on insomnia. Test yield is improved by selecting patients who are older, have neurologic findings, or whose problem is refractory to treatment.

This case illustrates several points from our discussion:

A Case Report

A 43-year-old man had been in excellent health without any sleep-related complaint until he developed persistent severe headaches. Brain imaging revealed a pituitary-hypothalamic mass. A cystic craniopharyngioma extending to the third ventricle was subsequently excised. There were no postoperative surgical complications, but an immediate change was apparent in the patient's vegetative drives—he lost his sex drive, and his appetite became ravenous. During the following 4 months the patient's weight increased from 165 to 220 pounds. His wife noted excessive sleep during the day. The patient denied any problem.

Upon presentation to our sleep clinic the patient appeared superficially normal except for frequent yawning and a healed craniotomy scar behind the hairline. He denied ancillary symptoms of narcolepsy. Our preliminary differential diagnoses included sleep apnea versus an unusual postsurgical hypersomnia related to the other obvious disturbances of hypothalamic function. We began the evaluation with a 24-hour ambulatory cassette recording.

During this recording the patient had more than 15 naps between noon and midnight accumulating to 3.5 hours' sleep. The patient denied having slept during the day. No sleep-onset REM periods were noted. During the nocturnal recording period, the patient gained an additional 7.5 hours' sleep fragmented by frequent apneas as detected by the single channel of thermistor. The thermistor was intermittently out of position, so a full assessment of severity was impossible. The patient subsequently completed a standard PSG, confirming position-dependent apnea with mild desaturation and an MSLT that revealed mean nap latency of 3.5 minutes and no REM. When the results were discussed with the patient, the finding of 3.5 hours' unremembered daytime sleep

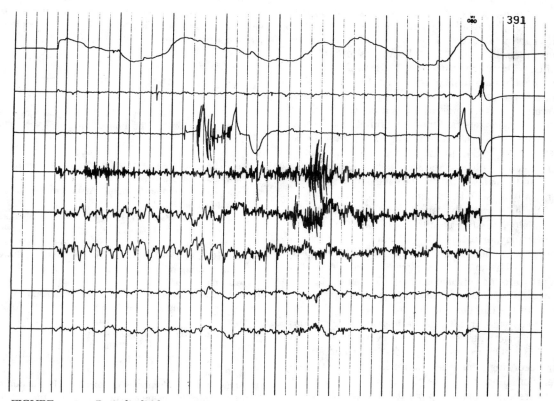

FIGURE 11-2. *Periodic limb movement with associated EEG arousal as recorded by ambulatory cassette PSG. PSG montage: channel 1, nasal-oral thermistor; 2, left anterior tibialis EMG; 3, right anterior tibialis EMG; 4, chin EMG; 5, C_3-M_2; 6, O_z-C_z; 7, left EOG; 8, right EOG.*

was the most important factor in the patient's acceptance of his diagnosis of sleep apnea and treatment.

This case underscores the following points: (1) Ambulatory PSG provides critical data on "daytime" functioning. (2) Ambulatory PSG may be sensitive in detecting severe apnea but is liable to technical problems and is less adequate for mild apnea. (3) The ambulatory and standard PSG each provide different, and complementary, types of clinical data.

RESEARCH IN THE FREE ENVIRONMENT

Perhaps the greatest contributions of ambulatory PSG will come in the field rather than in clinical assessment. The durable and portable Oxford Medilog recorders will document human physiology under adverse conditions that may only be speculated about in the fixed laboratory environment. Consider the 24-hour monitoring of nine mountaineers in Nepal as they ascended from 4115 to 6220 meters.[30] Twenty-nine recordings were completed, and all were interpretable. The study demonstrated decrements in slow-wave sleep with increasing altitude.

The dangers of sleep deprivation and shift work can be fully revealed only with ambulatory monitoring. Torsvall and coworkers conducted 24-hour Medilog recordings in 25 mill workers on rotating shifts.[31] During the night shift, 20% of the workers took involuntary naps of mean duration of 43 minutes. These dangers would be magnified for transportation workers such as cockpit crews. Rosekind and associates reported modification of the Medilog recorder to allow clean recording in the cockpit of a 747 jetliner.[32] Cockpit crew members who took a scheduled in-flight nap were subsequently more alert and took fewer involuntary naps than members who took no scheduled nap.[33]

We have recently reported on the continuous ambulatory cassette monitoring of two professional tennis players before, during, and after a world record marathon singles tennis match lasting 146 hours.[34] The match was played in Myrtle Beach, South Carolina between 8:10 A.M. September 25 and 10:10 A.M. October 1, 1988. The high temperatures were in the eighties and humidity was high. Technologists were in attendance to reapply electrodes and change batteries and tapes every 24 hours. A total of 356 hours' recording were made, and 99% of the recording time was interpretable despite the adverse circumstances. The players were allowed only 2 hours' scheduled sleep per day, which was virtually all slow-wave with minimal REM.

The players additionally succumbed to microsleeps during court changes, thus revealing their sleepiness. This study demonstrates the resiliency of ambulatory recording while confirming in a "real-world" situation many premises regarding sleep deprivation derived from laboratory work.

CONCLUSIONS

Ambulatory cassette PSG complements other standard laboratory assessments of sleep apnea, primary hypersomnias, and insomnia. In disorders of excessive daytime sleepiness its primary utility is in diagnosis of suspected severe sleep apnea, follow-up assessment after intervention for sleep apnea, or preliminary overnight PSG before MSLT. Ambulatory PSG may be used as the primary tool for evaluating insomnia. Its advantages include patient comfort and convenience, potential cost savings, elimination of the FNE, ease of sleep stage scoring with the auditory transformation of the EEG, and simplicity of data handling and storage. Success in achieving interpretable studies hinges on the diligence of the technician. Liabilities of the ambulatory PSG are the absence of a technician to make technical corrections and behavioral observations and the limited number of channels. Use of the ambulatory cassette PSG in the field may confirm laboratory models of real problems and provide new insights into socially relevant sleep-wake issues such as sleep deprivation.

REFERENCES

1. Wilkinson RT, Mullaney D. Electroencephalogram recording of sleep in the home. Postgrad Med 1976; 52:92–96.
2. Lemmi H. The use of computers in accredited centers and laboratories—a clarification. Assoc Prof Sleep Soc Newslett 1990;5(2):15.
3. Lemmi H. Accreditation notes. Assoc Prof Sleep Soc Newslett 1990;5(3):20.
4. Hoelscher TJ, McCall WV, Powell J, et al. Two methods of scoring with the Oxford Medilog 9000: Comparison to conventional paper scoring. Sleep 1989;12:133–139.
5. Erwin CW, Ebersole JS, Marsh GR. Combined auditory-visual scoring of polysomnographic data at 60 times real time. J Clin Neurophysiol 1987;4:214.
6. Hoelscher TJ, Erwin CW, Marsh GR, et al. Ambulatory sleep monitoring with the Oxford Medilog 9000: Technical acceptability, patient acceptance, and clinical indications. Sleep 1987;10:606–607.
7. Agnew HW, Webb WS, Williams RL. The first night effect: An EEG study of sleep. Psychophysiology 1966; 2:263–266.
8. Sharpley AL, Solomon RA, Cowen PJ. Evaluation of first night effect using ambulatory monitoring and automated sleep stage analysis. Sleep 1988;11:273–276.
9. Sharpley AL, Solomon RA, Cowen PJ. Sleep stability with home sleep recording and automated sleep stage analysis. Sleep 1990;13:538–540.

10. Edinger JD, Marsh GR, McCall WV, et al. Sleep variability across consecutive nights of home monitoring in older mixed DIMS patients. Sleep 1991;14:13–17.

11. Ancoli-Israel S. Ambulatory cassette recording of sleep apnea. In: Ebersole JS, ed. Ambulatory EEG Monitoring. New York: Raven Press, 1989;299–315.

12. Peter JH, Fuchs E, Kohler U, et al. Studies in the prevalence of sleep apnea activity (SAA): Evaluation of ambulatory screening results. Eur J Respir Dis 1986;69(suppl 146):451–458.

13. Lucas EA, Bradshaw CM, Burk JR, et al. Comparison of a 4-channel recorder to polysomnography (PSG) as a screening device in a sleep disorders center [Abstr]. Sleep Res 1990;19:369.

14. McDannold MD, Scharf MB, Fletcher MS, et al. A comparison of the Edentech 2700 multichannel recorder with polysomnography in patients with obstructive sleep apnea. Sleep Res 1990;19:372.

15. Cornwell AC, Weitzman ED, Marmarou A. Ambulatory and in-hospital continuous recording of sleep state and cardiorespiratory parameters in 'near miss' for the sudden infant death syndrome and control infants. Biotelemetry 1978;5:113–122.

16. Pierano P, Lacombe J, Kastler B, et al. Night sleep heart rate patterns recorded by cardioneumography at home in normal and at-risk for SIDS infants. Early Hum Dev 1988;17:175–186.

17. Broughton RJ. Ambulatory sleep-wake monitoring in the hypersomnias. In: Ebersole JS, ed. Ambulatory EEG Monitoring. New York: Raven Press, 1989;277–298.

18. De Groen JHM, Koper H, Bergs PPE, et al. Ambulatory sleep-wake polygraphy in narcolepsy. Electroencephalogr Clin Neurophysiol 1985;60:420–422.

19. Bennett T, Evans DF, Hosking DJ. A technique for monitoring penile erections during sleep as a basis for investigating the problem of erectile impotence. In: Stott FD, Raftery EB, Sleight P, et al., eds. ISAM 1987 Proceedings of the Second International Symposium on Ambulatory Monitoring. London: Academic Press, 1978;273–280.

20. McCall WV, Edinger JD, Krystal A, et al. Ambulatory polysomnographic differences in healthy and insomniac older men. J Ambulatory Monit (in press).

21. Soldatos CR, Kales A, Kales JD. Management of insomnia. Annu Rev Med 1979;30:301–312.

22. Kales A, Bixler EO, Soldatos CR, et al. Biopsychobehavioral correlates of insomnia, part 1: Role of sleep apnea and nocturnal myoclonus. Psychosomatics 1981;23:589–600.

23. Jacobs EA, Reynolds CF, Kupfer DJ, et al. The role of polysomnography in the differential diagnosis of chronic insomnia. Am J Psychiatry 1988;145:346–349.

24. Edinger JD, Hoelsher TJ, Webb MD, et al. Polysomnographic assessment of DIMS: Empirical evaluation of its diagnostic value. Sleep 1989;12:315–322.

25. McCall WV, Edinger JD, Marsh GR, et al. Neurologic findings in patients with periodic limb movements. Neuropsychiatry Clin Neurosci 1991;3:429–430.

26. Pollak CP, Coleman RM, Kokkoris CP, et al. New techniques for recording and displaying long term EMG data: Application to ambulatory patients with nocturnal myoclonus [Abstr]. Sleep Res 1979;8:271.

27. Ancoli-Israel S, Kripke DF, Mason W, et al. Comparisons of home sleep recordings and polysomnograms in older adults with sleep disorders. Sleep 1981;4:283–291.

28. Edinger JD, McCall WV, Marsh GR, et al. Variability of periodic movements of sleep in subjects studied with ambulatory technique [Abstr]. Sleep Res 1990;19:219.

29. Diagnostic Classification Steering Committee, Thorpy MJ. International Classification of Sleep Disorders: Diagnostic and Coding Manual. Rochester, Minn: American Sleep Disorders Association, 1990.

30. Finnegan TP, Abraham P, Docherty TB. Ambulatory monitoring of the electroencephalogram in high altitude mountaineers. Electroencephalogr Clin Neurophysiol 1985;60:220–224.

31. Torsvall L, Akerstedt T, Gillander K, et al. 24H ambulatory EEG recording of sleep/wakefulness in shift work [Abstr]. Sleep Res 1987;16:256.

32. Rosekind MR, Townsend B, Rountree M, et al. Modification of the Medilog 9000-II recorder to reduce 400 Hz noise in the cockpit environment [Abstr]. Sleep Res 1990;19:377.

33. Rosekind MR, Connel LJ, Dinges DF, et al. Preplanned cockpit rest: EEG sleep and effects on physiologic alertness. Sleep Res 1991;20:129.

34. Edinger JD, Marsh GR, McCall WV, et al. Daytime functioning and nighttime sleep before, during, and after a 146-hour tennis match. Sleep 1990;16:526–532.

12

Sleep Scoring Technique

Merrill M. Mitler
J. Steven Poceta
Barbara G. Bigby

Continuous recordings of electroencephalographic (EEG), electrooculographic (EOG), and electromyographic (EMG) activity are required for the modern classification of wakefulness, rapid eye movement (REM) sleep, and non-REM (NREM) sleep.

Since the first days of EEG recordings, EEG potentials were thought to depend somehow on electrical activity generated by brain cells. Exactly what brain cell activity, however, and the mechanisms by which electrical signals are picked up at the site of an electrode are not yet completely understood. It is now certain, however, that the relatively brief action potentials generated when a neuron fires are not significantly involved. Rather, EEG waves are thought to represent volume-conducted summations of the excitatory and inhibitory postsynaptic potentials (EPSPs and IPSPs) that constantly occur on cells of the cerebral cortex closest to the recording electrode. The most common neurons involved are thought to be the pyramidal cells found in layers III and V of the cerebral cortex. Pyramidal neurons have long apical dendritic structures projecting from above to the cell body as well as axons projecting below the cell body. Desynchronized or activated EEG patterns, then, are produced when the numbers of simultaneous EPSPs and IPSPs are relatively equal, yielding small and rapid changes in the voltages as recorded from the scalp. Synchronized or deactivated EEG patterns, by contrast, arise when the numbers of simultaneous EPSPs and IPSPs yield large, slow changes in the voltages as recorded from the scalp. In contrast with standard EEG procedures, polysomnographic (PSG) scoring into wakefulness, NREM stages 1 through 4, and REM sleep usually requires only the C_3-A_2 or C_4-A_1 and O_1-A_2 or O_2-A_1 derivations of the many derivations defined by the 10-20 system.

The EOG recording depends on the retinocorneal potential; that is, the back of the eye (retina) is electronegative relative to the front of the eye (cornea). When the eyeball moves, it is as if a battery (dipole) is moving in space. If the cornea is moving toward an electrode, it will register a positive potential, and vice versa. Typical EOG electrode sites for the active electrode in PSG are the outer canthi, and perhaps above and below each orbit. The usual reference electrode is the opposite ear lobe (A_1 or A_2).

The EMG recording depends on the summation of electrical potentials generated when individual muscle fibers contract. For sleep staging in PSG, selection of the muscle group to record is based on the presence of appropriate levels of muscle tone during NREM sleep, against which loss of tone can be documented during REM sleep. Other factors important in selection include ease of access and comfort for the patient. The overwhelming best choice are the muscle groups just below the chin; that is, the digastric and submental muscles. Because of unreliable tonus during NREM sleep, a poor second choice for humans is the muscles in the back of the neck. The EMG recordings in PSG are usually bipolar, with both electrodes positioned 2 to 4 cm apart over the muscle group to be recorded.

EARLY APPROACHES TO EEG STAGING

Soon after bioelectric potentials were recorded from the human scalp, attention was directed to how the patterns of EEG potentials correlate with behavior. Early investigators focused on EEG changes as humans went from wakefulness to sleep and were unaware of the existence of REM sleep. At Harvard University the group of Loomis, and at the University of Chicago the group of Blake, both devised systems to categorize EEG patterns by utilizing the frequency and amplitude of brain activity.[1,2] The Gibbs and Gibbs atlas (1950) also categorized the EEG along the dimension of depth.[3]

The discovery of REM sleep, previously referred to as paradoxical sleep, led to the routine recording of eye movements and muscle tension when monitoring sleep and required restructuring and reconceptualization of sleep staging. For example, the notion of sleep depth had to be operationally defined along some dimension of the intensity of the arousing stimulus, and measurements had to be taken in both NREM and REM sleep.

SCORING SYSTEMS

The Rechtschaffen and Kales System

In 1968, Rechtschaffen and Kales published guidelines for the standardization of terminology and sleep staging methods in humans.[4] This technique has been used since, and continues to be the standard by which sleep is analyzed.

Terminology and technique employ the international EEG 10-20 electrode placement system.[5,6] Based on EEG, chin muscle EMG, and eye movements measured by electrodes placed near the eyes, the following stages can be recognized, as well as their prominent features:

Stage wakefulness. The EEG contains alpha activity (8 to 13 Hz) and/or low-voltage, mixed-frequency activity.
Stage 1. A relatively low-voltage, mixed-frequency EEG without REMs.
Stage 2. Relatively low-voltage, mixed-frequency EEG background with 12 to 14 Hz sleep spindles and K complexes.
Stage 3. Moderate amounts of high-amplitude, slow-wave activity.
Stage 4. Large amounts of high-amplitude, slow-wave activity.
Stage REM. A relatively low-voltage, mixed-frequency EEG in conjunction with episodic REMs and low-amplitude EMG.

NREM sleep refers to stages 1 through 4. Some laboratories utilize the term *movement time* to refer to portions of the record where movement (muscle) artifact obscures the underlying brain potentials. Many laboratories that deal only with adult subjects consider such periods wakefulness.

For details of the technical aspects, the reader is referred to the Rechtschaffen and Kales manual.[4] In brief, the EEG recording should utilize a paper speed of at least 10 mm/sec, and most laboratories utilize this speed, though 15 mm/sec and 30 mm/sec allow for greater analysis of rapid EEG waveforms, especially epileptiform activity. Filter settings must allow an adequate pen response, and sensitivities should allow for a pen deflection of 7.5 to 10 mm for a 50-μV signal. The manual bases the sleep stages in part on EEG waveform amplitudes, and thus a standard electrode array must be utilized, namely, a central electrode (C_3 or C_4) referenced to the opposite ear (mastoid, A_2 or A_1). An occipital lead is useful for optimizing and recognizing the alpha rhythm. Bipolar montages and recording from other areas of the brain have specific applications but are not needed for routine scoring of sleep stages.

The Rechtschaffen and Kales system is an "epoch-by-epoch" approach to the scoring of human sleep. An epoch is a given amount of time chosen to be both convenient and realistic. Usually, an epoch is one page, and this one page may represent 20 or 30 seconds, depending on paper speed (15 or 10 mm/sec, respectively). In general, epochs are scored as one stage, depending on the majority of the epoch. Thus, short-lived changes may not enter into the analysis at all. For example, a person who is having repetitive arousals lasting 5 seconds and occurring every 25 seconds would be scored as having continuous sleep, and thus the total amount of "waking" time would be underestimated. Alternatively, a patient could show "sleep" records for 12 seconds and then arouse or move for, say, 18 seconds, and all epochs would show waking, thus underestimating the total sleeping time. These are more than just technical points, because these short-lived stage changes clearly have meaning for the restorative aspects of sleep, but the Rechtschaffen and Kales method cannot adequately analyze them, as it was developed principally for scoring normal sleep. When pathologic processes are present, certain modifications are necessary, and simply staging sleep does not give all the necessary information. The concept of *transitional sleep* was proposed recently, in an effort to quantify periods of sleep with very frequent stage transitions.[7] This method is not yet in common use but has the advantage of avoiding the rigidity of a fixed epoch scored as only one stage. Our laboratory also pays attention to short-lived sleep stage changes, mostly by counting the number and type of arousals and noting their relation to various other aspects of the PSG, such as stage preference and body position.

COMPUTERIZED METHODS OF EEG ANALYSIS AND SLEEP STAGE SCORING

Computerized methods have attempted to manage the large amount of analog data an overnight sleep study generates, as well as to minimize the amount of time required to accurately score and analyze a PSG study. Several commercially available systems appear adequate for the routine sleep staging of relatively normal sleepers, though when sleep EEG is disrupted, as by sleep apnea or drug-related spindling and fast activity, hand scoring is the only reliable method for sleep staging.

One important development is increasing availability of quantified EEG technology.[8] Utilizing digital transformation techniques, the EEG signal is transformed into individual frequency bands of varying power. Quantified EEG permits detailed analysis of the EEG power attributable to, for example, alpha wave activity or delta activity. Such analyses can be done to compare from night to night, from treatment condition to treatment condition, from patient to patient, or even from electrode to electrode.

CLINICAL METHOD

At our center, all PSGs are hand scored for both sleep stages and pathologic events such as apneas, periodic leg movements, abnormal REM structure, or unusual arousals.

Sleep Staging

We follow the Rechtschaffen and Kales guidelines exactly, and have summarized them below. We hand-score the records in 30-second epochs, and the scorer uses a worksheet on which are preprinted the epoch numbers, with two spaces next to the epoch number on which to record both the sleep stage and any pathologic event. The scorer records the sleep stage at any time there has been a change, and records each event, such as arousing apneas. Occasionally, when the record shows a monotonous pattern of repetitive apneas, we simply score a representative portion of the record for events and formal staging. The portions of the record scored, perhaps 60 to 120 minutes, should contain all sleep stages and sleeping positions the patient achieves.

As is well-known, sleep is staged into 20- or 30-second epochs, and these epochs are considered both independently and in the context of preceding and succeeding epochs. Sleep is a continuous and dynamic process; very few patterns change suddenly. Thus, our examination of sleep into 30-second epochs is somewhat artificial from the outset but is a practical, and reasonably realistic, means of describing the physiologic process.

Stage W, wakefulness, is scored when the EEG shows either an alpha rhythm or a lower-voltage, mixed-frequency EEG, perhaps with beta potentials (> 13-Hz activity). The stage can also usually be recognized because of the high chin EMG tone, frequent REMs and blinks, and sometimes frequent body movements. Sometimes the alpha rhythm is prominent and of high voltage, and sometimes it can barely be discerned. The major problem in subjects who have no well-defined alpha rhythm is deciding when to score stage 1. Usually, some slowing of the EEG can be seen in combination with rolling eye movements and lessening of the chin EMG.

Stage 1 sleep is scored when, by definition, there is a relatively low-voltage, mixed-frequency EEG with a prominence of activity in the 2- to 7-Hz range. This stage occurs most often in the transition from wakefulness to other sleep stages, or following a body movement or arousal. Usually, this stage is short lived, perhaps lasting only a few minutes. Vertex sharp waves and higher-voltage theta activity can be recognized, usually near the end of this stage, but scoring of stage 1 requires absence of K complexes and sleep spindles. Slow (rolling) eye movements are often recognized, both during drowsiness and wakefulness when an alpha rhythm is present and during early stage 1. Sometimes these movements are "fast," but they should never be truly saccadic, as in REM sleep or wakefulness. Usually, stage 1 is a transition stage from wakefulness to stage 2 or REM sleep, and is scored when more than 50% of the epoch is characterized by stage 1 features. Typically, one observes rolling eye movements and mild decreases in EMG muscle tone as the alpha rhythm "breaks up" and yields to the slower, lower-voltage theta patterns of stage 1 sleep.

Stage 2 sleep is defined by the presence of sleep spindles or K complexes and the absence of high-amplitude slow waves sufficient to define stages 3 and 4. The definition of a sleep spindle requires 12- to 14-Hz activity occurring for at least 0.5 second. K complexes are triphasic potentials defined as well-delineated negative sharp waves followed by a positive component and lasting more than 0.5 second. Certain definitions of the K complex require it to be immediately followed by spindle frequencies, but this is not part of the Rechtschaffen and Kales criteria. The K complex is maximal in the vertex region and is often associated with a potentially arousing stimulus such as a noise. Other EEG patterns that may be identified during this stage include lambdoid waves, also known as positive occipital sharp transients of sleep. Positive occipital sharp transients of sleep are not specific to stage 2, however, and may be seen during other NREM stages.

Because of the transient nature of the sleep spindle and K complexes, long intervals may occur between these events, and the definition of stage 2 sleep allows as much as 3 minutes of *stage 1 epochs* between spindles or K complexes. If more than 3 minutes of EEG patterns consistent with stage 1 sleep occur the area is to be scored as stage 1. If an arousal occurs during the 3 minutes between spindle and K complexes, then the epochs up to the arousal are scored as stage 2 and those after the arousal are scored independently (usually as wakefulness or stage 1). This rule, and similar guidelines for scoring REM sleep in long periods between eye movements, typify the fact that not all epochs can be scored independently and scoring often depends on their context.

Stage 3 and stage 4 sleep, also known as slow-wave or delta sleep, take their definition from the delta wave. These are EEG waveforms that usually begin late in stage 2 and are 2 Hz or slower with a minimum amplitude of 75 μV (peak to peak). They must be distinguished from K complexes. Stage 3 is scored when an epoch contains 20% to 50% slow waves, and stage 4 is scored when the epoch has more than 50% slow waves. In borderline epochs it is often necessary to actually measure (perhaps by underlining) the slow waves in the epoch. The definition refers to actual time during the slow waves, not to lower-amplitude portions between slow waves. Seed spindles and K complexes may or may not be present in these stages.

When scoring is performed carefully, fairly high interscorer reliability is reported for scoring slow-wave sleep, but in actual practice we find that the reliable scoring of stage 3 often depends on the experience of the scorer. It is not always practical to measure all borderline epochs, and thus in each laboratory a standard develops which, ideally, is quite close to the published Rechtschaffen and Kales guidelines. Another area that causes confusion is the amplitude criteria. It is well known that a variety of conditions affect the measured amplitude of EEG signals. Some of these include the local biophysical properties of the skull. Additionally, with aging there is a tendency for a decrement in amplitude of the slow waves seen in sleep, owing, at times to both pathologic and nonpathologic processes. If the minimum amplitude criterion is not applied, significantly more slow-wave sleep might be scored, as in the case of elderly persons who have some cerebral atrophy. The Rechtschaffen and Kales committee decided for a variety of reasons to retain the minimum amplitude criterion, in part to remain consistent with previous research and in part to force a more explicit and exact definition of these sleep stages. This does not disallow others from analyzing studies with other criteria, but such differences must be specifically noted.

Stage REM is identified by the appearance of a relatively low-voltage, mixed-frequency EEG, low chin EMG, and rapid (saccadic) eye movements. The EEG pattern resembles that of stage 1, though there should not be as many vertex sharp waves or other high-voltage waveforms. Notched theta waves, appearing in bursts (so-called sawtooth waves) are characteristic. Alpha activity may occur and may be more prominent than in stage 1.

The chin EMG level often causes problems in scoring REM. Obviously, this measurement is not quantitative, so relative levels are assessed. Ideally, chin tone is highest in wakefulness, lower in stage 1,

lower yet in stages 2, 3, and 4, and very low in stage REM. Sometimes this is not true, and chin tone can increase in sleep (e.g., with bruxism, tension headaches), but if REM sleep is to be scored, the *chin EMG cannot be relatively elevated;* that is, it must be as low as or lower than the EMG seen elsewhere in the record. Technically, a problem often develops if the gain setting is such that the chin EMG appears too low during wake or NREM. In that case, one may not be able to see the drop in tone that should occur during REM. Thus, it is important to keep the gain on the chin EMG amplifier as high as is practically possible during any NREM stage. This often necessitates changing gain just after the patient falls asleep, to minimize pen damage and ink splattering.

Certain problems occur in regard to scoring the beginning and ending of REM periods, sleep spindles, long periods without eye movements, and arousals within a REM period. As in the case of sleep spindles, the manual states that any section of record contiguous with stage REM in which the EEG shows relatively low voltage and mixed frequency is scored REM, regardless of whether REMs are present, provided the EMG remains at the REM level and there are no intervening arousals. However, if two spindles occur with no intervening eye movements, that portion of the record between the spindles can be considered stage 2 and is scored as such if the amount of time between spindles is sufficient to influence a full epoch or epochs. The problem with the beginnings and endings of REM periods is that the three determinants of the stage, EEG, EOG, and EMG, do not change simultaneously. Several possibilities thus exist, which are illustrated in detail in the Rechtschaffen and Kales manual.[4]

SLEEP EEG SCORING IN RELATION TO PATHOLOGIC EVENTS

The basic rules of Rechtschaffen and Kales pertain to the scoring of sleep stages, even if pathologic events such as apneas occur. Epochs are still scored by the majority of the epoch. In general, we score (pathologic) events only during sleep, though clearly many events, particularly periodic leg movements, occur during wakefulness. These events must be noted by the technician and taken into account when formulating a final diagnosis and treatment plan, but they are not counted by the technician or used in calculating indices (e.g., respiratory disturbance index).

Respiratory Events

When apnea occurs, the patient is usually in a state of sleep, though we have clearly seen snoring and apneas while the EEG continues to show alpha activity, albeit with rolling eye movements. Occasionally the apneas are brief enough that an entire epoch cannot be scored as sleep, despite repetitive apnea. This is a special situation about which one cannot make rules and that requires the judgment of a polysomnographer.

A respiratory event is scored when there is a decrease or cessation of airflow for 10 seconds or longer. In our laboratory, we consider the total loss of airflow to be an apnea, and a decrease of any other amount (subtotal) to be hypopnea. Most definitions require a decrease of at least 50% of resting, prehypopnea airflow, but we find this too strict, for three reasons. First, a thermistor is not a calibrated or quantitative measure of actual airflow. Second, we often utilize end-tidal carbon dioxide as our measurement. Last, even minimal decreases in airflow, especially if associated with a decline in oxyhemoglobin saturation, may be clinically significant. Both hypopneas and apneas are considered respiratory events and are used to calculate a respiratory disturbance index. We do not usually consider the significance of apneas to be different from that of hypopneas, in terms of pathology, arousal, and such; thus, we usually score them together. Our recent experience with nasal bilevel positive airway pressure (BIPAP) however, has illustrated the importance of distinguishing between the two for purposes of adjusting airway pressures while the patient sleeps. Again, any airflow, such as that which would produce a snoring noise, prohibits use of the term *apnea* and, so, is considered hypopnea.

Events are considered obstructive when respiratory effort continues during the decrement in airflow. Depending on the means by which one is measuring respiratory effort, and whether the event is an apnea or hypopnea, the effort may be increased or decreased. Usually, obstructive events have associated snoring and a "breakthrough" breath, which is the larger-amplitude hypopnea at the start of the postapneic breathing. Paradoxical effort is a good indicator of strong respiratory effort and upper airway resistance (occlusion), but "paradoxing" is often observed in normal persons during REM sleep. When normal, the paradoxing should not be associated with discrete respiratory events, arousals, or desaturation.

Obstructive apneas, by definition, have respiratory effort throughout the entire period of decreased airflow. Mixed apneas have a central component at the beginning of the event, followed by obstructive elements; however, in our experience most "obstructive" apneas (defined clinically and pathophysiologically) begin with a brief period of cessation of respiratory effort. This may be due to hypocarbia, which occurs at the end of the resuscitative breath-

ing, or may in part be a pharyngeal reflex, but in any case we do not bother to score as *mixed* apneas that have a *brief* central component followed by typical obstructive features. Thus, we score as obstructive apneas those in which the central component at the beginning of the apnea is less than about 25% of the time of the total apnea. We score an apnea as mixed when the central component is predominant, but several breaths of obviously obstructive effort then occur before the arousal. Thus, mixed apneas are those with a central component ranging from about 25% to 90% of the apnea, followed by clear signs of obstruction before the apnea ends (Fig. 12-1). This is somewhat arbitrary, but our clinical experience is overwhelming that there is a gradual transition in grading apneas from obstructive to mixed to central.

The scoring of central apneas often causes discussion. By definition, a central, or diaphragmatic apnea is one in which neither respiratory effort nor airflow occurs. Central apneas can often be recognized as one of two types. One has waxing and waning effort, commonly thought of as Cheyne-Stokes breathing, with no evidence at all of an obstructive component. Cheyne-Stokes breathing, with gradual onset and offset of respiratory effort, is easily recognized and is often associated with cardiac or central nervous system disease. The other type of central apnea appears more like a mixed apnea but with minimal or no terminal obstructive phase. We score this type of apnea as central when most of the apnea contains no respiratory effort at all, the terminal phase with effort is nonexistent or is very short (one or two breaths at most), and paradoxing is not evident. Offset and onset of breathing may be abrupt. We do not routinely record esophageal pressure, but at times it may be necessary to document the level of respiratory effort. Intercostal EMG can also be helpful as a supplemental measure of respiratory effort.

There is clearly a problem with making hard and fast rules about central versus obstructive events. Definition of the events for purposes of scoring may not represent the underlying pathophysiology. The pathophysiologic event observed and the scoring should coincide, but this is not always possible. For example, we have seen patients who have central apnea only when lying supine and others who have predominantly central apnea yet respond well to nasal continuous positive airway pressure (CPAP), as if upper airway obstruction could trigger a central apnea.[9] We allow for some component of measured obstruction when scoring central apneas, because even in a person whose upper airway anatomy does not produce frank apneas, a long central apnea might produce some minor upper airway floppiness and occlusion. Thus, when the central drive returns, some evidence of upper airway resistance may be seen, perhaps some snoring. We saw another example

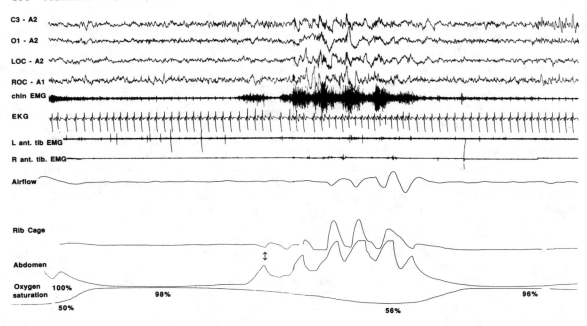

| C3 - A2 |
| O1 - A2 |
| LOC - A2 |
| ROC - A1 |
| chin EMG |
| EKG |
| L ant. tib EMG |
| R ant. tib. EMG |
| Airflow |
| Rib Cage |
| Abdomen |
| Oxygen saturation |

100%   98%   96%
50%   56%

FIGURE 12-1.   *A 60-second excerpt from a nocturnal PSG shows mixed apnea. Note significant central component (absence of respiratory effort) at onset of apnea and "paradoxing" of rib cage and abdomen near end of apnea (arrows). Paper speed 10 mm per second; EEG and EOG calibration 75 μV/cm (vertical extent of double arrow). Other gain settings are not standardized in our laboratory because they are adjusted for clarity throughout the night.*

recently, when a 35-year-old man with a history of loud snoring but no apnea developed a severe viral cardiomyopathy with congestive heart failure and Cheyne-Stokes breathing. His predisposition to snoring made many of the respiratory events appear as mixed or obstructive, but after application of nasal CPAP the "pure" central apneas (Fig. 12-2) were evident. Until a clear understanding of the pathophysiology of respiration and sleep emerges, and can account for the wide variety of clinical phenomena observed, all of our scoring and labeling is somewhat contrived.

Respiratory events can cause arousals, which may be of different types, as discussed in the section on arousals in general. We divide all respiratory events into one of three categories, based on the type and duration of the arousal. These are (1) no EEG change, (2) EEG changes without awakening, and (3) EEG changes with awakening. The first category is obvious and is characterized by events that do not appear to affect the EEG or produce other signs of arousal (such as significant chin muscle tension). The second category refers to arousals characterized as a change in stage of sleep (as from stage 3 to stage 1) or those with a change to alpha rhythm that lasts less than 15 seconds. The last category refers to a waking EEG pattern that lasts more than 15 seconds.

In summary, all respiratory events are recorded both by type (obstructive, mixed, central) and by arousal (none, less than 15 seconds, or waking).

Leg Movements

One can measure the electrical activity of many muscles, but in routine sleep recordings, both anterior tibialis muscles are usually monitored. Potentials occur from this muscle in many different circumstances. For example, with almost any body movement of the patient, during wakefulness or sleep, a potential is seen. Our laboratory follows the criteria originally outlined by Coleman to score periodic leg movements (nocturnal myoclonus).[10] Figure 12-3 is a representative sample showing periodic leg movements in sleep. Leg jerks are scored when a potential occurs in one or both anterior tibialis channels that cannot be attributed to an arousal from some other cause. To be scored as a leg jerk, a potential must last at least 0.5 seconds. We do not score potentials that occur during wakefulness, but these movements are important to note as a possible indicator of restless legs syndrome or other movement disorder.

Leg movements may occur in episodes that exhibit periodicity or randomly. For the purposes of calculating movement indices, we consider only those potentials that occur in episodes. We divide all leg potentials into one of three categories, as we do respiratory events. These are (1) no EEG changes, (2) EEG changes without awakening, and (3) EEG changes with awakening.

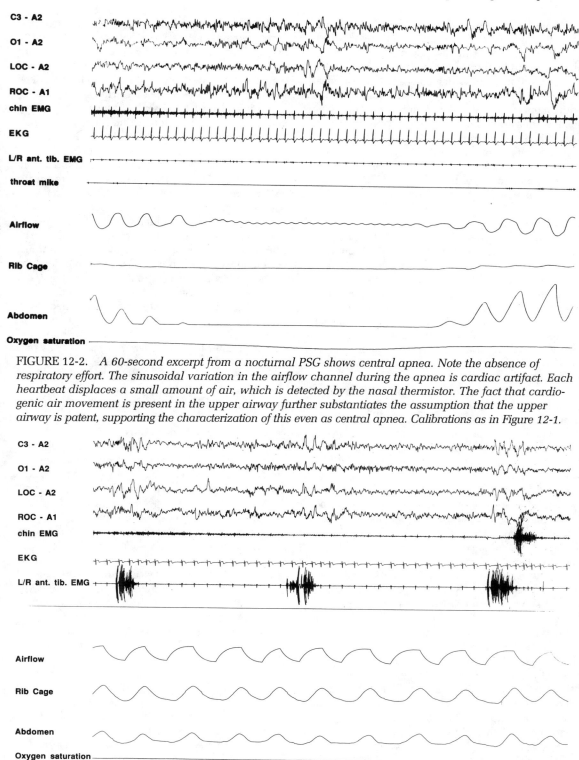

FIGURE 12-2. *A 60-second excerpt from a nocturnal PSG shows central apnea. Note the absence of respiratory effort. The sinusoidal variation in the airflow channel during the apnea is cardiac artifact. Each heartbeat displaces a small amount of air, which is detected by the nasal thermistor. The fact that cardiogenic air movement is present in the upper airway further substantiates the assumption that the upper airway is patent, supporting the characterization of this even as central apnea. Calibrations as in Figure 12-1.*

FIGURE 12-3. *A 60-second excerpt from a nocturnal PSG shows typical nocturnal myoclonus. We would score the final leg jerk as arousal because of the evident change in the EEG. Calibrations as in Figure 12-1, except that signals from the right and left legs are combined.*

When leg movements occur in an episode, the arousal may precede, occur simultaneously, or follow the beginning of the leg potential.[11] During an obvious episode, therefore, we do not try to make a fine distinction about which comes first, the arousal or the leg movement, but for arousals not associated with an episode, we do try to differentiate between a spontaneous arousal and one that is caused by a leg jerk. When scoring random arousals, if the leg potential occurs before the initial signs of arousal, we score this as an arousing leg jerk. If the K complex or other sign of arousal occurs before the leg potential, it is scored as a spontaneous arousal.

Arousals

There are many types of arousals. Usually, one defines arousals based on the EEG. Thus, although an increase in heart rate or respiratory rate may constitute a physiologic arousal in response to some event, these are not usually scored. One tries to describe both the nature and the cause of the arousal. We have discussed some of the causes of arousal, namely, respiratory events and leg movements. Often, however, arousals appear to be spontaneous, having no discernible cause. Not all arousals are pathologic, but for the purposes of sleep stage scoring and analysis, an attempt should be made to identify the cause of as many arousals as possible. In some cases of apparently spontaneous arousals, one can assume that the cause is an event in a system that is not being monitored, such as occult gastroesophageal reflux. Many spontaneous arousals are caused by intrinsic brain activity alone and are not triggered by any particular peripheral factor.

Careful analysis of each arousal is necessary before concluding that the arousal is spontaneous (produced purely by the central nervous system). For example, snoring can cause repetitive arousals in the absence of apneas, or hypopneas. For this reason we routinely record from a snoring microphone taped onto the neck. Similarly, very slight fluctuations in oxygen saturation can provoke arousal. In other instances, review of the videotape may reveal noise coming from adjoining rooms.

In general, we do not score as an arousal a simple sleep stage shift, such as from stage 3 to stage 2, unless there is some associated behavioral or neurophysiologic change. For example, an abrupt change from stage 4 to stage 1, with an increase in muscle tone and a light cry from the patient, is probably significant and should be scored. Also, when a patient is just entering sleep and is drowsing from wakefulness toward stage 1, we usually do not score arousals. Only if the shifts between wakefulness and stage 1 continue for a prolonged period would we describe them as pathologic arousals.

A commonly encountered arousal may take the form of a sudden return to a waking record, such as the alpha rhythm. There may be an increase in chin muscle tone, and evidence of movement. The arousal may be short lived or produce wakefulness. The arousals may be predominant during a certain stage of sleep and may be absent during another. They may be periodic or random. Such factors and patterns of arousals are recorded and used in later analysis of the PSG and the clinical situation.

As mentioned, a certain number of arousals from various causes is normal in sleep and they are always encountered when scoring a record. The scorer must have an appropriate threshold for scoring arousals, and this must be determined by the laboratory staff. For example, the K complex is often considered to be a brain response to some internal arousing stimulus, but obviously one cannot score all K complexes as arousals. At the other extreme, a scorer must not overlook brief arousals that might not be sufficient to cause stage changes but are sufficient to affect sleep in other ways.

A recent preliminary report from a task force of the American Sleep Disorders Association has provided some rules for the scoring of EEG arousals.[12] In this system, an EEG arousal is defined as an abrupt shift in EEG frequency, which may include theta, alpha, or frequencies greater than 16 Hz but not spindles, subject to various conditions, some of which will be mentioned. Subjects must be asleep, a state defined as 10 continuous seconds or more of the indication of any stage of sleep, before an EEG arousal can be scored. Thus, arousal scoring is independent of Rechtschaffen and Kales' epoch scoring. At least 10 continuous seconds of intervening sleep is necessary to score a second arousal. The EEG frequency shift must last 3 seconds or more to be scored as an arousal. Arousals in NREM sleep can occur without any increase in chin muscle tone, whereas arousals in REM sleep can be scored only if accompanied by an increase in submental EMG amplitude. Arousals are not scored only on the basis of chin muscle tone or on changes in respiration or heart rate. Also, K complexes or delta waves are not counted as arousals unless there is also the abrupt shift to higher frequencies, seen in at least one derivation.

Our laboratory is utilizing these criteria, defined in greater detail in the report,[12] and would add a few modifying rules to assist the technicians. First, the word *abrupt* is very important, because fast frequencies are often seen in various stages of sleep that should not be counted as arousals. Thus, we have had to emphasize that arousals need to be *distinguishable from the background rhythm* of the concurrent stage. Second, we prefer to score some arousals that are mostly in the form of K complexes. A series of high-voltage waves, probably representing K complexes, is a common response to any arousing stimulus. Such complexes are increasingly recognized as clinically significant entities, especially when they occur in a periodic fashion or are associated with non-restorative sleep.[13] A possibly related phenomenon is the *epileptic K complex*, in which sharp waves are intermingled with a series of K complexes.[14]

The task force recommendations require fast activity as a prerequisite to scoring an arousal. We consider as an arousal a series of at least three or four K-like complexes, especially if they occur in association with some identifiable event such as a contraction of the anterior tibialis muscle, an increase in chin EMG, or intrusion of alpha activity (Fig. 12-4). However, even if no events are associated with these complexes, such as EMG changes, we are more likely to score them and to consider them clinically significant if the complexes are periodic.

Alpha-Delta Sleep

Another common pattern of sleep EEG is delta sleep with alpha frequencies superimposed on or interposed with the slower delta waves.[15] This pattern is often seen in patients with chronic musculoskeletal pain and other patients with the complaint of non-restorative sleep. An epoch of alpha-delta sleep consists of 5% to 20% of delta activity interspersed with prominent alpha activity. This alpha activity is usu-

ally 1 to 2 Hz slower than the alpha rhythm typical of quiet waking. We score the record as stage 3 or 4, but make note of the overriding alpha activity (Fig. 12-5).

Sleep Stage Scoring in Patients with Central Nervous System Disease

Often, one must score the record of a patient with a brain disease that is likely to disrupt the normal patterns of activity, such as head injuries, degenerative neurologic diseases, prior brain surgery, or metabolic encephalopathy. One could also put patients with REM behavior disorder in this category. Often, there is no identifiable alpha rhythm, because the waking state is characterized by diffuse theta and delta wave activity. Sleep onset and offset are thus very difficult to delineate. Such cases require revision of the normal rules. For example, one must note eye movements at the beginning of the record, coupled with frequent body movements and a high chin EMG to determine that the EEG represents wakefulness. One can then determine the onset of sleep through other means, including behavioral correlates from the videotape, regularization of respiration, or the presence of rolling eye movements. At such times the EEG usually slows or increases in voltage, and this represents the person's initial sleep. Sometimes, stage 3 or 4 sleep is overscored in such patients because of an underlying tendency for (pathologic) delta activity. We have seen patients

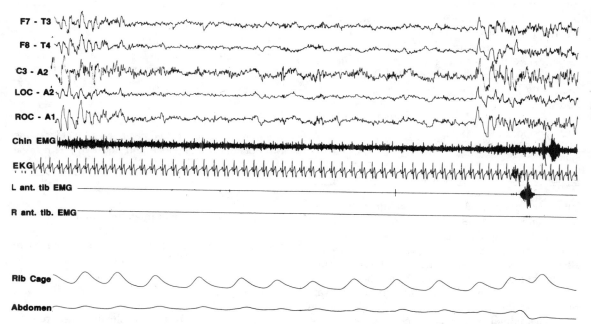

FIGURE 12-4. *A 60-second excerpt from a nocturnal PSG shows periodic K-alpha arousals in a 45-year-old man who had frequent nocturnal awakenings and complained of daytime sleepiness. He was successfully treated with Tegretol. Calibrations as in Figure 12-1.*

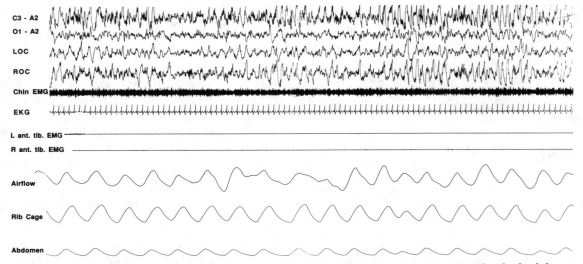

FIGURE 12-5.　*A 60-second excerpt from a nocturnal PSG shows alpha-delta sleep. Note that both alpha and delta frequencies are evident. Calibrations as in Figure 12-1.*

with a monotonous tendency for similar EEG patterns in waking and sleeping, and often the usual landmarks of stage 2 sleep are completely absent. All such patients must be recorded and scored on an empiric basis.

The REM behavior disorder should not now cause major problems in scoring REM, but we have clearly seen patients with Parkinson's disease who had almost no identifiable REM, and upon close review of the record, already complicated by the problems discussed above, we could identify probable REM of very short duration (less than 1 or 2 epochs), aborted by muscle activity and movement. Usually, however, the onset of REM periods in REM behavior disorder can be identified, but they are frequently interrupted by muscle artifact, arousals, and waking rhythms. The scorer must make special note of these arousals and score them within the REM period, as necessary.

SLEEP STUDIES IN NEWBORN INFANTS

The development of sleep and wakefulness begins in utero and continues throughout the perinatal period.[16] During this same period sleep begins to differentiate into two distinct states that are seen as REM and NREM stages. Because of these developmental changes, sleep studies in newborn infants require a unique set of interpretative tools, which are outlined in the infant counterpart of Rechtschaffen and Kales, edited by Anders and coworkers.[17] In this manual, four states of sleep and wakefulness are recognized in newborn infants: wakefulness, active-REM sleep, quiet sleep, and indeterminate sleep.

Assigning sleep states in infants requires consideration of external factors such as light, sound, and temperature, which have profound physiologic effects on newborns. In addition, respiratory monitoring is crucial because the pattern of breathing is the single most useful characteristic for sleep state scoring.

Useful categories to aid in coding observed behavior and PSG data include the following ones[17]:

Respiration

Breathing is called *regular* if the respiratory rate is less than 20 cycles per minute; breathing is called *irregular* if the respiratory rate is greater than 20 cycles per minute.

Eye movements

Eye movements are coded positive (+) if at least one REM occurs in the epoch and negative (−) if none occur.

Electromyogram

The muscles near the chin are recommended. Muscle tone is called *high* if more than half the epoch shows *tonic* muscle activity; it is called *low* if more than half the epoch shows suppression.

Patterns of EEG activity

Low-voltage, irregular (LVI): Voltage ranges from 14 to 35 μV, usually 20 to 30 μV. Record is dominated by theta activity (5 to 8 Hz), but slow waves (1 to 5 Hz) do occur.

Trace alternant (TA): Bursts of high-voltage, slow waves with occasional rapid, low-voltage waves superimposed and with sharp waves of 2 to 4 Hz interspersed between the slow waves.

High-voltage, slow (HVS): Continuous, moderately rhythmic, moderately high-voltage waves with an amplitude of 50 to 150 μV and a frequency of 0.5 to 4 Hz.

Mixed (M): Both high-voltage, slow and low-voltage components.

Miscellaneous activities

The miscellaneous category includes penile erections, sneezes, coughs, hiccoughs, yawns, burps, regurgitation, and flatus.

Interventions

External events that disturb the infant and may change the sleep recording include feeding and diaper changes.

Behavioral scales have been developed to supplement PSG findings because of the difficulty of determining sleep stage using EEG alone. One such scale, developed by Prechtl and Beintma,[19] identifies five behavioral states:

State 1. Eyes closed, regular respiration, no gross movements.
State 2. Eyes closed, irregular respiration.
State 3. Eyes open, no gross movement.
State 4. Eyes open, gross movements.
State 5. Eyes open or closed, vocal.

Criteria for Sleep State Scoring in Infants

In practice, sleep state scoring involves assessment of behavioral state along with EMG, EEG, and EOG recordings.[17–19]

To score an epoch as *wakefulness*, at least three of the following criteria must be fulfilled:

1. Sustained tonic EMG with active bursts.
2. Eyes open.
3. Within a given minute, breathing rate variation greater than 45 breaths per minute as measured by a respiratory tachometer.
4. Vocalization.
5. Sustained gross movement.

Active REM sleep

Chin EMG activity is absent (EMG is coded *low*) and at least three of the following criteria are observed:

1. At least one eye movement, independent of chin and gross body movement (EOG is +).

2. Within a given minute, breathing rate variation is greater than 25 breaths per minute as measured by a respiratory tachometer (respiration is *irregular*).
3. Presence of twitches and brief head movements.
4. Absence of EEG spindles or TA; EEG is usually LVI or M.

Other observations that help establish the state of REM include frequent facial movements, including grimaces, frowns, and bursts of sucking; limb movements and gross body movements are common; penile erections and brief vocalizations such as grunts and whimpers are present.

Quiet sleep

All of the following criteria must be fulfilled:

1. Within a given minute, breathing variation is no greater than 25 breaths per minute (respiration is *regular*).
2. Eyes closed. No more than one isolated eye movement (EOG is −).
3. Sustained EMG tonus (EMG is *high*), EEG spindles or tracé alternant or both (EEG is HVS, TA, or M).
4. No gross body movements.

Indeterminate sleep

Epochs in which the criteria for any stage are not fulfilled, such as epochs near sleep onset or sleep state changes can be scored as indeterminate sleep.

Sleep Scoring in Older Infants and Children

By approximately age three months, the presence of the rudimentary forms of REM and NREM sleep stages allows the use of a modified adult scoring system.[20] In children older than 2 years, the adult equipment setup can be used with little or no modification, and the Rechtschaffen and Kales method applied.[4]

TABULATION AND REPORT

Modern clinical practice of sleep disorders medicine is now so uniform from practice site to practice site that a standard format is the norm for sleep laboratory findings. At minimum, nocturnal sleep parameters should be tabulated to clearly present time in bed, total sleep time, and standard parameters relating to sleep structure (i.e., time spent in various stages and selected latencies). Following the tabulation of sleep parameters, a narrative summary (often with selected data tabulated) is prepared that incorporates relevant cardiopulmonary and movement data. Below is a sample report from our laboratory that we find adequate and representative of the standards of practice observed in North America. The sleep data are dictated into our template by the clinician relying on a computer program that reduces sleep stage data that have previously been entered in the form of page numbers and technologist-scored sleep staging. Several programs of this type are commercially available. The narrative conclusion aims to relate all sleep laboratory findings to a final diagnosis.

It is important to prepare the sleep laboratory report as a document that is distinct from the sleep disorders center consultation, which sets forth the clinical history, diagnosis, and treatment recommendations or management plan. In fact, many of our sleep laboratory reports are prepared by a physician who has no direct clinical knowledge of the patient. It is the consultation (rather than the sleep laboratory report) that should conform to local standards of medical practice and applicable laws, such as laws regarding reporting of disability and driving impairment (see Appendix 12-1).

APPENDIX 12-1. SAMPLE REPORT

SCRIPPS CLINIC
AND RESEARCH FOUNDATION
Division of Sleep Disorders
Sleep Disorders Center

Clinical Polysomnography Report

ATTENDING PHYSICIAN:
DIAGNOSIS: Sleep apnea.

Procedures:

Polysomnography was conducted on the night of 3/24/91. Recording began at 2211 and ended at 0635 for a total recording of 504 minutes.

Medical parameters monitored throughout the night were: left and right central electroencephalogram (EEG), left and right electrooculogram (EOG), digastric muscle electromyogram (EMG), respiratory airflow from sensors placed at the nasal and buccal orifices, and respiratory effort from sensors placed around the thorax and around the abdomen. Cardiac rhythm was monitored from electrodes placed on either clavicle, producing an all-night (8–12 hours) electrocardiographic (ECG) waveform similar to V2. An all-night audio and visual record of events was kept by means of continuous monitoring with an infrared video camera, a low-level microphone, and a videocassette recorder. A microphone was fixed on the neck to record respiratory sounds.

Additional parameters for the specific diagnostic purposes of this recording included EMG from both anterior tibialis muscles and all-night stress oxygenation with quantified ear oximetry.

Qualitative Description

The patient reported that the quality and quantity of sleep was much better than usual. He did not awaken with his hangover, headachy feeling. He did not awaken with nasal congestion. Respiratory sounds were heard as occasional snores. Respiratory airflow and effort measures disclosed 39 obstructive hypopneas, all of which caused arousal. Interestingly, the patient had significant desaturations in REM sleep that were not associated with discrete apneas or hypopneas, though there may have been a slight decrease in tidal volume over long periods of time during his REM periods, leading to desaturation. The study was not typical for obstructive sleep

PARAMETRIC ANALYSIS:

SLEEP PARAMETER	OBSERVED VALUE	LABORATORY NORMS
Sleep latency (3 epochs stage 1 sleep)	1 min.	0–60 min.
Patient's estimate of sleep latency	60 min.	5–60 min.
Estimation of error for sleep latency	+59 min.	−5–+20 min.
Sleep duration	332 min.	300–420 min.
Patient's estimate of sleep duration	420 min.	300–450 min.
Estimation error for sleep duration	+88 min.	−60–+30 min.
Sleep efficiency (% of time asleep)	65.9%	80–93%
Percent stage 1 NREM	7.7%	7–16%
Percent stage 2 NREM	60.5%	47–87%
Percent stage 3 NREM	11.5%	0–5%
Percent stage 4 NREM	5.4%	0–0%
Percent stage REM	14.9%	13–29%
Latency from first sleep to REM sleep	75 min.	10–210 min.

apnea syndrome, though occasional hypopneas were seen. Baseline oxygen saturation was 95%. The mean overnight was 92%, and the lowest value was 76%. The computer counted 44 desaturation events. The pattern of oximetry shows long desaturations to about 80% during each REM period, some of which are repetitive but many are simply stable desaturations. This pattern suggests that the patient is on the steep part of the oxyhemoglobin dissociation curve and has limited pulmonary reserve and that changes in tidal volume were occurring during REM sleep though it was difficult to measure. The steady-state heart rate was about 70 without significant change. The blood pressure was: h.s. 170/70 mmHg, a.m. 140/80 mmHg. The EMG recordings from both legs disclosed 215 contractions of the anterior tibialis muscle organized into several episodes, mostly in the middle and late portions of the night. These occurred during NREM sleep and were absent in REM sleep. The potentials have a period of about 30 seconds. Review of the videotape reveals mild movements of the ankles and knees, the details of which are obscured by the bed covers. The leg movements significantly fragment sleep and contribute to over 150 arousals.

Sleep structure was abnormal for this 80-year-old man. Sleep was deep at times but frequently fragmented. He has long periods of waking time. REM sleep in particular was fragmented. For reasons that were not quite clear, there was more slow-wave than expected.

Conclusion

The nocturnal polysomnographic data and accompanying audiovisual recording demonstrate:

1. Periodic leg movements of sleep (nocturnal myoclonus). This is moderately severe with a movement index of 39 and a movement arousal index of 27.
2. REM hypoxemia. This is not definitely obstructive in nature and appears to be on the basis of a central decrease in tidal volume in association with limited pulmonary reserve. The lowest saturation value obtained was 76% and the patient spent 9% of the sleeping time with saturation under 90%. The mean saturation overnight was 92%.
3. Occasional obstructive hypopneas in a number borderline for the diagnosis of obstructive sleep apnea. The Respiratory Disturbance Index is 7.
4. Subjectively, an extremely good night of sleep with the patient awakening without his usual headachy feeling and his usual sinus congestion. This could be due to the different sleeping environment.

REFERENCES

1. Davis H, Davis P, Loomis A. Human brain potentials during the onset of sleep. J Neurophysiol 1939;1:24–38.
2. Blake H, Gerard R. Brain potentials and depth of sleep. Am J Physiol 1937;119:692–703.
3. Gibbs F, Gibbs E. Atlas of Electroencephalography. I. Methodology and Normal Controls. Cambridge, Mass.: Addison-Wesley, 1950.
4. Rechtschaffen A, Kales A. A Manual of Standardized Terminology, Techniques and Scoring System for Sleep Stages of Human Subjects, Los Angeles: UCLA Brain Information Service/Brain Research Institute, 1968.
5. Jasper HH. The ten-twenty electrode system of the International Federation. Electroencephalogr Clin Neurophysiol 1958;10:371–375.
6. Brazier MAB, Cobb W, Fischgold H, et al. Preliminary proposal for an EEG terminology by the Terminology Committee of the International Federation of Electroencephalography and Clinical Neurophysiology. Electroencephalogr Clin Neurophysiol 1961;13:646–650.
7. McGregor P, Thorpy M, Schmidt-Nowara W, et al. T-sleep: An improved method for scoring breathing-disordered sleep. Sleep 1992;15:359–363.
8. American Psychiatric Association Task Force on Quantitative Electrophysiological Assessment. Quantitative electroencephalography: A report on the present state of computerized EEG techniques. Am J Psychiatry 1991;148:961–964.
9. Issa FG, Sullivan CE. Reversal of central sleep apnea using nasal CPAP. Chest 1986;90:165–171.
10. Coleman RM. Periodic movements in sleep (nocturnal myoclonus) and restless legs syndrome. In: Guilleminault C, ed. Sleeping and Waking Disorders. Indications and Techniques. Menlo Park, Calif: Addison-Wesley, 1982;265–295.
11. Kotagal P, Ferber RA, Mograss M. Relationship of EEG changes to periodic leg movements. Sleep Res 1990;19:224–224.
12. EEG arousals: Scoring rules and examples, a preliminary report from the Sleep Disorders Atlas Task Force of the American Sleep Disorders Association. Sleep 1992;15:174–184.
13. Hoelscher TJ, Ware JC, McBrayer RH. Insomnia with periodic EEG arousals in the absence of apnea and myoclonus. Sleep Res 1989;18:245–245.
14. Peled R, Lavie P. Paroxysmal awakenings from sleep associated with excessive daytime sleepiness: A form of nocturnal epilepsy. Neurology 1986;36:95–98.
15. Wittig RM, Zorick FJ, Blumer D, et al. Disturbed sleep in patients complaining of chronic pain. J Nerv Ment Dis 1982;170:429–431.
16. Guilleminault C. Sleep and Its Disorders in Children. New York: Raven Press, 1987.
17. Anders T, Emde R, Parmelee A. A Manual of Standardized Terminology, Techniques and Criteria for Scoring of Stages of Sleep and Wakefulness in Newborn Infants. Los Angeles: UCLA Brain Information Service, NINDS Neurological Information Network, 1971.

18. Prechtl HFR, Beintema D. The neurological examination of the full term newborn infant. In: Clin Develop Med 1964;12:74.

19. Hoppenbrouwers T. Electronic monitoring in the newborn and young infant: Theoretical considerations. In: Guilleminault C., ed. Sleeping and Waking Disorders. Indications and Techniques. Menlo Park, Calif: Addison-Wesley, 1982;17–59.

20. Coons S. Development of sleep and wakefulness during the first 6 months of life. In: Guilleminault C, ed. Sleep and Its Disorders in Children. New York: Raven Press, 1987;17–27.

13

Techniques for the Assessment of Sleep-Related Erections

Max Hirshkowitz
Ismet Karacan

WHAT IS NOCTURNAL PENILE TUMESCENCE?

Nocturnal penile tumescence (NPT) is a cyclic pattern of penile erections that occur in virtually all sexually potent men. More accurately called sleep-related erections, this naturally occurring cycle provides a measurable phenomenon for objectively indexing erectile function. The erections normally occur in close coordination with rapid eye movement (REM) sleep.

SLEEP-RELATED ERECTIONS, REM SLEEP, AND DREAMING

The discovery of REM sleep by Aserinsky and Kleitman[1] launched a new era in sleep research. Aserinsky[2] speculated that the penile erection cycle during sleep, previously described by Ohlmeyer and associates,[3] was possibly related to the periodic recurrence of REM sleep. Subsequent studies by Karacan[4] and Fisher and associates[5] confirmed this hypothesis. These two research groups, working independently, demonstrated a close temporal relationship between REM sleep and sleep-related nocturnal penile tumescence in deference to his advisors' suggestion that *penile erections in sleep* was too explicit in those more restrained times before the sexual revolution.

For many years, the postulated underlying psychosexual nature of dreams provided the basis for dream interpretation. The coupling of REM sleep and penile erections, given the close association between REM sleep and dreaming, revived interest in sexual dream content. In his investigations, Karacan[4] found that erotic dream content did not typically accompany NPT. By contrast, in a four-case series, Fisher[6] described sudden NPT increases related to overtly erotic dream content. More recent dream studies, however, demonstrate the paucity of erotic content in laboratory dream reports.[7,8] In fact, McCarley and Hoffman[9] found no erotic content in 104 dreams from 14 subjects they studied.

Use in the Diagnosis of Impotence

Karacan's keen interest in both sleep phenomena and sexual function led him in 1970 to suggest using sleep erection recordings to differentially diagnose impotence.[10] Motivated by the desire for an objective basis by which to distinguish psychogenic from organic impotence, Karacan and others began exploring the sleep erection cycle for biologic markers. The development of surgical treatments for erectile impotence increased the need for more reliable diagnostic techniques.

At the most basic level, the presence of an erection of normal circumference increase and rigidity confirms erectile capacity. Inability to volitionally produce a rigid erection during an office visit, can be due to either situational inhibitory factors or organic impotence. Similarly, if fantasy, erotica, or both, fail to elicit an adequate erection, the cause of impotence remains obscure. Sleep studies provide another opportunity to examine erectile capacity. Under the veil of sleep, any sexual inhibition present in wakefulness fades and an erection-promoting parasympathetic arousal state predominates during REM sleep. A penile erection of normal size and rigidity accompanying REM sleep establishes erectile capability. It must be emphasized, however, that polysomnographic (PSG) studies of sleep-related erections do not obviate the need for a thorough sexual history, genital neurovascular examination, psychometrics, medical history, and physical examination. In some cases, endocrine and nerve conduction studies are also required.

TRADITIONAL POLYSOMNOGRAPHIC TECHNIQUE

How Recordings Are Made

The traditional technique for evaluating sleep-related erections includes recording electroencephalographic (EEG) and electrooculographic (EOG) activity in conjunction with penile circumference increase.

Tracings are scored for sleep stages and wakefulness. The pioneer researchers never lost sight of the fact that the erection cycle was sleep dependent and principally a REM sleep phenomenon.

The standard laboratory approach to recording penile circumference increase involves placing mercury-filled strain gauges around the penis. During an erection, the column of mercury elongates and the tubing narrows, thus increasing the gauge's electrical resistance. Electrical resistance is transduced to direct current voltage by a bridge amplifier. The bridge amplifier output, when connected to the polygraph pen driver input, provides a continuous tracing of circumference change. Placing two gauges, one at the penile base and the other at the coronal sulcus, offers several advantages over using a single gauge placed at mid-shaft: redundancy, improved reliability, and greater sensitivity to erectile anomalies.

In addition to scoring sleep stages and penile circumference increases, contemporary laboratory NPT protocols should include evaluation of breathing patterns and leg movements. These data assist the interpretation of penile circumference recordings, because men with erectile dysfunction have a strikingly high prevalence of sleep apnea and periodic limb movement disorder.[11,12]

Preparation and calibration

Properly fitting gauges are key to accurate recording of sleep-related erections. If a gauge is loose on the penis, circumferential expansion occurs before it is registered by pen deflection on the polygraph. This results in underestimation of circumference increase or even failure to detect erectile episodes. If a gauge is too tight, the bridge amplifier may distort its output. Transduction amplifiers have an optimal range in which the input-output response is linear. Significantly elevated baseline input may drive the amplifier beyond its linear range when an erection occurs. Also, a tight gauge is more likely to break. Therefore, careful penile circumference measurement and an adequate supply of gauges of varying sizes are essential. One should carefully inspect each gauge before and after it is placed around the penis. It should fit snugly but not tightly; kinking or rolling the gauge must be avoided.

The electrical characteristics differ between strain gauges; therefore, each gauge requires careful nightly calibration. The ultimate purpose of calibration is to establish an invariant relationship between actual circumference increase and the amplitude of pen deflection on the polygraph. Different calibration procedures can attain this goal; however, we describe the one used at our sleep disorders and research center.

To calibrate, we simulate a 20-mm penile circumference increase using a calibration block. The block consists of two short cylinders mounted concentrically, one atop the other. We maintain a selection of calibration blocks, named according to the circumference of the smaller of the two cylinders (called the *small end*). Block small ends range from 50 to 150 mm, in increments of 5 mm. For all calibration blocks, the circumference of the larger cylinder (*large end*) exceeds the smaller by precisely 20 mm.

We perform calibration in four steps. First, the gauge is placed around the small end and the electrical baseline on the bridge amplifier is adjusted to align the pen with a polygraphic baseline. Second, we carefully move the gauge to the large end and adjust the amplifier gain so that the polygraph pen deflects 15 mm above pen baseline. Next, after moving the gauge back to the small end, we check that the pen returns to baseline. If the pen fails to return to baseline, the first two steps are repeated. In the final step we recheck the large end to ensure a 15-mm deflection. We use a 20-mm to 15-mm actual-polygraphic ratio to avoid pen blocking during robust erections recorded from volunteer research subjects. Many laboratories prefer a more intuitive one-to-one ratio, especially if they perform only clinical evaluations. Careful gauge handling (to avoid damage) and choosing appropriate-sized calibration blocks expedites calibration.

Once the properly calibrated gauges are placed on the patient, the pen should deflect several millimeters above baseline (assuming the patient does not have an erection). If the pen is below baseline, the gauge is too loose and should be replaced. A tight or stretched gauge producing a large pen deflection should also be replaced. With a properly fitting gauge, the small pen deflection present at the beginning of the record can be brought to baseline mechanically or with the balance control. Gain should never be altered after calibration. Barring unforeseen problems, this procedure enables the polygraph to produce a continuous, accurate tracing of penile circumference increase.

Measuring rigidity

To achieve vaginal penetration an erection must attain some degree of axial rigidity; circumferential increase alone is not enough. Therefore, the penile rigidity during a tumescence episode is the single most important measure for assessing erectile capacity. Although penile circumference increase and axial rigidity correlate fairly well in normal subjects, dissociation frequently occurs in men who complain of erectile failure. Karacan[13] first remarked on the need to assess rigidity in 1977, and other investigators soon followed with evidence documenting penile enlargement without rigidity.[14]

To measure rigidity, we awaken the patient during a representative sleep-related erection and apply a calibrated force to the tip of the penis. The force sufficient to buckle the penile shaft (penile buckling resistance) is the index of axial rigidity. If no buckling occurs with forces up to 1000 g, we terminate the procedure and assign the value 1000 g. Regrettably, some confusion has arisen because our original rigidity meter measured buckling in pressure (0 to 300 mm Hg). This device was a large syringe modified with a rubber cap on one end and a sphygmomanometer on the other. The devices in current use are electronic or spring-loaded force meters.

As part of the rigidity measurement procedure, we photograph the erect penis and ask the patient to estimate what percentage of a full erection he has. The technician also rates the erection for percentage of fullness. We find the photograph useful to document abnormalities in penile size and shape (e.g., the curvature associated with Peyronie's disease). For patients who elect prosthetic implantation, the photograph may help the surgeon select the proper-sized device. Finally, we carefully inspect each photograph to cross-validate rigidity measures.

What Can Be Measured?

Scoring sleep-related erections

At our center all tracings are manually scored to provide quantitative information about the nocturnal erections. For detailed scoring rules, the reader should see Karacan, Salis, and Williams[15] and Karacan.[16] Essentially, we score each tumescence episode for three phases of activity. The first tumescence phase scored is called *T-up*. Accompanied by arterial inflow, which produces penile swelling and increases intracorporeal pressure, T-up plateaus at some maximum circumference increase in normal subjects. The next phase, during which circumference remains at the maximum plateau, is called *T-max*. Detumescence (*T-down*) follows, characterized by venous outflow and decreasing penile circumference. *T-zero* marks the point at which detumescence reaches completion.

We score each tumescence episode by tabulating the polygraph page (30-second epoch) at which T-up, T-max, T-down, and T-zero begin. Using a laboratory computer, the scorer enters these data along with sleep stage scoring. Entry also includes demarcation of sleep interruption required for rigidity measurement, buckling force values, and the percentage of full erection estimates made by patient and technician. The computer then provides a graphic illustration of the sleep stages and sleep-related erection episodes (Figure 13-1) and a numerical summary.

Quantity, quality, and architecture of erections

Like most physiologic phenomena, sleep-related erections can be characterized along three quantitative dimensions: frequency, magnitude, and duration. The number of tumescence episodes indexes frequency. We most often represent magnitude by overall nightly maximum circumference increase; however, mean circumference increase per episode also provides useful information. Total tumescence time is the most common measure of duration.

Erectile quality is objectively assessed by measuring rigidity during one or more representative episodes of tumescence. Subjective estimates of erectile quality are also useful. These derive from the patient's and the technician's judgment of the percentage of a full erection that is present at the time rigidity is measured. Exaggerated patient underestimation of erection fullness suggests a psychogenic component in the erectile impotence.

Parameters of erectile architecture include the slopes of increasing tumescence (T-up) and the swiftness of detumescence (T-down). Additionally, abnormalities in the duration of each phase of erection help characterize pathophysiology. Duration of sustained maximal erection (T-max) is especially important, because many patients specifically complain about inability to sustain their erection during intercourse. Abnormal concordance between circumferential expansion at the penile base and at the coronal sulcus suggests vascular problems.

Coordination between sleep and erections

To fully appreciate a patient's sleep-related erectile pattern, data concerning the coordination between NPT and REM sleep are essential. The frequency, periodicity, and duration of tumescence episodes depend, to a large degree, on REM sleep. We often find it useful to normalize sleep erection measures according to the amount of sleep or REM sleep, for comparison with normative data. Furthermore, sleep data help determine the validity of a study by ruling out NPT decreases secondary to sleep fragmentation or insufficient REM sleep. Frequently non-REM (NREM) erections should alert the clinician to possible neurogenic problems.

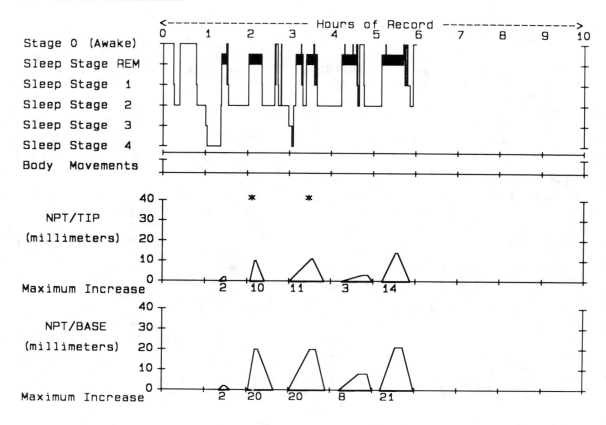

FIGURE 13-1.   *Sleep stages and NPT recorded from a healthy, 48-year-old, sexually potent research study volunteer. Penile circumference increases are shown for gauges placed at both the coronal sulcus (tip) and penile base (base). Asterisks indicate awakenings to record buckling resistance (rigidity). Maximum rigidity was greater than 1000 g. This subject had no history of medical or psychiatric illness, took no medication, and had no sleep-wake complaints or disturbances.*

OTHER RECORDING DEVICES AND WHAT THEY MEASURE

Stamps, Snap Gauges, and Felt Gauges

The desire to objectify diagnostic techniques fueled enthusiasm for using NPT testing in clinical practice. To avoid costly and labor-intensive laboratory sleep studies, a search began for less expensive, nonlaboratory alternatives.[17-25]

Encircling the penis with postage-type stamps at bedtime was perhaps the first shortcut sleep erection detection technique.[17] The patient is instructed to note upon morning awakening whether separation has occurred at the perforations between stamps. Stamp ring breakage is attributed to sleep-related erections, and conversely an intact ring is thought to verify organic impotence. In the original study, 22 potent men broke the stamp ring on 58 of 62 nights

compared to only 1 stamp breakage observed among 11 impotent patients tested for 30 nights. Subsequent studies by other investigators report less consistent results.[26,27]

More elaborate penile erection detection devices have also been developed. These include snap gauges, felt gauges, and expandable tubes. Again, initial validation study successes for some of these devices were followed by mixed results.[28] These approaches detect only the presence of an erection, providing no information about erectile frequency or duration. On the basis of direct experience attempting to develop such a device, Morales and colleagues[27,29] suggested that sleep-related movement could produce artifactual detection of tumescence. Therefore, false negative NPT results (the finding of normal NPT when the patient is organically impaired) represent a serious shortcoming of these assessment approaches.

Bedside Erection Monitors and RigiScan Device

The most sophisticated home NPT monitors record circumference change continuously during the night. Although brain and eye movement activities are not recorded, one can visualize the number, duration, and circumference increase of nocturnal erections. The presence of periodic episodes of tumescence provides useful diagnostic information; however, the absence of an erection cycle may indicate either organic impotence or disturbed sleep. Without information on the presence or absence of REM sleep, false positive tests (a finding of reduced NPT that is not produced by organic impotence) represent a major concern, especially when surgical treatment is considered.

Penile Buckling Resistance Versus Penile Compressibility

Some nonlaboratory devices measure penile compressibility. Although penile compressibility differs from buckling resistance, both are called *rigidity*. RigiScan assesses compressibility by tightening its penile loops and measuring penile resistance to compression. Snap gauges have embedded calibrated filaments that break upon reaching certain outward pressure. Felt gauges expand when the penis exceeds specific noncompressible expansion.

The original literature emphasizing the importance of penile rigidity refers specifically to penile buckling resistance (axial rigidity), not to compressibility. The manufacturer's advertisements citing our articles and those of Richard Allen[30] are, therefore, misleading. The quotations concerning the need for rigidity data, in addition to circumference increase data, are from discussions of penile buckling resistance and not compressibility.

Summary

Laboratory sleep studies clearly provide the most complete set of data characterizing sleep-related erections, including visual inspection and penile buckling resistance measures. Table 13-1 summa-rizes the parameters that can be examined with different recording devices. Bedside NPT monitors and the RigiScan Device continuously monitor penile circumference change, but they provide no information concerning sleep status. RigiScan also measures penile compressibility. The expandable and felt gauges can detect tumescence episodes and record the nightly maximum circumference increase. Finally, the least expensive device (stamp rings), at best, reveals only whether or not an erection has occurred during the sleep period. Like stamp rings, snap gauges detect circumference increase, but they also provide a crude measure of compressibility.

INTERPRETATION OF RESULTS

General Considerations

Relationship to aging

In the general population, studies indicate a generalized decline in erectile function with advancing age. It is not known whether these changes are secondary to pathology or are natural consequences of aging. The prevalence of prostate problems and use of medications that may adversely affect potency both increase with aging. The relationship between aging and sleep-related erections in sexually potent men has been ascertained by Karacan and associates[31,32] and replicated by independent research groups led by Reynolds[33] and Schiavi.[34] In our studies, subjects with significant mental or physical disease were excluded; therefore, the oldest groups (60 to 69 and 70 to 79 years) represent a specific subsample of the senior population.

Our most important observation was that all sexually potent men had penile erections during sleep.[31,32] *Modest* but statistically reliable declines were found for a number of specific parameters of sleep erections (total tumescence time, duration of REM sleep–related tumescence, number of REM erection episodes). Schiavi and colleagues[34] found greater NPT decline in their oldest group (aged 65 to

TABLE 13-1. NPT Recording Devices and What They Measure

Parameter	Sleep Studies	Bedside and RigiScan Monitors	Expandable and Felt Gauges	Snap Gauges and Stamp Rings
Presence/absence	Yes	Yes	Yes	Yes
NPT frequency	Yes	Yes	No	No
NPT magnitude	Yes	Yes	Yes	No
NPT duration	Yes	Yes	No	No
NPT architecture	Yes	Yes	No	No
REM sleep coordination	Yes	No	No	No
Sleep disruptions	Yes	No	No	No
Abnormal penile curvature	Yes	No	No	No
Penile bucking resistance	Yes	No	No	No

74 years). However, their sample included men with intermittent erectile failure, which occurred more often among those in the older groups. The research team led by Reynolds[33] found a small age-related decline in the number of episodes, the ratio of tumescence to sleep duration, and the proportion of REM sleep with tumescence. These authors indicated that age accounted for less than 15% of variance in their measures of sleep-related erections. Finally, the Pittsburgh group[33] found no decline for penile buckling resistance (rigidity) associated with aging. The empirical data from these investigations convincingly demonstrate the ubiquity of sleep-related erections and their persistence, aging notwithstanding, in healthy, sexually potent men.

Sources and use of normative data

Karacan[10] championed the idea that NPT testing could provide an objective basis for diagnosing male impotence. He immediately recognized, however, that achieving this goal required normative data. Projects followed to compile normative descriptions of the NPT cycle in young boys, young adults, middle-aged men, and elderly.[35-38] These data were further analyzed with respect to aging and published in the *American Journal of Psychiatry*[31] and the now defunct journal *Waking and Sleeping*.[32] A recent replication and extension of these data has been published by Reynolds and colleagues[33] in the journal *Sleep*.

Care must be exercised in comparing an individual's results to normative data. Normative descriptions are based on multinight PSGs recorded from men selected for good health whose sleep integrity and continuity are normal. Patients referred for sleep-related erection studies often have significant sleep disturbance. The dependency of NPT on REM sleep necessitates interpolation of normative values with respect to the characteristics of the patient's sleep. Although normalization of erection measures by REM sleep time or total sleep time can help, severely disturbed or fragmented sleep may render a study uninterpretable. The most common REM sleep disturbance results from first night adaptation to the laboratory setting. Additional nights of PSG usually remedy this nuisance. For patients with a sleep disorder, multinight PSG or therapeutic intervention (e.g., sleep restriction therapy to consolidate sleep) typically improves interpretability. Nonetheless, some studies may prove inconclusive, which, though disappointing, is certainly preferable to false positive or false negative interpretations.

Finally, it is of interest to note that presleep sexual activity and sexual arousal before sleep do not alter the patterns of sleep-related erections. Conversely, sexual abstinence in healthy volunteer subjects is not associated with changes in measures of sleep-related erections.[39,40]

Rigidity

The maximum penile buckling resistance is the most important measure obtained during NPT testing. The rationale for its use to infer erectile capacity is based on the results of several studies. Female volunteers performing vaginal insertions with variously sized, lubricated, Lucite rods needed an average minimum force of 500 g to achieve penetration.[41] In another study, during the rigidity measurement procedure we asked men whether their erection was adequate for sexual intercourse. We found that erections with buckling resistances below 500 g were seldom rated as sufficient to achieve penetration. Finally, in groups of sexually potent men, regardless of age, rigidity averages well above 500 g.[33] The vaginal insertion and penetration capability–rating studies, coupled with the normative rigidity data, have led many to regard a buckling resistance of 500 to 550 g as the critical minimum *cutting score* for erectile capacity.

Normal Sleep-Related Erections

Normal sleep-related erections with adequate rigidity suggest functional erectile capacity. Figure 13-2 illustrates the sleep stage and nocturnal penile tumescence recorded from a patient with psychogenic impotence. Before diagnosing psychogenic impotence in a man with normal NPT, the clinician should consider four conditions: (1) Peyronie's disease, (2) pelvic steal syndrome, (3) somatic nerve lesion or neuropathy, and (4) acute androgen deficiency. Though rare, these represent organic conditions that may be associated with normal sleep tumescence profiles. Misdiagnosis can be avoided by performing a neurovascular genital examination and complete rigidity measurement procedure (see Measuring Rigidity).

Men with Peyronie's disease have abnormal penile curvature that can impair penetration, even if circumferential expansion is normal. Surprisingly, some men are unaware of their condition. Visual observation and photographing the erection during the rigidity measurement procedure documents penile curvature and provides the basis for proper diagnosis.

Pelvic steal syndrome refers to the loss of an erection due to shunting of blood away from the pelvis during leg movement and thrusting. Measuring the effect of knee bending on penile arterial blood pressures help detect *steal syndrome*. A large, rapid blood pressure drop during this procedure alerts the clinician to the need for further urologic assessment.

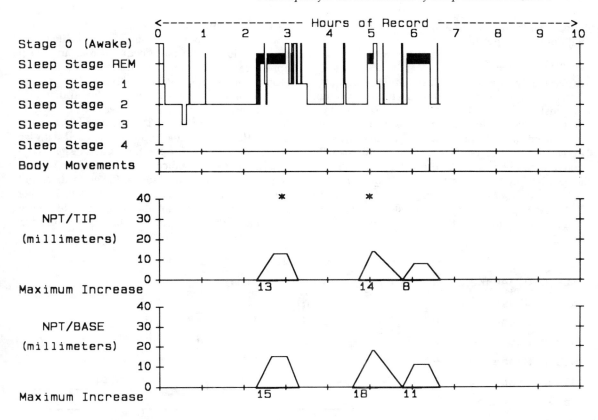

FIGURE 13-2. *Sleep stages and NPT recorded from a 56-year-old patient with psychogenic impotence. Sleep-related erections are well-coordinated with REM sleep and normal with respect to frequency, magnitude, and duration. Rigidity measured during the first erectile episode was 880 g. The patient grossly underestimated his percentage of a full erection (30%) compared to the technician's rating (70%). There was no evidence of pelvic steal syndrome. The patient's medical history is significant for alcohol abuse) duodenal ulcers, hypertension (treated with hydrochlorothiazide), and depression (after death of wife). Currently there are no sleep-wake complaints; however, combat-related posttraumatic stress disorder nightmares were noted in the past.*

Similarly, neurovascular genital examination of ascending sensory pathways may be needed to rule out neural lesions.

Ten years ago we reported diminished NPT in men with a subnormal testosterone level.[42] In a more recent study[43] we provoked androgen deficiency by discontinuing testosterone replacement therapy in a group of hypogonadal men. We observed significant decline in the frequency, magnitude, and duration of sleep-related erections after approximately 2 months, though most men still met minimum criteria for adequate erectile capacity. Therefore, a short but critical time frame exists during which endocrine evaluation is needed to rule out acute androgen deficiency in patients with an apparently psychogenic sleep erection profile.

If normal sleep erections occur and Peyronie's, steal, penile nerve problems, and acute androgen

deficiency are ruled out, psychogenic erectile dysfunction is diagnosed. It is incorrect to assume, however, that psychopathology invariably accompanies psychogenic impotence; psychometric test findings may be completely normal. The erectile failure may arise from specific behavior or relationship problems. Conversely, men with impotence of organic cause are not immune to psychological, psychiatric, or relationship problems. We commonly find significant psychopathology in men with clearly organic impotence.

Diminished Sleep-Related Erections

PSGs that indicate below-normal sleep-related erections require careful interpretation. The clinician must consider sleep integrity, drug effects, and comorbid factors. Figure 13-3 illustrates the sleep

Record Number: 00041715

stages and penile circumference increase in a man with organic impotence.

Sleep duration and integrity

A reasonably consolidated sleep period of adequate duration is the basic prerequisite for interpreting diminished sleep-related erections. Especially in elderly subjects, the duration of the sleep episode (time from sleep onset to final awakening) may have to exceed 6.5 hours. We have seen several sexually potent men older than 65 years who exhibited prolonged latency to the first erection. In one case, the patient's only erection occurred during the third REM sleep episode, after 5 hours' sleep. It was normal for magnitude, duration, and rigidity.

We frequently encounter sleep disorders during PSG of men referred for evaluation of erectile impotence. Periodic limb movement disorder and sleep apnea are the most common. In a recently published report, we described PSG data from 768 consecutively evaluated impotent men. We found that 54% had 15 or more leg movements per hour of sleep.[11] Many of these patients had disrupted sleep. Repeated REM sleep interruptions associated with leg movements rendered more than a few tests inconclusive. In some instances, therapeutic intervention reduced movement arousals sufficiently to permit interpretation of penile circumference data. In other cases, the great night-to-night variability in leg movements permitted interpretation of repeat recordings

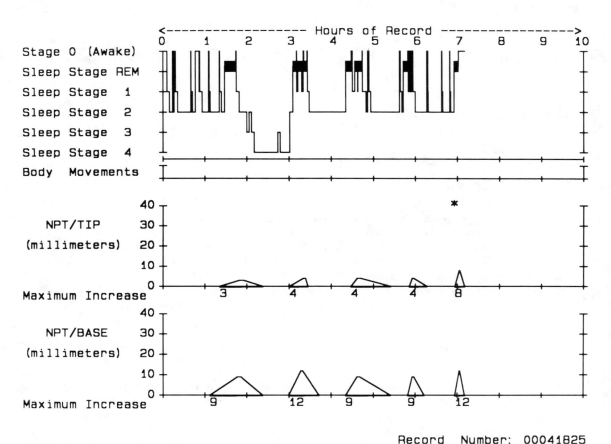

Record Number: 00041825

FIGURE 13-3.   *Sleep stages and NPT recorded from a 64-year-old patient with organic impotence. Notwithstanding a normal number of tumescence episodes, well-coordinated with REM sleep, circumference increase and rigidity were below normal. Maximum rigidity, measured during the patient's best erection was 220 g. The other recording night had a similar NPT profile. Past health was significant for diabetes (insulin-dependent). We found borderline prolonged bulbocavernosus reflex latency and reduced penile arterial blood pressures on the right side. Sleep efficiency (91%) and REM percent (16%) were within normal limits. REM sleep latency was 73 minutes (43 minutes on night 1) and all slow-wave sleep followed the first REM episode (also on night 1); however, we found no history or indication of depression. Significant periodic leg movements in sleep were revealed by PSG, for which the patient was subsequently treated. Although the patient had a small oropharynx and low-set soft palate, sleep-related breathing was normal.*

made on nights when the number of leg movements was fortuitously low.

We also investigated sleep-related breathing in 1025 men complaining of erectile dysfunction.[12] Forty-four percent had significant sleep apnea (five episodes or more per hour of sleep) and 20% had moderate to severe sleep apnea (15 or more apneas per hour). These two large-scale studies confirm previous reports of the prevalence of leg movement and apnea disorders in men suffering from impotence.[44,45] Direct evidence that occult sleep disorders can impede interpretation of simple penile circumference recordings is provided by Pressmen and colleagues.[45] Thus, in patients with concurrent sleep pathology, PSG is crucial for interpretation.

Nasal continuous positive airway pressure (CPAP) therapy for management of sleep-related breathing disorders is now generally available. CPAP affords the sleep center a unique opportunity to advance impotence diagnostic technique in men with sleep apnea. In our current impotence assessment protocol, we routinely titrate CPAP when PSG reveals a significant respiratory disturbance. In patients with apnea-related reductions in REM sleep, REM-rebound sometimes unmasks REM-disrupted reduced NPT. Thus, NPT is sometimes normalized by CPAP therapy (Figure 13-4A & B); moreover, self-reported erectile function may also improve.

Drug effects

Many drugs reportedly cause impotence.[15,46,47] The widespread use of antihypertensives makes them highly visible in the sexual dysfunction clinic. Prevalent estimates of sexual dysfunction range upward to 66% for β-blockers, 42% for α-andrenergics, and 36% for diuretics. Antidepressants, especially tricyclics with strong anticholinergic properties, produce erectile failure. Clinical reports also indicate impotence related to antipsychotic medications, most notably haloperidol and chlorpromazine. Finally, we frequently encounter an assortment of other impotence-producing drugs, including antiandrogens, cancer chemotherapy agents, cimetidine, digoxin, disulfiram, and atropine. Segraves and

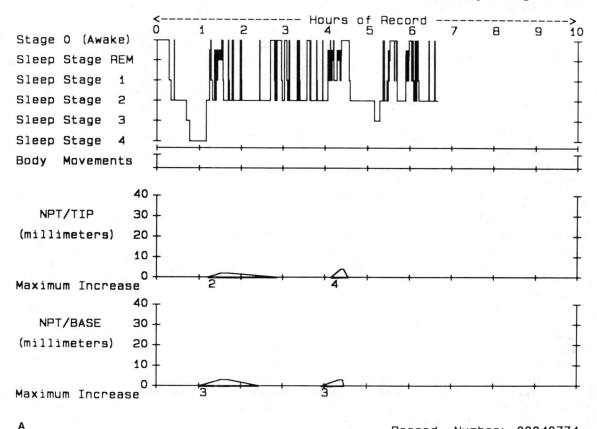

A

Record Number: 00040774

FIGURE 13-4(A). *Sleep stages and NPT recorded from a 48-year-old man with erectile failure and obstructive sleep apnea. Panel A illustrates the baseline night during which respiratory disturbance index (RDI) was 29 episodes per hour of sleep.*

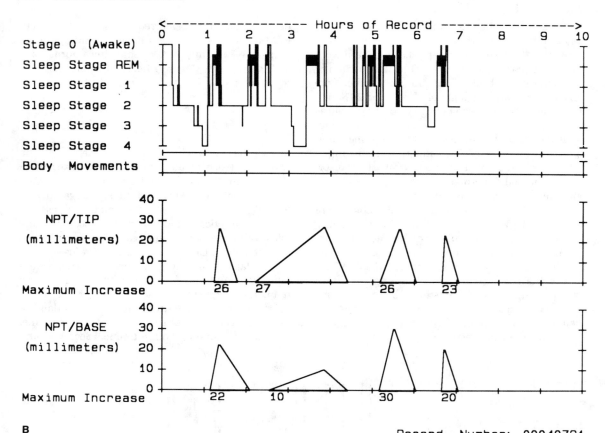

B

Record Number: 00040791

FIGURE 13-4(B).   *(Continued) Panel B shows the histogram for a night recorded during CPAP treatment (7 cm H$_2$O pressure); RDI was reduced to four episodes per hour. Sleep architecture, REM sleep, and sleep-related erections improved. The value of apnea detection and CPAP intervention as part of the diagnostic protocol are clearly evident.*

associates[46] provide an extensive review of the association between erectile dysfunction and pharmacologic agents.

Aside from their detrimental effects on sexual potency, some drugs adversely affect REM sleep. If a medication significantly suppresses or abolishes REM sleep, sleep-related erection testing may be inconclusive. Thus, acquiring a thorough drug history is essential. Tricyclic antidepressants, monoamine oxidase inhibitors, amphetamines, cocaine, barbiturates, and some benzodiazepines are particularly troublesome. When possible, we arrange for abstinence or reduction in medication before and during sleep evaluations. In some cases, data from the later portion of the night provide adequate information. For example, we occasionally see patients treated with antihypertensives who have no erections associated with their early REM sleep episodes. Toward morning, however, when drug levels decline, normal REM sleep–related tumescence occurs. Ware[48] reports a similar profile in his patients treated with cardiovascular medications.

Comorbidity factors

The clinical literature associates erectile impotence with a wide variety of cardiovascular, endocrine, genitourinary, neurologic, psychiatric, and other conditions. Those most often encountered at our clinic include: diabetes, hypertension, genital or pelvic trauma, hypogonadism, myocardial infarction, obstructive sleep apnea, chronic obstructive pulmonary disease, prostate conditions, chronic alcoholism, renal failure, spinal cord injury, multiple sclerosis, epilepsy, narcolepsy, Parkinson's disease, opiate and cocaine abuse, and major depressive disorders. Evidence for whether a disease is causally or casually related to impotence varies. Research has provided information concerning the mechanisms underlying organic impotence for some of these conditions (e.g., diabetes, hypertension, hypogonadism).

Sleep-related erection studies are available that compare a variety of patient groups to controls. Investigators have studied men with diabetes,[49–52] hypogonadism,[42,43] chronic obstructive pulmonary disease,[53] alcoholism,[54,55] spinal lesions,[56–58] end-stage renal disease,[59] hypertension,[60,61] and depression.[62,63]

In an early report by Karacan and colleagues,[64] data were presented indicating that sleep erections were diminished by dream anxiety. This finding was reiterated in subsequent reports,[10] and critics of NPT often cited this as evidence for sleep erection responsiveness to psychogenic phenomena. In the original study, however, dream reports were subjected to content analysis and indexed according to anxiety descriptor scores. Dreams were associated with normal erections, irregular erections, or no erections. Anxiety index scores did not differ between dreams associated with the different types of tumescence. In contrast, content analysis scores for anxiety were statistically higher in dreams with predominantly irregular erections than in dreams with normal erections. Irregular erections were those in which circumference fluctuated or detumescence began before the awakening made to gather dream reports. Irregular erection, in this study, by no means indicated that nightly values for sleep-related erection values were below normal limits.[65]

Advantages and Disadvantages of Different Techniques

Comparison of studies with and without polysomnography

Critical reviews of sleep-related erection testing frequently intermix laboratory PSG evaluations and nonlaboratory, nonpolygraphic procedures. This fuels the controversy over the reliability and validity of NPT testing for the differential diagnosis of impotence.

As nonlaboratory techniques became readily available, the type of patients referred for laboratory evaluation changed. Referrals for PSG study now frequently involve three special types of clinical cases. The first includes those difficult patients who have a complex, confusing history. The second is legal cases in which compensation or guilt hinges on erectile status. Finally, physicians, other health care workers, foreign dignitaries, and celebrities who need erectile function assessment are routinely referred for sleep studies at our center. Decisions on when and for whom laboratory NPT studies are ordered may reflect less clinical confidence in nonlaboratory techniques. Table 13-2 summarizes the susceptibility of various techniques to false positive and false negative interpretations.

Over the years we have encountered a significant number of patients who attempted to manipulate the test outcome. Their motivations ranged from psychopathology to intent to defraud. Men with Munchausen's syndrome seeking surgical procedures and psychogenically impotent men seeking a surgical quick fix can easily produce false positive test results when non-PSG techniques are used. Patients intentionally not wearing snap gauges or stamp rings, incorrectly reporting results of expandable gauges, or avoiding sleep by using stimulants represent a real problem to diagnosis by non-PSG evaluations. A patient accused of sexual assault may claim innocence based on erectile impotence. Others may seek compensation for job-related injury. By contrast, patients intentionally breaking snap gauges (faking having a good erection) to avoid surgery or obtain anxiolytics, though rare, does occur. With proper sleep laboratory evaluation, maneuvers to produce false positive or false negative tests do not succeed.

Comparison with visual sexual stimulation

If videotaped erotic materials evokes penile tumescence of normal circumference increase and adequate rigidity, erectile capacity is established. In a patient with erectile failure a normal response to visual erotica suggests psychogenic impotence. As

TABLE 13-2. Comparison of Nonlaboratory and Laboratory Recording Procedures for Susceptibility to Artifact and Tampering*

	Sleep Studies	Bedside & RigiScan Monitors*	Expandable & Snap Gauges, & Stamp Rings*
Body movement artifact	OK	OK‡	False −
Reflex spasm erection	OK	OK‡	False −
Short sleep period	OK	OK	False +
Disrupted sleep	OK	False +	False +
Disrupted REM sleep	OK	False +	False +
Clinical sleep disorders	OK	False +	False +
Tampering/faking good	OK	OK‡	False −
Tampering/faking bad	OK	False +	False +

*A false positive (+) test erroneously supports the diagnosis of organic impotence. A false negative (−) test erroneously supports the diagnosis of psychogenic impotence.

‡Very careful inspection of tracings by an experienced scorer looking for sudden baseline changes can help avoid false negative conclusions; however, research has shown that the addition of simultaneous EMG tracings improves overall accuracy.[66]

when normal NPT is found, Peyronie's disease, steal syndrome, neuropathy, and acute androgen deficiency must be ruled out and factors such as performance anxiety would need further investigation. In these situations, however, PSG can still add information when the erectile complaint specifically involves inability to sustain erections.

By contrast, a partial, nonrigid erection in response to visual sexual stimulation contributes no information diagnostically. It is equally probable that the lack of arousal has an organic or a psychogenic basis. Sexual preference mismatch between the patient and the video subject matter, sexual inhibition, and situational anxiety are all confounding factors. Therefore, in clinics with a referral base of predominantly organically impotent men, visual sexual stimulation does little more than add another procedure. In clinics that assess a large proportion of men with psychogenic impotence, however, the visual stimulation paradigm could serve as an economical triage tool.

Comparison with vasodilator injection technique

Penile injection of vasodilators (phentolamine, papaverine, prostaglandin E_1, individually or in combination) has become a popular technique for managing impotence. Some urologists inject regardless of whether the problem is organic or psychogenic. Injections appear less effective in patients with severe vasculogenic impotence, whereas patient with a neurogenic dysfunction may be hypersensitive. Reports indicate injection may fail to produce an erection in some psychogenically impotent men.[67] The diagnostic utility of vasodilator injection requires further, and more systematic, study. At present, vasodilator injection is more of a therapeutic *challenge procedure* than a diagnostic test. The effects of long-term use of penile vasodilator injections are not known, but reports of complications and adverse reactions are increasing.

Clinical Importance of Proper Diagnosis

Selection of treatment

Years ago, when treatment options were limited, making a specific causal diagnosis was less crucial, but with the advent of treatment options, ranging from psychotherapy to surgical intervention, information concerning cause became more important. The development of an implantable penile prosthesis intensified the need for more accurate diagnostic techniques. Currently, therapeutic options for impotence include psychotherapy, marriage counseling, behavior therapy, psychiatric treatment of depression, revascularization surgery, penile arterial bypass, prosthetic implantation, testosterone injection, vacuum device, and vasodilator injection.

Importance to the patient

As it is one of the basic biologic drives, the importance of sexuality should never be underestimated. We already know that patients may fail to comply when a medication's side effects include impotence.[68,69] For some men sexual potency fills an essential psychological need. Self-image, job performance, and interpersonal adjustment can all be destroyed by impotence. An erroneous diagnosis of psychogenic impotence can lead to ineffective behavioral or psychological treatment. The resulting increase in frustration level can make a bad situation worse. Misdiagnosis of organic impotence may lead to surgical procedures that destroy normal penile physiology.

Importance to the patient's sexual partner

Erectile failure affects not only the patient but also his sexual partner. Improper treatment of impaired sexual function can provoke frustration, guilt, and marital discord. By contrast, the dramatic improvement in mental outlook among couples for whom accurate diagnosis led to proper treatment is tremendously gratifying. The importance of sexuality to intimate relationships is immortalized in the popular maximum "couples fight about money, family, and sex." This is truly an instance where last is not least.

REFERENCES

1. Aserinsky E, Kleitman N. Regularly occurring periods of eye motility and concomitant phenomena during sleep. Science 1953;118:273–274.
2. Aserinsky E. Ocular Motility during Sleep and Its Application to the Study of Rest-Activity Cycles and Dreaming. Doctoral dissertation, University of Chicago, 1953.
3. Ohlmeyer P, Brilmayer H, Hullstrung H. Periodische Vorgange im Schlaf. Pflugers Arch 1944;248:559–560.
4. Karacan I. The Effect of Exciting Presleep Events on Dream Reporting and Penile Erections during Sleep. Doctoral thesis, State University of New York, Downstate Medical Center, Brooklyn, 1965.
5. Fisher C, Gross J, Zuch J. Cycle of penile erection synchronous with dreaming (REM) sleep. Arch Gen Psychiatry 1965;12:29–45.
6. Fisher C. Dreaming and sexuality. In: Loewenstein RM, Newman LM, Schur M, et al. eds. Psychoanalysis—A General Psychology. New York: International Universities Press, 1966;537–569.
7. Snyder F. The phenomenology of dreaming. In: Madow L, Show LH, eds. The Psychodynamic Implications of the Physiological Studies on Dreams. Springfield, Ill: Charles C Thomas, 1970.

8. Gaillard JM, Moneme A. Modification of dream content after preferential blockade of mesolimbic and mesocortical dopaminergic systems. J Psychiatr Res 1977; 13:247–256.

9. McCarley RW, Hoffman E. REM sleep dreams and the activation-synthesis hypothesis. Am J Psychiatry 1981;138:904–912.

10. Karacan I. Clinical value of nocturnal erection in the prognosis and diagnosis of impotence. Med Aspects Hum Sexuality 1970;4:27–34.

11. Hirshkowitz M, Karacan I, Arcasoy MO, et al. The prevalence of periodic limb movements during sleep in men with erectile dysfunction. Biol Psychiatry 1989; 26:541–544.

12. Hirshkowitz M, Karacan I, Arcasoy MO, et al. Prevalence of sleep apnea in men with sexual dysfunction. Urology 1990;36:232–234.

13. Karacan I. Advances in the psychophysiological evaluation of male erectile impotence. In: Flach FF, ed. Weekly Psychiatry Update Series, 43. New York: Biomedia, 1977;43:1–6.

14. Wein AJ, Fishkin R, Carpiniello VL, et al. Expansion without significant rigidity during nocturnal penile tumescence: A potential source of misinterpretation. J Urol 1981;126:343–344.

15. Karacan I, Salis PJ, Williams RL. The role of the sleep laboratory in the diagnosis and treatment of impotence. In: Williams RL, Karacan I, eds. Diagnosis and Treatment. New York: John Wiley & Sons, 1978;353–382.

16. Karacan I. Evaluation of nocturnal penile tumescence and impotence. In: Guilleminault C, ed. Sleeping and Waking Disorders: Indications and Techniques. Menlo Park, Calif: Addison-Wesley, 1982;343–371.

17. Barry JM, Blank B, Boileau M. Nocturnal penile tumescence monitoring with stamps. Urology 1980;15:171–172.

18. Kenepp D, Gonick P. Home monitoring of penile tumescence for erectile dysfunction. Initial experience. Urology 1979;14:261–264.

19. Procci WR, Martin DJ. Preliminary observations of the utility of portable NPT. Arch Sex Behav 1984;13:569–580.

20. Bradley WE, Timm GW, Gallagher JM, et al. New method for continuous measurement of nocturnal penile tumescence and rigidity. Urology 1985;26:4–9.

21. Virag R, Virag H, Lajujie J. A new device for measuring penile rigidity. Urology 1985;25:80–81.

22. Bertini J, Boileau MA. Evaluation of nocturnal penile tumescence with Potentest. Urology 1986;27:492–494.

23. Bradley WE. New techniques in evaluation of impotence. Urology 1987;29:383–388.

24. Kessler WO. Nocturnal penile tumescence. Urol Clin North Am 1988;15:81–86.

25. Slob AK, Blom JHM, van der Werff ten Bosch JJ. Erection problems in medical practice: differential diagnosis with relatively simple method. J Urol 1990;143:46–50.

26. Imagawa A, Kawanishi Y. NPT monitoring with stamps: Actual intracavernous pressure at separation. Impotence 1986;1:64.

27. Morales A, Condra M, Reid K. The role of penile tumescence monitoring in the diagnosis of impotence: A review. J Urol 1990;143:441–444.

28. Allen R, Brendler CB. Snap-gauge compared to a full nocturnal penile tumescence study for evaluation of patients with erectile impotence. J Urol 1990;143:51–54.

29. Morales A, Marshall PG, Surridge DH, et al. A new device for diagnostic screening of nocturnal penile tumescence. J Urol 1983;129:288–290.

30. Allen RP. Erectile impotence: Objective diagnosis from sleep-related erections (nocturnal penile tumescence). J Urol 1981;126:353.

31. Karacan I, Williams RL, Thornby JI, et al. Sleep-related penile tumescence as a function of age. Am J Psychiatry 1975;132:932–937.

32. Karacan I, Salis PJ, Thornby JI, et al. The ontogeny of nocturnal penile tumescence. Waking Sleeping 1976; 1:27–44.

33. Reynolds CF, Thase ME, Jennings JR, et al. Nocturnal penile tumescence in healthy 20- to 59-year-olds: A revisit. Sleep 1989;12:368–373.

34. Schiavi RC, Schreiner-Engel P, Mandeli J, et al. Healthy aging and male sexual function. Am J Psychiatry 1990;147:766–771.

35. Karacan I, Hursch CJ, Williams RL, et al. Some characteristics of nocturnal penile tumescence during puberty. Pediatr Res 1972;6:529–537.

36. Karacan I, Hursch CJ, Williams RL, et al. Some characteristics of nocturnal penile tumescence in young adults. Arch Gen Psychiatry 1972;26:351–356.

37. Hursch CJ, Karacan I, Williams RL, et al. Some characteristics of nocturnal penile tumescence in early middle-aged males. Comp Psychiatry 1972;13:539–548.

38. Karacan I, Hursch CJ, Williams RL, et al. Some characteristics of nocturnal penile tumescence in elderly males. J Gerontol 1972;27:39–45.

39. Karacan I, Williams RL, Salis PJ. The effect of sexual intercourse on sleep patterns and nocturnal penile erections. Psychophysiology 1970;7:338–339.

40. Karacan I, Ware JC, Salis PJ, et al. Sexual arousal and activity: Effect on subsequent nocturnal penile tumescence patterns. Sleep Res 1979;8:61.

41. Karacan I, Moore CA, Sahmay S. Measurement of pressure necessary for vaginal penetration. Sleep Res 1985;14:269.

42. Cunningham GR, Karacan I, Ware JC, et al. The relationships between serum testosterone and prolactin levels and nocturnal penile tumescence (NPT) in impotent men. J Androl 1982;3:241–247.

43. Cunningham GR, Hirshkowitz M, Korenman SG, et al. Testosterone replacement therapy and sleep-related erections in hypogonadal men. J Clin Endocrinol Metab 1990;70:792–797.

44. Schmidt HS, Wise HA. Significance of impaired penile tumescence and associated polysomnographic abnormalities in the impotent patient. J Urol 1981;126:348–352.

45. Pressman MR, DiPhillipo MA, Kendrick JI, et al. Problems in the interpretation of nocturnal penile tumescence studies: Disruption of sleep by occult sleep disorders. J Urol 1986;136:595–598.

46. Segraves RT, Madsen R, Carter CS, et al. Erectile dysfunction associated with pharmacological agents. In:

Segraves RT, Schoenberg HW, eds. Diagnosis and Treatment of Erectile Disturbances: A Guide for Clinicians. New York: Plenum, 1985;23–63.

47. Murray FT, Klimberg IW, Cohen MS. Organic impotence. In: Kassirer JP, ed. Current Therapy in Internal Medicine. Philadelphia: BC Decker, 1991;3:1375–1386.

48. Ware JC. Suppression of NPT during the first REM sleep period. Sleep Res 1984;13:71.

49. Karacan I, Scott FB, Salis PJ, et al. Nocturnal erections, differential diagnosis of impotence, and diabetes. Biol Psychiatry 1977;12:373–380.

50. Karacan I, Salis PJ, Ware JC, et al. Nocturnal penile tumescence and diagnosis in diabetic impotence. Am J Psychiatry 1978;135:191–197.

51. Karacan I. Diagnosis of erectile impotence in diabetes mellitus. An objective and specific method. Ann Intern Med 1980;92:334–337.

52. Hirshkowitz M, Karacan I, Rando KC, et al. Diabetes, erectile dysfunction, and sleep-related erections. Sleep 1990;13:53–68.

53. Fletcher EC, Martin RJ. Sexual dysfunction and erectile impotence in chronic obstructive pulmonary disease. Chest 1982;81:413–421.

54. Karacan I, Moore CA. Sexual dysfunction in alcoholic men. In: Wheatley D, ed. Psychopharmacology and sexual disorders. British Association for Psychopharmacology Monograph #4. Oxford: Oxford University Press, 1983;113–122.

55. Snyder S, Karacan I. Effects of chronic alcoholism on nocturnal penile tumescence. Psychosomat Med 1981;43:423–429.

56. Karacan I, Dimitrijevic M, Lauber A, et al. Nocturnal penile tumescence (NPT) and sleep stages in patients with spinal cord injuries. Sleep Res 1977;6:52.

57. Karacan I, Dervent A, Salis PJ, et al. Spinal cord injuries and NPT. Sleep Res 1978;7:261.

58. Halstead LS, Dimitrijevic M, Karacan I, et al. Impotence in spinal cord injury: Neurophysiological assessment of diminished tumescence and its relation to supraspinal influences. Curr Concepts Rehab Med 1984;1:8–14.

59. Karacan I, Dervent A, Cunningham G, et al. Assessment of nocturnal penile tumescence as an objective method for evaluating sexual functioning in ESRD patients. Dialysis Transplant 1978;7:872–876, 890.

60. Karacan I, Salis PJ, Hirshkowitz M, et al. Erectile dysfunction in hypertensive men: Sleep-related erections, penile blood flow, and musculovascular events. J Urol 1989;142:56–61.

61. Hirshkowitz M, Karacan I, Gurakar A, et al. Hypertension, erectile dysfunction, and occult sleep apnea. Sleep 1989;12:223–232.

62. Thase ME, Reynolds CF, Glanz LM, et al. Nocturnal penile tumescence in depressed men. Am J Psychiatry 1987;144:89–92.

63. Thase ME, Reynolds CF, Jennings JR, et al. Nocturnal penile tumescence is diminished in depressed men. Biol Psychiatry 1988;24:33–46.

64. Karacan I, Goodenough DR, Shapiro A, et al. Erection cycle during sleep in relation to dream anxiety. Arch Gen Psychiatry 1966;15:183–189.

65. Kaya N, Moore C, Karacan I. Nocturnal penile tumescence and its role in impotence. Psychiatr Ann 1979; 9:426–431.

66. Marshall P, McGrath P, Schillinger J. Importance of electromyographic data in interpreting nocturnal penile tumescence. Urology 1983;22:153–156.

67. Allen RP, Brendler CB. Nocturnal penile tumescence predicting response to intracorporeal pharmacological erection testing. J Urol 1988;140:518–522.

68. Gillin JC, Horowitz D, Wyatt RJ. Pharmacologic studies of narcolepsy involving serotonin, acetylcholine, and monoamine oxidase. In: Guilleminault C, Dement WC, Passouant P, eds. Narcolepsy. New York: Spectrum, 1976;585–604.

69. Hogan MJ, Wallin JD, Baer RM. Antihypertensive therapy and male sexual dysfunction. Psychosomatics 1980;21:234–237.

III

Clinical Aspects

14

An Approach to a Patient with Sleep Complaints

Sudhansu Chokroverty

Several epidemiologic studies have clearly shown that sleep complaints are very common in the general population.[1-10] Two important multiple-center studies were conducted by Colemen and others.[8,9] The first study,[8] conducted over a two-year period (1978 to 1980), included (PSG) 4698 patients, each of whom underwent a polysomnographic (PSG) study. The proportions of diagnostic categories in those with sleep complaints, after those evaluated for impotency are excluded are 51% with hypersomnia, 31% with insomnia, 15% with parasomnia, and 3% with sleep-wake schedule disorders. A subsequent report by Coleman[9] on 3085 patients over a 1-year period (1981 to 1982) showed remarkable consistency with the results of the first study. The most frequent disease categories included in these surveys were sleep apnea, narcolepsy, and insomnia related to psychiatric or psychophysiologic disorders. The 1979 Institute of Medicine[7] study concluded that about one-third of all adults in USA had some sleep disturbances. Some important epidemiologic factors identified in various studies include these[11]: old age, female sex, poor education and socioeconomic status, recent stress, alcohol, and drug abuse. It is important for physicians to be aware of this high prevalence of sleep disturbances, which cause considerable physical and psychological stress.

An approach to a sleep complaint must begin with a clear understanding of the various sleep disorders listed in the International Classification of Sleep Disorders[12] (see also Chapter 15). Briefly, this classification includes four categories: dyssomnias, parasomnias, medical or psychiatric sleep disorders, and proposed sleep disorders.

Dyssomnias include intrinsic, extrinsic, and circadian rhythm sleep disorders. Intrinsic disorders result from causes within the body; extrinsic disorders are secondary to external causes. Circadian rhythm disorders result from disruption of sleep-wake circadian rhythm.

The two major sleep complaints in the category of dyssomnia are insomnia and hypersomnia. Insomnia includes idiopathic and psychophysiologic insomnia, insomnia with central sleep apnea syndrome, and insomnia with restless legs syndrome–periodic limb movement disorder (RLS-PLMS).

Hypersomnia includes narcolepsy, obstructive sleep apnea syndrome (OSAS), central sleep apnea syndrome, alveolar hypoventilation syndrome, idiopathic, recurrent, and posttraumatic hypersomnia, and sometimes RLS-PLMS.

Parasomnias are disorders of arousals and sleep-wake transition disorders that are not primary sleep disorders but intrude into sleep. These consist of arousal and sleep-wake transition disorders, rapid eye movement (REM)–related parasomnias, and others.

Medical or psychiatric sleep disorders include disorders secondary to medical, psychiatric, and neurologic disorders.

Proposed sleep disorders include those about which we have inadequate information.

Physicians should also have an understanding of the severity of the two major sleep complaints. Sleepiness (hypersomnia) and sleeplessness (insomnia) can be mild, moderate, or severe.[12] Multiple sleep latency tests (MSLTs) show a mean sleep onset latency of 10 to 15 minutes for mild hypersomnia, 5 to 10 minutes for moderate hypersomnia, and less than 5 minutes for severe hypersomnia. Mild insomnia causes little or no functional impairment, moderate insomnia and mild to moderate impairment, and severe sleeplessness severe impairment. An understanding of this severity of hypersomnia and insomnia is important for designing of tests, therapeutic intervention, follow-up, and prognosis.

CLINICAL CHARACTERISTICS OF THE TWO MAJOR COMPLAINTS

Details are given in several chapters in this book and are briefly summarized here.

Insomnia

The general complaints of insomnia may include all or some of these[11]: difficulty falling asleep, frequent awakening, early morning awakening, insufficient or total lack of sleep, daytime fatigue, tiredness or sleepiness, lack of concentration, irritability, anxiety, and sometimes depression. Some patients may be preoccupied with psychosomatic symptoms such as aches and pains.

Hypersomnia

Hypersomnolent patients may complain of excessive daytime sleepiness (EDS), falling asleep in an inappropriate place and under inappropriate circumstances (e.g., while driving, at school, at work, at social activities), a lack of relief of symptoms following additional sleep at night, daytime fatigue, morning headache, inability to concentrate and remain alert, impairment of motor skills and cognition, and listlessness. Additional symptoms that may help make an etiologic diagnosis include snoring, cessation of breathing at night as reported by the bed partner, obstructive sleep apnea syndrome and waking up at night fighting for breath as noted in obstructive sleep apnea syndrome (OSAS). Attacks of cataplexy, hypnagogic hallucinations, sleep paralysis, and automatic behavior may be observed in patients with narcolepsy.

ETIOLOGIC DIAGNOSIS

Insomnia and hypersomnia are symptoms and do not constitute a specific diagnosis. Every attempt should be made to find a cause for these complaints. The causes are described in several chapters in this book and are briefly enumerated here.

Insomnia may be secondary to a variety of psychiatric (e.g., depression, anxiety), medical, or neurologic disorders, pain anywhere in the body, or drug or alcohol abuse, or associated with RLS-PLMS. It may be a manifestation of circadian rhythm sleep disorders (e.g., jet lag, delayed sleep phase syndrome, irregular sleep-wake schedule disorders). Shift workers may suffer nighttime sleep disturbances and daytime fatigue and sleepiness. Finally, for some, insomnia is a lifelong condition and no cause is found (idiopathic insomnia). Yet other patients have subjective complaints of sleeplessness but no objective evidence (e.g., normal PSG findings).

The etiologic differential diagnosis of hypersomnia may include the following conditions: OSAS, central sleep apnea and primary alveolar hypoventilation syndrome, narcolepsy, a variety of psychiatric, medical, and neurologic illnesses, drug or alcohol abuse, idiopathic central nervous system (CNS) hypersomnolence, periodic somnolence (e.g., Kleine-Levin syndrome, menstrual cycle–associated). Occasionally patients with RLS-PLMS complain of EDS.

METHOD OF CLINICAL EVALUATION

A physician equipped with this background knowledge should attempt to make a clinical diagnosis based on the history and physical examination of a patient who complains of sleep disturbance. PSG study, MSLT, and other laboratory tests must be confirmatory and subservient to the clinical diagnosis, which depends on a multifactorial analysis of many facets of a sleep complaint.

HISTORY

The first step in the diagnosis and assessment of a sleep-wakefulness disturbance is a careful evaluation of the sleep complaints. The history should seek information on sleep habits, drugs and alcohol consumption, psychiatric, medical, and neurologic illnesses, history of previous illness, and family history.[13-16]

Sleep History[13-16]

The sleep history is fundamentally important and is the first step in identifying the nature of the sleep disorder. Symptoms during the entire 24 hours should be evaluated, not just those that occur at sleep onset or during sleep at night. In addition to intrinsic and extrinsic dyssomnias, 24-hour symptomatic evaluation helps diagnose and manage circadian rhythm sleep disorders. The clinician should pay attention to symptoms that occur in the early evening or at sleep onset (e.g., paresthesias and uncontrollable limb movements of RLS); during sleep at night (e.g., repeated awakenings, snoring, and cessation of breathing in OSAS); on awakening in the morning (e.g., feeling exhausted and sleepy as in OSAS); in late morning and afternoon (e.g., daytime fatigue and excessive somnolence as in OSAS and irresistible desire to have brief sleep as in narcolepsy). Early morning awakening may be noted in insomnia due to depression. Abnormal motor activities may be associated with REM behavior disorder (RBD), other parasomnias, and in patients with seizures.

In evaluating sleep history, Kales and coworkers[13-15] enumerated these important principles: (1) Define the specific sleep problem. (2) Assess the clinical course. (3) Differentiate between various sleep disorders. (4) Evaluate sleep-wakefulness patterns. (5) Question the bed partner. (6) Evaluate the impact of the disorder on the patient.

One should analyze the onset, frequency, duration, and severity of the sleep complaint, its progression, evolution, and fluctuation over time, and any events that could have initiated it.[17] An analysis of these factors may differentiate transient disorders from persistent ones. The physician should inquire about the patient's functional status and mood during the daytime, any medicines and their effects on the sleep complaint, and about sleep hygiene.

Finally, psychological, social, medical, and biologic factors and their interactions should be considered, in order to understand the patient's problem.[17] An interview with the bed partner, caregiver, and, in case of a child, a parent, is important for diagnosis of abnormal movements (PLMS or other body movements), abnormal behavior (parasomnias, nocturnal seizures), and breathing disorders during sleep. The bed partner may also be able to answer questions about the patient's sleeping habits, past drug use, psychosocial problems (e.g., stress at home, work or school), and changes in sleep habits.

Sleep Questionnaire

A sleep questionnaire containing a list of pertinent questions relating to sleep complaints, sleep hygiene, sleep patterns, medical, psychiatric, and neurologic disorders, and drug or alcohol use, may be filled out by the patients to save time during the history taking.

Sleep Log or Sleep Diary

A sleep log kept over a 2-week period would be a valuable indicator of sleep hygiene, and it can also be used to monitor progression following therapeutic intervention. Such a log should capture information on bedtime, arising time, daytime naps, amount of time needed to go to sleep, number of nighttime awakenings, total sleep time, and feelings on arousal (e.g., refreshed or drowsy).

Drug and Alcohol History[13-15]

The physician should inquire about drugs that could cause insomnia (e.g., CNS stimulants, bronchodilators, B-blockers, corticosteroids, sedative-hypnotics) or hypersomnolence, about alcohol consumption and alcohol dependence, and about insomnia related to drug withdrawal (e.g., intermediate- or short-acting benzodiazepines, nonbenzodiazepine hypnotics). Caffeine consumption and smoking should also be considered as contributing factors to insomnia.

Psychiatric History[13-16]

Attention should be paid to signs of possible psychiatric or psychophysiologic disorders (e.g., depression, anxiety, psychosis, obsession, life stress situation, personality traits). If sleep disorders are secondary to a psychiatric illness, treating it allevi-

ates the sleep disturbance in most cases. If the sleep complaint persists following such treatment an additional cause or a primary sleep disorder should be suspected.

Medical and Neurologic History

Pertinent inquiry should be directed to possible symptoms of a variety of medical and neurologic illnesses (see Chapters 20 and 22). These symptoms direct attention to secondary sleep disorders.

History of Past Illnesses

The history may yield clues to significant past medical, psychiatric, or neurologic disorders that could be responsible for the present sleep disturbance. It is also important to evaluate the premorbid personality by inquiring into the history. Finally, a history of a drug or alcohol habit or use of street drugs may reveal the role of these agents in the sleep complaint.

Family History[13]

In certain sleep disorders family history is very important. A family history is found in about a third of patients with narcolepsy and RLS. OSAS, with or without obesity, has also been described in other family members. There is a high prevalence of sleepwalking, sleep terrors, and primary enuresis in other family members. Many neurologic disorders, including fatal familial insomnia, have a family history. Currently, an intensive search is going on for a gene specific for narcolepsy and RLS.

PHYSICAL EXAMINATION

It is essential to conduct a thorough physical examination of every patient with a sleep complaint. It may uncover clues to important medical disorders involving respiratory, cardiovascular, gastrointestinal, or endocrine systems; or a neurologic disease, especially one affecting neuromuscular, cervical spinal cord, or brain stem region, which may cause sleep-related breathing disorders as well as insomnias. In OSAS, physical examination may uncover upper airway anatomic abnormalities, which may need surgical correction if medical and continuous positive airway pressure (CPAP) treatment fail to relieve the symptoms. Examination may reveal systemic hypertension, which is a risk factor for sleep apnea.

CLINICAL PHENOMENOLOGY

In this section clinical characteristics of some common sleep disorders are briefly described. Details are given in several other chapters.

Obstructive Sleep Apnea Syndrome

OSAS is much more common in men than women, and onset of symptoms generally occurs after age 40 years. The symptoms are of two kinds: those that occur during sleep and those that occur during the waking hours (see Chapter 16). Nocturnal sleep symptoms include loud snoring, choking during sleep, cessation of breathing, sitting up fighting for breath, abnormal motor activities during sleep disruption, sometimes esophageal reflux, nocturia and nocturnal enuresis (noted mostly in children), and occasionally profuse sweating at night. The daytime symptoms include excessive daytime somnolence, which is characterized by sleep attacks lasting a half hour to 2 hours and occurring mostly when the patient is sitting down, for example to watch television. The prolonged duration and the nonrefreshing nature of the sleep attacks differentiates them from narcoleptic sleep attacks. The other diurnal events include personality changes such as impairment of memory, irritability, impairment of motor skills, morning headache, sometimes hypnagogic hallucinations, and automatic behavior with retrograde amnesia. In men, impotence is often associated with severe and longstanding cases of OSAS. Physical examination may reveal obesity in about 50% of the cases, in addition to anatomic abnormalities in the upper airway. In severe cases, polycythemia, and evidence of cardiac failure, pulmonary hypertension, and cardiac arrhythmias may be noted.

Narcolepsy

The sleep attacks of narcolepsy generally begin in the second or third decade of life, and in about 30% of some cases a family member has a history of similar attacks. The classical sleep attack consists of an irresistible desire to fall asleep at inappropriate times and lasts some few minutes to as long as 20 to 30 minutes. These attacks are often accompanied by cataplexy, during which there is transient loss of tone in the somatic muscles, often triggered by an emotional outburst. The patient may momentarily fall to the ground, or the head may simply slump forward for a few seconds. Three additional manifestations (e.g., hypnagogic hallucinations, sleep paralysis, and disturbed night sleep) are part of the narcolepsy pentad. It is a lifelong condition and is generally less severe in persons of advanced years. Sometimes patients with narcolepsy also have sleep apnea (central, obstructive, or mixed).

Insomnia

Insomnia may occur at any age when the patient complains of difficulty initiating or maintaining sleep. A large percentage of insomnia patients suffer from psychiatric illness, and a common cause of insomnia is depression. In this condition, early morning awakening is characteristic. Insomnia may be associated with a variety of psychiatric, medical, and neurologic illnesses or maybe drug induced. Sometimes, no cause can be found.

Restless Legs Syndrome

The fundamental problem is a complex sensorimotor disorder characterized by paresthesias or dysesthesias, predominantly in the legs, and motor restlessness during periods of repose and relaxation. This may begin at any age but often does in childhood or adolescence. Once started, it continues throughout life with periodic fluctuations, and sometimes it is severe in patients after age 50 years. Approximately a third of the patients will give a family history of a similar condition, suggesting a dominant mode of inheritance. Some patients may also have dyskinesias during relaxed wakefulness, and most patients have PLMS. Sleep disturbances, in particular sleep-onset insomnia, is a major problem. Because of nocturnal insomnia, the patient may have daytime hypersomnolence, and occasionally also sleep apnea.

Parasomnias

Parasomnias are a variety of abnormal movements and behaviors that occur during sleep.

Sleepwalking

Somnambulism is common in children and occurs at sleep onset during non-REM (NREM) sleep stages 3 and 4. Patients either do not remember or have a vague dreamlike memory of the events. Episodes may last a few seconds to 30 minutes. Electroencephalography (EEG) may show characteristic high-voltage synchronous delta waves at the onset, resembling hypnagogic hypersynchrony.

Sleep Terror

Night terrors or Pavor Nocturnus also occurs during NREM stage 3 and 4 sleep. They are common in childhood, somnambulism and sleep terror may occur together. Again, patients have no recollection or a vague memory of the events.

Nightmares

Nightmares occur during REM sleep and are vivid, frightening dreams followed by awakening and vivid recall.

REM Behavior Disorder

RBD is common in elderly persons and occurs during REM sleep. A characteristic feature of this syndrome is the intermittent loss of REM-related muscle hypotonia and appearance of a variety of abnormal motor activities during REM sleep. The violent motor behavior during sleep may pose a risk to the bed partner. The condition may be idiopathic or may be secondary to some neurologic disorder.

Head Banging

Head banging (Rhythmic Movement Disorder or Jactatio Capitis Nocturna) is characterized by rhythmic forward and backward or lateral, and occasionally rocking, head and body movements lasting up to an hour or so. It is more common in infants and may occur at any stage of sleep.

LABORATORY INVESTIGATIONS

Polysomnography

PSG is an invaluable laboratory test for the diagnosis and treatment of sleep disorders, particularly in patients with hypersomnia. All-night PSG, rather than a single daytime nap study, is required. A daytime single-nap study generally misses REM sleep, and most severe cases of obstructive sleep apneas are noted during REM sleep. Maximum oxygen desaturation also occurs at this stage. With a daytime study the severity of the symptoms cannot be assessed. Because treatment—and particularly treatment with CPAP—might be adversely affected, an all-night sleep study is essential. To determine the optimal level of the CPAP, both REM and NREM sleep recordings are required. The indications for PSG in persons who complain of EDS are not controversial. Such patients should have a PSG unless their hypersomnolence is a transient phenomenon secondary to misuse or use of sedatives or hypnotics. To monitor the efficacy of treatment with CPAP and to observe the results of CPAP treatment for OSAS, an all-night PSG study is necessary. It should be noted that, following the first night of nasal CPAP, the following important changes are noted in the PSG[18]: an increase in the amount of slow-wave sleep, an increase in the amount of REM sleep, a decrement of sleep fragmentation, and increased sleep continuity. The last factor may be responsible for improvement of daytime functioning in these patients.

Some patients with narcolepsy may also have sleep apnea, and for them a PSG study is necessary, which should be followed by the MSLT.

Indications for PSG in patients with insomnia are somewhat controversial. Hauri[16] listed the following indications for PSG to investigate insomnia: (1) to rule out sleep apnea or PLMS that may be associated with or the cause of insomnia; (2) to exclude sleep epilepsies that may cause insomnia; (3) to document sleep latency, sleep efficiency, total sleep, and sleep architecture; (4) to document atypical PSG features (e.g., alpha intrusion into NREM sleep, frequent "mini-arousals"); (5) to compare the subjective with the objective assessment of sleep efficiency and sleep latency; and (6) to document the patient's behavior during sleep at night and at sleep onset.

Sleep fragmentation, as documented by PSG, is an important consequence of OSAS and may also be secondary to PLMS. Sleep fragmentation (fluctuation in sleep stages due to NREM-REM cycling throughout the night)[18] in part, may determine daytime behavior and thus should be measured.[18] Fragmentation depends on the number of such sleep stage shifts.

Another controversy about PSG study in insomnia is how many studies are necessary. According to Hauri,[16] 1 night of PSG is adequate to rule out sleep apnea, PLMS, and atypical PSG features, and at least 2 nights of PSG is required to study the amount of sleep in a patient who has subjective complaints but no objective findings. Hauri also stated that if sleep apnea or nocturnal epilepsy is suspected or observed a follow-up PSG study is needed to evaluate it further.[16] Full EEG montages using multiple channels are required for recordings in such patients.

Ideally, two nights of PSG studies should be performed. The first night's study documents the extent and severity of the sleep apnea, but the so-called first-night effect and night-to-night variability are the confounding factors. On the second night, CPAP is administered to patients with OSAS, but because of the expense involved, in many centers a single night's recording is performed and during the latter part of the recording CPAP is administered to document optimal pressure and its effect on PSG findings. It should be noted that it is highly unlikely that moderate to severe cases of OSAS will be missed by a single night's recording.

Sometimes PSG is useful in sleep disorders caused by certain psychiatric illnesses, for example, depression, psycho-physiologic insomnia, or sleep-wake schedule disturbances.

Multiple Sleep Latency Test

The MSLT is essential for documenting pathologic sleepiness and for diagnosing narcolepsy. (see Chapter 10).

Video-Polysomnographic Study

Parasomnias are generally diagnosed on the basis of the clinical history, but sometimes PSG, and particularly video-PSG,[19] is required to document the condition. Because certain parasomnias mimic seizure disorders, PSG, and again, particularly video-PSG, is essential when seizure disorder[19] is suspected. For nocturnal epilepsy video-PSG utilizing multiple-channel EEG and multiple montages is required. Ideally, if sleep epilepsy is suspected the video-PSG recording should have the capability for EEG analysis at the standard EEG speed of 30 mm per second, to identify epileptiform discharges.[19]

Standard Electroencephalographic Study

EEG is necessary to investigate suspected epilepsy.

Ambulatory Electroencephalography or Polysomnography

Ambulatory EEG or PSG is required for patients with suspected sleep epilepsy and may be useful for understanding the circadian variation and for studying circadian rhythm sleep disorders.

Neuroimaging Study

Neuroimaging is essential when a neurologic illness is suspected of causing a sleep disturbance.

Other Laboratory Tests

Blood and urinalysis, electrocardiography (ECG), Holter ECG, chest radiography, and other investigations to rule out gastrointestinal, pulmonary, cardiovascular, endocrine, and renal disorders should be conducted to diagnose insomnia or hypersomnia caused by a variety of medical disorders. In rare cases, when autonomic failure causes a sleep disturbance or sleep-related breathing disorder, autonomic function tests may be required for diagnosis of the primary condition. Finally, with some patients suspected of having a sleep disturbance of psychiatric or psychological cause, the Minnesota Multiphasic Personality Inventory may be required.

In conclusion, this chapter has given an outline for an approach to a patient with a sleep complaint. This should begin with a careful clinical analysis of the patient's symptom, keeping in mind the classification of sleep disorders and its pertinent manifestations along with the underlying basic science foundations of such disorders. In most cases, diagnosis can be made on clinical grounds with minimal laboratory investigations, to minimize the patient's suffering and expenses. In this way, we honor the Hippocratic oath by comforting patients and causing no harm.

REFERENCES

1. McGhie A, Russell SM. The subjective assessment of normal sleep patterns. J Ment Sci 1962;108:642–654.

2. Hammond EC. Some preliminary findings on physical complaints from a prospective study of 1,064,004 men and women. Am J Public Health 1964;54:11–23.

3. Tune G. Sleep and wakefulness in 509 normal adults. Br J Med Psychol 1969;42:75–80.

4. Johns MWW, Egan P, Gay TJ, et al. Sleep habits and symptoms in male medical and surgical patients. Br Med J 1970;2:509–512.

5. Karacan I, Thornby JI, Anch M, et al. Prevalence of sleep disturbance in a primarily urban Florida county. Soc Sci Med 1976;10:239–244.

6. Bixler EO, Kales A, Soldatos CR, et al. Prevalence of sleep disorders in the Los Angeles Metropolitan Area. Am J Psychiatry 1979;136:1257–1262.

7. Institute of Medicine. Sleeping pills, insomnia and medical practice. Washington, DC: National Academy of Sciences, 1979.

8. Coleman RM, Roffwarg HP, Kennedy SJ, et al. Sleep-wake disorders based on a polysomnographic diagnosis. A national cooperative study. JAMA 1982;247:997–1003.

9. Coleman RM. Diagnosis, treatment and follow-up of about 8000 sleep/wake disorder patients. In: Guilleminault C, ed. Sleep/Wake Disorders: Natural History, Epidemiology and Long-Term Evaluation. New York: Raven Press, 1983; 87–97.

10. Gislason T, Almqvist M. Somatic diseases and sleep complaints: An epidemiological study of 3201 Swedish men. Acta Med Scand 1987;221:475–481.

11. Aldrich MS. Cardinal manifestations of sleep disorders. In: Kryger MN, Roth T, Dement WC, eds. Principles and Practice of Sleep Medicine. Philadelphia: WB Saunders, 1989;313–319.

12. Diagnostic Classification Steering Committee. The International Classification of Sleep Disorders: Diagnostic and Coding Manual. Rochester, Minn: American Sleep Disorders Association, 1990;259–280.

13. Kales A, Soldatos CR, Kales JD. Taking a sleep history. Am Fam Physician 1980;22:101–108.

14. Kales A, Kales JD. Evaluation and Treatment of Insomnia. New York: Oxford University Press, 1984.

15. Kales JD, Carvell M, Kales A. Sleep and sleep disorders. In: Cassel CK. Riesenberg DE, Sorensen LB, et al. eds. Geriatric Medicine. New York: Springer-Verlag, 1990; 562–579.

16. Hauri PJ. Evaluating disorders of initiating and maintaining sleep (DIMS). In: Guilleminault C, ed. Sleeping and Walking Disorders: Indications and Techniques. Menlo Park, Calif: Addison-Wesley, 1982;225–244.

17. Liebmann RC, et al. The assessment of sleep-wakefulness. In: Peter JH, Podszus T, Von Wichert P, eds. Sleep-Related Disorders and Internal Diseases. New York: Springer-Verlag, 1987;30.

18. Rothenberg SA. Measurement of sleep fragmentation. In: Peter JH, Podszus T, Von Wichert P, eds. Sleep-Related Disorders and Internal Diseases. New York: Springer-Verlag, 1987;63.

19. Aldrich M, Jahnke B. Diagnostic value of video-EEG polysomnography. Neurology 1991;41:1060–1066.

15

Classification of Sleep Disorders

Michael J. Thorpy

The symptom-based sleep disorders classifications of the past formed the basis for the modern classifications. In 1990, the most recent, widely used classification, the International Classification of Sleep Disorders (ICSD), was produced following a lengthy 5-year process initiated by the American Sleep Disorders Association (Table 15-1).[1-156] The ICSD classification was developed in association with the three major international sleep societies, the European Sleep Research Society, The Japanese Society of Sleep Research, and the Latin American Sleep Society. The resulting publication is the comprehensive text, *The International Classification of Sleep Disorders (ICSD): Diagnostic and Coding Manual.*[157]

The ICSD lists 84 sleep disorders, each with descriptive details, specific diagnostic, severity, and duration criteria. In addition there is coding information for clinical and research purposes. The ICSD has four major categories: *dyssomnias,* disorders of initiating and maintaining sleep and disorders of excessive sleepiness; *parasomnias,* disorders that primarily do not cause a complaint of insomnia or excessive sleepiness; the *disorders associated with medical or psychiatric disorders;* and the *proposed sleep disorders,* that is, disorders for which insufficient information is available to confirm their acceptance as definitive sleep disorders. The *proposed* sleep disorders category was required because of the rapid advances of sleep medicine, which have resulted in the discovery of several new sleep disorders.

DYSSOMNIAS

The dyssomnias, disorders that produce either insomnia or excessive sleepiness, are the major (primary) sleep disorders associated with either disturbed nighttime sleep or impaired wakefulness.

The dyssomnias contain a heterogeneous group of sleep disorders that have their origin in different body systems. For example, a disorder of the central nervous system (CNS) is believed to be the cause of narcolepsy,[7,8] whereas a physical obstruction in the upper airway may be the sole cause of obstructive sleep apnea syndrome.[14,15]

The dyssomnias are divided into three major groups: the intrinsic sleep disorders, the extrinsic sleep disorders, and the circadian rhythm sleep disorders. The divisions are based, in part, on pathophysiologic mechanisms. Because the circadian rhythm sleep disorders share a common chronophysiologic basis, they were kept as a single group. Both intrinsic and extrinsic factors may be involved in some of the circadian rhythm sleep disorders, so some of them, such as delayed sleep phase syndrome, are subdivided into intrinsic and extrinsic types.

Intrinsic Sleep Disorders

The intrinsic sleep disorders are primary sleep disorders that originate or develop in the body or arise from causes in the body. This section contains only those disorders that are included in and defined by the designation *dyssomnias.* Some sleep disorders due to processes arising in the body are not listed in the intrinsic section but are listed in the parasomnias, medical-psychiatric, or proposed sleep disorder sections.

The intrinsic sleep disorders include various types, some of which, such as psychophysiologic insomnia,[1,2] sleep state misperception,[3,4] restless legs syndrome,[22,23] and idiopathic insomnia,[5,6] are primarily disorders that produce insomnia. Psychophysiologic insomnia, a common form of insomnia, is a disorder of somatized tension and learned sleep-preventing associations that result in a complaint of insomnia and associated decreased functioning during wakefulness. *Sleep state misperception* is a relatively new term for a disorder in which a complaint of insomnia or excessive sleepiness occurs in the absence of objective evidence of sleep disturbance. Restless legs syndrome is well-known, but the term *idiopathic insomnia* indicates a lifelong inability to obtain adequate sleep that presumably is due to an abnormality of the neurologic control of the sleep-wake system.

Narcolepsy,[7,8] recurrent hypersomnia,[9,10] idiopathic hypersomnia,[11,12] and posttraumatic hypersomnia[13] are principally disorders of excessive sleepiness. Narcolepsy is a disorder of unknown cause that is characterized by excessive sleepiness

TABLE 15-1.   The International Classification of Sleep Disorders

	Recommended
1. Dyssomnias	ICD-9-CM No.
A. Intrinsic sleep disorders	
1. Psychophysiological insomnia[1,2]	307.42-0
2. Sleep state misperception[3,4]	307.49-1
3. Idiopathic insomnia[5,6]	780.52-7
4. Narcolepsy[7,8]	347
5. Recurrent hypersomnia[9,10]	780.54-2
6. Idiopathic hypersomnia[11,12]	780.54-7
7. Posttraumatic hypersomnia[13]	780.54-8
8. Obstructive sleep apnea syndrome[14,15]	780.53-0
9. Central sleep apnea syndrome[16,17]	780.51-0
10. Central alveolar hypoventilation syndrome[18,19]	780.51-1
11. Periodic limb movement disorder[20,21]	780.52-4
12. Restless legs syndrome[22,23]	780.52-5
13. Intrinsic sleep disorder NOS	780.52-9
B. Extrinsic sleep disorders	
1. Inadequate sleep hygiene[24,25]	307.41-1
2. Environmental sleep disorder[26,27]	780.52-6
3. Altitude insomnia[28,29]	993.2
4. Adjustment sleep disorder[30,31]	307.41-0
5. Insufficient sleep syndrome[32,33]	307.49-4
6. Limit-setting sleep disorder[34]	307.42-4
7. Sleep-onset association disorder[35]	307.42-5
8. Food allergy insomnia[36,37]	780.52-2
9. Nocturnal eating (drinking) syndrome[38,39]	780.52-8
10. Hypnotic-dependent sleep disorder[40,41]	780.52-0
11. Stimulant-dependent sleep disorder[42,43]	780.52-1
12. Alcohol-dependent sleep disorder[44]	780.52-3
13. Toxin-induced sleep disorder[45]	780.54-6
14. Extrinsic sleep disorder NOS	780.52-9
C. Circadian rhythm sleep disorders	
1. Time zone change (jet lag) syndrome[46,47]	307.45-0
2. Shift work sleep disorder[48,49]	307.45-1
3. Irregular sleep-wake pattern[50,51]	307.45-3
4. Delayed sleep phase syndrome[52,53]	780.55-0
5. Advanced sleep phase syndrome[54,55]	780.55-1
6. Non-24 hour sleep-wake disorder[56,57]	780.55-2
7. Circadian rhythm sleep disorder NOS	780.55-9
2. Parasomnias	
A. Arousal disorders	
1. Confusional arousals[58,59]	307.46-2
2. Sleepwalking[60,61]	307.46-0
3. Sleep terrors[62,63]	307.46-1
B. Sleep-wake transition disorders	
1. Rhythmic movement disorder[64,65]	307.3
2. Sleep starts[66,67]	307.47-2
3. Sleep talking[68,69]	307.47-3
4. Nocturnal leg cramps[70,71]	729.82
C. Parasomnias usually associated with REM sleep	
1. Nightmares[72,73]	307.47-0
2. Sleep paralysis[74,75]	780.56-2
3. Impaired sleep-related penile erections[76,77]	780.56-3
4. Sleep-related painful erections[78,79]	780.56-4
5. REM sleep-related sinus arrest[80]	780.56-8
6. REM sleep behavior disorder[81,82]	780.59-0
D. Other Parasomnias	
1. Sleep bruxism[83,84]	306.8
2. Sleep enuresis[85,86]	780.56-0

TABLE 15-1.   *(continued)*

	Recommended
3. Sleep-related abnormal swallowing syndrome[87]	780.56-6
4. Nocturnal paroxysmal dystonia[88,89]	780.59-1
5. Sudden unexplained nocturnal death syndrome[90,91]	780.59-3
6. Primary snoring[92,93]	780.53-1
7. Infant sleep apnea[94,95]	770.80
8. Congenital central hypoventilation syndrome[96,97]	770.81
9. Sudden infant death syndrome[98,99]	798.0
10. Benign neonatal sleep myoclonus[100,101]	780.59-5
11. Other Parasomnia NOS	780.59-9
3. Sleep Disorders Associated with Medical/Psychiatric Disorders	
A. Associated with mental disorders	290-319
1. Psychoses[102,103]	292-299
2. Mood disorders[104,105]	296-301
3. Anxiety disorders[106,107]	300
4. Panic disorder[108,109]	300
5. Alcoholism[110,111]	303
B. Associated with neurological disorders	320-389
1. Cerebral degenerative disorders[112]	330-337
2. Dementia[113,114]	331
3. Parkinsonism[115,116]	332-333
4. Fatal familial insomnia[117,118]	337.9
5. Sleep-related epilepsy[119,120]	345
6. Electrical status epilepticus of sleep[121,122]	345.8
7. Sleep-related headaches[123,124]	346
C. Associated with other medical disorders	
1. Sleeping sickness[125,126]	086
2. Nocturnal cardiac ischemia[127,128]	411-414
3. Chronic obstructive pulmonary disease[129,130]	490-494
4. Sleep-related asthma[131,132]	493
5. Sleep-related gastroesophageal reflux[133,134]	530.1
6. Peptic ulcer disease[135,136]	531-534
7. Fibrositis syndrome[137,138]	729.1
4. Proposed sleep disorders	
1. Short sleeper[139,140]	307.49-0
2. Long sleeper[141,142]	307.49-2
3. Subwakefulness syndrome[143]	307.47-1
4. Fragmentary myoclonus[145]	780.59-7
5. Sleep hyperhidrosis[145,146]	780.8
6. Menstruation-associated sleep disorder[147,148]	780.54-3
7. Pregnancy-associated sleep disorder[149,150]	780.59-6
8. Terrifying hypnagogic hallucinations[151]	307.47-4
9. Sleep-related neurogenic tachypnea[152]	780.53-2
10. Sleep-related laryngospasm[153,154]	780.59-4
11. Sleep choking syndrome[155,156]	307.42-1

Reproduced by permission of the American Sleep Disorders Association from Diagnostic Classification Committee. Thorpy MJ, Chairman. International Classification of Sleep Disorders: Diagnostic and Coding Manual. Rochester, Minn.: American Sleep Disorders Association, 1990.

that typically is associated with cataplexy and other rapid eye movement (REM) sleep phenomena such as sleep paralysis and hypnagogic hallucinations. Recurrent hypersomnia is characterized by recurrent episodes of hypersomnia that typically occur weeks or months apart, one form of which is the Kleine-Levin syndrome. Idiopathic hypersomnia, which can be confused clinically with narcolepsy, is a disorder of presumed CNS cause that is associated with a normal or prolonged major sleep episode and excessive sleepiness in the daytime with prolonged (1 to 2-hour) sleep episodes of non-REM (NREM) sleep. Posttraumatic hypersomnia is hypersomnia that occurs as a result of a traumatic event that involves the CNS.

The next four disorders, obstructive sleep apnea syndrome,[14,15] central sleep apnea syndrome,[16,17] central alveolar hypoventilation syndrome,[18,19] and periodic limb movement disorder,[20,21] are sleep-related breathing disorders that can produce a complaint of either insomnia or excessive sleepiness.

The term *intrinsic* implies that the primary cause of the disorder is an internal (endogenous) abnormality in physiology within the body. It is clear, however, that for some disorders external factors are important in either precipitating or exacerbating the disorder. The following examples are given to help explain the rationale for organizing the disorders under the group heading of *intrinsic*.

Posttraumatic hypersomnia[13] is an example of an intrinsic disorder that could not exist without an external event that produced the head injury. The primary cause of the hypersomnia, however, is of CNS origin and is listed in the *intrinsic* section, as the disorder persists after the traumatic event has terminated. Obstructive sleep apnea syndrome can be induced by an external factor such as consumption of alcohol, but the syndrome would not be possible without the internal factor of upper airway obstruction and a physiologic predisposition to develop the disorder.

Extrinsic Sleep Disorders

The extrinsic sleep disorders include those that originate or develop from causes outside the body. External (exogenous) factors are integral in producing these sleep disorders, and removal of the external factors leads to resolution of the sleep disorder. Internal factors may be important in the development or maintenance of the sleep disorder, just as external factors can be important in the development or maintenance of an intrinsic sleep disorder. The internal factors would not, by themselves, have produced the sleep disorder in the absence of an external factor.

Although there appears to be overlap between some disorders, for example, alcohol-dependent sleep disorder,[44] environmental sleep disorder,[26,27] and inadequate sleep hygiene,[24,25] the ICSD text and diagnostic criteria highlight the differences. Some explanation may be helpful.

Inadequate sleep hygiene[24,25] is a sleep disorder that is due to daily habits that are inconsistent with the maintenance of good quality sleep and full daytime alertness. It is a sleep disorder that develops out of normal behavioral practices that for another person usually would not disturb sleep. For example, an irregular bedtime or waketime that might not be associated with sleep disturbance in one person may produce a sleep disturbance in another. Though environmental factors can produce a disorder of inadequate sleep hygiene, the diagnosis of an environmental sleep disorder is made only when the environmental factors are particularly abnormal and not under the patient's own control, such as excessive noise or extreme lighting effects that would produce sleep disturbance in most people. Caffeine consumed in coffee or sodas can produce a disorder of inadequate sleep hygiene if the amount consumed is within the limits of common use, whereas taking stimulants in amounts considered excessive by normal standards can lead to a diagnosis of a stimulant-dependent sleep disorder.[42,43] Similarly, sleep that is disrupted by drinking what would be considered a socially normal amount of alcohol can lead to a diagnosis of inadequate sleep hygiene, whereas sleep disrupted by drinking what most people consider an excessive amount of alcohol taken primarily to induce sleep can lead to a diagnosis of alcohol-dependent sleep disorder.[44]

Altitude insomnia,[28,29] also known as acute mountain sickness, is an acute insomnia, usually accompanied by headache, loss of appetite, and fatigue, that follows ascent to high altitudes. Insomnia may be the sole manifestation of altitude insomnia, whereas the term *acute mountain sickness* usually applies when other physiologic disturbances predominate.

Some of the extrinsic sleep disorders have internal factors that are important for the expression of the sleep disturbance, but external factors are essential for the continuation of the sleep disturbance, but external factors are essential for the continuation of the sleep disturbance. When they are removed, the sleep disturbance resolves. For example, the extrinsic disorder, adjustment sleep disorder,[30,31] represents sleep disturbance that is temporarily related to acute stress, conflict, or environmental change that causes emotionally induced arousal. Because it is due to psychologically stressful factors it could be considered to be internally generated, but an external event causes the sleep disturbance and if it is removed the disorder resolves. If the sleep disorder continues after removal of the external factor, an intrinsic sleep disorder may have developed, such as psychophysiologic insomnia.[1,2]

Limit-setting sleep disorder[34] is primarily a childhood disorder characterized by inadequate enforcement of bedtime by a caretaker, with resultant stalling or refusal to go to bed at an appropriate time. Another predominantly childhood sleep disorder is sleep-onset association disorder,[35] which occurs when sleep onset is impaired by the absence of a certain object or set of circumstances such as sucking on a pacifier.

Circadian Rhythm Sleep Disorders

The circadian rhythm sleep disorders comprise the third section of the dyssomnias and are grouped together because they share an underlying chrono-physiologic basis. The major feature of these disorders is a misalignment between the timing of the patient's sleep pattern and that which is desired or regarded as the societal norm. The underlying problem in the majority of circadian rhythm sleep disorders is that the patient cannot sleep when sleep is desired, needed, or expected. The waking hours can occur at undesired times as a result of sleep episodes that occur at inappropriate times. Therefore, the patient may complain of insomnia or excessive sleepiness. For several of the circadian rhythm sleep disorders, once sleep is initiated the major sleep episode is of normal duration and has normal REM-NREM cycling. Intermittent sleep episodes can occur in some disorders, such as the irregular sleep-wake pattern.[50,51]

The first two circadian rhythm sleep disorders, time zone change (jet lag) syndrome[46,47] and shift work sleep disorder,[48,49] are disorders in which the sleep episodes occur at a time that is not synchronized with the underlying circadian rhythms of such measures as temperature or biochemical variables. Delayed sleep phase syndrome,[52,53] advanced sleep phase syndrome,[54,55] and non–24-hour sleep-wake syndrome[56,57] are disorders in which the timing of sleep is synchronized with underlying circadian rhythms. Delayed sleep phase syndrome is a disorder in which the major sleep episode is delayed in relation to the desired clock time, a delay that results in symptoms of sleep-onset insomnia or difficulty awakening at the desired time. Advanced sleep phase syndrome is similar, but the sleep episode is advanced in relation to the desired clock time and symptoms are compelling evening sleepiness, early sleep onset, and awakening earlier than desired. The non–24-hour sleep-wake syndrome is a rare disorder that consists of a chronic steady pattern of 1 to 2-hours daily delays in the sleep onset and awaking times.

It should be pointed out that the appropriate timing of sleep within the 24-hour day can be disturbed in many other sleep disorders, particularly those associated with the complaint of insomnia. Patients with narcolepsy[7,8] can have a pattern of sleepiness identical to that due to an irregular sleep-wake pattern.[50,51] Because, however, the primary sleep diagnosis is narcolepsy, the patient should not receive a second diagnosis of a circadian rhythm sleep disorder unless the disorder is unrelated to the narcolepsy. For example, a diagnosis of time zone change (jet lag) syndrome could be stated along with a diagnosis of narcolepsy, if appropriate. Similarly, patients with mood disorders[104,105] or psychoses[102,103] can, at times, have a sleep pattern similar to that of delayed sleep phase syndrome.

Some disturbance of sleep timing is a common feature in patients who have a diagnosis of inadequate sleep hygiene.[24,25] Only if the timing of sleep is the predominant cause of the sleep disturbance, and is outside the societal norm, is the diagnosis circadian rhythm sleep disorder. Limit-setting sleep disorder[34] is also associated with an altered time of sleep within the 24-hour day, but the timing of sleep in this disorder is not within the patient's control, nor is it intrinsically induced. If the setting of limits is a function of the caretake, then the sleep disorder is more appropriately diagnosed within the extrinsic subsection of the dyssomnias; that is, as a limit-setting sleep disorder.[34]

Three circadian rhythm sleep disorders have intrinsic and extrinsic subtypes: delayed sleep phase syndrome, advanced sleep phase syndrome, and non–24-hour sleep-wake syndrome. These disorders can be socially or environmentally induced or can be due to an abnormal circadian pacemaker or its entrainment mechanism.

PARASOMNIAS

The parasomnias consist of sleep disorders that are not abnormalities of the processes responsible for sleep and wakefulness per se but are undesirable phenomena that occur predominantly during sleep. The parasomnias are disorders of arousal, partial arousal, and sleep stage transition. Many of the parasomnias are manifestations of CNS activation. Autonomic nervous system changes and skeletal muscle activity are the predominant features. The parasomnias are subdivided into the arousal disorders, the sleep-wake transition disorders, the parasomnias associated with REM sleep, and other parasomnias.

The *arousal* disorders consist of the classic disorders of sleepwalking[60,61] and sleep terrors[62,63] and a newly described disorder, confusional arousals.[58,59]

The *sleep-wake transition* disorders include those that occur in the transition from wakefulness to sleep or from sleep to wakefulness, such as sleep starts[66,67] and sleep talking.[68,69] This group does not include disorders that are clearly associated with REM sleep, such as sleep paralysis.[74,75] Although some of the sleep-wake transition disorders can occur during sleep or even in wakefulness, such as rhythmic movement disorder (jactatio capitis nocturna),[64,65] the most typical occurrence of these disorders is in the transition from wakefulness to sleep. Restless legs syndrome[22,23] could be considered a sleep-wake transition disorder, but it is not a parasomnia, as it is associated primarily with a complaint of insomnia and therefore is listed in the dyssomnias.

The parasomnias usually associated with REM sleep include six disorders that have a close association with the REM sleep stage.

The fourth subsection contains parasomnias that are not classified in the previous three sections. The *other parasomnias* include disorders such as sleep bruxism[83,84] and sleep enuresis.[85,86] The infant sleep-related breathing disorders are listed here, as they do not produce complaints of insomnia or excessive sleepiness and are most typically regarded as parasomnias. Sudden infant death syndrome (SIDS) is listed, as it most commonly occurs during sleep and appears likely to have a sleep-related mechanism.

Disorders of Arousal

The disorders of arousal are disorders associated with impaired arousal from sleep. Onset in slow-wave sleep is a typical feature. Confusional arousals,[58,59] newly described though they were alluded to in the original description of the disorders of arousal, consist of confusion during and following arousal from sleep, most typically from deep sleep in the first part of the night. These episodes are more prevalent in children who sleepwalk[60,61] or have sleep terrors[62,63] and may be partial manifestations of those disorders. Confusional arousals can occur as an isolated sleep disorder.

Sleep-Wake Transition Disorders

The sleep-wake transition disorders occur in the transition from wakefulness to sleep, sleep to wakefulness, or, more rarely, at sleep stage transitions. All commonly occur in otherwise healthy persons and thus are regarded as physiologic alterations rather than pathologic conditions. Each can occur with exceptionally high frequency or severity that can lead to discomfort, pain, embarrassment, anxiety, or disturbance of a bed partner's sleep.

Rhythmic movement disorder[64,65] is the preferred term for head banging or jactatio capitis nocturna, as several forms of rhythmic activity can occur without predominant head banging. Although this disorder occurs in sleep stages it more commonly is associated with drowsiness during sleep onset or in the transition from wakefulness to sleep. Rhythmic movement disorder also can occur during full wakefulness and alertness, particularly in persons who are mentally retarded. Sleep starts (hypnic jerks)[66,67] are included as a disorder because they can cause a sleep onset insomnia. Sleep talking[68,69] does not usually have any direct consequences to the patient, though it can be embarrassing and disturb the sleep of the bed partner.

Parasomnias Usually Associated with REM Sleep

The parasomnias associated with REM sleep are grouped together because some common underlying pathophysiologic mechanism related to REM sleep may underlie all of them.

The term *nightmares* applies to REM sleep phenomena. Thus, there is little chance of confusing this disorder with that associated with slow-wave sleep, the sleep terror.[62,63] Two newly described sleep disorders are included in this section: REM sleep–related sinus arrest[80] and REM sleep behavior disorder.[81,82] REM sleep–related sinus arrest is a rare cardiac rhythm disorder that is characterized by sinus arrest during REM sleep in otherwise healthy persons. REM sleep behavior disorder is characterized by the intermittent loss of REM sleep electromyographic (EMG) atonia and by the appearance of elaborate motor activity associated with dream mentation. This latter disorder is being recognized more often, particularly in elderly persons and those with neurologic disorders, and sometimes in association with other sleep disorders such as narcolepsy.

Other Parasomnias

The terms *sleep bruxism*[83,84] and *sleep enuresis*[85,86] are preferred over the terms nocturnal bruxism and nocturnal enuresis used previously, as they denote the association with sleep rather than time of day. A new entry, primary snoring,[92,93] is included because snoring may be associated with altered cardiovascular status, and can be a forerunner to the development of the obstructive sleep apnea syndrome.[14,15] Primary snoring not only can lead to impaired health, but can be a cause of social embarrassment and can disturb the sleep of a bed partner. Snoring associated with obstructive sleep apnea syndrome is not diagnosed as primary snoring. The sleep-related abnormal swallowing syndrome[87] is retained in this classification, though it is noted that there have been few additional reports since it was first described. Nocturnal paroxysmal dystonia[88,89] is characterized by repeated dystonia or dyskinetic (ballistic, choreoathetoid) episodes that are stereotyped and occur during NREM sleep. A sleep-related frontal lobe epileptic focus is considered to be responsible for the disorder in some patients. Because this disorder is solely a sleep phenomena, it is classified here rather than as a sleep disorder associated with neurologic disease.

Sudden unexplained death syndrome[90,91] is also a relatively newly described syndrome that has a specific association with sleep and therefore is classified here. Benign neonatal sleep myoclonus[100,101] is a disorder of muscle activity that occurs solely during sleep in infants.

Included in this group are SIDS[98,99] and the infant sleep-related breathing disorders infant sleep apnea[94,95] and congenital central hypoventilation syndrome.[96,97] Insomnia or excessive sleepiness is not a predominant complaint, and usually the disorders are associated with a sudden event noticed to occur during sleep. Thus, they are listed in the parasomnias section. The inclusion of these infant breathing disorders as sleep disorders requires further explanation.

Newborns and young infants sleep a great portion of the day, and the majority of apneas and related respiratory disorders are observed during sleep. Apnea, hypoventilation, and periodic breathing are intrinsic features of infancy, reflecting immaturity of the respiratory system rather than disease. The respiratory instability during sleep may predispose some infants to SIDS.[98,99] The majority of SIDS cases happen while the infant is presumed to be asleep, but even though infant sleep apnea has been implicated as a precursor to SIDS, there is no definitive evidence by which to establish a direct link. SIDS is therefore discussed separately.

MEDICAL OR PSYCHIATRIC SLEEP DISORDERS

Many medical and psychiatric disorders are associated with disturbances of sleep and wakefulness. The division into medical and psychiatric is somewhat arbitrary. This section is divided into three subsections. The first is a listing of the psychiatric disorders that are commonly associated with disturbed sleep or wakefulness, the second indicates the importance of neurologic disorders and their effect upon the sleep and wakefulness states, and the third is a list of disorders that fall into other medical specialty areas.

Only medical disorders commonly seen in the practice of sleep disorders medicine are listed in the medical-psychiatric section. It is recognized that a large number of medical and psychiatric disorders are associated with disturbances of sleep and wakefulness, but an exhaustive list is not provided in the classification.

Sleep Disorders Associated with Mental Disorders

Although most psychiatric disorders can have an associated sleep disturbance, the psychoses,[102,103] mood disorders,[104,105] anxiety disorders,[106,107] panic disorders,[108,109] and alcoholism[110,111] are presented here because they are common in patients who present with sleep complaints and they need to be considered in the differential diagnosis. Panic disorder,[108,109] one of the anxiety disorders, can produce only a sleep complaint.

Sleep Disorders Associated with Neurologic Disorders

Neurologic disorders that are commonly associated with sleep disturbance are cerebral degenerative disorders,[112] dementia,[113,114] and Parkinson's

disease.[115,116] Fatal familial insomnia[117,118] is a rare progressive disorder that begins with difficulty initiating sleep and leads within a few months to total lack of sleep and later to spontaneous lapses from quiet wakefulness into a sleep state with enacted dreams (oneiric stupor). This disorder is associated with autonomic and thalamic degeneration and ultimately leads to death.

Epilepsy can be exacerbated by a sleep disturbance, and there can be epileptic phenomena that occur predominantly during sleep; thus the term *sleep-related epilepsy.*[119,120] Because of its pure association with NREM sleep, electrical status epilepticus of sleep[121,122] is listed separately. Electrical status epilepticus of sleep is characterized by continuous and diffuse spike–and–slow wave complexes that persist through NREM sleep.

Some forms of headache, particularly migraine and cluster headaches, can occur predominantly in sleep and are listed under sleep-related headaches.[123,124]

Sleep Disorders Associated with Other Medical Disorders

A variety of additional medical disorders have features that occur during sleep or cause sleep disturbance. Sleeping sickness[125,126] is included, as it is common in Africa, though rarely in other continents. Encephalitis lethargica is not included because it has rarely occurred in recent years.

Cardiac ischemia during sleep can lead to myocardial infarction or cardiac arrhythmias and may not be symptomatic. Nocturnal cardiac ischemia[127,128] is presented in the classification because of its importance to the health of the population and in the hope of stimulating further research on the causes. Myocardial infarction during sleep is not listed, as it rarely is seen in the practice of sleep medicine and rarely needs to be included in the differential diagnosis of a sleep complaint.

Chronic obstructive pulmonary disease[129,130] and sleep-related asthma[131,132] are common enough in the population to warrant inclusion. Other pulmonary disorders can have sleep-related features but rarely present because of sleep disturbances. Many respiratory disorders produce disturbed breathing during sleep that can lead to the development of the central sleep apnea syndrome.[16,17]

Two gastrointestinal disorders are included in this section, sleep-related gastroesophageal reflux[133,134] and peptic ulcer disease.[135,136] The discomfort associated with peptic ulcer disease commonly occurs during the major sleep episode. Although the incidence of peptic ulcer disease appears to be declining in the United States, in some countries, notably Japan, it is very high.

Fibrositis syndrome,[137,138] also known as fibromyositis syndrome, is included because it is associated with disturbed sleep and an abnormal electroencephalographic pattern during sleep, called alpha sleep.

PROPOSED SLEEP DISORDERS

The fourth section of the ICSD, proposed sleep disorders, includes disorders for which insufficient or inadequate information is available to substantiate unequivocally the existence of the disorder. Some of these disorders are newly described, such as sleep-related laryngospasm,[153,154] and some are the subject of controversy as to whether they are disorders in their own right or are at the extreme end of the range of normal physiology, such as short sleeper.[139,140]

Short sleepers and *long sleepers*[141,142] are persons whose sleep episodes are either shorter or longer than is considered normal, but whose sleep is not disturbed. They present with either an inability to sleep or excessive sleepiness, and thus are important in the differential diagnosis of these symptoms. It is necessary to describe them to provide appropriate diagnostic information for clinical purposes.

The subwakefulness syndrome,[143] also known as the subvigilance syndrome, has been described for many years, although it is little known. It consists of a complaint of inability to sustain alertness despite the fact that evidence of nocturnal sleep disruption or severe excessive sleepiness cannot be documented by polysomnography. It is unclear whether this is a variant of another disorder of excessive sleepiness such as idiopathic hypersomnia[11,12,143] or represents a manifestation of a psychological state.

Fragmentary myoclonus,[144] a newly described disorder associated with excessive sleepiness, consists of frequent brief myoclonic jerks that occur during NREM sleep at random in many muscle groups. It may be a variant of the normal phasic muscle activity that typically is seen at sleep onset, but insufficient information is currently available.

Sleep hyperhidrosis,[145,146] night sweats, can be due to a variety of underlying disorders, such as neurologic disease and the obstructive sleep apnea syndrome. An idiopathic form of this disorder occurs, but it has rarely been described in the literature.

Sleep disturbance characterized by either insomnia or excessive sleepiness can be associated with the menstrual cycle, menopause (menstrual-associated sleep disorder),[147,148] or pregnancy (pregnancy-associated sleep disorder).[149,150] Although well-recognized as common, reports of the sleep characteristics of these menstrual states are rare and the underlying cause of the sleep disturbances is unclear. Whether these disorders are due to a specific and primary effect on sleep mechanisms or to another disorder, such as premenstrual stress syndrome or back pain related to pregnancy, is not known.

Terrifying hypnagogic hallucinations[151] are intensely frightening hallucinatory phenomena that occur at sleep onset. Though sometimes associated with other sleep disorders such as narcolepsy,[7,8] they can occur in an idiopathic form. Terrifying hypnagogic hallucinations have rarely been described, and they have not been clearly differentiated from unpleasant sleep-onset dreams.

Sleep-related neurogenic tachypnea[152] is characterized by a sustained increase in respiratory rate during sleep. It occurs at sleep onset, is maintained throughout sleep, and reverses immediately on return to sleep. Although it is rarely described as an idiopathic form of tachypnea, it can be associated with an underlying neurologic disorder.

Sleep-related laryngospasm[153,154] and the sleep choking syndrome are associated with a complaint of sleep-related breathing difficulty. Sleep-related laryngospasm is an episode of abrupt awakening from sleep with an intense sensation of inability to breathe and stridor. The sleep choking syndrome is a disorder of unknown cause characterized by frequent episodes of awakening with a choking sensation. Patients with these disorders present because of symptoms similar to those of the obstructive sleep apnea syndrome.[14,15]

The proposed sleep disorders are described in anticipation that additional information will be forthcoming in the medical literature to establish their nature more clearly.

REFERENCES

1. Hauri PJ, Fischer J. Persistent psychophysiological (learned) insomnia. Sleep 1986;9:38–53.
2. Reynolds CF, Taska LS, Sewitch DE, et al. Persistent psychophysiologic insomnia: Preliminary research diagnostic criteria and EEG sleep data. Am J Psychiatry 1984;141:804–805.
3. Beutler LE, Thornby JI, Karacan I. Psychological variables in the diagnosis of insomnia. In: Williams RL, Karacan I, eds. Sleep Disorders: Diagnosis and Treatment. New York: John Wiley, 1978;61–100.
4. Carskadon M, Dement W, Mitler M, et al. Self-report versus sleep laboratory findings in 122 drug free subjects with the complaint of chronic insomnia. Am J Psychiatry 1976;133:1382–1388.
5. Hauri PJ, Olmsted E. Childhood onset insomnia. Sleep 1980;3:59–65.
6. Regestein QR, Reich P. Incapacitating childhood onset insomnia. Compr Psychiatry 1983;24:244–248.
7. Guilleminault C. Narcolepsy and its differential diagnosis. In: Guilleminault C, ed. Sleep and Its Disorders in Children. New York: Raven Press, 1987;181–194.

8. Mitler MM, Hajdukovic R, Erman M, et al. Narcolepsy. J Clin Neurophysiol 1990;7:93–118.

9. Reynolds CF, Kupfer DJ, Christianson CL. Multiple sleep latency test findings in Kleine-Levin syndrome. J Nerv Ment Dis 1984;172:41–44.

10. Takahashi Y. Clinical studies of periodic somnolence. Analysis of 28 personal cases. Psychiatr Neurol (Jpn) 1965;853–889.

11. Billiard M. Other hypersomnias. In: Thorpy MJ, ed. Handbook of Sleep Disorders. New York: Marcel Dekker, 1990;353–371.

12. Poirier G, Montplaisir J, Lebrun A, et al. HLA antigens in narcolepsy and idiopathic hypersomnolence. Sleep 1986;9:153–158.

13. Guilleminault C, Faull KM, Miles L, et al. Posttraumatic excessive daytime sleepiness: a review of 20 patients. Neurology 1980;33:1584–1589.

14. Brouillette RT, Fernbach SK, Hunt CE. Obstructive sleep apnea in infants and children. J Pediatr 1982;100:31–40.

15. Guilleminault C. Clinical features and evaluation of obstructive sleep apnea. In: Kryger MH, Roth T, Dement WC, eds. Principles and Practice of Sleep Medicine. Philadelphia: WB Saunders, 1989; 552–558.

16. Guilleminault C, Kowall J. Central sleep apnea in adults. In: Thorpy MJ, ed. Handbook of Sleep Disorders. New York: Marcel Dekker, 1990; 337–351.

17. Guilleminault C, Quera-Salva MA, Nino-Murcia G, et al. Sleep apnea and partial obstruction of the airway. Ann Neurol 1987;21:465–469.

18. Plum F, Leigh RJ. Abnormalities of central mechanisms. In: Hornbein TF, ed. Regulation of Breathing, Part II. Lung Biology in Health and Disease. New York: Marcel Dekker, 1981;17:989–1067.

19. Sullivan CE, Issa FG, Berthon-Jones M, et al. Pathophysiology of sleep apnea. In: Saunders NA, Sullivan CE, eds. Sleep and Breathing. Lung Biology in Health and Disease. New York: Marcel Dekker, 1984;21:299–364.

20. Coleman R. Periodic movements in sleep (nocturnal myoclonus) and restless legs syndrome. In: Guilleminault C, ed. Sleeping and Waking disorders: Indications and Techniques. Menlo Park, Calif.: Addison-Wesley, 1982;265–295.

21. Coccagna G. Restless legs syndrome/periodic leg movements in sleep. In: Thorpy MJ, ed. Handbook of Sleep Disorders. New York: Marcel Dekker, 1990; 457–478.

22. Ekbom KA. Restless legs syndrome. Neurology 1960;10:868–873.

23. Coccagna G. Restless legs syndrome/periodic leg movements in sleep. In: Thorpy MJ, ed. Handbook of Sleep Disorders. New York: Marcel Dekker, 1990;457–478.

24. Bootzin RR, Nicassio PM. Behavioral treatments for insomnia. In: Hersen M, Eisler RM, Miller PM, eds. Progress in Behavior Modification. New York: Academic Press, 1978;6:1–45.

25. Spielman AJ. Assessment of insomnia. Clin Psychol Rev 1986;6:11–25.

26. Haskell EH, Palca JW, Walker JM, et al. The effects of high and low ambient temperatures on human sleep stages. Electroencephalogr Clin Neurophysiol 1981;51:494–501.

27. Thiessen GJ, Lapointe AC. Effect of continuous traffic noise on percentage of deep sleep, waking, and sleep latency. J Acoust Soc Am 1983;73:225–229.

28. Nicholson AN, Smith PA, Stone BM, et al. Altitude insomnia: Studies during an expedition to the Himalayas. Sleep 1988;11:354–361.

29. Weil JV. Sleep at high altitude. In: Kryger M, Roth T, Dement WC, eds. Principles and Practice of Sleep Disorders Medicine. Philadelphia: WB Saunders, 1989; 269–275.

30. Agnew H, Webb W, Williams RL. The first night effect: An EEG study of sleep. Psychophysiology 1966;7:263–266.

31. Beutler L, Thornby J, Karacan I. Psychological variables in the diagnosis of insomnia. In: Williams RL, Karacan I, eds. Diagnosis and Treatment. Sleep Disorders. New York: John Wiley, 1978;61–100.

32. Carskadon M, Dement W. Effects of total sleep loss on sleep tendency. Percept Mot Skills 1979;48:495–496.

33. Roehrs T, Zorick F, Sickelsteel R, et al. Excessive daytime sleepiness associated with insufficient sleep. Sleep 1983;6:319–325.

34. Ferber R. Sleeplessness in the child. In: Kryger MH, Roth T, Dement W, eds. Principles and Practice of Sleep Medicine. Philadelphia: WB Saunders, 1989; 633–639.

35. Ferber R. Sleeplessness in the child. In: Kryger MH, Roth T, Dement WC, eds. Principles and Practice of Sleep Medicine. Philadelphia: WB Saunders, 1989; 633–639.

36. Kahn A, Mozin MJ, Casimir G, et al. Insomnia and cow's milk allergy in infants. Pediatrics 1985;76:880–884.

37. Kahn A, Mozin MJ, Rebuffat E, et al. Difficulty in initiating and maintaining sleep associated with cow's milk allergy in infants. Sleep 1987;10:116–121.

38. Ferber R. The sleepless child. In: Guilleminault C, ed. Sleep and Its Disorders in Children. New York: Raven Press, 1987;141–163.

39. Stunkard AJ, Grace WJ, Wolfe HG. The night eating syndrome. Am J Med 1955;7:78–86.

40. Gillin JC, Spinwebber CL, Johnson LC. Rebound insomnia: A critical review. J Clin Psychopharmacol 1989;9:161–172.

41. Kales A, Soldatos CR, Bixler EO, et al. Rebound insomnia and rebound anxiety: A review. Pharmacology 1983;26:121–137.

42. Oswald I. Sleep and dependence on amphetamine and other drugs. In: Kales A, ed. Sleep: Physiology and Pathology. Philadelphia: JB Lippincott, 1969;317–330.

43. Watson R, Hartmann E, Shildkraut J. Amphetamine withdrawal: Affective state, sleep patterns and MHPG excretion. Am J Psychiatry 1972;129:263–269.

44. Pokorny AD. Sleep disturbances, alcohol, and alcoholism: A review. In: Williams RL, Karacan I, eds. Sleep Disorders: Diagnosis and Treatment. New York: John Wiley, 1978;233–260.

45. Friedman PA. Poisoning and its management. In: Braunwald E, Isselbacher KJ, Peterdorf RG, Wilson JD, eds. et al., Harrison's Principles of Internal Medicine, ed. 11. New York: McGraw-Hill, 1987.

46. Graeber RC. Sleep and wakefulness international aircrew. Aviat Space Environ Med 1986;57 (Suppl):12.

47. Winget CM, DeRoshio CW, Markley CL, et al. A review of human physiological and performance changes associated with desynchronosis of biological rhythms. Aviat Space Environ Med 1984;55:1085–1095.

48. Torsvall L, Akerstedt T. Sleepiness on the job: Continuously measured EEG changes in train drivers. Electroencephalogr Clin Neurophysiol 1987;66:502–511.

49. Walsh JK, Tepas DI, Moss PD. The EEG sleep of night and rotating shift workers. In: Johnson LC, Tepas DI, Colquhoun WP, et al., eds. Biological Rhythms, Sleep and Shift Work. New York: SP Medical, 1981;347–356.

50. Okawa M, Takahashi K, Sasaki H. Disturbance of circadian rhythms in severely brain-damaged patients correlated with CT findings. J Neurol 1986;233:274–282.

51. Wagner D. Circadian rhythm sleep disorders. In: Thorpy MJ, ed. Handbook of Sleep Disorders. New York: Marcel Dekker, 1990;493–527.

52. Thorpy MJ, Korman E, Spielman AJ, et al. Delayed sleep phase syndrome in adolescents. J Adolesc Health Care 1988;9:22–27.

53. Weitzman ED, Czeisler CA, Coleman RM, et al. Delayed sleep phase syndrome, a chronobiological disorder with sleep-onset insomnia. Arch Gen Psychiatry 1981;38:737–746.

54. Kamei R, Hughes L, Miles L, et al. Advanced-sleep phase syndrome studied in a time isolation facility. Chronobiologia 1979;6:115.

55. Moldofsky H, Musisi S, Phillipson EA. Treatment of advanced sleep phase syndrome by phase advance chronotherapy. Sleep 1986;9:61–65.

56. Kokkoris CP, Weitzman ED, Pollak CP, et al. Longterm ambulatory monitoring in a subject with a hypernychthemeral sleep-wake cycle disturbance. Sleep 1980; 2:347–354.

57. Weber AL, Cary MS, Conner N, et al. Human non-24-hour sleep-wake cycles in an everyday environment. Sleep 1980;2:347–354.

58. Ferber R. Sleep disorders in infants and children. In: Riley TL, ed. Clinical Aspects of Sleep and Sleep Disturbance. Boston: Butterworths, 1985;113–158.

59. Thorpy MJ. Disorders of arousal. In: Thorpy MJ, ed. Handbook of Sleep Disorders. New York: Marcel Dekker, 1990; 531–549.

60. Kales A, Soldatos CR, Bixler EO, et al. Hereditary factors in sleep walking and night terrors. Br J Psychiatry 1980;137:111–118.

61. Thorpy MJ. Disorders of arousal. In: Thorpy MJ, ed. Handbook of Sleep Disorders. New York: Marcel Dekker, 1990;531–549.

62. Fisher C, Kahn E, Edwards A, et al. A psychophysiological study of nightmares and night terrors: Physiological aspects of the stage 4 night terror. J Nerv Ment Dis 1973;157:75–98.

63. Thorpy MJ. Disorders of arousal. In: Thorpy MJ, ed. Handbook of Sleep Disorders. New York: Marcel Dekker, 1990;531–549.

64. Sallustro F, Atwell CW. Body rocking, head banging and head rolling in normal children. J Pediatr 1978;93:704–708.

65. Thorpy MJ. Rhythmic movement disorder. In: Thorpy MJ, ed. Handbook of Sleep Disorders. New York: Marcel Dekker, 1990;609–629.

66. Broughton R. Pathological fragmentary myoclonus, intensified sleep starts and hypnagogic foot tremor: Three unusual sleep-related disorders. In: Koella WP, ed. Sleep 1986. Stuttgart: Fischer-Verlag, 1988;240–243.

67. Oswald I. Sudden bodily jerks on falling asleep. Brain 1959;82:92–93.

68. Aarons L. Evoked sleep talking. Percept Mot Skills 1970;31:27–40.

69. Arkin AM. Sleep talking: A review. J Nerv Ment Dis 1966;143:101–122.

70. Jacobsen JH, Rosenberg RS, Huttenlocher PR, et al. Familial nocturnal cramping. Sleep 1986;9:54–60.

71. Weiner IH, Weiner HL. Nocturnal leg muscle cramps. JAMA 1980;244:2332–2333.

72. Fisher CJ, Byrne J, Edwards T, et al. A psychophysiological study of nightmares. J Am Psychoanal Assoc 1970; 18:747–782.

73. Hartman E. The Nightmare. New York: Basic Books, 1984.

74. Goode GB. Sleep paralysis. Arch Neurol 1962;6:228–234.

75. Hishikawa Y. Sleep paralysis. In: Guilleminault C, Dement WC, Passouant P, eds. Narcolepsy. New York: Spectrum, 1976;97–124.

76. Fisher C, Schavi RC, Edwards A, et al. Evaluation of nocturnal penile tumescence in the differential diagnosis of sexual impotence; A quantitative study. Arch Gen Psychiatry 1979;36:431–437.

77. Karacan I, Howell JW. Impaired sleep-related penile tumescence. In: Thorpy MJ, ed. Handbook of Sleep Disorders. New York: Marcel Dekker, 1990;631–640.

78. Karacan I. Painful nocturnal penile erections. JAMA 1971;215:1831.

79. Matthews BJ, Crutchfield MB. Painful nocturnal penile erections associated with rapid eye movement sleep. Sleep 1987;10:184–187.

80. Guilleminault C, Pool P, Motta J, et al. Sinus arrest during REM sleep in young adults. N Engl J Med 1984;311:1006–1010.

81. Schenck CH, Bundlie SR, Ettinger MG, Mahowald MW. Chronic behavioral disorders of human REM sleep: A new category of parasomnia. Sleep 1986; 9:293–306.

82. Mahowald MW, Schenck CH. REM-Sleep behavior disorder. In: Thorpy MJ, ed. Handbook of Sleep Disorders. New York: Marcel Dekker, 1990;567–594.

83. Funch DP, Gale EN. Factors associated with nocturnal bruxism and its treatment. J Behav Med 1980;3:385–397.

84. Ware JC, Rugh J. Destructive bruxism: Sleep stage relationship. Sleep 1988;11:172–181.

85. Mikkelsen EJ, Rapoport JL. Enuresis: Psychopathology, sleep stage, and drug response. Urol Clin North Am 1980;7:361–377.

86. Brown L. Nocturnal enuresis. In: Thorpy MJ, ed. Handbook of Sleep Disorders. New York: Marcel Dekker, 1990;595–608.

87. Guilleminault C, Eldridge FL, Phillips JR, et al. Two occult causes of insomnia and their therapeutic problems. Arch Gen Psychiatry 1976;33:1241–1245.

88. Lugaresi E. Nocturnal paroxysmal dystonia. In: Thorpy MJ, ed. Handbook of Sleep Disorders. New York: Marcel Dekker, 1990;551–565.

89. Lugaresi E, Cirignotta F, Montagna P. Nocturnal paroxysmal dystonia. J Neurol Neurosurg Psychiatry 1986;49:375–380.

90. Baron RC, Thacker SB, Gorelkin L, et al. Sudden death among Southeast Asian refugees. JAMA 1983; 250:2947–2951.

91. Otto CM, Tauxe RV, Cobb LA, et al. Ventricular fibrillation causes sudden death in Southeast Asian immigrants. Ann Intern Med 1984;100:45–47.

92. Lugaresi E, Cirignotta F, Montagna P. Snoring: Pathogenic, clinical, and therapeutic aspects. In: Kryger MH, Roth T, Dement WC, eds. Principles and Practice of Sleep Medicine. Philadelphia: WB Saunders, 1989; 494–500.

93. Waller PC, Bhopal RS. Is snoring a cause of vascular disease? An epidemiological review. Lancet 1989; 1:143–146.

94. Durand M, Cabal L, Gonzalez F, et al. Ventilatory control and carbon dioxide response in preterm infants with idiopathic apnea. Am J Dis Child 1985;139:717–720.

95. Henderson-Smart DJ. The effect of gestational age on the incidence and duration of recurrent apnea in newborn babies. Aust Paediatr J 1985;17:273–276.

96. Fleming PJ, Cade D, Bryan MH, et al. Congenital central hypoventilation and sleep state. Pediatrics 1980;66:425–428.

97. Paton JY, Swaminathan S, Sargent CW, et al. Hypoxic and hypercapneic ventilatory responses in awake children with congenital central hypoventilation syndrome. Am Rev Respir Dis 1989;140:368–372.

98. Hoppenbrouwers T, Hodgman JE. Sudden infant death syndrome (SIDS): An integration of ontogenetic, pathologic physiologic and epidemiologic factors. Neuropediatrics 1982;13:36–51.

99. Merritt TA, Valdes Dapena M. SIDS research update. Pediatr Ann 1984;13:193–207.

100. Coulter DL, Allen RJ. Benign neonatal sleep myoclonus. Arch Neurol 1982;39:191–192.

101. Resnick TJ, Moshe SL, Perotta L, et al. Benign neonatal sleep myoclonus: Relationship to sleep states. Arch Neurol 1986;43:266–268.

102. Ganguli R, Reynolds CF, Kupfer DJ. EEG sleep in young, never-medicated, schizophrenic patients: A comparison with delusional and nondelusional depressives and with healthy controls. Arch Gen Psychiatry 1987;44:36–44.

103. Zarcone VP. Sleep and schizophrenia. In: Williams RL, Karacan I, Moore CA, eds. Sleep Disorders: Diagnosis and Treatment. New York: John Wiley, 1988;165–188.

104. Gillin JC, Duncan W, Pettigrew KD, et al. Successful separation of depressed, normal, and insomniac subjects by EEG sleep data. Arch Gen Psychiatry 1979;36:85–90.

105. Reynolds CF, Kupfer DJ. Sleep research in affective illness: State of the art circa 1987. Sleep 1987;10:199–215.

106. Reynolds CF, Shaw DM, Newton TF, et al. EEG sleep in outpatients with generalized anxiety: A preliminary comparison with depressed outpatients. Psychiatry Res 1983;8:81–89.

107. Rosa RR, Bonnett MM, Kramer M. The relationship of sleep and anxiety in anxious subjects. Biol Psychol 1983;16:119–126.

108. Hauri PJ, Friedman M, Ravaris CL. Sleep in patients with spontaneous panic attacks. Sleep 1989;12:323–337.

109. Mellman TA, Unde TW. Electroencephalographic sleep in panic disorder. Arch Gen Psychiatry 1989;46:178–184.

110. Porkny AD. Sleep disturbances, alcohol and alcoholism: A review: In: Williams RL, Karacan I, eds. Sleep Disorders: Diagnosis and Treatment. New York: John Wiley, 1978;389–402.

111. Wagman A, Allen R. Effects of alcohol ingestion and abstinence on slow wave sleep of alcoholics. In: Gross MM, ed. Alcohol Intoxication and Withdrawal, II. New York: Plenum Press, 1975;453–466.

112. Aldrich M. Sleep and degenerative neurological disorders involving the motor system. In: Thorpy MJ, ed. Handbook of Sleep Disorders. New York: Marcel Dekker, 1990;673–692.

113. Evans LK. Sundown syndrome in institutionalized elderly. J Am Geriatr Soc 1987;35:101–108.

114. Vitiello MV, Prinz PN. Sleep/wake patterns and sleep disorders in Alzheimer's disease. In: Thorpy MJ, ed. Handbook of Sleep Disorders. New York: Marcel Dekker, 1990;703–718.

115. Mouret J. Difference in sleep in patients with Parkinson's disease. Electroencephalogr Clin Neurophysiol 1975;38:563–567.

116. Nausieda PA. Sleep in Parkinson's disease. In: Thorpy MJ, ed. Handbook of Sleep Disorders. New York: Marcel Dekker, 1990;719–735.

117. Lugaresi E, Medori R, Montagna P, et al. Fatal familial insomnia and dysautonomia with selective degeneration of thalamic nuclei. N Engl J Med 1986;315:997–1003.

118. Lugaresi E. Fatal familial insomnia. In: Thorpy MJ, ed. Handbook of Sleep Disorders. New York: Marcel Dekker, 1990;479–489.

119. Degan R, Niedermeyer E, eds. Epilepsy, Sleep and Sleep Deprivation. Amsterdam: Elsevier, 1984.

120. Montplaisir J. Epilepsy and sleep: Reciprocal interactions and diagnostic procedures involving sleep. In: Thorpy MJ, ed. Handbook of Sleep Disorders. New York: Marcel Dekker, 1990;643–662.

121. Patry G, Lyagoubi S, Tassinari CA. Subclinical "electrical status epilepticus" induced by sleep in children. Arch Neurol 1971;24:242–252.

122. Tassinari CA, Bureau M, Dravet C, et al. Epilepsy with continuous spikes and waves during sleep. In: Roger J. Dravet C. Bureau M, et al. eds. Epileptic Syndromes in Infancy, Childhood and Adolescence. London: John Libbey Eurotext, 1985;194–204.

123. Dexter JD. Relationship between sleep and headaches. In: Thorpy MJ, ed. Handbook of Sleep Disorders. New York: Marcel Dekker, 1990;663–671.

124. Kayed K, Godtlibsen OB, Sjaastad O. Chronic paroxysmal hemicrania IV: "REM sleep locked" nocturnal headache attacks. Sleep 1978;1:91–95.

125. Bert J, Collomb H, Fressy J, Gastaut H. Etude electrographique du sommeil nocturne. In: Fischgold H, ed. Le Sommeil de Nuit Normal et Pathologique. Paris: Masson, 1965;334–352.

126. Schwartz BA, Escande C. Sleeping sickness: Sleep study of a case. Electroencephalogr Clin Neurophysiol 1970;3:83–87.

127. Muller J, Ludmer PL, Wellick SN, et al. Circadian variation in the frequency of sudden cardiac death. Circulation 1987;75:131–138.

128. Nowlin JB, Troyer WG Jr, Collins WS, et al. The association of nocturnal angina pectoris with dreaming. Ann Intern Med 1965;63:1040–1046.

129. Fleetham J, West P, Mezon B, et al. Sleep, arousals and oxygen desaturation in chronic obstructive pulmonary disease. The effect of oxygen therapy. Am Rev Respir Dis 1982;126:429–433.

130. Flenley C. Chronic obstructive pulmonary disease. In: Kryger M, Roth T, Dement WC, eds. Principles and Practice of Sleep Medicine. Philadelphia: WB Saunders, 1989;601–610.

131. Douglas NJ. Asthma. In: Kryger M, Roth T, Dement WC. Principles and Practice of Sleep Medicine. Philadelphia: WB Saunders, 1989;591–600.

132. Montplaisir J, Walsh J, Malo JL. Nocturnal asthma features of attacks, sleep and breathing patterns. Am Rev Respir Dis 1982;125:18–22.

133. Orr WC. Gastrointestinal disorders. In: Kryger M, Roth T, Dement WC. Principles and Practice of Sleep Medicine. Philadelphia: WB Saunders, 1989;622–629.

134. Orr WC, Johnson LF, Robinson MG. The effect of sleep on swallowing, esophageal peristalsis, and acid clearance. Gastroenterology 1984;86:814–819.

135. Segawa K, Nakazawa S, Tsukamoto Y, et al. Peptic ulcer is prevalent among shift workers. Dig Dis Sci 1987;32:449–453.

136. Stacher G, Presslich B, Starker H. Gastric acid secretion and sleep stages during natural night sleep. Gastroenterology 1975;68:1455–1499.

137. Moldofsky H, Saskin P, Lue FA. Sleep and symptoms in fibrositis syndrome after a febrile illness. J Rheumatol 1988;15:1701–1704.

138. Saskin P, Moldofsky H, Lue FA. Sleep and posttraumatic rheumatic pain modulation disorder (fibrositis syndrome). Psychosomatic Med 1986;48:319–323.

139. Hartmann E, Baekeland F, Zwilling GR. Psychological differences between short and long sleepers. Arch Gen Psychiatry 1972;26:463–468.

140. Webb WB. Are short and long sleepers different? Psychol Rep 1979;44:259–264.

141. Hartmann E, Baekeland F, Zwilling GR. Psychological differences between short and long sleepers. Arch Gen Psychiatry 1972;26:463–468.

142. Webb WB. Are short and long sleepers different? Psychol Rep 1979;44:259–264.

143. Roth B. Narcolepsy and Hypersomnia. Basel: Karger, 1980.

144. Broughton R, Tolentino MA, Krelina M. Excessive fragmentary myoclonus in NREM sleep: A report of 38 cases. Electroencephalogr Clin Neurophysiol 1985;61:123–309.

145. Geschickter EH, Andrews PA, Bullard RW. Nocturnal body temperature regulation in man: a rationale for sweating in sleep. J Appl Physiol 1966;21:623–630.

146. Lea MJ, Aber RC. Descriptive epidemiology of night sweats upon admission to a university hospital. South Med J 1985;78:1065–1067.

147. Billiard M, Guilleminault C, Dement WC. A menstruation-linked periodic hypersomnia. Neurology 1975;25:436–443.

148. Ho A. Sex hormones and the sleep of women. Sleep Res, 1972;1:184.

149. Errante J. Sleep deprivation or postpartum blues? Top Clin Nurs 1985; 6:9–18.

150. Karacan I, Williams RL, Hursh CJ, et al. Some implications of the sleep pattern of pregnancy for postpartum emotional disturbances. Br J Psychiatr 1969; 115:929–935.

151. Broughton R. Neurology and dreaming. Psychiatr J Univ 157, Ottawa 1982;7:101–110.

152. Willmer JP, Broughton RJ. Neurogenic sleep related polypnea—a new disorder? Sleep Res 1989;18:322.

153. Kryger MH, Acres JC, Brownell L. A syndrome of sleep, stridor and panic. Chest 1981;80:768.

154. Thorpy MJ, Aloe F. Sleep-related laryngospasm. Sleep Res 1989;18:313.

155. Arnold GE. Disorders of laryngeal function. In: Paparella MM, Shumrick DA, eds. Otolaryngology. Philadelphia: WB Saunders, 1973;3:638.

156. Thorpy MJ, Aloe FS. Choking during sleep. Sleep Res 1989;18:314.

157. Diagnostic Classification Steering Committee. Thorpy MJ, Chairman. International classification of sleep disorders. Diagnostic and coding manual. Rochester, Minn.: American Sleep Disorders Association, 1990.

16

Obstructive Sleep Apnea Syndrome

Mindy B. Cetel

Christian Guilleminault

DEFINITION

Obstructive sleep apnea syndrome (OSAS) is an insidious condition of repetitive upper airway closure during sleep characterized by a constellation of symptoms and objective findings.[1] The most common presenting complaints are infamously loud snoring, along with unrefreshing sleep and daytime somnolence. OSAS may long remain undetected because the breathing disturbances occur at night but the consequences are reflected in impaired daytime functioning. Amazingly, patients with even severe sleep apnea of many decades' duration often remain unaware of the cause of their difficulties. Bed partners are invaluable informants in describing frightening cessations of breathing, choking sounds, and stridorous gasps when breathing resumes. The course is gradually progressive; thus, the delineation of normal from abnormal daytime functioning becomes obscured over the years. Sleepiness is typically misperceived as "growing old."

Complete closure of the upper airway is termed *obstructive apnea*; partial closure, *hypopnea*. When measured by polysomnographic (PSG) recording, obstructive apneas are defined as total cessation of airflow at the nose and mouth lasting at least 10 seconds, associated with ongoing thoracic and abdominal efforts to inspire. Hypopneas are seen as greater than 50% decreases in airflow lasting at least 10 seconds associated with continued respiratory efforts. They are usually associated with a drop in blood oxygen saturation.[1] Gould and coworkers[2] have suggested defining hypopnea differently by focusing more on thoracoabdominal effort. Using inductive plethysmography, hypopnea would be defined as a decrease in effort of at least 50%.[2] Both apneas and hypopneas are terminated with a large inspiratory breath. Central apneas are seen on PSG study as episodes of cessation of thoracic and abdominal respiratory efforts as well as nasal-oral airflow, lasting at least 10 seconds. Longstanding obstructive apnea may result in disturbances of central and peripheral respiratory reflexes, which are one cause of central apneas. Mixed apneas are comprised of central and obstructive components.

The number of apneas and hypopneas are separately totalled, then divided by the hours of total sleep time to yield an apnea index (AI) and hypopnea index (HI). The AI and HI are summed to give the respiratory disturbance index (RDI), which is the average number of respiratory disturbances per hour of sleep.[3]

Controversy exists concerning the exact RDI and AI indices that constitute a mild disorder as opposed to normal sleep.[4] Individual patients manifest varying degrees of symptoms for any given RDI. The correlations between RDI severity and long-term morbidity are not precisely delineated. These relationships are confounded by night-to-night fluctuations in the RDI, the degree of oxygen desaturation, and the proportion of time spent under reduced oxygen saturation. With these disclaimers in mind, AI over 5 and RDI over 10 are most commonly considered to lie in the pathologic range, for clinical purposes.[5]

The obstructive sleep apnea syndrome lies along a continuum of nocturnal obstructive upper airway disorders. In order of increasing severity, this spectrum encompasses pure snoring without daytime sleepiness, the newly described *upper airway resistance syndrome*, which may be present without associated snoring and is associated with daytime sleepiness,[6] and progressive degrees of obstructive apnea based on RDI and oxyhemoglobin desaturations.

The specific pathophysiology of these respective syndromes is discussed later in this chapter. As little is known about the incidence and prevalence of the recently reported upper airway resistance syndrome, most of the presentation focuses on the well-known OSAS.

EPIDEMIOLOGY

Apnea frequency increases with age and is strongly correlated with obesity and male gender.[7-9] Prevalence reaches a maximum between the fifth and seventh decades.[10] Postmenopausal women tend to lose their gender-associated protective effect. Various studies attempted to measure the prevalence of OSAS in the general population using surveys and PSGs of a limited number of subjects. All are limited by biases that tend to underestimate the actual prevalence. Surveying 1502 healthy male Israelis by questionnaire, 78 of whom underwent PSG, Lavie estimated the minimal prevalence of people with sleepiness and an AI greater than 10 to be 0.7% of the adult male population.[11] By sampling healthy men and setting the AI above 10, a minimizing bias is attained. Gislason and coworkers surveyed 3201 Swedish males, aged 30 to 69 years, and polysomnographically evaluated 61 of those with severe snoring and sleepiness.[12] Of those so evaluated, AI was greater than 5 for 18%, 10 for 11%, and greater than 20 for 3%. RDIs of 5, 10, and 20 were found in 23%, 15%, and 5% respectively, of those studied, yielding a minimum estimate of OSAS of 1.3%

Schmidt-Nowara[13] conducted a population-based survey of 1195 adults by questionnaire, of whom 275 men and women participated in home monitoring using a carbon dioxide detecting apnea monitor. Of the 47 subjects with more than 20 events per hour 32 underwent PSG. In conjunction with information gathered from the larger population, the estimated minimal prevalence of OSAS based on an RDI of at least 10 was 2.3% for men and 1.1% for women aged 40 or older.

MORBIDITY AND MORTALITY

Cardiovascular System

Systemic and pulmonary hemodynamics undergo acute and chronic changes as a consequence of obstructive apnea, most of which reverse after successful treatment of the upper airway obstruction. Significant increases in systemic arterial pressure occur cyclically with episodes of apnea, and maximal elevations follow the resumption of ventilation. In a study of 10 moderately to severely apneic subjects, during apneas systolic and diastolic pressures rose about 25% from baseline values (i.e., from 126 to 159 mm Hg systolic and 65 to 83 mm Hg diastolic).[14] With apneas occurring in very close clusters continuously throughout the night, often in association with very severe oxygen desaturations, elevations may be extreme, exceeding 200 mm Hg systolic and 120 mm Hg diastolic.[15]

Evidence implicates several mechanisms that contribute to these cyclic increases in blood pressure. Falling PaO_2 and acidosis signal the carotid chemoreceptors to trigger vasomotor center–mediated arteriolar constriction, leading to increased systemic vascular resistance. Increased effort against a closed upper airway leads to significant right-to-left interventricular septal shifts and decreased cardiac output. Left ventricular "collapse" can occur with very negative inspiratory pressures. With resumption of ventilation, and the abrupt shift from sleep to wakefulness, there is a release of vagal predominance and heightened sympathetic tone. Pulmonary stretch reflexes induce tachycardia, which increases cardiac output. Changes in preload and afterload due to the repetitive Müller's (and at times Valsalva's) maneuvers are also factors in the cardiac output changes. Elevated sympathetic nervous system activity is evidenced by increased urinary catecholamine levels, which return to normal after treatment of apnea.[16]

Untreated OSAS is associated with a prevalence of chronic hypertension of at least 50%,[17] whereas about 30% of all idiopathic hypertensives have obstructive sleep apnea.[18,19] Although a direct causal role for OSAS in the development of chronic hypertension has not been proven, following treatment of apnea, hypertension has also improved.[20]

Recently, increased release of atrial natriuretic peptide (ANP) during sleep has been shown in sleep apnea, associated with increases in urine and sodium output.[21] ANP suppresses the renin-angiotensin-aldosterone system, and plasma renin activity curves have been found to be abnormally flattened in apneics during sleep.[22] These changes serve to reduce blood volume and lower blood pressure, and may play a protective or compensatory role against blood pressure increases in OSAS. Treatment of apnea normalizes ANP, thereby diminishing diuresis and natriuresis, and increases renin and aldosterone release.

Moderate to severe increases in pulmonary arterial pressure occur with each apneic episode. Maximal pulmonary pressures are generated during rapid eye movement (REM) sleep. They coincide with maximal hypoxemic and hypercapnic values[20] and probably reflect hypoxic pulmonary vasoconstriction. When pressure gradients between the pulmonary artery lumen and thoracic cavity are evaluated, -transpulmonary artery pressure decreases during the first 25 seconds of apnea, increases until breathing returns, and then transiently rises more rapidly.[23] Another hemodynamic change involved reductions in cardiac output of up to one-third of baseline values with apneas that lasted longer than 35 seconds.[24]

The development of persistent pulmonary hypertension and cor pulmonale may be caused by severe hypoxemia during sleep,[25,26] but it is more likely in the setting of daytime hypoxemia.[27] Treatment of apnea amelioriates pulmonary artery hypertension and right-sided heart failure.[28,29]

Cardiac arrythmias occurring exclusively during sleep are exceedingly common in apneics. Sinus arrythmia accompanies each obstructive respiratory cycle, where rate diminishes with the cessation of airflow and accelerates when breathing resumes. These changes can be mild or severe, resulting in repetitive cycles of bradycardia and tachycardia fluctuating from under 30 beats per minute to more than 120 beats per minute.[30] Severe sinus bradycardia (less thasn 30 beats per minute) affects about 10% of sleep apneics and is usually seen in the setting of severe hypoxemia.[31–33] These aberrations of rate, combined with hypoxemia, predispose to conduction defects, malignant arrythmias, and perhaps sudden death. Asystoles of up to 13 seconds, second-degree atrioventricular (AV) block, premature ventricular contractions, and runs of ventricular tachycardia are among documented apnea-related abnormalities.

Proposed mechanisms of bradycardia, Mobitz I AV block, and asystole involve vagal nerve activation due to both Müller's maneuver and hypoxemic carotid body stimulation. EEG arousal with airway reopening and lung expansion triggers cardiac acceleration. Increased sympathetic tone due to hypoxemia and acidosis may be expressed after vagal influence is withdrawn, leading to premature ventricular contractions (PVCs), sinus tachycardia and ventricular tachycardia. PVC frequency and other ventricular arrhythmias were shown to correlate with severity of oxygen desaturation, increasing threefold with desaturations below 60% as compared to 90%.[34]

From a global perspective, many of these physiologic changes to asphyxia may be viewed as an attempt to preserve perfusion to the critical cerebral and coronary systems. Increased systemic pressure selectively perfuses these critical central vasculatures, while bradycardia decreases myocardial oxygen consumption. Upon return of ventilation, cardiac rate and output rise in the setting of sympathetic dominance and decreased systemic resistance. The demand for myocardial oxygen to accomplish this work precedes the supply of reperfused blood, rendering the myocardium vulnerable to malignant arrhythmias.[35]

Surprisingly, in spite of the strong cerebral vasodilating effects of hypercapnia and the protective mechanisms discussed above, cerebral blood flow during sleep is more decreased in apneics than in normals.[36,37] Especially interesting is the finding that global and regional cerebral perfusion is decreased in apneics during wakefulness.[37,38] This suggests altered cerebral autoregulatory mechanisms.

Sleep apnea, and even snoring, has been epidemiologically linked to increased incidences of myocardial infarction and stroke.[39,40] In a study comparing cumulative survival after 5 years for untreated and treated patients with an AI greater than 20, cumulative survival was roughly 75% in the untreated group as compared to almost 100% for the treated group.[41] Cardiovascular death was also significantly increased compared to that in the general U.S. population data in another study. Peak age of death in sleep apneics was between 55 and 64 years, compared to 72 years in a general U.S. male population.[42]

Other systemic abnormalities implicated in association with OSA include early renal dysfunction, characterized by an increased incidence of proteinuria.[43] Proteinuria was found in 26% of 50 patients with an RDI above 5, compared with none of an equal number of patients with other types of sleep disorders.[44]

PATHOPHYSIOLOGY

The upper airway includes regions made up of bone and cartilage (nose, larynx and extrathoracic trachea) and regions made up of soft tissues (nasopharynx, oropharynx, and hypopharynx). It is in the latter regions that most airway closures occur during sleep. In the early 1970s, there was disagreement as to whether decreased patency of the upper airway during sleep was related to an active contraction at the velopharyngeal sphincter[45] or to inability of the upper airway muscles to oppose a sucking maneuver during inspiration.[46] Weitzman and colleagues[45] presented videotapes indicating that occlusion occurred mainly at the velopharyngeal "sphincter," a finding recently re-emphasized by Remmers and colleagues[47] with fiberoptic endoscopy. However, the Stanford team and their respective coworkers (Hill and Guilleminault)[46,48] performed similar fiberoptic evaluations, continuously filming and simultaneously recording the electromyographic (EMG) activity of many different upper airway muscles. These authors concluded that there was no active contraction. At sleep onset there was a decrease in EMG activity in the upper airway muscles, not only at the level of the velopharyngeal sphincter but also in many dilator muscles. The first breaths following sleep onset or a return to sleep after arousal were associated with closure of the upper airway, as indicated by endoscopy.

Since this early work the pathophysiology of upper airway occlusion during sleep has been elucidated. The size of the pharyngeal upper airway depends on a balance of forces between the upper airway dilators, which maintain upper airway patency, and the negative pharyngeal intraluminal pressure created by thoracic expansion during inspiration. Thus, upper airway patency requires the coordination of upper airway dilators and inspiratory muscles. Bernouilli's principle dictates that narrowing of any segment while airflow is maintained increases the velocity of airflow in that segment. This decreases intraluminal pressure and further narrows the segment, favoring its collapse. Incoordination of inspiratory muscles and upper airway dilators leads to upper airway occlusion during sleep. This was reported as early as 1978 by Guilleminault and Motta[49] in an investigation of patients with post-poliomyelitis syndrome who had been treated with cuirass ventilator. These patients developed negative intrathoracic pressure that could not be counteracted by the upper airway dilators; the pressure led to the development of obstructive sleep apnea. These findings were later confirmed by Hyland and colleagues[50] and by Simonds and Branthwaite.[51] Lack of coordination in reflexes does not seem to be the first step in most cases of obstructive sleep apnea.

Recently it has been demonstrated in adult men that with sleep onset there is an increase in resistance due to a decrease in upper airway muscle tone.[52] This increased resistance has no known consequences though in snorers it increases further with each snore. In response to this increased resistance, many subjects are able to increase their inspiratory effort and maintain normal tidal volume. Increased effort is demonstrated by esophageal pressure (P_{es}) monitoring,[53] which may reach peak inspiratory nadirs of minus 12 to minus 15 cm H_2O. The effort is constant over time, without any impact on sleep electroencephalogram (EEG) or oxygen saturation. In other cases,[53] the upper airway dilators are unable to oppose the negative pharyngeal intraluminal pressure enough to maintain minute ventilation and normal gas exchange. Then, inspiratory efforts are increased. This increase is translated to an increase in P_{es} nadir. With increasing inspiratory efforts the width of the upper airway decreases, as upper airway dilators are unable to exactly match the inspiratory negative pressure.

Several mechanisms can be used by the subject to maintain normal minute ventilation. One well-demonstrated method consists in a prolongation of inspiratory time (T_i) associated with a decrease in expiratory time (T_e). (Total respiratory cycle [T_{tot}] is unchanged.[53]) At some point an abnormally negative P_{es} pressure is reached, tidal volume is reduced for one to three breaths owing to further narrowing of the upper airway, and an arousal response is triggered. This response is transient and short (as short as two seconds by visual EEG scoring).

The transient EEG arousal response leads to reopening of the upper airway. It also fragments sleep.[53] Initially these intermittent changes are not recognized as "obstructive sleep apnea," owing to monitoring techniques; however, pharyngeal sleep deprivation has been shown to slowly blunt the responses of many reflexes. In addition, this initial, intermittent sleep fragmentation probably plays a role in the progressive development of full-blown OSAS.

Interestingly, a large percentage of obstructive sleep apnea patients exhibit subtle craniofacial abnormalities such as a high arched high palate, a long soft palate placed low, and redundant tissues and a moderately retroplaced mandible.[54] It has recently been found that these abnormalities may be responsible for obstructive apnea during the first weeks of life in certain subjects.[55] These abnormalities are related to genetic factors, and we have investigated several families in which a small upper airway has been passed down for generations.[56]

The upper airway begins at the nares and includes the nasal vestibule, nasopharynx, oropharynx, and hypopharynx. The pharynx is an especially vulnerable portion of the upper airway, because it serves both digestive and respiratory functions. It must be sufficiently floppy to contract and guide food into the esophagus, while alternately it must maintain sufficient muscle dilation to keep from being sucked by the inspiratory negative pressure and closed.

Nasal obstruction from any cause, including allergic congestion, swollen lymphoid tissue, or septal deviation, can initiate obstructive nocturnal respiratory conditions by rerouting breathing through the mouth. Mouth breathing predisposes to abnormal airway dynamics that favor pharyngeal collapse and backward displacement of the base of tongue. The dilating genioglossus and geniohyoid muscles become mechanically disadvantaged, and airway resistance is increased.

The next potential level of obstruction arises at the nasopharynx and oropharynx, owing to enlarged adenoidal, tonsillar, and soft palate tissues. Such enlargement is secondary to hereditary and acquired factors. Allergies and recurrent upper respiratory infections cause lymphoid tissues to enlarge. Snoring itself renders the uvula more edematous because of suction and trauma, which further compromises the small oropharyngeal space. Macroglossia may be due in part to obesity and is implicated in OSAS.[57]

As mentioned earlier, a constellation of jaw malformations are associated with OSAS; these include a highly-arched hard palate and Class II dental occlusion (overjet). The position of the mandible relative to the maxilla determines the posterior extension of the tongue. Because the genioglossus muscle inserts on the mandible, with retrognathia or micrognathia the genioglossus originates on a backward displaced mandible and thus extends farther posteriorly, predisposing to hypopharyngeal obstruction. During sleep in the supine position, gravity pulls the tongue farther into the pharyngeal lumen, and varying degrees of decreased muscle tone additionally relax the tongue dorsally.

Chronic nasal obstruction during childhood, which results in mouth breathing, may induce craniofacial changes that predispose to sleep apnea later in life. This has been shown in rhesus monkeys with experimentally partially occluded nostrils, which developed mandibular deficiency relative to paired controls. Oral breathing changed EMG activity in facial muscle groups, leading to altered forces on the developing facial skeleton.[58-60] Partial improvement in these changes occurred if the obstruction was relieved early enough. Upper airway obstruction from enlarged adenoids in children has been shown to lead to decreased mandibular size and retrognathia, among other craniofacial changes.[61,62]

Adiposity compromises the upper airway not only by the direct mass effect of a double chin externally compressing the pharynx in the supine position, but also by internally infiltrating the parapharyngeal structures, displacing airspace with adipose tissue. Pharyngeal dilator muscle mechanics may be compromised by this loading.

Male gender theoretically contributes to upper airway obstruction because of ill-understood hormonal influences. Evidence implicates testosterone as the main factor. A study of seven obese males and seven obese females showed OSAS in only six of the males; the spared one was hypogonadal.[63] Theoretically, testosterone may contribute to obstruction by inducing more parapharyngeal muscle bulk and more centripetal fat distribution. Perhaps this explains the common observation that snoring commences at puberty or during the immediate postpubertal period. It should be emphasized that morbid obesity is not a requirement for OSAS. Even a few kilograms of excessive weight can tip the balance toward upper airway obstruction in anatomically vulnerable patients.

Morbid obesity further degrades waking and sleeping ventilation, beyond its impact upon upper airway dynamics. Adipose deposition around the abdomen, diaphragm, and ribs reduces thoracic cage compliance, requiring increased work to breathe.[64] Functional residual capacity is decreased and atelectasis of dependent airways may create ventilation and perfusion mismatch with hypoxemia.[65] In the supine position, the abdominal weight creates additional load, which increases hypoxemia.[66] During REM sleep, muscle atonia renders accessory respiratory muscles such as the intercostals and upper airway dilators functionally paralyzed. Thus, the diaphragm contributes mostly to inspiration against the load created by the heavy chest mass, leading to profound oxygen desaturations seen during REM in some obese patients.

Summary

Partial or complete upper airway occlusion is related to the development of subatmospheric intrathoracic pressure during inspiration. This subatmospheric pressure is transmitted to the pharyngeal region, creating "suction" on the soft tissues that are the major constituents of the pharyngeal airway. To prevent closure, reflexes are normally activated at least 500 msec before the beginning of inspiration, to activate contraction of upper airway dilator muscles in opposition to this subatmospheric intrathoracic pressure.

During sleep, many of the upper airway dilator muscles have much less contractile power than the diaphragm. The genioglossus and geniohyoid muscles in particular are affected. This physiologic change allows the development of abnormal inspiratory upper airway resistance, which may result in partial or complete occlusion. If abnormalities of the upper airway (abnormal anatomic features, functional defects) reduce its size below a critical level or limit the capabilities of upper airway dilator muscles, during sleep, a more or less pronounced collapse occurs in this very flexible region.

The obesity hypoventilation syndrome with increased $PaCO_2$ has been described during the awake state. It is felt to result from reduced hypoxic and hypercapnic ventilatory drive and is not attributed to weight-related mechanical factors.[67]

Neural factors that relate to state changes from wakefulness to sleep, or across sleep stages, also figure in the genesis of OSAS. During sleep, the waking-related contribution to ventilatory drive is lost. This *wakefulness stimulus*[68] consists of factors that are independent of metabolic and voluntary components. With sleep onset, autonomic integration of acid-base and oxygen homeostasis is believed to occur in the medulla. Inputs to this regulator include peripheral chemoreceptors for partial pressure of carbon dioxide (PCO_2) and partial pressure of oxygen (PO_2), central chemoreceptors for pH and PCO_2, and stretch receptors in the lung, thoracic wall, and upper airway. Ventilatory responses to both hypercapnia and hypoxia are decreased in all stages of sleep,[69,70] but more profound decrements usually occur during phasic REM than in non-REM (NREM) states. However, a REM sleep–related obesity hypoventilation syndrome may be seen, indicating that state-related changes produce further blunting of hypoxic and hypercapnic drives. REM sleep–related decrements in muscle tone, which lead to changes in thoracoabdominal mechanics with distortion of the thoracoabdominal wall, are further increased in obese persons. During sleep, PO_2, tidal volume, and minute ventilation are decreased, while PCO_2 increases some 2 to 6 mm Hg. These changes are attributed to resetting of the carbon dioxide set point and a depressed ventilatory drive per given level of PCO_2 compared to wakefulness. For unknown reasons, males have a reduced ventilatory response to carbon dioxide, compared to females.[71]

The upper airway dilator muscles are accessory respiratory muscles that are partially controlled by chemoreceptors for arterial blood gases. They also receive input from thoracic, mouth, and jaw proprioceptors. Upper airway obstruction may occur when there is a mismatch in timing between neural signals that trigger the inspiratory pump muscles (of which the diaphragm predominates) and those that activate the upper airway dilator muscles.[72] Diaphragmatic inspiratory effort prior to activation of the dilator muscles would tend to suck the upper airway closed. Such a phenomenon is seen experimentally when normal sleeping humans are passively hyperventilated and then are allowed to resume spontaneous breathing. Hypocapnia causes transient central apnea, which may be terminated with an obstructive apnea.[73]

With sleep onset, sensitivity of the central carbon dioxide set point to the peripheral chemoreceptors is reduced. This results in central apnea or a reduction in diaphragmatic effort and a decrease in tidal volume (central hypopnea), which allows PCO_2 to rise. If resumption of breathing induces obstruction by the mismatched timing mechanism discussed above, a brief arousal may be triggered. Arousal resets the PCO_2 to the awake set point and increases ventilation. With the resumption of sleep, a cycling of central apnea, obstructive apnea, and arousal occurs.[74] This is commonly observed in the mixed apneas typically of obstructive sleep apneics. Any cause of sleep fragmentation, such as periodic limb movements, may produce the unstable respiratory state productive of this commonly observed type of sleep-onset apneas in predisposed individuals.

In addition to the chemoreceptor influences described above, pressure-sensitive reflexes exert a more rapid influence on upper airway patency. Located throughout its extent,[75] they coordinate the interplay of forces between inspiratory pump muscles and dilator muscles in a breath-to-breath fashion. When suction pressure produced by the diaphragm is registered, these reflexes increase genioglossus muscle activity, moving the tongue anteriorly and prolonging the inspiration. Longer inspiratory times reduce the peak suction pressure, facilitating patency of the airway.

These reflexes are normally reduced during sleep but may be defective or ineffectual in patients with sleep apnea. Sullivan and coworkers found upper airway closure to occur at abnormally low inspiratory pressures in patients with sleep apnea during a study where the nasal airway was occluded.[76]

Even when peripheral chemoreceptor drive was added (which should normally facilitate patency), there was no augmentation in activation of the dilator muscles as measured by closing pressure.

The degree of hypercapnia in sleep apnea is influenced by input from the peripheral chemoreceptors upon upper airway dilators and the inspiratory pump and by the ability of these reflexes to trigger arousal with resumption of ventilation.

Most obstructive sleep apnea patients are normocapnic while awake. However, a limited population of severe sleep apneics display hypercapnia while awake, which is not attributable to pulmonary disease or obesity. The hypercapnia in these patients indicates hypoventilation due to downward resetting of chemoreceptor reflex sensitivity. Sullivan et al[76] showed that these patients had decreased carotid body responses to hypoxemia and also failed to develop normal augmentation of response to superimposed arterial hypercarbia. Elevated levels of carbon dioxide were required to produce a ventilatory response. These patients demonstrated long periods of obstructive apnea or hypopnea, concomitant with sustained arterial oxygen desaturations and arterial carbon dioxide elevations.

Such resetting of chemoreceptors may allow a patient to endure longer apneic events while asleep without being aroused. Because the chemoreceptor responses are depressed, they do not lead to increased inspiratory efforts (as would normally occur with sensitive reflexes); thus the partially occluded upper airway is not sucked entirely closed. Diminished inspiratory efforts through a narrow upper airway cause reduced total ventilation, with oxyhemoglobin desaturation and carbon dioxide elevation.

Nightly treatment with nasal (continuous positive airway pressure) (CPAP) normalized the "awake" hypercapnia, leading to the conclusion that the sleep apnea was a major factor in its development.

Snoring

Snoring is a noise that can be produced by vibration occurring at several levels of the upper airway. It may be associated with various degrees of upper airway resistance. It may be heard following a complete airway obstruction (OSA), with a significant hypopnea, or with hypoventilation, leading to a cohort of symptoms. It may be associated with a limited and intermittent drop in tidal volume and be associated with isolated sleepiness. It may be present without other clinical symptoms. The notion that snoring itself may engender cardiovascular risk was questioned recently. Past studies of snorers probably failed to separate out subpopulations with upper airway resistance syndrome (see below) or situational apneics favored by such behavioral eliciters as alcohol or sedative use. Although more research is required, it is likely that heavy chronic snorers eventually evolve into patients with clinically significant syndromes of obstruction.[77] Snoring, however, is not a prerequisite for partial upper airway occlusion that leads to clinical symptoms.

Upper Airway Resistance Syndrome
(see Figure 16-1)[6]

Upper airway resistance syndrome causes a chronic complaint of excessive daytime sleepiness (EDS), which is objectively confirmed by abnormal scores on the Multiple Sleep Latency Test (MSLT). A retrospective study selected 54 patients previously diagnosed at Stanford with idiopathic hypersomnolence based on pathologic MSLT scores, who were also snorers. The mean group MSLT score was 6.1 minutes; an abnormal score was defined as less than 8 minutes. These patients did not fit standard criteria for OSAS in terms of RDI, significant oxygen desaturation, or both.

In 14 patients (9 women, 5 men) nocturnal sleep showed fragmentation with repetitive 3- to 14-second alpha EEG arousals, with a mean of 49 ± 11 arousals per hour of sleep. When they were studied by

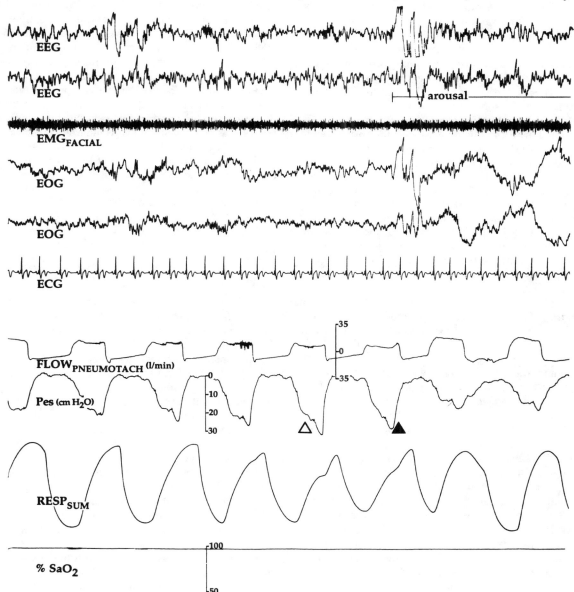

FIGURE 16-1. *PSG recording showing an example of upper airway resistance syndrome. Key: EEG, electroencephalogram; EMG$_{Facial}$; Facial muscle electromyogram; EOG, electrooculogram (right and left); ECG, electrocardiogram; FLOW$_{pneumotach}$, pneumotachometer to quantify airflow; Pes, esophageal manometry to record esophageal pressure; RESP$_{sum}$, respiratory effort. Note peak increase in effort is associated with a small drop in peak flow and tidal volume triggering a transient EEG arousal indicated by the solid arrowhead.*

esophageal balloon manometry (a technique that reflects intrathoracic inspiratory efforts as negative "suction" pressure) and a pneumotachometer with face mask to quantify airflow, a pattern emerged. Progressively increasing inspiratory efforts were demonstrated by excessively negative P_{es} nadirs between -13 and -51 cm H_2O (normal is > -8), accompanied by decreasing peak flow and tidal volume one to three breaths before the arousals. These sequences were punctuated by repeated arousals. Since the arousals and snoring would have been the only abnormalities identifiable by standard PSG recordings, these patients would not have met standard criteria for obstructive sleep apnea based on oxygen desaturation or scorable apneas and hypopneas.

These 14 patients underwent CPAP titration to eliminate the snoring and alpha arousals. At 3-week follow-up, subjective complaints of EDS were eliminated in all 14 patients, MSLT scores normalized to a group mean of 13 ± 3 minutes, and arousals were reduced to eight per hour of sleep.

In a prospective study of patients with EDS, 48 patients fulfilling PSG and MSLT criteria for idiopathic hypersomnia (RDI less than 5 and MSLT no more than 8) were studied with home ambulatory monitoring, including evaluation of snoring, several nocturnal PSG recordings, and subsequent nocturnal P_{es} polygraphic monitoring. Fifteen subjects (eight women, seven men) with sleep fragmentation and peak P_{es} nadirs below -12 cm H_2O were restudied with P_{es} in conjunction with quantitative airflow measurement via pneumotachometer and face mask. Mean body mass index (BMI) was 22.7 ± 2.1 kg/m^2 for the women and 24.3 ± 4.0 kg/m^2 for the men. Snoring was continuous in ten, intermittent in four, and absent in two. Mean RDI was 2.1 ± 1.7. Mean SaO_2 nadir was $91.4 \pm 2.1\%$. These patients showed abnormal breathing periods where progressive increases of P_{es} nadir, associated with decreases in peak flow and tidal volume, were interrupted by alpha EEG arousal.

The subjects were adapted to nasal CPAP for two nights. On the second night, P_{es} measurement was obtained and optimal CPAP pressure eliminated the abnormal P_{es} nadirs, snoring, and sleep fragmentation. Follow-up MSLT results showed an improved mean of 13.5 ± 2.1 and subjective disappearance of EDS. Thus, approximately one third of patients given the standard diagnosis of idiopathic hypersomnia at a major sleep disorders center had a treatable form of upper airway obstruction.

Secondary Apnea

A variety of medical conditions and craniofacial malformations are commonly associated with OSA. Patients with congenital syndromes of micrognathia such as the Pierre Robin, Crouzon's, Hunter's, and Treacher-Collins syndrome present in childhood; children with cleft palates repaired by a pharyngeal flap have developed iatrogenic obstruction. Cranial base abnormalities associated with OSA include achondroplasia, Arnold-Chiari, and Klippel-Feil malformations. Down's syndrome patients have large tongues and retrognathia that predispose to upper airway obstruction. Children with Prader-Willi syndrome may suffer OSA owing to morbid obesity.

Endocrine abnormalities that cause OSA include hypothyroidism with myxedema, which causes macroglossia and parapharyngeal tissue infiltration. Acromegaly is a known cause of macroglossia.

Neurologic disorders associated with OSA include the Shy-Drager syndrome of multisystem degeneration (central and obstructive apnea) and neuromuscular diseases involving facial and thoracoabdominal muscles such as poliomyelitis and myotonic and muscular dystrophy. Secondary kyphoscoliosis worsens nocturnal respiratory function. Lesions of the temporomandibular condyle leading to retrognathia may be developmental or acquired secondary to rheumatoid arthritis, osteomyelitis, or trauma.

EVALUATION

History

Pertinent symptoms of OSAS fall into daytime and nighttime categories. Loud, gutteral snoring, worst in the supine position, punctuated by choking sounds followed by cessation of breathing is virtually pathognomonic. Although snoring commonly starts around the time of puberty, presentation to a physician is typically prompted by a recent increase in snoring intensity associated with weight gain. The sleep of the bed partner is compromised by the patient's high-amplitude snoring and restless sleep. The volume may be so loud as to exceed standards set by the Occupational Safety and Health Administration for workplace safety.[77] The apneic phase can last seconds to more than a minute. These respiratory cessations may be frightening to bed partners, who often remain vigilant to wake the patient to resume breathing. Partners often begin sleeping in separate rooms, which may stress the relationship.

Restless sleep stems in large part from sleep fragmentation caused by airway obstruction. Repetitive EEG arousals lasting seconds are seen to terminate many apneic episodes, thus allowing restoration of "wakeful" muscle tone observed on the chin EMG. This facilitates a restorative breath, allowing the cycle to repeat. Behavioral arousals accompany some of these EEG arousals, resulting in position changes, abrupt raising of the upper torso off the bed, and large flailing limb movements. Some of these movements appear to be agitated, with concomitant groaning or crying out of short, dysphoric phrases such as, Oh, God. The vast majority of brief arousals are not consciously recalled on awakening, though the patient may appreciate that the quality of sleep has been poor. Clues to restless sleep are provided by asking the patient if their bedcovers are very disturbed, and how many times they recall awakening at night.

It is surprisingly infrequent that the patient awakens with actual awareness of an asphyxia sensation such as choking or gasping. When this does occur, it may be accompanied by what is described as a feeling of dying, and the patient may run to a window or sit up at the edge of the bed. Rarely, they are still unable to draw an inspiratory breath, but they usually can do so after coughing. It is believed that this may be due to adhesion of the uvula to the posterior pharynx.

There appears to be a subpopulation of sleep apneics whose presenting complaint is sleep maintenance insomnia. A proportion of their arousals trigger full awakenings that last at least several minutes. Because patients remain unaware of the respiratory antecedents of these awakenings, OSAS should be part of the differential diagnosis of patients who have chronic difficulty maintaining sleep.

Symptoms related to snoring are a dry mouth or sore throat on awakening. Morning headaches that resolve within an hour of awakening should be sought in the history, as they may be clues to nocturnal hypercarbia. They are typically generalized or bifrontal. The occurrence of nocturnal confusion spells, such as watering the plants with milk, may be due to either hypoxemia or slow-wave sleep parasomnia triggered by an arousal induced by an abnormal breathing event.

Polyuria—multiple trips to the lavatory—has recently been related to elevated plasma levels of ANP and catecholamines.[78] Following the first night of treatment with nasal CPAP, a return to normal levels with concomitant decrease in urine volume to approximately 50% of pretreatment amounts has been reported. This helps explain why enuresis is more common in children with OSAS and was reported in 7% of 120 apneic adults. Confusion and raised intraabdominal pressures from inspiratory attempts against a closed upper airway may also contribute.

Nocturnal esophageal acid reflux and heartburn are facilitated when excessively negative intrathoracic pressure exerts upward suction on abdominal contents and increased abdominal pressure expels the contents.

Bruxism may be noted and may be a clue to dental malocclusion resulting from the common jaw misalignment etiologically related to obstructive sleep apnea. A history of dental braces to correct an overjet is common.

History of seasonal or environmental allergies should be sought, as these are common causes of nasal obstruction in adults and adenotonsillar enlargement in children. Nasal obstruction with mouth breathing during childhood has been suggested to be etiologically related to subsequent mandibular growth insufficiency, in studies of rhesus monkeys with chronic and temporary nasal obstruction.[59,60]

Nocturnal perspiration may be associated with the increased effort required to inspire against resistance over the course of a night. Increased calorie expenditure to breathe may also account for a subpopulation of sleep apneics who have difficulty gaining weight.

Ethanol and other sedatives used before bedtime worsen OSA by at least two mechanisms. They greatly diminish the contraction of the upper airway dilators and interfere with the organization of reflexes that coordinate upper airway dilators with the contraction of inspiratory muscles.[80] A history of increased snoring or development of any of these symptoms in association with sedating substances should raise the index of suspicion for OSA. In elderly patients with AI greater than 5, sedative use or sleep deprivation escalates the AI significantly, into the pathologic range.[81]

The cardinal daytime symptom of OSAS is EDS, which manifests as a tendency to inadvertently fall asleep during quiet or boring situations, to take intentional naps, or to present short but repetitive attention lapses during monotonous tasks. Such sleepiness is the consequence of sleep fragmentation. Patients usually mistakenly attribute their dozing off to the characteristics of the situation (i.e., boredom) rather than an abnormal intrinsic degree of somnolence. It helps to inform patients that quiet settings do not produce sleepiness but merely unmask it. Patients often forget or deny episodes of daytime sleepiness, which may be better elicited from household members who observe frequent episodes of dozing while watching television or reading. Momentary lapses into sleep while driving are a potentially lethal consequence of somnolence and should always be sought by inquiring about motor vehicle accidents due to sleepiness or inadvertently dozing at the wheel or swerving into another lane. Such incidents are particularly likely on long or monotonous trips. Affirmative answers require rapid treatment interventions.

Cognitive complaints resulting from EDS are common and may be the only clue to EDS in persons who misperceive their sleepiness. Symptoms include poor memory and difficulty concentrating or making decisions. Automatic behavior—an action performed but subsequently not recalled—is an extreme manifestation of such cognitive impairment. Increased errors and poor judgment may place patients at risk for losing their jobs.[82] Severe morning confusion and disorientation, termed *sleep drunkenness*, may be a sequela of preceding hypoxemia.

Sleep fragmentation may produce personality changes that are often first noted by family members. These include irritability, anxiety, aggression, and depression. More marked personality changes involving irrational behavior, jealousy, and suspiciousness are reported.[82] Sleepy patients report less enjoyment from previously engaging activities. They are typically misperceived as unmotivated or lazy, descriptors that they come to believe if the underlying cause remains undiscovered. Diminished libido or impotence is not uncommon, even in patients who are not elderly.

In taking the medical history, inquiries regarding systemic sequelae must be sought. These include the existence and duration of borderline or elevated blood pressure, angina, symptoms of right-sided heart failure including peripheral edema, and transient cerebrovascular ischemic symptoms.

Examination

Patient evaluation begins with observing the patient in the waiting room for sleeping or snoring. The height and weight provide a body mass index (expressed in kilograms per square meter) by which to assess the degree of obesity; the upper limit of normalcy for American males is 28 kg/m^2. The distribution of weight should be noted, as more midline deposition favors nocturnal respiratory disorders. In particular, adiposity or muscularity of the neck predisposes to upper airway obstruction, while severe abdominal obesity may additionally predispose to alveolar hypoventilation. A nasal voice is a clue to nasal obstruction, and mild hoarseness is often noted in heavy snorers. The lateral facial profile should be inspected for retrognathia or micrognathia, keeping in mind that the relevant site is the indentation below the lip, which identifies the genial tubercle, where the tongue takes insertion on the mandible. The patient should bite down to demonstrate dental occlusion. Overjet is recorded in millimeters, and underbite is noted as well. The temporomandibular joint is palpated with wide jaw opening for subluxation or a click—further evidence of jaw malalignment. The oral cavity is inspected for dental prostheses, size of tongue, and soft palate size and appearance. Soft palate edema and erythema may be due to snoring. A soft palate positioned inferiorly behind the tongue may be due to chronic excessive suction from snoring. Tonsillar hypertrophy is noted. The hard palate is checked for a high arch, which correlates with OSAS.

Evidence of upper airway obstruction is obtained by evaluating breathing while the patient lies supine with the jaw slacked slightly open and nares occluded, to simulate mouth breathing during sleep. If snoring or labored breathing results, this is good evidence that even greater difficulties occur during sleep.

The nose is assessed for septal deviation, polyps, flaring of the nostrils, and patency of either vestibule with the opposite naris occluded. The thyroid is palpated.

Blood pressure, pulse, and a general physical examination are performed, with an eye to signs of cardiac dysrhythmia or failure. Lung auscultation provides clues to pulmonary disease which would exacerbate oxygen desaturation caused by upper airway obstruction. Complete neurologic evaluation may uncover neuromuscular disorders that affect upper airway patency and respiratory muscle function. A complete physical examination rules out generalized diseases, particularly those that induce lymph node enlargement or mucosal infiltration that may reduce the upper airway lumen.

History and evaluation should reveal possible secondary causes of OSAS. These include a search for a local tumor in the upper airway. Suspicion is raised in the presence of rapid emergence of obstructive symptoms unassociated with weight gain, throat pain, constant hoarseness, or other vocal cord dysfunction, prominent difficulty swallowing, or nasal regurgitation. Such symptoms should prompt otolaryngologic evaluation.

Laboratory Evaluation

Polysomnography

A full night's PSG study in the sleep laboratory is the main method of evaluation. The study devotes various channels to the electroencephalogram (EEG) (i.e., C$_4$-A$_1$, C$_3$-A$_2$, O$_1$-O$_2$), electrooculogram (EOG), chin and limb (usually anterior tibialis) noninvasive EMG, qualitative measurements of oronasal airflow, thoracic and abdominal respiratory efforts, electrocardiogram (ECG), and pulse oximetry. An entire night's study is recommended, as opposed to a partial night's, as substantial changes in respiratory disturbance typically occur from one sleep cycle to another throughout the night. Because REM sleep predominates toward the end of the night, REM-related respiratory disturbances might easily be missed without a full night's study.

PSG allows quantification of various factors disturbed in sleep apneics, including the RDI, oxygen desaturations, sleep stage percentages, and sleep efficiency. Sleep fragmentation can be assessed as awakenings of variable length or EEG arousals lasting only several seconds. PSG helps determine the causes of arousals—apnea or unsuspected factors such as periodic limb movements or primary insomnia.

Associations of sleep stage and positional influences on respiratory disturbance can be made. Cardiac dysrhythmias and their relationship to oxygen desaturation and sleep stage are identified.

Relatively invasive techniques for measuring upper airway pressure may have more limited clinical utility. The upper airway resistance syndrome may be suspected only because of transient alpha EEG arousals on the standard PSG, warranting additional investigation using esophageal manometry. Catheter systems that allow measurement of differential pressures at different levels of the upper airway may also help determine the level of collapse to which surgical intervention should be addressed.[83-85]

Newer technologies are rapidly emerging that allow in-home sleep monitoring. These offer the benefits of reduced cost and increased accessibility to larger segments of the population. Current disadvantages include less information, especially reliable EEG evaluation vital to the detection of brief arousals. It is likely that these drawbacks will be circumvented in the near future.

The Multiple Sleep Latency Test (MSLT)[86]

The MSLT is considered an objective meaure of excessive daytime somnolence. A series of daytime naps (usually five) of 20 minutes' duration at 2-hour intervals is performed to determine time to sleep onset (sleep latency). The latencies are averaged. In the absence of confounding factors (such as insufficient preceding nocturnal total sleep time, or hypnotic medication use), scores under 8 minutes are generally regarded as abnormal. REM sleep during naps is also noted. Because demonstration of EDS is not required for the diagnosis of obstructive sleep apnea, MSLTs are not mandatory for the evaluation of OSA; however, if a PSG for suspected OSA is negative, MSLT performed the next day may help reveal a different sleep disorder of excessive somnolence.

When complaints of somnolence persist after adequate treatment is instituted, an MSLT may reveal an unsuspected second sleep disorder that requires a separate treatment approach.

Imaging studies

As an adjunct to clinical evaluation, particularly when surgical treatment is contemplated, various imaging procedures can help identify the site of upper airway obstruction. The interested reader is referred to a recent comprehensive overview.[87] Imaging is also imperative when the history raises suspicion that a mass lesion is the cause of upper airway obstruction. It should be kept in mind that procedures performed on an awake patient do not reveal the actual anatomy during sleep, when postural and state-related changes in muscle tone alter the relationships observed during wakefulness.

Cephalometric radiographs provide a midline view of relevant cranial base and facial bones and their soft tissue appendages. Maxillary or mandibular deficiency can be calculated, and awake posterior airway space measured as the distance between the base of the tongue and the posterior pharyngeal wall. Soft palate and lymphoid tissue extent are identified.

Fiberoptic endoscopy of the upper airway performed in the seated and supine positions provides further assessment of the possible sites of collapse down to the vocal cords. The patient can perform Valsalva's and Müller's maneuvers to elicit collapse, though the predictive value for identifying candidates for surgical success following uvulopalatopharyngoplasty is limted.[88-90] Fiberoptic endoscopy should be systematically performed to eliminate secondary causes of upper airway obstruction.

Computed tomography (CT) provides detailed surveys of cross-sectional levels of the upper airway, and magnetic resonance imaging (MRI) can capture multiple planes. They have been used mainly as research tools, owing to their expense. Newer techniques such as fast CT may prove to have prognostic clinical utility in selecting candidates for a successful surgical outcome. The 50-msec scan time, as compared to 2 to 5 seconds for conventional CT, is sufficiently rapid to show dynamic dimensional changes across various levels of the upper airway during the respiratory cycle. Fast CT can potentially be used to investigate the patient while asleep.

Video fluoroscopy of the pharynx, in anteroposterior and lateral views, offers another means for observing dynamic anatomic changes in the upper airway during ventilation. Its clinical utility is limited owing to the significant radiation exposure.

Other studies

Pulmonary function tests, including spirometry and arterial blood gases, are a useful adjunct to investigation. Patients with daytime hypoxemia or carbon dioxide retention due to intrinsic lung disease might be expected to show severe oxygen desaturation with the addition of obstructive sleep pathology and may require cautious addition of low-flow oxygen to nasal CPAP. Those with restrictive pulmonary dynamics based on morbid obesity might require special treatment with BIPAP, Bilevel Positive Airway Pressure (BiPAP[TM], Respironics, Inc.) or intermittent positive-pressure ventilation (see below). Reactive airway disease can be detected and treated. Arterial blood gas values provide the most relevant information for a sleep evaluation when they are obtained after the patient lies supine for 20 minutes. This helps detect insufficent ventilation associated with the supine position. A special request to the laboratory is required.

Thyroid function screening excludes hypothyroidism as a cause of apnea and daytime somnolence. Polycythemia without known lung disease should prompt consideration of sleep apnea.

TREATMENT

Behavioral Recommendations

Once OSA is diagnosed, treatments can be suggested based on evaluation of contributing factors and severity of disease. In overweight patients without obvious fixed anatomic considerations such as retrognathia, weight loss might result in eventual cure. For most patients, nasal CPAP should be instituted along with weight loss measures. When applicable, a program of exercise is facilitated after daytime somnolence is ameliorated by CPAP. For patients who will not be completely cured by weight loss alone, significant weight reduction often allows lowering of the CPAP pressure requirement or increases the likelihood of a surgical cure. After a large loss the lowest adequate pressure should be retitrated.

Eliminating central nervous system depressants such as ethanol or sedatives from the bloodstream at bedtime reduces the severity of OSA. When a strong positional relationship is discovered and obstruction is associated only with the supine position, the patient is advised to sleep on one side or prone. By sewing a golf or tennis ball into a sock attached to the back of the pajamas, patients can learn to avoid the supine position. Recently a buzzer-type training device was introduced that sounds when the patient lies supine for a brief time. In mild cases, attention to position may suffice.

Elevating the bed about 30 degrees by placing blocks under the head may help in mild cases or until definitive treatment is implemented.

Pharmacologic

Tricyclic antidepressants such as protryptilline have been used to increase muscle tonus and diminish REM time in cases where OSA was mild or REM related. Progesterone acts as a respiratory stimulant in obese patients but has no impact on an obstructed airway. Unfortunately, pharmacologic approaches have been largely unsuccessful.

CPAP and BIPAP (See also Chapter 28)

An enormous advance in the treatment of OSA began in the early 1980s, with the first commercially available continuous positive-pressure generators. These bedside machines compress room air and chan-

nel it through a soft vinyl or silicone nasal mask or endonasal cushions at a given pressure. CPAP serves as a pneumatic splint to keep the upper airway patent. Pressure requirements must be established for each patient during sleep. Optimal pressure is the lowest one that completely eliminates obstructive apneas, hypopneas, and snoring. Patients who routinely consume ethanol in the evening are most accurately titrated to CPAP after consuming their usual intake, which raises the pressure requirement.

BIPAP, bilateral Positive Airway Pressure (BiPAP^{TM}, Respironics, Inc.) differs from CPAP in that it employs separate inspiratory and expiratory pressures. The machine times itself to patient-initiated breathing. By reducing the pressure on expiration, it lowers the resistance against which the patient must exhale. This is advantageous for patients with severely restrictive pulmonary dynamics such as those with emphysema or morbid obesity, as well as those with neuromuscular weakness. Patients with normal lungs who could not tolerate CPAP might feel more comfortable on BIPAP, especially those who require higher CPAP pressure, in the range of 12 to 17 cm H_2O. Those with severe discomfort due to drying of the mucosae could benefit from the overall decrease in airflow relative to CPAP. BIPAP also offers a higher range of respiratory pressures than CPAP, with maximum pressures of 23 cm H_2O. It can assist ventilation of patients who also hypoventilate during sleep, despite the fact that pressure ventilators are less efficacious than volume ventilators. Intermittent positive-pressure ventilation may be more useful in some patients with sleep-related hypoventilation.

Ideally, PSG study to titrate CPAP or BIPAP pressure should be performed over 1 or 2 nights, to allow adequate assessment. By the end of the first night the optimal pressure is approximated, and on the second night this pressure can be checked for adequacy throughout all stages and positions. It is especially critical to evaluate the patient in the supine position, where the pressure requirement is maximal. With severe apnea, a rebound of unusually long and misscheduled REM and slow-wave sleep occurs once adequate airway patency is attained. REM-sleep rebound shows unusually prominent phasic activity, while the slow-wave sleep episodes may show exceptionally high voltages. A rare but dangerous sequela of REM rebound has been seen in severe apnea: it is the development of CO_2 retention when CPAP pressures are titrated at a moderate to low level with carbon dioxide retention under slightly suboptimal pressure. During a long rebound, arousability is suppressed, and if partial upper airway closure persists, dangerous hypoxemia may result.[91]

Treatment with nasal CPAP or BIPAP offers advantages of safety and ensured efficacy over surgical approaches. They offer immediate and complete treatment for OSA and are less costly than extensive surgical approaches. They can be used temporarily while weight loss is accomplished or surgery is contemplated. Positive pressure eliminates risk factors for associated morbidity along with daytime somnolence. Modern CPAP units are small, portable, and quiet. Some gradually adjust the pressure upward to the preset pressure, allowing sleep onset to occur at more comfortable lower pressures.

Disadvantages of CPAP lie in psychological resistance to ongoing nightly reliance on a machine. Patients may feel claustrophobic or perceive an obstacle to intimacy with their bed partner, restriction of their movement in bed, or a reminder of their mortality. Those who travel frequently may find it inconvenient. Generally, young adults or those who are dating find this treatment to have an unacceptable social impact.

Common physical difficulties encountered include reactive nasal congestion or rhinitis, drying of the nasal-oral mucosa, discomfort or skin trauma from an ill-fitting mask, and allergic or contact dermatitis from the mask. Nasal symptoms usually subside after the first few months and can be ameliorated with nasal steroid inhalers. Dryness can be treated with saline nasal sprays or in-line or room humidifiers. Comfort issues and dermatitis should be closely supervised, with trials of various mask adaptors and styles, or by altering the mode of delivery via nasal cushions. Psychological distress is minimized with support from the entire sleep laboratory team, with reassurance and understanding at the time of initiation, and with close follow-up. Sleep apnea support groups in many areas help with coping and compliance. Occasionally, a brief course of bedtime anxiolytics is required, but the patient is made to fully understand that the apnea will worsen if the medication is used without the CPAP. Flow leaks through an open mouth can be minimized by use of a chin strap.

Long-term compliance has been only fair: 60% to 85% of patients, it is estimated, still use their machine regularly after 1 year.[92,93] Compliance has been found to be associated with the severity of daytime hypersomnolence prior to CPAP but not with pretreatment disease severity as indicated by the respiratory disturbance index or oxygen saturation nadir. Intellectual understanding of the benefits of nightly use, (i.e., to decrease cardiovascular risk factors) appears to be insufficient to motivate long-term compliance.

For patients who do not desire the extensive surgery that might be required to produce a complete cure, selective surgery to relieve nasal obstruction can reduce pressure requirements and improve tolerance to CPAP.

For patients with more than mild oxygen desaturation on diagnostic testing (i.e., less than 85%) who elect surgical treatment, CPAP initiation may be contemplated preoperatively to decrease the postoperative risk of further desaturation due to edema. Preoperative CPAP also reduces soft palate edema due to snoring and improves overall health status. Weight loss achieved prior to surgery and while using CPAP increases the chance of successful cure by creating more airway space through parapharyngeal tissue reduction.

Surgical Approaches

Surgery is individually tailored to overcome upper airway obstruction after a thorough analysis of the three main levels of potential obstruction: the nose, soft palate, and the base of tongue. Often, more than one level must be treated, either sequentially or simultaneously. Patients must understand that surgical treatment is an extensive and more costly process and has greater risks than medical treatment. In addition, surgery carries no guarantees of cure for any given patient; only statistical cure rates are available.

Nasal obstruction can be corrected with septoplasty, polypectomy or turbinate reduction. Soft palate resection via uvulopalatopharyngoplasty (UPPP) carries approximately a 50% cure rate.[54] The most common postoperative adverse sequelae include severe pain for about 2 weeks, transient nasal reflux and nasal speech due to palatal incompetence, minor loss of taste, and tongue numbness. Major complications involve permanent nasal reflux or nasal speech due to permanent velopharyngeal incompetence and scarring with retraction leading to palatal stenosis.

Because this procedure ameliorates snoring due to vibration of the uvula without addressing potential obstruction behind the base of the tongue, a major sign of ongoing residual obstruction may be masked. It is therefore imperative to follow-up on all surgeries with a postoperative sleep study. Ideally, the study should be delayed at least 4 months after surgery to allow thorough resolution of edema and readjustment of respiratory reflexes. Those with moderate to severe apnea can be maintained on CPAP in the interim and withdrawn 2 weeks before the study to allow expression of airway changes from potential residual obstruction.

Geniotubercle advancement via inferior sagittal osteotomy is a technique pioneered at Stanford[95] to address the retroposition of the tongue by advancing the insertion point of the genioglossus. It involves a small mandibular incision at the geniotubercle, pulling the bone segment through the jaw and allowing the fracture to heal. This is usually performed in conjunction with UPPP. Common complications are minor and consist of transient dental nerve anesthesia. Mandibular fracture may occur if the incision extends into the alveolus. Hyoidotomy with subhyoid myotomy and anterior superior repositioning with a fascia graft is now commonly performed in association with geniotubercle advancement. Based on 55 patients followed up postoperatively, the combined success rate of the surgical procedure consisting of geniotubercle advancement with inferior sagittal osteotomy and hyoid myotomy with resuspension associated with UPPP is approximately 70%.[96] Midface advancement involving Le Fort I mandibular ostetomy and a maxillary ostetomy is specifically reserved for patients whom other treatments have failed and who do not want to be treated with nasal CPAP. Patients undergoing midface advancement have previously had the other surgeries discussed above and have not shown adequate improvement at 4- to 6-month follow-up, which includes clinical evaluation and polygraphic monitoring. A study of 30 patients who underwent such surgery revealed no significant differences in efficacy, as compared to curative treatment with nasal CPAP, on indices of oxygen saturation nadir, RDI, and normalization of sleep architecture.[94]

Dental Appliances

Different types of dental devices have been tried in the recent past. These devices have the same goal as inferior sagittal osteotomy with geniotubercle advancement, though much less space is gained than by surgical procedures. The most commonly used devices are the Esmarch appliance, the Bionator, and the tongue-retaining device. Objective studies reporting results at 1 year follow-up are few. In mild cases, these devices may be helpful.

OBSTRUCTIVE SLEEP APNEA IN CHILDREN

OSA occurs in premature and full-term infants and in children. In very young patients, the apnea usually becomes apparent through color change and bradycardia; in children, a constellation of clinical symptoms signals the condition. At different ages, different symptoms are emphasized. Post-pubertal teenagers do not differ from young adults, but younger children often present a different clinical picture.

Clinical Features

OSAS can be associated with a series of daytime and nighttime signs and symptoms that may not be obvious at an initial evaluation.[97,98] The daytime symptoms include (1) EDS so severe that school authorities suggest medical consultation and (2) abnormal daytime behavior ranging from aggressiveness and hyperactivity to pathologic shyness and social withdrawal. Children may exhibit learning problems, morning headaches, frequent upper air-

way infections, failure to thrive, or obesity. Nocturnal symptoms include difficulty breathing while asleep, heavy snoring, apneic episodes, restless sleep, heavy sweating, nightmares, night terrors, and enuresis.

Reasons for seeking consultation tend to vary with age. In children younger than 5 years, difficulty breathing while asleep, heavy snoring, sleep apneic episodes observed by parents, restless sleep, nightmares, and night terrors are the most frequent reasons for consultation. This may be because parents check young children's sleep often and young children fall asleep early, allowing parents to note abnormal sleep behavior. In children older than 5 years, EDS (associated with complaints of tiredness and daytime fatigue), abnormal daytime behavior, learning disabilities, frequent morning headaches, nocturnal enuresis, and major discipline problems are common reasons for consultation. A few children are referred at a late stage of the syndrome; they not only exhibit significant failure to thrive but also may have had hospitalizations for unexplained acute cardiac failure or unexplained development of systemic hypertension. The cardiac failure often occurred when the child contracted a cold or bronchopneumopathy, which may not have been severe but which in combination with the chronic nocturnal problem led to the acute failure.

The clinical evaluation of children should be as thorough as for adults, and suspicion of obstructive sleep apnea should lead to polygraphic monitoring during sleep.

Polygraphic Testing

Although repetitive apneas may be as frequent in children as in adults, most commonly the PSG test indicates only intermittent apneas. Sometimes no apneas are monitored even when florid symptoms are observed.[99]

Prepubescent children have a greater tendency to present complete apneas during REM sleep. During NREM sleep they snore loudly. Documented by a sonogram, snoring is commonly associated with an increase in respiratory rate. The degree of tachypnea is very variable within a given age group, and sometimes within a given subject during the night. The increase in breathing frequency compensates for the decrease in tidal volume (V_T) and allows maintenance of normal minute ventilation with an appropriate level of oxygen saturation. However, partial upper airway obstruction leads to great enhancement of respiratory efforts, very obvious when one observes the very laborious, noisy mouth breathing during sleep. Measurement of esophageal pressure (P_{es}) demonstrates the increase in respiratory efforts. P_{es} nadir may reach -35 to -40 cm H_2O without induction of a complete collapse of the upper airway in 5- to 6-year-old children. Increased efforts may also be demonstrated by monitoring intercostal and diaphragmatic EMG. Surface electrodes placed 10 mm apart near the eighth right intercostal space, between the axillary and mamillary lines, permit collection of the EMG activity of the inspiratory muscles. The signal can be integrated, and, depending on the calibration procedures used, semiquantitative or quantitative measurements may be obtained. Measurement (and integration) of abdominal muscle activity during expiration, again with use of surface electrodes, may demonstrate the degree of active expiratory effort that some of these children have to perform. Despite the increase in respiratory efforts associated with snoring and increased upper airway resistance, children may not present very fragmented sleep. The short alpha EEG arousals seen with increased upper airway resistance in adults may be much more uncommon here; however, breathing may appear laborious, and increased efforts are often demonstrated by perspiration and sweat (at the head and neck or generalized). This suggests that the daytime sleepiness observed in these children, in spite of near normal sleep structure and absence of microarousals cannot be explained by sleep fragmentation alone.

It may be hypothesized that some changes in the child's metabolism may also be involved in daytime fatigue and sleepiness. These children sometimes exhibit failure to thrive, and usually they are slim and have difficulty gaining weight in spite of a normal appetite. They also may be shorter than expected. Nocturnal secretion of growth hormone in children with repetitive apneas has been shown to be abnormally low, and we have noted a similar decrease with heavy snoring. Polygraphic monitoring must thus focus not only on the presence or absence of apnea (with the knowledge that absence of apnea may be very misleading) but also on increase in respiratory effort, increase in breathing frequency and the importance of thoracoabdominal mechanical changes.

The repetitive inspiratory efforts expended during complete or, more often, partial upper airway obstruction lead to abnormal septal motion with leftward shift of the interventricular septum and the development of pulsus paradoxus.[100] Cardiac arrhythmias, particularly asystole and secondary AV block, may be seen, and intermittent increase in systolic blood pressure may be noted. Finally, systemic hypertension has been observed in association with OSA. Systemic hypertension in prepubertal children disappears completely with tracheostomy. To date, the only cases of systemic hypertension of recent origin that were found to be clearly "idiopathic" and in which treatment of OSA led to complete and long-term normalization of blood pressure were in prepubertal and pubertal children.

Asthma and Upper Airway Obstruction During Sleep

In children, a relationship exists between these two syndromes. Allergic reactions very early in life lead to mucosal swelling and enlargement of the pharyngeal region. There is a well-known interaction between the size of the upper airway and craniofacial development, particularly development of the mandible, during early childhood. Presence of upper airway allergies thus limits maxillo-mandibular growth and causes a decrease in the size of the upper airway. Small upper airways are often associated with increased upper airway resistance during sleep, leading to increased respiratory efforts and the development of snoring during sleep. Increased upper airway resistance and nocturnal snoring worsen asthma, causing increased risk of a nocturnal asthma attack.

Orthodontic Complications and Upper Airway Obstruction During SLeep

Children with partial or complete upper airway obstruction during sleep frequently have maxillomandibular growth retardation. Abnormal orthodontic features are common. Class II malocclusion is frequently seen, but it is not the only orthodontic problem. As 60% of facial development is complete by age 4 years, and 90% by 11 years, it is important to recognize the orthodontic involvement and also to understand that inappropriate orthodontic treatment, which further impairs maxillomandibular growth, may catalyze snoring and significantly increase upper airway resistance during sleep. Abnormal maxillomandibular development may be responsible for nocturnal snoring and bruxism.

TREATMENT

Age also has an impact on therapeutic approaches.

Tonsillectomy and Adenoidectomy

Nasal obstruction is rarely the only factor in the development of apnea, but it can be a contributing factor. In such cases, correcting the obstruction can alleviate, if it does not cure, the OSAS. If there are markedly enlarged tonsils or adenoids with no other abnormal factors, the child should undergo tonsillectomy alone or tonsillectomy and adenoidectomy (T/A). Too often, however, not enough attention is paid to problems that may be associated with enlarged tonsils and adenoids—abnormally long soft palate, retroposition of the mandible, or soft tissue infiltration behind the base of the tongue—which may explain residual apnea after tonsillectomy. Furthermore, if T/A is performed during the prepubertal years in boys, there is a chance that the extensive soft tissue growth that occurs during puberty may cause reappearance of OSAS in those whose airway space is already compromised by malocclusion (e.g., mild to moderate retroposition of the mandible). Fiberoptic endoscopy must be performed systematically in association with one imaging test to determine how much soft tissue surgery is needed, but the classic UPPP is not recommended for children.

Tracheostomy

In the past, tracheostomy was a frequent treatment when T/A was insufficient. Tracheostomy resolves the OSAS, but it may cause secondary problems such as depression in children following surgery, and families commonly have difficulty accepting the surgery and caring for the stoma. Nevertheless, tracheostomy is clearly beneficial in many cases. The need for tracheostomy can be alleviated by the use of nasal CPAP.

Nasal Continuous Positive Airway Pressure

Prepubertal children as young as 6 months have been treated with nasal CPAP at Stanford since 1984[101]; long-term treatment has been successful. Several U.S. and foreign manufacturers (Respironics, in Pennsylvania, USA; Healthdyne, in Georgia, USA; SEFAM in Vandoeuvre les Nancy, France) currently supply nasal CPAP for young children, and Respironics provides masks for infants and very young children.

The complications and problems associated with this treatment have been related to (1) difficulty for the children, many of whom were mentally retarded, in understanding how the mask and CPAP equipment functioned; (2) difficulty getting parents to collaborate with the medical team to train the child to keep the nasal mask on; (3) air leaks at the edge of the mask causing reappearance of apnea and eye irritation; and (4) skin allergy to the mask in small children. Problems 1 and 2 were responsible for some children's abandoning nasal CPAP treatment; problems 3 and 4 were occasionally bothersome but never led to interruption of therapy. The theoretical risk of stomach dilation due to incorrect administration or other mishap has never been reported. No system has an alarm to indicate complete displacement of the mask, so for very young children, hand restraint during sleep may be necessary to adapt the child to the apparatus.

Orthodontic and Maxillomandibular Surgery

Children with OSAS often have a retroposition of the mandible, a steep mandibular plane, or an abnormally arched palate, abnormalities that are not necessarily obvious. No one overlooks Pierre Robin syndrome, but specialists will not appreciate the mandibular problem, and orthodontists may not be aware of the impact on the upper airway of a moderately abnormal mandible. Orthodontic approaches may help redirect growth and may, in certain children, prevent the reappearance of snoring and sleep apnea, particularly in post-pubertal boys.

When maxillofacial abnormalities are clearly related to the presence of OSAS in children, maxillofacial surgery may be considered. Piecuch[102] reported a child treated with maxillofacial surgery for OSAS. Kuo and coworkers[103] have reported two cases and Bear and Priest[104] three cases of OSAS that were resolved by maxillofacial surgery; the largest series of patients (teenagers and adults) treated with maxillofacial surgery to date was reported by Riley and colleagues.[95,96] Though good results have been reported with surgery in pubertal children, we recommend investigating orthodontic approaches before considering it for prepubertal children.

SUMMARY

OSAS is distressingly common and must be considered a disease with diverse adverse systemic consequences, including cardiovascular risk. As such, inquiries into the existence of snoring and excessive daytime somnolence should be part of the physicians' review of systems. Because daytime somnolence appears in many guises, such as fatigue and cognitive difficulties, a high index of suspicion for this condition must be maintained. Sleep apnea diminishes the restorative effects of the one third of life we spend sleeping, thus degrading the quality of the wakeful two thirds. Evaluation and treatment are now readily available at sleep disorders centers. Treatment recommendations can be tailored to the patient's problems, taking into consideration individual preference, age, personality, life style, and objective findings at PSG.

REFERENCES

1. American Sleep Disorders Association. Obstructive sleep apnea syndrome. In: The International Classification of Sleep Disorders, Diagnostic and Coding Manual. 1990:52–58:342
2. Gould GA, Whyte KF, Rhind GB, et al. The sleep hypopnea syndrome. Am Rev Respir Dis 1990; 142:295–300.
3. American Sleep Disorders Association. The International Classification of Sleep Disorders. Diagnostic and Coding Manual. 1990:346.

4. Berry DTR, Webb WB, Block AJ. Sleep apnea syndrome: A critical review of the apnea index as a diagnostic criterion. Chest 1984;86:529–531.

5. Guilleminault C, van den Hoed J, Mitler M. Clinical overview of the sleep apnea syndromes. In: Guilleminault C, Dement W, eds. Sleep Apnea Syndromes. New York: Alan R. Liss, 1978:1–12.

6. Guilleminault C, Stoohs R, Clerk A, et al. From obstructive sleep apnea syndrome to upper airway resistance syndrome. Sleep 1992;15:513–516.)

7. Bixler E, Kales A, Soldatos C, et al. Sleep apneic activity in a normal population. Res Commun Chem Pathol Pharmacol 1982;36:141–52.

8. Block AJ, Boysen PG, Wynne JW, et al. Sleep apnea, hypopnea, and oxygen desaturation in normal subjects: A strong male predominance. N Engl J Med 1979;300;513–17.

9. Guilleminault C, Quera-Salva MA, Partinen M, et al. Women and obstructive sleep apnea. Chest 1988;93:104–109.

10. Coleman RM, Roffwarg HP, Kennedy SJ, et al. Sleep-wake disorders based on a polysomnographic diagnosis. A national cooperative study. JAMA 1982;247:997–1003.

11. Lavie P. Incidence of sleep apnea in a presumably healthy working population: A significant relationship with excessive daytime sleepiness. Sleep 1983;6:312–18.

12. Gislason T, Almqvist M, Eriksson G, et al. Prevalence of sleep apnea syndrome in Swedish men—an epidemiological study. J Clin Epidemiol 1988;41;571–576.

13. Schmidt-Nowara, W, Jennum P. Epidemiology of sleep apnea. In: Guilleminault C, Partinen M, eds. Obstructive Sleep Apnea Syndrome. Clinical Research and Treatment. New York: Raven Press, 1990:1–8.

14. Shepard JW Jr, Garrison M, Grither D, et al. Hemodynamic responses to O_2 desaturation in obstructive sleep apnea [Abstr]. Am Rev Respir Dis 1985; 131:A106.

15. Schroeder JS, Motta J, Guilleminault C. Hemodynamic studies in sleep apnea. In: Guilleminault C, Dement W, eds. Sleep Apnea Syndromes. New York: Alan R. Liss, 1978:177–196.

16. Fletcher E, Miller J, Schaaf J, et al. Fletcher J: Urinary catecholamines before and after tracheostomy in obstructive sleep apnea. Sleep Res 1985;14:154.

17. Guilleminault, C van den Hoed J, Mitler MM. Clinical overview of the sleep apnea syndromes. In: Guilleminault C, Dement W, eds. Sleep Apneas Syndromes. New York: Alan R. Liss, 1978:1–12.

18. Lavie P, Ben-Yosef R, Rubin AE. Prevalence of sleep apnea among patients with essential hypertension. Am Heart J 1984;107:543–548.

19. Williams AJ, Houston D, Finberg S, et al. Sleep apnea syndrome and essential hypertension. Am J Cardiol 1985;55:1019–1022.

20. Coccagna G, Mantovani M, Brignani F, et al. Continuous recording of the pulmonary and systemic arterial pressure during sleep in syndromes and hypersomnia with periodic breathing. Bull Physiopathol Respir 1972;8:1159–1172.

21. Krieger J, Laks L, Wilcox I, et al. Atrial natriuretic peptide release during sleep in patients with obstructive sleep apnea before and during treatment with nasal continuous positive airway pressure. Clin Sci 1989;77:407–411.

22. Follenius M, Krieger J, Krauth MO, et al. Obstructive sleep apnea treatment: Peripheral and central effects on plasma renin activity and aldosterone. Sleep 1991;14:211–217.

23. Krieger J, Reitzer B, Weitzenblum E, et al. Transmural pulmonary arterial pressure during obstructive sleep apneas. Sleep Res 1987;16:375.

24. Guilleminault C, Motta J, Mihm F, et al. Obstructive sleep apnea and cardiac index. Chest 1986;89:331–334.

25. Krieger J, Weitzenblum E. Determinants of respiratory insufficiency in obstructive sleep apnea patients. Dur Respir J 1988:1:96s.

26. Leech JA, Onal E, Givan V, et al. Right ventricular dysfunction relates to nocturnal hypoxemia in patients with sleep apnea syndrome [Abstr]. Am Rev Respir Dis 1985;131:A104.

27. Bradley TD, Rutherford R, Grossman RF, et al. Role of daytime hypoxemia in the pathogenesis of right heart failure in the obstructive sleep apnea syndrome. Am Rev Respir Dis 1985;131:835–839.

28. Bland JW Jr, Edwards KF, Brinsfield D. Pulmonary hypertension and congestive heart failure in children with chronic upper airway obstruction. Am J Cardiol 1969;22:830–837.

29. Tilkian RG, Guilleminault C, Schroeder JS, et al. Hemodynamics in sleep-induced apnea. Ann Intern Med 1976;85:714–719.

30. Tilkian AG, Motta J, Guilleminault C. Cardiac arrhythmias in sleep apnea. In Guilleminault C, Dement W, eds. Sleep Apnea Syndromes. New York: Alan R. Liss, 1978:197–210.

31. Miller WP. Cardiac arrhythmias and conduction disturbances in the sleep apnea syndrome. Am J Med 1982;73:317–321.

32. Guilleminault C, Connolly SJ, Winkle RA. Cardiac arrhythmia and conduction disturbances during sleep in 400 patients with sleep apnea syndrome. Am J Cardiol 1983;52:490–494.

33. Shepard JW Jr, Garrison MW, Grither DA, et al. Relationship of ventricular ectopy to nocturnal O_2 desaturation in patients with obstructive sleep apnea. Chest 1985;88:335–340.

34. Shepard JW Jr. Cardiorespiratory changes in obstructive sleep apnea. In: Kryger MH, Roth T, Dement WC, eds. Principles and Practice of Sleep Medicine. Philadelphia: WB Saunders, 1989;537–551.

35. Derman S, Karacan I, Hartse KM, et al. Changes in local cerebral blood flow measured by CT scan during wakefulness and sleep in patients with sleep apnea syndrome and narcolepsy [Abstr]. Sleep Res 1981;10:190 [Abstr].

36. Meyers JS, Sakai F, Karacan I, et al. Sleep apnea, narcolepsy and dreaming: Regional cerebral hemodynamics. Ann Neurol 1980;7:479–485.

37. Giombetti RJ, Kneisley LW, Miller BL, et al.: Waking cerebral blood flow abnormality in sleep apnea syndrome. Sleep Res 1990;19:229.

38. Kneisley LW, Daly J, Giombetti RJ, et al. Partial reversal of abnormal waking cerebral blood flow in patients with sleep apnea. Sleep Res 1990;19:243.

39. Palomaki H, Partinen M, Juvela S, et al. Snoring as a risk factor for sleep related brain infarction. Stroke 1989;20:1311–1315.

40. Lugaresi E, Cirignotta F, Coccagna G, et al. Some epidemiological data on snoring and cardiocirculatory disturbances. Sleep 1980;3:221–224.

41. He J, Kryger MH, Zorck FJ, et al. Mortality and apnea index in obstructive sleep apnea. Experience in 385 male patients. Chest 1988;94:9–14.

42. Partinen M, Jamison A, Guilleminault C: Long-term outcome for obstructive sleep apnea: Mortality. Chest 1988;94:1200–1204.

43. Chaudhary BA, Sklar AH, Chaudhary TK, et al. Sleep apnea, proteinuria, and nephrotic syndrome. Sleep 1988;1:69–73.

44. Seliger M, Mendelson WB. Renal function in obstructive sleep apnea. APSS Annual Meeting Abstract Toronto 1991; 138.

45. Weitzman ED, Pollack CP, Borowiecki B, et al. The hypersomnia sleep apnea syndrome: Site and mechanism of upper airway obstruction. In Guilleminault C, Dement WC, eds. Sleep Apnea Syndromes. New York: Alan R. Liss, 1978:235–248.

46. Hill MW, Guilleminault C, Simmons FB. Fiberoptic and EMG studies in hypersomnia sleep apnea syndrome. In Guilleminault C, Dement WC, eds. Sleep Apnea Syndromes. New York: Alan R. Liss, 1978:249–258.

47. Remmers JE, Launois S, Feroah T, et al. Mechanics of the pharynx in patients with obstructive sleep apnea. In: Issa FG, Suratt PM, Remmers JE, eds. Sleep and Respiration. Prog Clin Biol Res 345, pp. 261–271. New York: Wiley-Liss, 1991.

48. Guilleminault C, Hill MW, Simmons FB, et al. Obstructive sleep apnea: Electromyographic and fiberoptic studies. Exp Neurol 1978;62:48–67.

49. Guilleminault C, Motta J. Sleep apnea syndrome as a long-term sequela of poliomyelitis. In: Guilleminault C, Dement WC, eds. Sleep Apnea Syndromes. New York: Alan R. Liss, 1978:309–315.

50. Hyland RH, Hutcheon MA, Perl A, et al. Upper airway occlusion induced by diaphragmatic pacing for primary alveolar hypoventilation: Implications for the pathogenesis of obstructive sleep apnea. Am Rev Respir Dis 1981;124:180–184.

51. Simonds AK, Branthwaite MA. Efficiency of negative ventilatory equipment. Thorax 1985;40:213.

52. Skatrud JB, Dempsey JA. Airway resistance and respiratory muscle function in snorers during NREM sleep. J Appl Physiol 1985;59:328–335.

53. Stoohs R, Guilleminault C. Snoring during NREM sleep: Respiratory timing, esophageal pressure behavior, and EEG arousal. Respir Physiol 1991;85:151–167.

54. Jamieson A, Guilleminault C, Partinen M, et al. Obstructive sleep apneic patients have craniomandibular abnormalities. Sleep 1986;9:469–477.

55. Guilleminault C, Stoohs R. From "apnea of infancy" to obstructive sleep apnea syndrome in the young child. Chest (in press).

56. Guilleminault C, Heldt G, Powell N, et al. Small upper airway: A familial risk for apnea in near-miss SIDS and their parents. Lancet 1986;i:402–407.

57. Larsson S-G, Gislason T, Lindholm C-E. Computed tomography of the oropharynx in obstructive sleep apnea. Acta Radiol 1988;29:401–405.

58. Vargervik K, Miller AJ, Chierici G, et al. Morphologic response to changes in neuromuscular patterns induced by altered modes of respiration. Am J Orthod 1984;85:115–124.

59. Miller AJ, Vargervik K, Chierici G, et al. Experimentally induced neuromuscular changes during and after nasal airway obstruction. Am J Orthodont 1984;85:385–392.

60. Vargervik K, Harvold E. Experiments on the interaction between orofacial function and morphology. Ear Nose Throat J 1987;66:201–208.

61. Linder-Aronson S. Adenoids. Their effect on mode of breathing and nasal airflow and their relationship to characteristics of the facial skeleton and the dentition. Acta Otolaryngol Suppl (Stockh) 1970;265:1–132.

62. Solow B, Siersbaek-Nielsoen S, Greve E. Airway adequacy, head posture, and craniofacial morphology. Am J Orthodont 1984;86:214–223.

63. Harmon E, Wynne JW, Block AJ: Sleep-disordered breathing and oxygen desaturation in obese patients. Chest 1981;79:256–260.

64. Naimark A, Cherniack RM. Compliance of the respiratory system and its components in health and obesity. J Appl Physiol 1960;15:377–382.

65. Holley HS, Milic-Emili J, Becklake MR, et al. Regional distribution of pulmonary ventilation and perfusion in obesity. J Clin Invest 1967;46:475–481.

66. Tucker DH, Sieker HO. The effects of change in body position on lung volumes and intrapulmonary gas mixing in patients with obesity, heart failure and emphysema. J Clin Invest 1960;39:787–791.

67. Zwillich CW, Sutton FO, Pierson DJ, et al. Decreased hypoxic ventilatory drive in the obesity-hypoventilation syndrome. Am J Med 1975;59:343–347.

68. Fink BR. Influence of cerebral activity in wakefulness on regulation of breathing. J Appl Physiol 1961;16:15–20.

69. Berthon-Jones M, Sullivan CE. Ventilatory and arousal responses to hypoxia in sleeping humans. Am Rev Respir Dis 1982;125:632–639.

70. Douglas NJ. Control of ventilation during sleep. Chest Clin North Am 1985;6:563–575.

71. Weill J, White DP, Douglas NJ, et al. Ventilatory control during sleep in normal humans. In: West JB, Lahiri S, eds. High Altitude and Man. Bethesda, Md.: American Physiological Society, 1984;91–100.

72. Hwang JC, St John WM, Bartlett D Jr. Afferent pathways for hypoglossal and phrenic responses to changes in upper airway pressure. Respir Physiol 1984;55:341–354.

73. Skatrud JB, Dempsey JA. Interaction of sleep state and chemical stimuli in sustaining rhythmic ventilation. J Appl Physiol 1983;55:813–822.

74. Dempsey JA, Skatrud JB. A sleep-induced apneic threshold and its consequences. Am Rev Respir Dis 1986;133:1163–1170.

75. Widdicombe J, Sant'Ambrogio G, Mathew OP. Nerve receptors of the upper airway. In Mathew OP, Sant'Ambrogio G. Respiratory Function of the Upper Airway. New York: Marcel Dekker, 1988:193–231.

76. Sullivan CE, Grunstein RR, Marrone O, et al. Sleep apnea—pathophysiology: Upper airway and control of breathing. In: Guilleminault C, Partinen M, eds. Obstructive Sleep Apnea Syndrome: Clinical Research and Treatment. New York: Raven Press, 1990:49–69.

77. Lugaresi E, Cirignotta F, Coccagna G, et al. Clinical significance of snoring. In: Saunders NA, Sullivan CE, eds. Sleep and Breathing. New York: Marcel Dekker, 1984:283–298.

78. Guilleminault C. Obstructive sleep apnea syndrome: A review. Psychiatr Clin North Am 1987;4:607–621.

79. Baruzzi A, Riva R, Cirignotta F, et al. Atrial natriuretic peptide and catecholamines in obstructive sleep apnea syndrome. Sleep 1991;1:83–86.

80. Issa FG, Sullivan CE. Alcohol, snoring and sleep apnea. J Neurol Neurosurg Psychiatry 1982;45:353–359.

81. Guilleminault C, Silvestri R, Mondini S, et al. Aging and sleep apnea: Action of benzodiazepine acetazolamide, alcohol and sleep deprivation in a healthy elderly group. J Gerontol 1984;39:655–661.

82. Guilleminault C, van den Hoed, Mitler MM. Clinical overview of the sleep apnea syndrome. In: Guilleminault C, Dement WE, eds. Sleep Apnea Syndromes. New York: Alan R. Liss, 1978;1–12.

83. Hudgel DW. Variable site of airway narrowing among obstructive sleep apnea patients. J Appl Physiol 1986;61:1403–1409.

84. Chaban R, Cole P, Hoffstein V. Site of upper airway obstruction in patients with idiopathic obstructive sleep apnea. Laryngoscope 1988;98:641–647.

85. Shepard JW Jr, Thawley SE. Localization of upper airway collapse during sleep in patients with obstructive sleep apnea. Am Rev Respir Dis 1990;141:1350–1355.

86. Carskadon MA, Dement WE, Mitler MM, et al. Guidelines for the Multiple Sleep Latency Test (MSLT): A standard measure of sleepiness. Sleep 1986;9:519–524.

87. Shepard JW, Gefter WB, Guilleminault C, et al. Evaluation of the upper airway in patients with obstructive sleep apnea. Sleep 1991;4:361–371.

88. Sher AE, Thorpy MJ, Shprintzen RJ, et al. Predictive value of Mueller maneuver in selection of patients for uvulopalatopharyngoplasty. Laryngoscope 1985;95:1483.

89. Wittig R, Fujita S, Fortier J, et al. Results of uvulopalatopharyngoplasty in patients with both oropharyngeal and hypopharyngeal collapse on Mueller maneuver. Sleep Res 1988;17:269.

90. Katsantonis GP, Maas CS, Walsh JK. The predictive efficacy of the Mueller maneuver in uvulopalatopharyngoplasty. Laryngoscope 1989;99:677–680.

91. Krieger J, Weitzenblum E, Manassier JP. Dangerous hypoxemia during continuous positive airway pressure treatment of obstructive apnea. Lancet 1983;2:1429–1430.

92. Waldhorn RE, Herrick TW, Nguyen MC, et al. Long-term compliance with nasal continuous positive airway pressure therapy of obstructive sleep apnea. Chest 1990;97:33–38.

93. Nino-Murcia G, McCann CC, Bliwise DL, et al. Compliance and side effects in sleep apnea patients treated with nasal continuous positive airway pressure. West J Med 1989;150:165–169.

94. Riley RW, Powell NB, Guilleminault C. Maxillofacial surgery and nasal CPAP. A comparison of treatment for obstructive sleep apnea syndrome. Chest 1990;98:1421–1425.

95. Riley R, Powell NB, Guilleminault C, et al. Maxillary, mandibular, and hyoid advancement: An alternative to tracheostomy in obstructive sleep apnea syndrome. Otolaryngol Head Neck Surg 1986;94:584–588.

96. Riley RW, Powell NB, Guilleminault C. Maxillofacial surgery and obstructive sleep apnea: Review of 80 patients. Otolaryngol Head Neck Surg 1989;101:353–361.

97. Guilleminault C, Eldridge FL, Simmons FB, et al. Sleep apnea in eight children. Pediatrics 1976;58:28–31.

98. Guilleminault C, Korobkin K, Winkle R. A review of 50 children with obstructive sleep apnea syndrome. Lung 1981; 159:275–281.

99. Guilleminault C, Winkle R, Korobkin R, et al. Children and nocturnal snoring: Evaluation of the effects of sleep-related respiratory resistive load and daytime functioning. Eur J Pediatr 1982;139:165–171.

100. Guilleminault C, Shiomi T, Stoohs R, et al. Echocardiographic studies in adults and children presenting with obstructive sleep apnea or heavy snoring. In: Gaultier C, Escourrou P, Curzi-Dascalova L, eds. Sleep and Cardiorespiratory Control. Paris: Collogue INSERM/John Libbey Eurotext, 1991;217:95–103.

101. Guilleminault C, Nino-Murcia G, Heldt G, et al: Alternative treatment to tracheostomy in obstructive sleep apnea: Nasal CPAP in children. Pediatrics 1986;78:797–802.

102. Piecuch JF: Costo-chondral grafts to temporomandibular joints [Abstr 38]. In: Abstracts and Proceedings of the Annual Meeting of the American Association of Oral and Maxillofacial Surgeons, Chicago, 1978.

103. Kuo PC, West RR, Bloomquist DS, et al. The effect of mandibular osteotomy in 3 patients with hypersomnia sleep apnea. Oral Surg 1979; 48:385–392.

104. Bear SE, Priest JH: Sleep apnea syndrome: Correction with surgical advancement of the mandible. J Oral Surg 1980;35:543–549.

17

Insomnia

James K. Walsh
Paul G. Hartman
James P. Kowall

DEFINITIONS

Insomnia is a condition of subjectively inadequate or nonrestorative sleep. Virtually everyone experiences occasional nights of poor sleep, whether they are caused by temporary stress or by excitement or worry over recent events. An occasional night of poor sleep does not in most instances engender severe consequences. In contrast, persistent insomnia often has profound detrimental effects on a person's life. Insomniacs frequently complain of impaired daytime function, including fatigue, irritability, mood disturbance, poor concentration, reduced work performance, and daytime sleepiness.

Insomnia may be experienced as difficulty falling asleep (sleep onset insomnia), frequent or prolonged awakenings from sleep (sleep maintenance insomnia), or nonrestorative sleep. Many persons with insomnia have two or more of these features.[1] Probably the most important issue guiding the diagnosis and treatment of insomnia is the duration of the complaint.[2] A sleep disturbance that lasts one to several nights in an isolated period is termed *transient insomnia* and is most often caused by an acute situational stress or travel across multiple time zones. Disturbed sleep that lasts several nights to a month is considered *short-term insomnia* and is usually associated with a more persistent stressful situation (for example, a new job or an illness in the family) or environmental factors (for example, noise). *Persistent insomnia* lasts a month or more and may be caused by any of a large number of conditions, including psychiatric disorders, medical disorders, and primary sleep disorders such as periodic leg movements during sleep, sleep apnea, or a circadian rhythm disturbance. In many cases, transient or short-term insomnia recurs, and if bouts of poor sleep become relatively frequent, this represents a form of persistent insomnia.

Perhaps because insomnia is such a pervasive problem, it appears to be accepted as a normal part of life. One in three adults reports at least occasional insomnia, and approximately 10% to 15% of the population considers insomnia a serious problem in their lives.[3] Yet a national survey found that physicians recorded a diagnosis of insomnia in only 0.42% of office visits.[4] A 1991 Gallup poll revealed that most persons who experience insomnia more than 2 nights per week never report it to their physician and are never asked about sleep by that physician. This survey indicated that only 5% of insomniacs visit a physician specifically to discuss their sleep problem, and 26% discuss insomnia during a visit made primarily for another problem.[5] Even when recognized by a physician, insomnia is likely to be assessed and treated inappropriately.[6] Nevertheless, direct costs associated with medical care and self-treatment for insomnia in the United States were recently estimated (in 1990 dollars) to be more than $11 billion annually.[7] The lack of effective health care for insomnia reflects principally the inadequate training in sleep medicine most health professionals receive. A major goal of this chapter is to provide a core of information about the characteristics and treatment of insomnia.

EPIDEMIOLOGY

Prevalence and Demographics

Of all sleep-related complaints, insomnia is the most prevalent, affecting more than 60 million American adults each year. As noted above, approximately 30% to 35% of adults report difficulty sleeping, and 10% to 15% report severe or chronic problems with sleep.[1,3,5,8–13] Table 17-1 summarizes the results of major American surveys of the prevalence of insomnia.

Demographic factors associated with the prevalence of insomnia among adults include age, gender, socioeconomic status, and marital status. As shown in Table 17-2, the prevalence of insomnia among adults rises with age[3]; however, more recent representative sample studies suggest that the age-associated increase is less dramatic than is often stated.[5,13] In addition, women are more likely to have insomnia than men; typical prevalence rates are approximately 40% and 30%, respectively. Insomnia also appears to be more common in people of low socioeconomic status.[1,9] Finally, divorced, widowed, or separated persons are more likely to report insomnia than those who are single or married,[1,9] but age may account in part for these findings.

TABLE 17-1.   Studies of Insomnia Prevalence in the United States

Investigators, Date	Sample	Prevalence (%)	Severity
Karacan et al[9] 1976	1645 adults, north Florida	35.4	13.4% severe, 22.0% moderate
Bixler et al[10] 1979	1006 adults, Los Angeles	32.2	
Karacan et al[1] 1983	2347 adults, Houston, Tex.	> 40 (males) > 53 (females)	
Welstein et al[11] 1983	6340 persons, San Francisco	30.7	
Mellinger et al[3] 1985	3161 adults, United States	35.0	17.0% serious
Gallup Organization[8] 1986	1015 adults, United States	16.6	4.7% totally dissatisfied, 11.9% somewhat dissatisfied
Ford and Kamerow[12] 1989	7954 adults, Baltimore, Md., Durham, N.C., and Los Angeles	10.2	
Gallup Organization[5] 1991	1000 adults, United States	36.0	9.0% chronic, 27.0% occasional
Balter and Uhlenhuth[13] 1991	5011 adults, United States	34.0	15% serious, 9% chronic

The relative prevalence in the United States of transient and short-term insomnia versus persistent insomnia is unknown. In a Swiss study of 20- and 21-year-old persons,[14] approximately 15% had occasional episodes of transient insomnia, another 16% had recurrent episodes of transient insomnia, and 9% reported persistent insomnia. Follow-up studies of these subjects at 2 and 7 years found that more than half the subjects with occasional episodes of transient insomnia had developed either recurrent or persistent insomnia. In addition, the majority of subjects with persistent or recurrent insomnia at baseline continued to have either persistent or recurrent insomnia at follow-up. These findings suggest that persistent insomnia is a relatively permanent disorder and that transient insomnia often evolves into persistent insomnia. Whether treatment of transient insomnia early in its course can prevent the development of persistent insomnia remains an important unanswered question.

Treatment

Whereas the majority of insomniacs never speak to a health professional about their sleep problem, many persons with insomnia attempt some form of self-treatment. Some of the more common methods used by persons dissatisfied with their sleep are watching television, reading, use of nonprescription medication, and drinking alcohol.[5,8] Alcohol is used by 28% of insomniacs to promote sleep, and nonprescription medication is used by 29%.[5] These figures are disconcerting, as neither alcohol nor nonprescription medications are effective for insomnia, and adverse effects are not uncommon.

Physicians' treatment of insomnia is quite limited, owing primarily to their lack of training in this area. Of the 2.67 million office visits in 1985 associated with a presenting complaint of insomnia, prescription medication for sleep was given in about 887,000 visits, or about one-third of the time.[4] As other treatments appear to be employed rarely, it is likely that no treatment was provided in a large percentage of cases.

Undertreatment of insomnia may in part represent a response to reports in the media of overuse and misuse of prescription hypnotics. However, these reports appear to have been overstated. The 1991 Gallup poll[5] indicated that only 21% of all insomniacs had ever taken prescription medication for sleep. Furthermore, the overall prevalence rate of prescription hypnotic use has consistently been reported to be less than 3% of adults in the United States, and the majority (64%) of users take the drug no more than 30 times per year.[3,15,16] Regular nightly use for a year or more is reported by 11% of all prescription hypnotic users.[3]

TABLE 17-2.   Prevalence and Severity of Trouble Falling Asleep or Staying Asleep, by Age

	Age Group (Yr.)				
	18–34	35–49	50–64	65–79	Total
Had trouble and was bothered					
A lot (%)	14	15	20	25	17
Not that much (%)	17	19	18	20	18
Used to have trouble (%)	15	15	10	6	12
Never had trouble (%)	54	51	52	49	52
Total	100	100	100	100	100

From Mellinger GD, Balter MD, Uhlenhuth EH: Insomnia and its Treatment: Prevalence and correlates. Arch Gen Psychiatry 1985; 42:225–232.

Consequences and Correlates

Several studies have shown that persons with insomnia report that sleep difficulty impairs their daytime functioning.[1,5,8,11,14] In the 1986 Gallup study,[8] more than 27% of all surveyed felt that their daytime activities were affected by poor sleep at least two days per week. When one considers only those dissatisfied with their sleep, this percentage jumps to 70%. The 1991 Gallup study[5] found that insomniacs reported memory and concentration problems, poor performance at work, and a higher incidence of automobile accidents caused by fatigue than did noninsomniacs. A longitudinal study of Navy personnel found that poor sleepers earned fewer promotions, were more likely to remain at lower pay grades, and were less frequently recommended for reenlistment than were good sleepers.[17] These findings support the complaint of impaired daytime function by insomniacs and possibly contribute to the association of insomnia with lower socioeconomic status.

Persons with insomnia are also more likely than good sleepers to have medical and psychological problems. Mellinger and coworkers found that 53% of persons with insomnia reported multiple health problems whereas two or more health problems were reported by only 24% of persons who never had insomnia.[3] Ford and Kamerow[12] found that people with insomnia were significantly more likely to utilize medical and psychological services than were persons who had no sleep complaint. In addition, a high prevalence of insomnia among general medical patients has been reported;[22-24] one report indicated that 56% of 500 consecutive patients in a family practice clinic had a sleep problem.[23]

Finally, a small number of laboratory studies of insomniacs have occasionally shown objective deficits in semantic memory,[18] impaired daytime vigilance,[19] and impaired gait and balance[20]; however, other investigations find no clear performance impairment in groups of insomniacs, perhaps because of extreme interindividual variability in the performance of insomniacs.[21]

Insomnia and Medical Disorders

Disturbed sleep has been reported to be associated with various medical conditions, including disorders of cardiovascular, respiratory, gastrointestinal, renal, and musculoskeletal systems.[25] Most epidemiologic research into the relationship of sleep disturbances to somatic disorders has been conducted in Europe. In a representative sample of 591 young Swiss adults, insomnia was associated with stomach disorders, appetite problems, sexual problems, exhaustion, respiration problems and heart problems.[26] Similarly, among 3201 Swedish men aged 30 to 69 years, various sleep problems were significantly more prevalent among those who had somatic disorders; for example, severe sleep maintenance insomnia was reported by 22% of men with diabetes, 19% of those with bronchitis or asthma, 16% of men with joint or low back pain, and 14% of hypertensives, compared with 7.5% of the entire sample.[27] Lastly, a Finnish study found that difficulty falling asleep and difficulty remaining asleep were significantly more prevalent in patients with myocardial infarction and in paraplegic patients than in controls.[28]

Recent research has begun to examine whether insomnia may play a role in the development of medical disorders. For example, epidemiologic studies have found that insomnia complaints may be predictive of increased risk for future cardiovascular disease. In a study of 10,778 males and females aged 35 to 59 years, poor sleepers were more than twice as likely as good sleepers to have ischemic heart disease in the next 6 years. Male poor sleepers' increased risk for heart disease remained significantly higher after controlling for the effects of age, neuroticism, and life satisfaction.[29]

Disturbed sleep may also be related to the occurrence of gastrointestinal disorders. In 100 patients with irritable bowel syndrome 28% of patients (versus 5% of controls) complained of poor sleep, and 63% of patients (versus 20% of controls) complained of constant tiredness.[30] In an epidemiologic study of 14,102 Norwegian adults, persons with insomnia were twice as likely as good sleepers to have one or more symptoms of irritable bowel syndrome.[31] Peptic ulcer has been found to be more prevalent among shift workers, who often have disturbed sleep, than in daytime workers. Patients with peptic ulcer have also been found to be more likely than controls to have insomnia.[32]

Lastly, sleep disturbance may be a factor in the fibrositis syndrome. Patients with fibrositis have widespread musculoskeletal pain, localized areas of tenderness, and chronic fatigue, but no apparent structural damage or disease. Most patients with fibrositis describe their sleep as light, restless, and not refreshing.[33] Objective sleep recording in fibrositis patients indicates a pattern of alpha waves in the EEG which persists throughout most non-rapid eye movement (NREM) sleep.[33] Inducing an analogous alpha sleep abnormality in normal persons by disturbing NREM sleep with periodic noises has been reported to cause fibrositis-like symptoms on awakening.[34] Furthermore, pharmacologic treatment of the sleep abnormality in fibrositis patients was reported to alleviate musculoskeletal symptoms.[33] The alpha sleep abnormality has also been found in some rheumatoid arthritis patients and osteoarthritis patients with fibrositis symptoms,[33,35] which suggests that alpha sleep is not specific to fibrositis. Some form of sleep disturbance may contribute to the common complaint of fatigue in arthritis.

In some, initial research findings suggest that insomnia may play a role in the development or continuation of dysfunction in various physiological systems. Further studies are needed to define these associations and to determine the physiological processes that link sleep and physical disorders. More information is also needed on the role of sleep in recovery from medical disorders, especially as modifiable elements in the hospital environment may disturb the sleep of recovering patients.[25] Finally, research is needed to determine the effectiveness of insomnia treatment for patients with co-existing medical disorders, and to determine whether treating insomnia in these patients has beneficial effects on their medical disorders.

Insomnia and Psychological Disorders

Psychological disorders are two to three times more prevalent in insomniacs than in others. This association is particularly strong for depression which is at least four times more prevalent in insomniacs.[3,12] Traditionally, insomnia in persons with psychological disorders has been attributed to emotional and physiological arousal associated with psychological distress.[36] More recently, neurophysiological investigations of sleep and depression suggest that certain pathophysiological mechanisms may underlie both depression and some types of sleep disturbance.[37,38]

Furthermore, recent epidemiologic research suggests that insomnia may be an early marker or a contributing factor to psychological disorders. In a large-scale longitudinal survey performed by Ford and Kamerow,[12] people who reported insomnia at baseline and 1 year later were four times as likely as noninsomniacs to have a psychological disorder at the end of the year. In contrast, subjects whose insomnia had resolved within the year were only slightly more likely than controls to develop a psychological disorder. Persons with insomnia at the followup interview were particularly at risk for symptoms of major depression, compared to persons who did not have insomnia or whose insomnia was resolved at followup. The risk for developing anxiety disorders and alcohol abuse was also greater for insomniacs than noninsomniacs. An important question raised by this study is whether early treatment for insomnia might reduce the risk of developing psychological disorders.

Insomnia and Mortality

Reported habitual short sleep duration, which occurs in some insomniacs, has been found to be associated with increased mortality risk, according to a large-scale longitudinal study by the American Cancer Society.[39] Sleeping less than 4 hours per night was associated with a relative increase in mortality risk of 2.8 for men and 1.5 for women, in comparison to men and women who slept 7 to 8 hours per night. Similarly, the Human Population Laboratory of the California State Department of Health found that persons who slept 6 hours or less per night had a 70% higher mortality rate over a 9-year period than those who slept 7 to 8 hours; long habitual sleep length was also associated with increased mortality risk.[40,41] In both studies, the increased mortality risk associated with habitual short sleep was present after controlling for other known risk factors.

The relationship between sleep and mortality risk is of special interest in the elderly, who obviously have a higher mortality rate than other age groups. In a study of 1855 non-institutionalized elderly people, elderly men who reported having severe insomnia were 3.15 times as likely to die over the next 3.5 years as those with only mild insomnia; interestingly, those who reported no insomnia were also somewhat more likely to die than those with mild insomnia.[42] In this study, self-reports of long or short sleep duration were also significantly associated with increased mortality risk, but this relationship may have been secondary to the associations of sleep length and mortality with other factors. In another study, elders whose objectively recorded sleep time deviated at least 2 hours from average for this age group had a 50% higher mortality risk over the next several years than those whose sleep length was within 1 hour of average.[43] Sleep length was a stronger predictor of mortality than history of smoking, cardiac disease, or hypertension, and remained a significant risk factor for mortality even after statistical control for the influence of age, body mass index, and physical endurance.

In summary, epidemiological studies suggest that both insufficient sleep and excessive sleep appear to be risk factors for mortality. These associations have not yet been adequately explained.

CONCEPTUAL MODEL OF INSOMNIA

Sleep is an essential physiological process, the adequacy of which reflects a person's medical, psychological, social, and environmental status. Insomnia may result from factors in any one or a combination of these domains. The large number of potential contributing factors to insomnia requires an organizational structure for information relevant to the diagnosis and treatment of insomnia. In one such scheme, based on work by Spielman and colleagues,[44] insomnia is conceptualized as the result of constitutional, precipitating, and perpetuating factors.

Constitutional Factors

Many factors contributing to insomnia appear to be constitutional i.e., relatively permanent features of an individual's physical makeup and functional processes. The quality of a person's sleep may reflect strengths or deficiencies in the neurological mechanisms underlying sleep and circadian processes. For example, Morris and colleagues[45] have shown that sleep-onset insomniacs have delayed core body temperature rhythms suggesting a circadian mechanism abnormality, either hereditary or acquired. Studies utilizing large twin cohorts[46,47] indicate that genetic factors may have a significant influence on sleep quantity and quality. In some forms of insomnia, such as restless legs syndrome, genetic factors may predominate.[48]

Constitutional factors also include the psychological makeup of an individual. Psychiatric disorders are often conceptualized as reflecting relatively constant personality characteristics or neurochemical dysfunction. Even in the absence of psychopathology, stable psychological characteristics such as excessive rumination, or internalization and somatization of stress, may contribute to poor sleep.

A constitutional predisposition to insomnia may be related to long-standing medical conditions, including chronic obstructive pulmonary disease, chronic renal insufficiency, duodenal ulcer, or other conditions that cause pain or physical discomfort.

Age is an important constitutional factor, in that the basic mechanisms of sleep appear to deteriorate with age. Furthermore, various disorders associated with insomnia occur more commonly in the elderly.

Within the present conceptual scheme, constitutional factors alone are not likely to produce insomnia, though this may occur in idiopathic insomnia. In most cases, rather, constitutional factors represent a predisposition or susceptibility that manifests as insomnia in the presence of sufficiently strong precipitating and perpetuating factors.

Precipitating Factors

It is assumed that precipitating factors are more likely to cause insomnia in persons who have a constitutional predisposition to poor sleep. In such cases, the onset of insomnia is often temporally contiguous with a specific change in a person's life. Healy and colleagues found that 74% of poor sleepers linked the onset of insomnia with a stressful life event.[49] Another study found that major events associated with the onset of insomnia most often concerned interpersonal relationships, loss of a significant person because of death or a move to a distant location, change in occupational or educational status, or a medical condition.[50] Such major events may produce psychological stress, leading to physiological and cognitive arousal that delay the onset and disrupt the continuity of sleep.

Insomnia may also be precipitated by a shift from a daytime to a nighttime work schedule, owing to the resulting mismatch between the body's circadian propensity to sleep and the time of day available for sleep. In addition, conditions of the sleeping environment, such as noise or an uncomfortable temperature, can hinder sound sleep. Other precipitating factors include pain or discomfort due to acute medical conditions or the onset of a psychiatric condition such as depression. It should be noted that a medical or psychiatric disorder that precipitates insomnia may occur in the context of a constitutional predisposition for the disorder. In many cases, insomnia remits following remission of the precipitating factors; in other cases, however, insomnia may persist because of the development of perpetuating factors.

Perpetuating Factors

Factors that maintain an insomnia condition are often different from those associated with its onset. Poor sleep and consequent problems in daytime functioning may engender an excessive concern about sleep, thereby increasing physiologic and cognitive arousal at bedtime and, paradoxically, inhibiting sleep. After insomnia has continued more than a few nights, associations may be learned that link bedtime and the sleeping environment with worry and difficulty sleeping rather than with a relaxed state conducive to sleep. Both performance anxiety and learned (conditioned) factors can perpetuate insomnia after precipitating factors have abated. Moreover, the person who experiences insomnia may develop poor sleep hygiene practices, such as taking long naps, extending time in bed, ingesting excessive caffeine during the day, or using alcohol as a hypnotic, all of which can maintain or exacerbate insomnia.

Insomnia may also be perpetuated by psychosocial factors that reinforce the insomniac's role as a "sick" person.[36] In some cases, the insomnia condition can become associated with secondary gain, providing an excuse to avoid unwanted work responsibilities or family interactions. Insomnia complaints may also generate reinforcing nurturance and concern for the patient from significant others.

Insomnia Threshold

Consistent with the model of Spielman and colleagues,[44] insomnia may occur if a critical threshold, termed the "*insomnia threshold*," is exceeded by the combination of effects due to constitutional, precipitating, and perpetuating factors. The relative importance of these factors varies among and within insomnia diagnostic classifications; for example, perpetuating factors are relatively more important in psychophysiological insomnia than in idiopathic insomnia, in which constitutional factors dominate. In addition, the relative weight of the three types of factors may change over the course of an insomnia condition (Figure 17-1).[44] In the representative insomnia case depicted in Figure 17-1 constitutional factors predispose the patient to insomnia but are not sufficient to cause it. A precipitating factor (e.g., a change in work status) added to the constitutional factor causes the onset of insomnia. As the insomnia continues, perpetuating factors develop that maintain the insomnia even after the stress that precipitated the insomnia is reduced.

In sum, a complete evaluation and treatment plan for insomnia requires consideration of constitutional, precipitating, and perpetuating factors. A rational treatment plan is based on the relative weight of these factors, as well as their amenability to treatment in a given patient.

DIAGNOSTIC CLASSIFICATION

The International Classification of Sleep Disorders (ICSD)[51] distinguishes three main categories of sleep disorders: dyssomnias, which result in insomnia or excessive sleepiness; parasomnias, i.e., abnormal behaviors during sleep; and sleep disorders associated with medical or psychiatric disorders. Dyssomnias are subdivided into intrinsic sleep disorders, extrinsic sleep disorders, and circadian rhythm disorders. Each of these categories includes a number of disorders that may result in the complaint of insomnia.

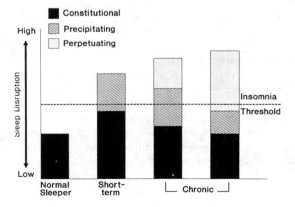

FIGURE 17-1.   *Conceptual factors contributing to insomnia. Accurate diagnosis and effective treatment require consideration of these three factors. (Adapted from Spielman AJ, Caruso LS, Glovinsky PB. A behavioral perspective on insomnia treatment. Psychiatr Clin North Am 1987;10:541–553.)*

The classification system itself is fully described in Chapter 15 of this text. This section describes the various disorders that are associated with insomnia.

It is again important to emphasize that chronic insomnia often results from multiple factors, as is clear from the conceptual issues just reviewed. The clinician cannot lose sight of this fact, despite the apparently conflicting emphasis on specific diagnosis in the forthcoming descriptions of various diagnostic entities. Multiple diagnoses are common, and treatment and management decisions often are also multifaceted. Diagnostic precision includes the need to prioritize diagnosis, and thus to implement treatments in their order of importance for each patient.

Intrinsic Sleep Disorders

Psychophysiological insomnia

In this common type of insomnia, patients demonstrate excessive worry about sleep, have cognitive and physiological overarousal at bedtime, and complain of impaired daytime functioning. For these patients, the bedroom, bedtime, and pre-sleep activities become increasingly associated with difficulty falling asleep rather than with the onset and maintenance of sleep.[36,52] In the terminology of classical conditioning theory, bedtime-related circumstances become conditioned stimuli that produce conditioned responses (e.g., hyperarousal) incompatible with sleep.

Psychophysiological insomnia often begins during an episode of situational stress, and becomes persistent as a result of performance anxiety and conditioning factors. Learned sleep-inhibiting associations may be formed after several nights of poor sleep, and they seem most likely to occur in persons with a constitutionally weak sleep-wake system. Patients often describe themselves as "light sleepers" who are sensitive to environmental disturbances. Many patients with psychophysiological insomnia have also learned to be overconcerned about sleep, leading to excessive efforts to fall asleep, which paradoxically increase arousal and inhibit sleep. Nights of poor sleep, of course, provide reinforcement of associations between sleep-related stimuli and anxiety about sleep, thus maintaining a cycle in which insomnia begets insomnia.[52]

Patients with psychophysiologic insomnia report long-term stability in their symptoms, but frequently fall asleep with less difficulty in environments other than their own bedroom (such as a hotel room or a sleep laboratory) or when engaged in activities other than trying to sleep (as while watching television). The latter observation suggests that these persons are not filling their sleep requirement. These patients also complain of daytime fatigue and difficulty functioning during the day[52] though they do not appear to be sleepier than noninsomniacs on standard measures of daytime sleep tendency.[19]

Overnight polysomnography (PSG) reveals objectively prolonged sleep latency, increased wakefulness after sleep onset, and elevated stage 1 sleep in persons with psychophysiologic insomnia. These objective findings distinguish psychophysiological insomnnia from sleep state misperception (see below).[51] Psychophysiological insomnia is not diagnosed if there is evidence of an underlying psychiatric or medical disorder, circadian rhythm disturbance, inadequate sleep hygiene, or extrinsic factors, even though somatized tension and learned associations can develop as contributing factors in these conditions.

Psychophysiological insomnia accounted for approximately 15% of the insomnia cases seen at sleep disorders centers in the late 1970s and early 1980s.[53] A larger percentage of the total population of insomniacs is suspected to have psychophysiologic insomnia, as a strong selection bias is present in sleep center patient populations for insomnias more directly associated with physical or psychiatric causes.

Treatment for psychophysiologic insomnia should typically include a combination of sleep hygiene instructions, behavioral techniques, and, in some instances, adjunctive use of hypnotic medication. Relaxation training, stimulus control therapy, and sleep restriction therapy are behavioral methods designed to alter the patient's response to the sleep environment; the latter two treatments may also increase sleep drive. Intermittent use of hypnotic medication may provide immediate relief for distressed patients, and in some cases may break the vicious cycle of performance anxiety or conditioning factors. Behavioral approaches and hypnotic therapy are discussed in greater detail later in this chapter.

Sleep state misperception

Some persons report insomnia that is not confirmed by objective recording of their sleep. In one study, PSG recording indicated an objective sleep latency of less than 15 minutes for 44% of insomniacs who reported habitual sleep latency of 60 minutes or more.[54] This discrepancy between subjective complaint and objective findings in some insomniacs may be caused by their misperception of electroencephalography (EEG)-defined sleep as wakefulness. When insomniacs and noninsomniacs were awakened from sleep after specific amounts of various EEG sleep stages, insomniacs were generally more likely than noninsomniacs to report having been awake immediately prior to the experimental awakenings.[55,56]

The cause of sleep state misperception is unknown. Persons with sleep state misperception have not been found to differ from good sleepers on measures of psychopathology[58] or in auditory awakening threshold.[56,59] One study has found that people with sleep state misperception have impaired daytime vigilance, compared to good sleepers and to other insomniacs (most of whom probably had psychophysiologic insomnia).[19] Some authors[60] have suggested that these patients may have a sleep abnormality that is not detected by current methods of recording and scoring sleep. It is interesting that sleep state misperception responds in a similar manner to behavioral treatments[61] and hypnotics[60] as insomnia with objective findings. Mendelson[62] suggested that hypnotics may decrease the likelihood that EEG-defined sleep is perceived as wakefulness.

The diagnosis of sleep state misperception requires a credible complaint of chronic insomnia, PSG evidence of normal sleep (in terms of latency, sleep duration, and the number or duration of arousals), and the patient's report of significantly disturbed sleep on the nights of PSG studies. In addition, sleep state misperception is not diagnosed for patients who have a psychiatric disorder or a sleep disorder (e.g., periodic leg movements in sleep) that could result in the perception of inadequate sleep. The ICSD[51] estimates that fewer than 5% of patients who present with insomnia have sleep state misperception. Trinder[63] has recently cast doubt on the validity of this diagnostic category. Trinder argues that, as insomnia is most often an intermittent condition, the laws of probability may account for most or all of patients with an insomnia complaint who sleep well during laboratory testing. However, in most cases there is a marked discrepancy between the length of EEG-defined sleep (e.g., 7 hours) and the immediate postsleep subjective estimate of sleep time (e.g., 2 hours), which strongly implies a disorder in the perception of sleep or an abnormality of sleep not detected by standard recording techniques.

Idiopathic insomnia

Patients with idiopathic insomnia have histories of difficulty sleeping since childhood, and in some cases, since birth. This classification, therefore, previously was labeled *childhood-onset insomnia*.[64] Assumed to be attributable primarily to constitutional factors that have not yet been determined, this type of insomnia probably results from various pathophysiologic mechanisms.[65] Theoretically, patients with this disorder may simply have weak neurophysiologic or neurochemical mechanisms of sleep. Alternatively, a lesion or defect in sleep-wake mechanisms might be involved.

Compared to patients with other forms of insomnia, patients with idiopathic insomnia tend to have more severe objective sleep disturbance, with longer latency to sleep onset and less sleep time.[64] Some patients with idiopathic insomnia have marked abnormalities in PSG-recorded sleep, such as very short sleep time, low sleep efficiency, or poor definition of sleep stages. Eye movements during REM have been reported to be less frequent in patients with idiopathic insomnia than in other insomniacs, suggesting that some idiopathic insomniacs may have neurochemical or anatomic defects in brainstem regions that control eye movements and regulate sleep and wakefulness.[64] In addition, patients with idiopathic insomnia may show "soft" neurological signs, such as attention and concentration difficulties, dyslexia, and mild diffuse electroencephalographic abnormalities.[64] The constellation of signs and symptoms tends to vary substantially among patients with idiopathic insomnia, which lends support to the idea that this classification encompasses a number of different pathophysiological processes.

The long-standing sleep disturbance that characterizes idiopathic insomnia usually leads to complicating factors such as poor sleep hygiene or learned sleep-inhibiting associations; however, the onset of the insomnia clearly predates these factors. Insomnia in these patients cannot be linked with any known medical, psychiatric, or circadian rhythm disorder, and is not dramatically affected by the degree of psychological stress. This disorder appears to be quite rare; idiopthic insomnia was diagnosed in only 0.3% of 1214 insomnia cases in a sleep center case series study.[66] Effective treatment for patients with idiopathic insomnia is not well-established; usually, a series of empirical trials with a variety of different medications (tried in various doses) is necessary before an appropriate drug regimen is found for a particular patient.[67,68]

Sleep apnea syndromes and sleep-related breathing disorders

Insomnia caused by disordered breathing during sleep is most likely in elderly persons.[69,70] The most common disorder of this type, obstructive sleep apnea (OSA), usually is associated with a history of loud snoring and daytime sleepiness.[71] However, a minority of patients with OSA complain predominantly about disturbed sleep, especially sleep maintenance difficulties. These patients report frequent awakenings that are most often unexplained, but sometimes may be associated with dyspnea, choking, or a snorting sensation.[71]

Central sleep apnea may present with a complaint of sleep onset or maintenance insomnia.[72] Often the patient is unaware of a ventilatory disorder during sleep. Central apnea may occur in an idiopathic form or may be associated with neurological lesions or cardiovascular disorders such as congestive heart failure.[73]

Treatment of obstructive sleep apnea requires elimination of the upper airway obstruction that occurs during sleep, as by surgery or use of nasal continuous positive airway pressure (CPAP).[71] Central sleep apnea may also sometimes respond to treatment with nasal CPAP, or it may require other therapeutic modalities such as supplemental oxygen or respiratory stimulants.[73] Further details regarding the diagnosis and treatment of sleep apnea syndromes may be found in Chapter 16.

Sleep-related breathing can also be disturbed by cardiac, pulmonary, or neurologic disorders. Congestive heart failure can result in either paroxysmal nocturnal dyspnea or periodic breathing in a pattern of Cheyne-Stokes respiration, both resulting in sleep maintenance insomnia. Chronic pulmonary disease can also lead to insomnia, due to repeated awakenings triggered by hypoxia, hypercapnia, airway resistance changes, or airway irritation and cough. Hypoxemia and alveolar hypoventilation are usually most severe during REM sleep. Patients with chronic pulmonary disease may benefit from treatment with supplemental oxygen to correct sleep-related hypoxemia. Patients with neuromuscular disorders that cause sleep-related hypoxemia and alveolar hypoventilation may also complain of disturbed or disrupted sleep. These patients may require assisted nocturnal ventilation. Further details regarding sleep and breathing in medical and neurologic disorders may be found in Chapters 20 and 22.

The identification of sleep-related breathing disorders in patients who complain of insomnia is important, as treatment with hypnotic medication may blunt arousal responses to respiratory stimuli and potentially worsen ventilation during sleep.[74] This is especially a concern in the elderly population, as patients in this group frequently complain of sleep maintenance difficulties and have a high incidence of sleep-related breathing disorders.

Periodic limb movements of sleep disorder
(See also Chapter 19.)

Patients with periodic limb movements of sleep (PLMS) disorder have episodes of repetitive and stereotyped PLMs during sleep that often result in brief awakenings. Typically, PLMs consist of extensions of the big toe and dorsiflexions of the ankle, sometimes with flexions of the knee and hip. Each movement lasts 0.5 to 5.0 seconds and is usually followed by another limb movement in 20 to 40 seconds.[75] The movements can also occur in the upper limbs, but this is much less common.[76] The etiology of Periodic

Limb Movement Disorder (PLMD) is unknown, but a number of causal factors have been postulated, including chronic sleep-wake disturbance,[77] loss of supraspinal inhibition of the pyramidal tracts during sleep,[78] inadequate peripheral blood perfusion,[79] compression of the lumbosacral spinal canal,[80] abnormalities in the endogenous opiate system,[81] and alterations in central dopaminergic transmission.[75]

A diagnosis of PLMD requires a complaint of insomnia (or excessive daytime sleepiness) and evidence of frequent repetitive PLMs, usually five or more per hour. As most patients with PLMS are unaware of the limb movements, a diagnosis usually requires PSG recording that includes surface electrodes on the legs.[87] The number of PLMs can vary from night to night. Many asymptomatic persons have PLMs, but the diagnosis of PLMD is not usually applied to persons who do not have a sleep-related complaint.

PLMD was the primary diagnosis for 13.3% of insomnia patients who presented at sleep disorders centers,[85] but the prevalence of PLMD in the general population is unknown. PLMs are very common in elderly persons[70] and also appear to be associated with a number of other sleep disorders. PLMs occur in almost all patients with restless legs syndrome (RLS), which appears to be a more serious variant of PLMD.[75] Patients with narcolepsy[86] and, possibly, sleep apnea[77] also have a high prevalence of PLMs. Lastly, PLMs may occur during periods of sedative-hypnotic withdrawal or treatment with tricyclic or nontricyclic antidepressants.[51]

A variety of treatments have been used for PLMD. Clonazepam and other benzodiazepines have been found to reduce arousals associated with the limb movements, though not the frequency of limb movements themselves.[88] Small doses of opioids have been found to be effective for PLMs, but concern over their abuse potential may limit their usefulness.[81] Recent studies have found that L-dopa together with a peripheral decarboxylase inhibitor significantly reduced PLMs.[89,90] Montplaisir and Godbout[75] recommend that benzodiazepines be used in milder cases of PLMS and L-dopa for more severe cases or when benzodiazepines may be contraindicated, as for persons likely to have disordered breathing during sleep.

Restless legs syndrome (See also Chapter 19)

Patients with RLS complain of an unpleasant paresthesia or dysesthesia in their legs when they are awake but inactive. This sensation is often described as a creeping or crawling sensation in the legs associated with an irresistible urge to move them. Temporary relief is obtained from voluntary leg movements, but the complaints return with the inactivity necessary for sleep onset.[91] Almost all patients with RLS also have PLMS. In addition, irregular leg movements are observed during wakefulness while the patient is at rest.[92] Sleep onset is typically delayed owing to the combination of subjective symptoms and leg movement.

RLS is thought to be much less common than PLMS, but the pathophysiologic mechanisms of the respective conditions are believed to be related.[75] A positive family history of RLS is often reported, and genetic studies have indicated autosomal dominant inheritance with incomplete penetrance.[93,94] Conditions that have been associated with RLS include pregnancy, iron deficiency anemia, folate deficiency, uremia, peripheral neuropathy, and various other disorders.[75,92]

Treatment for RLS is similar to that for PLMD. A combination of L-dopa and a peripheral decarboxylase inhibitor[75,92,95] has been found to be very effective. When resistance to L-dopa develops, use of a dopaminergic agonist such as bromocriptine[96] may be effective. Narcotics, such as oxycodone[81] have also proven very effective but carry the risk of dependency. Clinical studies have also shown benefit from clonazepam and carbamezepine.[75,92] Owing to the excellent response, L-dopa may be considered the drug of choice for RLS; benzodiazepines such as clonazepam may be effective for milder cases. If resistance develops to L-dopa, a dopaminergic agonist may be considered. For severe cases that are unresponsive to these measures, opioids may be indicated.[75]

Extrinsic Sleep Disorders

Inadequate sleep hygiene

Insomnia may be precipitated or perpetuated by behavior that is inconsistent with good sleep. Adhering to an irregular sleep-wake schedule (especially staying up later than usual and sleeping-in the next morning) is a common behavior that leads to insomnia. Other behaviors that disturb sleep include daytime napping; excessive time in bed; excessive use of caffeine, alcohol, or nicotine; vigorous exercise or mental activity near bedtime; habitual use of the bedroom for waking activities; and inadequate maintenance of a comfortable sleep environment (with respect to temperature, light, noise). Almost all patients with insomnia can benefit from a discussion of how to develop good sleep hygiene, and for some patients such instructions are curative. The diagnosis of inadequate sleep hygiene applies when one or more behaviors incompatible with sleep are the predominant cause of insomnia.[51] (See Table 17-3 for sleep hygiene instuctions.)

TABLE 17-3.　Sleep Hygiene Recommendations

1. Maintain a regular bedtime and awakening time. For most people, nightly time in bed should be no longer than 8 hours, since excessive time in bed may fragment sleep. Get out of bed at the regular time even if sleep was poor, as "sleeping-in" can disturb sleep the following night.
2. Do not nap during the day, as this results in poorer sleep at night. (However, persons who appear unable to obtain adequate sleep at night [e.g., elderly or shift workers] may benefit from regularly scheduled naps in the afternoon.)
3. Do not drink alcoholic beverages in the evening, as this disturbs sleep at night.
4. Avoid caffeinated beverages after noontime, as caffeine disturbs sleep. Limit total caffeine consumption to no more than two beverages per day.
5. Do not smoke just before bedtime or during the night, as this disturbs sleep.
6. Exercise regularly during the day, but avoid exercise in the evening within 3 hours of bedtime.
7. Do not use the bed or bedroom for anything other than sleep and sexual activity. If the bedroom is used for nonsleep activities (such as balancing the checkbook or watching television) it may become a stimulus for alertness, rather than for sleep.
8. Establish a relaxing routine in preparation for sleep. Engaging in frustrating activities or excessive worry close to bedtime may result in arousal and prevent sleep.
9. Maintain a comfortable temperature in the bedroom.
10. Keep the bedroom dark and quiet. Try to screen out any disturbing noise or light.

Drug- or alcohol dependency sleep disorders

This section describes insomnia due to dependency on hypnotics, stimulants, or alcohol. Insomnia associated with drug or alcohol dependence accounted for approximately 10% of insomnia cases at sleep disorders centers from 1978 to 1982,[53] but the prevalence of these types of insomnia in the general population is unknown. It should be noted that insomnia may be an adverse side effect of a variety of medications other than hypnotics and stimulants. Commonly prescribed medications that may produce insomnia as a side effect include beta blockers (such as propranolol), anticonvulsants (such as phenytoin), xanthines (such as theophylline), L-dopa, α-methyldopa, reserpine, clonidine, sympathomimetic agents (such as pseudoephedrine), and corticosteroids.[97]

Hypnotic dependency insomnia

Since the late 1970s, insomnia has been treated predominantly with drugs from the benzodiazepine class.[62] Before benzodiazepines, insomnia had been treated primarily with barbiturates and other rapidly addicting hypnotics. These agents were far more likely to result in tolerance and produce dependency. Nevertheless, with daily use, tolerance may be reported to the hypnotic effects of benzodiazepines, though pharmacological tolerance has not been demonstrated in sleep laboratory studies of a few weeks' duration.[98,99] The return of insomnia symptoms may prompt dose escalation in a small number of patients, but this appears to be quite rare.[13] Upon withdrawal from benzodiazepines, certain patients may experience a night or two of rebound insomnia, i.e., insomnia more severe than that before drug treatment began. It is theorized that some patients become dependent on hypnotics while attempting to avoid rebound insomnia.[100,101] The risk of rebound insomnia during drug withdrawal appears to be greater with large doses and with short-acting hypnotics, and it can be reduced by tapering the dose over a few nights rather than abruptly discontinuing the drug.

Hypnotic dependency insomnia is diagnosed in patients who have used a hypnotic on a daily (or almost daily) basis for at least 3 weeks and who experience serious exacerbation of insomnia when they attempt to withdraw from the hypnotic drug.[51] Patients with hypnotic dependency insomnia may also experience daytime symptoms of hypnotic withdrawal, such as increased anxiety, muscle tension, nausea, and aches. Hypnotic-dependency insomnia is not diagnosed if other medical or psychiatric disorders can account for the insomnia. Often, insomnia persists beyond the period of withdrawal from hypnotics, and the causal factors that led to drug use then need to be determined.

Stimulant dependency insomnia

A large variety of substances are central nervous system stimulants, including caffeine, theophylline, nicotine, sympathomimetic drugs, amphetamine, methylphenidate, pemoline, and cocaine. Medical uses of stimulants include appetite suppression, treatment of attention deficit disorder, and decongestion and bronchodilation. The effects of stimulants on sleep include increased sleep latency, reduced sleep time, increased number of awakenings during sleep, and alterations in sleep stages, particularly decreased REM sleep time.[102] The diagnosis of stimulant dependency insomnia depends on determining a temporal association between insomnia symptoms and the use of a stimulant. In addition, withdrawal from the stimulant may be associated with symptoms of excessive sleepiness. Abuse of stimulants may also cause psychiatric symptoms, such as periods of hypomania, paranoid ideation, and hallucinations.

Alcohol dependency insomnia

Many people drink alcoholic beverages at least occasionally to promote sleep.[5,8] Alcohol ingestion near bedtime decreases sleep latency but increases awakenings later in the night. Presleep alcohol also causes decreased REM sleep and increased delta sleep early in the night, and increased REM sleep later in the night.[102] The chronic use of alcohol as a hypnotic rapidly leads to tolerance to its sleep-inducing effects. Furthermore, when alcohol consumption is reduced or eliminated, withdrawal effects include fragmented sleep and awakenings with vivid dream recall, headache, and dry mouth. Severe sleeplessness may occur if a chronic user of presleep alcohol suddenly stops drinking it.

The diagnosis of alcohol dependency insomnia applies to persons with a sleep complaint who have consumed alcohol prior to sleep on nearly a nightly basis for at least the past month.[51] When they are drinking, patients usually awaken frequently from sleep, and they suffer severe exacerbation of insomnia if they discontinue alcohol. Alcohol dependency insomnia is not diagnosed if the patient meets standard criteria for alcoholism.

Adjustment sleep disorder

Adjustment sleep disorder refers to a complaint of insomnia that is temporally associated with an acute stress, conflict, or environmental change that causes emotional distress and arousal. The insomnia must develop in association with the stressor and resolve if either the stressor abates or the person's level of adaptation improves. Most people experience a one- or two-night episode of adjustment sleep disorder many times in their lives. Others have several episodes per year, each lasing a few days to a few weeks. These persons may be conceptualized as being close to their insomnia threshold owing to constitutional factors and to require little in the way of precipitating factors to disturb sleep. In this pattern, adjustment sleep disorder is a persistent, intermittent condition.

Other extrinsic sleep disorders

Many other external factors may lead to insomnia in addition to inadequate sleep hygiene, drug or alcohol dependency, and stress of adjustment.

Environmental sleep disorder refers to a complaint of insomnia that is temporally linked to a physical stimulus or environmental circumstance that disturbs sleep. Removal of the environmental condition results in a reduction in insomnia and eventual restoration of normal sleep. A variety of environmental conditions may cause insomnia, including noise, light, and uncomfortable temperatures as well as hospitalization, activity of the bed partner, responsibility for a newborn infant or invalid, and a situation that is perceived as potentially dangerous.

Altitude insomnia is an acute condition that occurs in association with ascent to high altitude (usually above 4000 m). The insomnia may be associated with other symptoms occurring at high altitudes, such as headache, nausea, tachycardia, and fatigue. This condition is caused by periodic breathing during sleep, which results from instability in the control of respiration owing to hypoxemia and hypocapnia at high altitude. Arousals occur during the hyperpneic phase of ventilation. Altitude insomnia can be effectively treated with acetazolamide.[103]

Sleeplessness in children may be associated with a number of disorders, including limit-setting sleep disorder, sleep-onset association disorder, food allergy insomnia, and nocturnal eating (drinking) syndrome.[51] Further details of sleep disorders in childhood may be found in Chapter 26.

Circadian Rhythm Sleep Disorders

Insomnia may be a symptom of several circadian rhythm disturbances, including time zone change (jet lag), shift work, irregular sleep-wake pattern, delayed sleep phase syndrome (DSPS), advanced sleep phase syndrome (ASPS), and non–24-hour sleep-wake disorder.[51] In this section, ASPS and DSPS are briefly reviewed, as they are important diagnostic considerations in patients with chronic insomnia. Further details of circadian rhythm physiology and sleep disorders may be found in Chapter 23.

Patients with DSPS report difficulty falling asleep and awakening at desired times.[104] These difficulties occur because the sleep phase of the endogenous sleep-wake rhythm begins hours after the desired bedtime and ends hours after the desired time for awakening. When patients delay bedtime by several hours and sleep until they awaken spontaneously, sleep is essentially normal. This syndrome is more common in adolescents and young adults. Bright light therapy in the morning[105] and chronotherapy[106] have been reported to be effective treatments for this disorder.

Patients with ASPS complain of difficulty staying awake in the later evening and inability to sleep past the early morning hours. In contrast to the DSPS, the circadian sleep phase occurs too early with respect to desired hours for sleep. It is important to distinguish the early morning awakenings of ASPS from those caused by depression, in which awakening usually occurs 3 to 5 hours after sleep onset, regardless of bedtime. ASPS is thought to be a rare disorder though more common in elderly persons. Bright light therapy[107] in the evening may help delay the sleep phase of the circadian rhythm. Reverse chronotherapy has also been proposed for treatment of ASPS,[108] however, neither treatment has been validated experimentally.

Insomnia Associated with Medical and Psychiatric Disorders

Insomnia may be a symptom of many diverse medical and psychiatric disorders.[97,109] When insomnia is a symptom of medical illness, it frequently is caused by nonspecific factors such as pain or breathing difficulties. Nonspecific factors may also play a role when insomnia is associated with neurological disorders, but here the possibility of abnormal or lesioned central nervous system sleep-wake mechanisms should be considered.

Insomnia associated with psychiatric disorders is common, occurring in approximately one-third of insomnia patients seen at sleep disorders centers.[53] This type of insomnia may reflect altered sleep mechanisms caused by the same pathophysiological processes that underlie the psychiatric illness.[37,38] Endogenous depression is the prototypical psychiatric disorder that is associated with insomnia. A classical symptom of depression is early morning awakening, but patients often report sleep onset and maintenance problems as well. PSG shows prolonged sleep latency, frequent awakenings with poor sleep efficiency, reduced delta sleep, and shortened REM latency.[37,110] REM time and phasic REM activity during the first half of the night are often increased.[37]

Insomnia associated with medical or psychiatric disorders is diagnosed when the sleep disturbance is temporally associated with a medical, neurologic, or psychiatric illness. Both improvement and worsening of insomnia are expected to follow a time course similar to that of the underlying illness. Psychiatric disorders are diagnosed when symptoms meet criteria as described in the Diagnostic and Statistical Manual of Mental Disorders, 3rd edition, revised.[111] Other possible causes of the insomnia, including PLMD, sleep apnea, circadian disorders, and drug or alcohol use, must be ruled out or judged to be subordinate to the medical or psychiatric disorder as a factor in the insomnia. The main focus of treatment is the medical or psychiatric disorder, but adjunctive pharmacological or behavioral treatment for insomnia may also be helpful in certain cases. Treatment with sedating tricyclic antidepressants, giving the major dose at bedtime, may be particularly effective for insomnia associated with depression.[112] Further information concerning sleep in medical and neurologic disorders may be found in Chapters 20 and 22 and regarding insomnia in psychiatric disorders may be found in Chapter 21.

EVALUATION

Insomnia, the most common of all sleep-related complaints, is associated with a wide variety of conditions; therefore, accurate diagnosis is critical before specific therapy can be offered. It is important for the clinician to dismiss the stereotype that all or nearly all insomnia complaints are psychogenic. One feature common to many insomniacs that has fostered this stereotype is the report of rumination prior to sleep onset or during awakenings at night. Such a history is considered evidence that psychological stress or worry, is the cause of the patient's sleep disturbance. Rumination, however, commonly occurs in sedentary situations (e.g., waiting for an appointment) when the human mind is not engaged in an ongoing activity; thus rumination may be a result of insomnia rather than its cause.

History and Physical Examination

The most important element in the evaluation of insomnia is the clinical history. If a medical or psychiatric condition is suspected as a major etiologic factor for the sleep complaint, initial treatment should be directed at this underlying condition. In some instances, ongoing treatment may need to be enhanced even if most symptoms associated with the disorder are controlled during wakefulness. For example, certain asthma patients experience asthma attacks during sleep though daytime attacks are effectively treated by antiasthma drugs.

Though the exact reason for these sleep-related asthma episodes is not clear, possible explanations include the normal increase in airway resistance during sleep; autonomic nervous system changes, particularly in REM; and the patient's inability to self-medicate as quickly during sleep. Regardless of the cause, adjustment of dose, timing, or type of antiasthma medication may be adequate to prevent nocturnal awakening.

Iatrogenic insomnia also deserves consideration, as many pharmacologic agents are known to disturb sleep. If the onset of an insomnia complaint appears to be temporally synchronous with initiation of pharmacotherapy (or a change in dose or timing) adjustment of medication, dose, or administration schedule may reduce insomnia. Table 17-4 contains a list of medications that commonly contribute to sleep disturbance.

The following decision tree analysis[113] is recommended for evaluation of insomnia in the primary care setting, based on the responses to four basic questions (Figure 17-2). We assume in this discussion that any medical or psychiatric disorders have been adequately assessed and optimally treated. This assumption is critical, as insomnia may result from a

TABLE 17-4. Medications That Commonly Cause Insomnia

β-Blockers
Corticosteroids
Bronchodilators (e.g., metaproterenol)
Respiratory stimulants (e.g., theophylline)
Stimulating antidepressants
   (e.g., protriptyline, fluoxetine, buproprion)
Methyldopa
Thyroid supplements
Central nervous system stimulants
Decongestants
Phenytoin

variety of such conditions. The four basic questions relate to the duration, stability, timing, and consequences of the insomnia. The answers to these four

questions narrow the diagnostic possibilities, and logically lead to decisions about assessment and treatment options.

The duration of the insomnia has specific diagnostic implications and often suggests the initial therapeutic approach. The definitions of transient, short-term, and persistent insomnia are discussed in the introduction to this chapter, along with common diagnostic considerations (see also Figure 17-2).

The stability of the insomnia from night to night may indicate the underlying cause. When associated with medical or psychiatric disorders, the severity of insomnia may fluctuate over weeks to months, usually in tandem with the course of the underlying illness. Many patients with frequent, intermittent episodes of insomnia have an adjustment sleep disorder, displaying sleep difficulty at times of stress, medical illness, or excitement. In contrast, patients

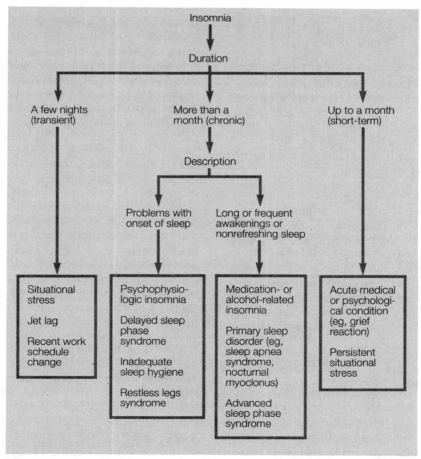

FIGURE 17-2. *A flow diagram illustrates a diagnostic approach to insomnia after exclusion of medical and psychiatric causes. (Published with permission from Walsh JK, Mahowald MW. Avoiding the blanket approach to insomnia. Postgrad Med 1991; 90:211–224.)*

with psychophysiological insomnia report long-term stability, except that some may sleep better in unaccustomed sleep environments. Relative stability is also a characteristic of delayed or advanced sleep phase syndrone, RLS, and sleep apnea syndromes.

The timing of the sleep disturbance provides important information for the differential diagnosis of persistent insomnia. Patients who complain principally about difficulty falling asleep often suffer from psychophysiologic insomnia, delayed sleep phase syndrome, inadequate sleep hygiene, or RLS. Patients who complain primarily about sleep maintenance difficulty or nonrefreshing sleep may suffer from sleep apnea, PLMS, drug- or alcohol-related sleep disorder, or advanced sleep phase syndrome. Early morning awakening raises the possibility of depression.

The consequences of the insomnia are manifested in the patient's daytime functioning. A distinction should be made between excessive daytime sleepiness (EDS) and daytime fatigue or tiredness. Complaints of fatigue, tiredness, lack of energy, irritability, reduced work performance, and difficulty with concentration are common in insomniacs, but symptoms of true EDS are much less so. When present, EDS usually indicates fragmented sleep, like that seen in sleep apnea or PLMS, or chronic insufficient sleep, as may occur with a circadian or schedule disturbance.

Other factors that may affect the onset and progression of the sleep disturbance should also be assessed, including medical and psychiatric disorders, psychosocial stressors, medication and drug use, and sleep hygiene factors.

As an adjunct to the patient's history, an interview with the bed partner should be performed whenever possible. A significant proportion of insomniacs have an inaccurate perception of their sleep, and the bed partner may be able to provide a more objective assessment of the problem. The bed partner may also provide information about symptoms that the patient typically is unaware of, such as snoring, apnea, or limb movements during sleep.

Lastly, a sleep diary often provides useful information, both for the patient and the physician. A 2-week diary gives an overview of the pattern of sleep and affords a baseline against which change with treatment can be measured. Patients often gain insight into their problem from the diary, such as an awareness of a relationship between daytime events and nights of disturbed sleep, or a realization that they have been focusing exclusively on their worst nights. The following minimal information should be obtained for each day of a 2-week period:

Bedtime and awakening time
Estimate of time to fall asleep

Number and duration of awakenings during night
Estimate of total time asleep
Medication, caffeine, and alcohol use
Subjective measure of daytime functioning and symptoms
Number and time of naps

The majority of insomniacs have unremarkable physical examinations. Nevertheless, neurological, endocrine, cardiac, and pulmonary disorders must be considered. Clinical laboratory assessment should be performed if indicated (e.g., screening for anemia, uremia and polyneuropathy, if symptoms of RLS are present). Similarly, psychiatric disorders must be carefully considered, and psychometric testing is often useful.

The Role of the Sleep Medicine Specialist

Referral to a sleep medicine specialist should be considered for patients with persistent insomnia that has been resistant to treatment and whenever a primary sleep disorder—periodic limb movements, RLS, sleep apnea, circadian rhythm disorder—is suspected. In most instances, referral initiates a consultation visit during which the consulting specialist determines the most appropriate diagnostic and treatment approach. Once again, the clinical sleep history is paramount and determines the need for completion of a sleep diary, psychological evaluation, medical assessment, PSG, or other diagnostic procedures. Alternatively, the clinical presentation of some cases directly suggests a treatment trial, the results of which may confirm or refute a preliminary diagnosis.

Many patients with insomnia probably do not need to undergo sleep laboratory testing, though there is uncertainty about the indications for PSG in the evaluation of insomnia.[114] A conservative approach would be to consider PSG for patients with a persistent, primarily sleep maintenance problem, especially if there are symptoms or risk factors for sleep apnea or PLMS. In general, PSG is more likely to produce clinically useful information on middle-aged and older adults,[115] at least in part because primary sleep disorders are more common in this age group.[70] The presence of symptoms of EDS should also be considered an indication for PSG.

TREATMENT

Treatment efficacy for insomnia is determined by improvement in sleep and in daytime functioning. When possible, treatment for insomnia should be directed toward reversing its underlying cause, which again indicates the importance of accurate diagnosis. Treatment strategies also vary depending on the duration of the insomnia (see Figure 17-2). The major distinction to be made is that between transient or short-term insomnia and persistent insomnia.

Treatment of Transient and Short-Term Insomnias

These temporary sleep disturbances are usually associated with acute situational stress or a sudden change in the sleep-wake schedule, and by definition they resolve spontaneously in less than a month. Thus, they may not warrant treatment, and unless episodes become recurrent treatment is not likely to be sought. Nevertheless, if significant psychic distress or daytime impairment occurs, treatment may be necessary.

Treatment for transient insomnia may be requested when the sleep disturbance recurs in a predictable fashion. Hypnotic medication appears to be the most effective and rational therapy unless it is contraindicated (see below). Patients typically require no more than a few nights' treatment, as the insomnia resolves spontaneously within a few days. Using the smallest effective dose of a rapidly eliminated benzodiazepine is recommended. In most patients, use as needed may be recommended when a consistent trigger for the insomnia is identified (e.g., jet lag, anxiety related to business meetings).

Short-term insomnia may be treated with hypnotic medication, as outlined above for transient insomnia, or a behavioral approach may be attempted. Instructions in sleep hygiene (see Table 17-3) or stimulus control therapy (discussed later) are simple behavioral approaches that may be considered. Treatment with benzodiazepine hypnotics usually provides more rapid relief than behavioral therapy. Patients should be instructed that hypnotic medication will be used as a short-term (no longer than a few weeks) treatment while the situation causing the insomnia runs its course. If the insomnia persists following a trial of pharmacotherapy or behavioral therapy, the causal factors should be reassessed in the context of persistent insomnia.

Treatment of Persistent Insomnia

Effective treatment of persistent insomnia depends on the precision of the diagnostic process. As outlined in the section on diagnostic classification, once a diagnosis is made specific therapy aimed at reversing the underlying cause of the insomnia may be offered. Specific therapy for each disorder is reviewed under the appropriate diagnostic sections.

In the remainder of this chapter therapies available for treating psychophysiologic insomnia, insomnia that has a large psychophysiologic component, and adjustment sleep disorders characterized by frequent, intermittent episodes of insomnia are discussed.

Behavioral Treatment

Most patients with persistent insomnia benefit from instruction in sleep hygiene. These instructions, which encourage habits that lead to better sleep, should be offered to nearly all patients. A number of other behavioral approaches have been developed,[44] two of which, stimulus control therapy[116] and sleep restriction therapy,[117] are reveiwed here. Both methods are directed at reversing the learned associations and negative conditioning factors that develop in persistent insomnia.

Stimulus control therapy is a technique aimed at promoting the association of the bedroom environment with sleep instead of wakefulness. The essential instructions to prevent sleep-inhibiting learned associations include going to bed only when sleepy and getting out of bed if sleep has not occurred within 10 to 20 minutes, both at the beginning of the night and during middle of the night awakenings. Patients are instructed to leave the bedroom and engage in a mundane, nonreinforcing activity and to return to bed only when they feel sleepy. This procedure is repeated throughout the night as often as necessary until the patient is able to fall asleep quickly upon going to bed. Morning wake-up time remains constant, regardless of the amount of sleep that has occurred. A more thorough review of stimulus control can be found in a chapter by Bootzin and coworkers.[116]

Sleep restriction therapy is a technique that limits time in bed, creating a degree of sleep deprivation. This technique, described fully by Spielman and coworkers,[117] is based on the assumption that partial sleep deprivation results in deeper, more continuous sleep, which helps reverse negative conditioning factors that perpetuate the insomnia and is somewhat more restorative. After a period of data gathering (collected in a sleep diary) insomniacs are instructed to limit their time in bed to the average amount of sleep they subjectively estimate they obtain each night, though not less than 5 hours. Sleep efficiency (SE) (total time asleep/total time in bed) is subjectively estimated each night. When SE rises above 90%, the time in bed is slowly increased, usually in 15- to 30-minute increments. This is repeated every time SE remains above 90% for several consecutive nights. EDS may occur when time in bed is significantly limited and is a potential disadvantage of this therapy.

Other behavioral techniques that may be effective treatment for persistent insomnia include several methods of relaxation training.[44,97] These techniques attempt to reduce the tension-anxiety component of insomnia. Methods include biofeedback, meditation and deep breathing exercises, guided imagery, and progressive muscle relaxation. Psychological therapies have also been described, including insight-oriented psychotherapy, cognitive therapy, and paradoxical intention.[97] An excellent text on the various treatment methods for chronic insomnia was recently published.[118]

Pharmacologic Treatment

Most investigators and clinicians agree that hypnotic medication should not be the sole form of treatment for the vast majority of chronic insomnia patients.[119] There are uncommon insomnia conditions, however, for which long-term hypnotic therapy provides significant relief (e.g., idiopathic insomnia, restless legs syndrome) and for which few, if any, alternatives are available.[67,75] For most chronic insomniacs, however, hypnotic medications play an adjunctive therapeutic role and specific treatment of the underlying etiologic factors is the primary therapeutic strategy. Persons with a history that suggests conditioning factor or performance anxiety is instrumental in their insomnia may derive benefit from a brief course of hypnotics, which may break the reinforcing cycle of nightly insomnia, thus reducing important perpetuating factors.

Hypnotic medication is most appropriate for chronic intermittent insomnia that has not responded to sleep hygiene or behavioral strategies. This type of insomnia most often takes the form of an adjustment sleep disorder; i.e., a susceptible person (due to constitutional factors) experiences insomnia at times of stress or excitement (precipitating factors). There is evidence that the majority of persons with persistent insomnia have such an intermittent pattern.[5] For them, use of a hypnotic for a few nights to a few weeks seems very helpful. Further, there is evidence that the majority of hypnotic users take medications periodically rather than nightly for months or years.[3]

Still, even when hypnotic medication would seem to be indicated, there is a global reluctance among physicians to prescribe sleeping pills. To some degree, patients also seem reluctant to submit to pharmacotherapy for insomnia. It is likely that these behaviors are the result of the perceptions that (1) the benefits of hypnotics do not outweigh the risks and (2) insomnia is a relatively benign complaint that has little associated morbidity. Recent studies suggest that both of these are misperceptions. Earlier, we reviewed accumulating evidence that the correlates and consequences of insomnia are far from trivial. Extensive epidemiological data collected by

Balter and Uhlenhuth[120] indicate that treating insomnia with prescription hypnotics as compared to no treatment or over-the-counter products, was reported to decrease many of the nighttime and daytime symptoms of insomniacs. Further, they find prescription hypnotics are associated with only infrequent adverse effects. Finally, though risk of dependency on benzodiazepines has been emphasized by some,[121] evidence has accumulated to suggest that the risk has been overstated and is less a property of the drug class than a reflection of user characteristics. For example, in controlled studies, users do not escalate drug doses on their own, and subjects escalate the dose of placebo as readily as that of active drug.[122,123] Further, of all hypnotic users, only 10% take the drugs nightly for more than a month. Thus, two signs of dependency behavior, dose escalation and frequency of use, are not common to most benzodiazepine hypnotic users. This suggests that risk of dependency is more closely related to the individual characteristics of the patient than to the medication itself.

Once the decision has been made to use a hypnotic for symptomatic treatment, typically a benzodiazepine is prescribed. Benzodiazepines have a very favorable therapeutic index and interact only with other central nervous system depressants. The selection of the specific drug should be based on the pharmacokinetic properties of the various available compounds and their relation to desired clinical effects. For example, rapidity of sleep onset is determined primarily by the drug's rate of absorption, assuming dose is held constant. Duration of hypnotic action (again holding dose constant) is determined by distribution and elimination properties, though the degree of distribution becomes much less important with drugs that accumulate with repeated dosing.

Some general recommendations and precautions apply, regardless of what hypnotic is used. First, therapy should be instituted with a small dose and maintained at the smallest effective dose. Second, the patient must follow instructions to take the medication (1) 30 minutes before bedtime, (2) only on the nights instructed, and (3) only at the recommended dose. Finally, whenever possible, combining multiple benzodiazepines for hypnotic or anxiolytic purposes should be avoided. If anxiolytic treatment is needed in addition to a hypnotic, a long-acting drug at bedtime or multiple doses of a single compound should be used. This makes assessment of efficacy much simpler.

Before hypnotic medication is prescribed, contraindications should be ruled out. These include a history of loud snoring or known sleep apnea, pregnancy, situations that require alertness upon awakening during the night, and a history of substance abuse. Special precautions apply in other situations, as with elderly patients or those with liver disease, because drug metabolism is prolonged. Usually, lowering the prescribed dosage is adequate to prevent problems of toxicity.[124] Caution is also needed in patients who have severe pulmonary disease, which may be worsened by sedation, and in some psychiatric patients, particularly those who are psychotic.

Rebound insomnia may develop when hypnotic medication is withdrawn abruptly.[100,101] This is most likely with larger dosages, and perhaps with prolonged nightly use of short-acting agents. Withdrawal effects can generally be avoided by using small doses and gradually tapering the dose when the drug is discontinued.[125]

Five benzodiazepines are now approved for use as sedative-hypnotics in the United States. Important features of these medications are mentioned briefly. More thorough discussions of the pharmacologic treatment of insomnia are published elsewhere.[126]

Flurazepam (Dalmane) was the first benzodiazepine marketed for insomnia. Although it is generally effective for initiating and maintaining sleep, it has substantial daytime carryover effects,[127] owing to the slow elimination of its major active metabolite (half-life 40 to 90 hours). If given in small doses there may also be a delay of one night in its efficacy for sleep-onset problems, until an effective plasma concentration is reached.

Temazepam (Restoril) is absorbed less rapidly than other benzodiazepines in its hard capsule formulation. The average time to peak plasma concentration may be more than 2 hours, making it less effective for sleep-onset insomnia, particularly in smaller doses. There appears to be little tendency to accumulate, since the elimination half-life ranges from 10 to 15 hours.[128] Thus, residual sedation is not common, but it increases with the dose. Rebound insomnia may occur after abrupt discontinuation of large doses of temazepam.

Triazolam (Halcion) is the most widely prescribed hypnotic. Its rapid elimination (half-life 2 to 4 hours) and rapid absorption are ideal for treatment of sleep-onset insomnia with avoidance of residual sedation. Rebound insomnia following discontinuation of treatment has been reported more frequently with triazolam, than with other benzodiazepine hypnotics primarily when recommended doses are exceeded.[100,101] There have also been reports of memory loss associated with its use,[129] and objective evidence of memory impairment has been documented in controlled clinical studies with most benzodiazepines.[130] However, one large epidemiologic study indicates that the potential for triazolam to produce anterograde amnesia is quite low and only slightly greater than for flurazepam, temazepam, or over-the-counter drugs.[120] Memory impairment with benzodiazepine use may be due in part to their hypnotic effect, as sleepiness at the time of learning disrupts memory consolidation, rather than a specific effect of these medications.[131] Because of anecdotal claims of bizarre behavior (e.g., disassociation, hallucinations, paranoia) in a small proportion of patients taking Halcion, a Food and Drug Administration (FDA) advisory panel reviewed safety and efficacy data in 1992. In sum, the panel concluded that triazolam is safe and effective when used at recommended doses. The panel also recommended strengthening cautions to avoid long-term use and large doses.

Quazepam (Doral) is the most lipophilic benzodiazepine, and readily crosses the blood-brain barrier and redistributes to peripheral tissue. The major active metabolite of quazepam is identical to that of flurazepam, resulting in a similar long elimination time, and the potential for accumulation and carryover effects with repeated dosing.[132] The high tissue distribution volume limits the duration of action when single doses are employed, thus reducing, to some degree, risk of residual sedation in this situation.

Estazolam (ProSom) is rapidly absorbed and has an intermediate elimination half-life (12 to 18 hours). Carryover sedation is more likely than with rapidly eliminated compounds (particularly with nightly use, as the drug accumulates) but less marked than with slowly eliminated drugs. Risk of rebound insomnia seems to be lower than with short-acting compounds.[133]

SUMMARY

Insomnia is a complaint or symptom that is usefully conceptualized as the result of constitutional, precipitating, and perpetuating factors. Growing evidence suggests significant morbidity is associated with this common symptom. Effective treatment requires an understanding of the differential diagnosis and available treatment options, both of which span the medical, psychiatric, behavioral, and pharmacological domains.

REFERENCES

1. Karacan I, Thornby JI, Williams RL. Sleep disturbance: A community survey. In: Guilleminault C, Lugaresi E, eds. Sleep/Wake Disorders: Natural History, Epidemiology, and Long-Term Evolution. New York: Raven Press, 1983;37–60.

2. Gillin JC, Byerley WF. Drug therapy: The diagnosis and management of insomnia. N Engl J Med 1990;322:239–248.

3. Mellinger GD, Balter MB, Uhlenhuth EH. Insomnia and its treatment: Prevalence and correlates. Arch Gen Psychiatry 1985;42:225–232.

4. Unpublished data from the 1985 National Ambulatory Care Survey, Division of Health Care Statistics, National Center for Health Statistics.

5. Gallup Organization. Sleep in America. Princeton, NJ: The Gallup Organization, 1991.

6. Everitt DE, Avorn J, Baker MW. Clinical decision making in the evaluation and treatment of insomnia. Am J Med 1990;89:357–362 [erratum, Am J Med 1990;89:838].

7. Walsh JK, Engelhardt CL. The Cost of Insomnia to America. Unpublished position paper written for the National Commission for Sleep Disorders Research, 1991.

8. Addison RG, Thorpy MJ, Roehrs TA, et al. Sleep/wake complaints in the general population. Sleep Res 1991;20:112.

9. Karacan I, Thornby JI, Anch M, et al. Prevalence of sleep disturbance in a primarily urban Florida county. Soc Sci Med 1976;10:239–244.

10. Bixler EO, Kales A, Soldatos CR, et al. Prevalence of sleep disorders in the Los Angeles metropolitan area. Am J Psychiatry 1979;136:1257–1262.

11. Welstein L, Dement WC, Redington D, et al. Insomnia in the San Francisco Bay area: A telephone survey. In: Guilleminault C, Lugaresi E, eds. Sleep/Wake Disorders: Natural History, Epidemiology, and Long-Term Evolution. New York: Raven Press, 1983;73–85.

12. Ford DE, Kamerow DB. Epidemiologic study of sleep disturbances and psychiatric disorders: An opportunity for prevention. JAMA 1989;262:1479–1484.

13. Balter MB, Uhlenhuth EH. Personal communication.

14. Angst J, Vollrath M, Koch R, Dobler-Mikola A. The Zurich Study—VII. Insomnia: Symptoms, classification and prevalence. Eur Arch Psychiatry Neuro Sci 1989;238:285–293.

15. Mellinger GD, Balter MB. Psychotherapeutic drugs: A current assessment of prevalence and pattern of use. In: Morgan JP, Kagan DV, eds. Society and Medication: Conflicting Signals for Prescribers and Patients. Lexington, Ky: D.C. Heath, and Co. 1983;137–154.

16. Parry HJ, Balter MB, Mellinger GD, et al. National patterns of psychotherapeutic drug use. Arch Gen Psychiatry 1973;28:769–783.

17. Johnson LC, Spinweber CL. Quality of sleep and performance in the Navy: A longitudinal study of good and poor sleepers. In: Guilleminault C, Lugaresi E, eds. Sleep-Wake Disorders: Natural History, Epidemiology, and Long-Term Evolution. New York: Raven Press, 1983;13–28.

18. Mendelson WB, Garnett D, Gillin JC, et al. The experience of insomnia and daytime and nighttime functioning. Psychiatr Res 1984;12:235–250.

19. Sugerman JL, Stern JA, Walsh JK. Daytime alertness in subjective and objective insomnia: Some preliminary findings. Biol Psychiatry 1985;20:741–750.

20. Mendelson WB, Garnett D, Linnoila M. Do insomniacs have impaired daytime functioning? Biol Psychiatry 1984;19:1261–1263.

21. Linnoila M, Erwin CW, Logue PE. Efficacy and side effects of flurazepam and a combination of amobarbital and secobarbital in insomniac patients. J Clin Pharmacol 1980;20:117–123.

22. Bixler EO, Kales A, Soldatos CR. Sleep disorders encountered in medical practice: A national survey of physicians. Behav Med 1979;6:1–6.

23. Coleman RM, Zarcone VP, Redington DJ, et al. Sleep-wake disorders in a family practice clinic. Sleep Res 1980;9:192.

24. Martin C, Zarcone V, LaBarber G, et al. Insomnia as presented to the private practice of a general physician. Sleep Res 1979;8:201.

25. Moore CA, Karacan I, Williams RL. Sleep in various medical and surgical conditions. In: Roessler R, Decker N, eds. Emotional Disorders in Physically Ill Patients. New York, Human Sciences Press, 1986;119–149.

26. Vollrath M, Wicki W, Angst J. The Zurich Study—VIII. Insomnia: Association with depression, anxiety, somatic syndromes, and course of insomnia. Eur Arch Psychiatry Neuro Sci 1989;239:113–124.

27. Gislason T, Almqvist M. Somatic disease and sleep complaints: An epidemiological study of 3,201 Swedish men. Acta Med Scand 1987;221:475–481.

28. Hyyppa MT, Kronholm E. Quality of sleep and chronic illnesses. J Clin Epidemiol 1989;42:633–638.

29. Partinen M. Stress and the heart: The sleep factor. Stress Med 1988;4:253–363.

30. Whorwell PJ. McCallum M, Creed FH, et al. Noncolonic features of irritable bowel syndrome. Gut, 1986;27:37–40.

31. Johnsen R, Jacobsen B, Forde OH. Associations between symptoms of irritable colon and psychological and social conditions and lifestyle. Br Med J 1986;292:1633–1635.

32. Segawa K, Nakazawa S. Tsukamoto Y, et al. Peptic ulcer is prevalent among shift workers. Dig Dis Sci 1987;32:449–453.

33. Moldofsky H. Sleep and fibrositis syndrome. Rheu Dis Clin North Am 1989;15:91–103.

34. Moldofsky H, Scarisbrick P. Induction of neurasthenic musculoskeletal pain syndrome by selective sleep state deprivation. Psychosomat Med 1976;38:35–44.

35. Mahowald MW, Mahowald ML, Bundlie SR, et al. Sleep fragmentation in rheumatoid arthritis. Arthritis Rheum 1989;32:974–983.

36. Kales A, Kales JD. Evaluation and Treatment of Insomnia. New York: Oxford University Press, 1984.

37. Reynolds CF, Kupfer DJ. Sleep in depression. In Williams RL, Karacan I, Moore CA, eds. Sleep Disorders: Diagnosis and Treatment, ed 2. New York: John Wiley & Sons, 1988;147–164.

38. Healy D. Rhythm and blues. Neurochemical, neuropharmacological and neuropsychological implications of a hypothesis of circadian rhythm dysfunction in the affective disorders. Psychopharmacology 1987;93:271–285.

39. Kripke DF, Simons RN, Carfinkel L, et al. Short and long sleep and sleeping pills: Is increased mortality associated? Arch Gen Psychiatr 1979;36:103–116.

40. Berkman LF, Breslow L. Health and Ways of Living: The Alameda County Study. New York: Oxford University Press, 1983.

41. Wingard DL, Berkman LF. Mortality risk associated with sleeping patterns among adults. Sleep, 1983;6:102–107.

42. Pollack CP, Perlick D, Linsner JP, et al. Sleep problems in the community elderly as predictors of death and nursing home placement. J Commun Health 1990;15:123–135.

43. Kripke DF, Ancoli-Israel S, Fell RL, et al. Health risk of insomnia. In: Peter JH, et al. eds. Sleep and Health Risk. New York: Springer-Verlag, 1991;547–554.

44. Spielman AJ, Caruso LS, Glovinsky PB. A behavioral perspective on insomnia treatment. Psychiatr Clin North Am 1987;10:541–553.

45. Morris M, Lack L, Dawson D. Sleep-onset insomniacs have delayed temperature rhythms. Sleep 1990;13:1–14.

46. Heath AC, Kendler KS, Eaves LJ, et al. Evidence for genetic influences on sleep disturbance and sleep pattern in twins. Sleep 1990;13:318–335.

47. Partinen M, Kaprio J, Koskenvuo M, et al. Sleeping habits, sleep quality, and use of sleeping pills: A population study of 31,140 adults in Finland. In: Guilleminault C, Lugaresi E, eds. Sleep/Wake Disorders: Natural History, Epidemiology, and Long-Term Evolution. New York: Raven Press, 1983.

48. Boghen D, Peyronnard J-M. Myoclonus in familial restless legs syndrome. Arch Neurol 1976;33:368–370.

49. Healey ES, Kales A, Monroe LJ, et al. Onset of insomnia: Role of life-stress events. Psychosomat Med 1981;43:439–451.

50. Kales JD, Kales A, Bixler EO, et al. Biopsychobehavioral correlates of insomnia, V: Clinical characteristics and behavioral correlates. Am J Psychiatry 1984;141:1371–1376.

51. Diagnostic Classification Steering Committee. International Classification of Sleep Disorders: Diagnostic and Coding Manual. Rochester, Minn: American Sleep Disorders Association, 1990.

52. Hauri P, Fisher J. Persistent psychophysiologic (learned) insomnia. Sleep 1986;9:38–53.

53. Coleman RM. Diagnosis, treatment and follow-up of about 8,000 sleep/wake patients. In: Guilleminault C, Lugaresi E, eds. Sleep/Wake Disorders: Natural History, Epidemiology, and Long-Term Evolution. New York: Raven Press,1983;87–97.

54. Carskadon MA, Dement WC, Mitler MM, et al. Self-reports versus sleep laboratory findings in 122 drug-free subjects with complaints of chronic insomnia. Am J Psychiatry 1976;133:1382—1388.

55. Borkovec TD, Lane TW, Vanoot PH. Phenomenology of sleep among insomniacs and good sleepers: Wakefulness experience when cortically asleep. J Abnorm Psychol 1981;90:607–609.

56. Mendelson WB, James SP, Garnett D, et al. A psychophysiological study of insomnia. Psychiatry Res 1986;19:267–284.

57. Hauri PJ, Olmstead E. What is the moment of sleep onset for insomniacs? Sleep 1983;6:10–15.

58. Beutler LE, Thornby JI, Karacan I. Psychological variables in the diagnosis of insomnia. In: RL Williams, I Karacan, eds. Sleep Disorders: Diagnosis and Treatment. New York: John Wiley & Sons, 1978:61–100.

59. Haynes SN, Fitzgerald SG, Shute G, et al. Responses of psychophysiologic and subjective insomniacs to auditory stimuli during sleep: A replication and extension. J Abnorm Psychol 1985;94:338–345.

60. Hauri PJ, Esther MS. Insomnia. Mayo Clin Proc 1990;65:869–882.

61. Borkovec TD, Grayson JB, O'Brien GT, et al. Relaxation treatment of pseudoinsomnia and idiopathic insomnia: An electroencephalographic evaluation. J Appl Behav Anal 1979;12:37–54.

62. Mendelson WB. Human Sleep: Research and Clinical Care. New York: Plenum Medical, 1987.

63. Trinder J. Subjective insomnia without objective findings: A pseudo diagnostic classification. Psychol Bull 1988;103:87–94.

64. Hauri PJ, Olmsted E. Childhood onset insomnia. Sleep 1980;3:59–65.

65. Regestein QR, Reich P. Incapacitating childhood-onset insomnia. Compr Psychiatry 1983;24:244–248.

66. Coleman RM, Roffwarg HP, Kennedy SJ, et al. Sleep-wake disorders based on a polysomnographic diagnosis: A national cooperative study. JAMA 1982;247:997–1003.

67. Regestein QR. Specific effects of sedative-hypnotic drugs in the treatment of incapacitating chronic insomnia. Am J Med 1987;83:909–915.

68. Hauri P. Primary insomnia. In: Kryger MH, Roth T, Dement WC, eds. Principles and Practice of Sleep Medicine. Philadelphia: WB Saunders, 1989;442–447.

69. Kales A, Bixler EO, Soldatos CR, et al. Biopsychobehavioral correlates of insomnia, Part 1. Role of sleep apnea and nocturnal myoclonus. Psychosomatics 1982;23:589–600.

70. Ancoli-Israel S. Epidemiology of sleep disorders. Clin Geriatr Med 1989;5:347–362.

71. Guilleminault C. Clinical features and evaluation of obstructive sleep apnea. In: Kryger MH, Roth T, Dement WC, eds. Principles and Practice of Sleep Medicine. Philadelphia: WB Saunders, 1989;552–558.

72. Guilleminault C, Eldridge FL, Dement WC. Insomnia with sleep apnea: A new syndrome. Science 1973; 181:856–858.

73. White DP. Central sleep apnea. In: Kryger MH, Roth T, Dement WC, eds. Principles and Practice of Sleep Medicine. Philadelphia: WB Saunders, 1989;513–524.

74. Robinson RW, Zwillich CW. The effects of drugs on breathing during sleep. In: Kryger MH, Roth T, Dement WC, eds. Principles and Practice of Sleep Medicine. Philadelphia: WB Saunders, 1989;501–512.

75. Montplaisir J, Godbout R. Restless legs syndrome and periodic movements during sleep. In: Kryger MH, Roth T, Dement WC, eds. Principles and Practice of Sleep Medicine. Philadelphia: WB Saunders, 1989;402–409.

76. Lugaresi E, Coccagna G, Berti Ceroni G, et al. Restless legs syndrome and noctural myoclonus. In: Gastaut H, Lugaresi E, Berti-Ceroni G (eds) The Abnormalities of Sleep in Man. Bologna: Aulo Graggi, 1968;285–294.

77. Coleman RM, Pollak CP, Weitzman ED. Periodic movements in sleep (nocturnal myoclonus): Relation to sleep disorders. Ann Neurol 1980;8:416–421.

78. Smith RC. Relationship of periodic movements in sleep (nocturnal myoclonus) and the Babinski sign. Sleep 1985;8:239–243.

79. Ancoli-Israel S, Seifert AR, Lemon M. Thermal biofeedback and periodic movements in sleep: Patients' subjective reports and a case study. Biofeedback Self Regul 1986;11:177–188.

80. Dzvonik ML, Kripke DF, Klauber M, et al. Body position changes and periodic movements in sleep. Sleep, 1986;9:484–491.

81. Walters A, Hening W, Cote L, et al. Dominantly inherited restless legs with myoclonus and periodic movements of sleep: A syndrome related to the endogenous opiates? In: Fahn S, Marsden CD, Van Woert MH, eds. Myoclonus. Advances in Neurology Vol. 43. New York: Raven Press, 1986;309–319.

82. Rosenthal L, Roehrs T, Sicklesteel J, et al. Periodic movements during sleep, sleep fragmentation, and sleep-wake complaints. Sleep 1984;7:326–330.

83. Saskin P, Moldofsky H, Lue FA. Periodic movements in sleep and sleep-wake complaint. Sleep, 1985;8:319–324.

84. Bixler EO, Kales A, Vela-Bueno A, et al. Nocturnal myoclonus and nocturnal myoclonic activity in a normal population. Res Commun Chem Pathol Pharmacol 1982;36:129–140.

85. Coleman RM, Bliwise DL, Sajben N, et al. Epidemiology of periodic movements during sleep. In: Guilleminault C, Lugaresi E, eds. Sleep/Wake Disorders: Natural History, Epidemiology and Long-Term Evolution. New York: Raven Press, 1983;217–229.

86. Mosko SS, Shampain DS, Sassin JF. Nocturnal REM latency and sleep disturbance in narcolepsy. Sleep 1984;7:115–125.

87. Coleman RM. Periodic movement in sleep (nocturnal myoclonus) and restless legs syndrome. In: Guilleminault C, ed. Sleeping and Waking Disorders, Indications and Techniques. Menlo Park, Calif: Addison-Wesley, 1982;265–295.

88. Mitler MM, Browman CP, Menn SJ, et al. Nocturnal myoclonus: Treatment efficacy of clonazepam and temazepam. Sleep 1986;9:385–392.

89. Guilleminault C, Mondini S, Montplaisir J, et al. Periodic leg movements, L-dopa, 5-hydroxytryprophan, and L-tryptophan. Sleep 1987;10:393–397.

90. Brodeur C, Montplaisir J, Godbout R, et al. Polygraphic features of L-dopa in restless legs syndrome (RLS) and periodic movements during sleep (PMS): A double-blind controlled study. Sleep 1988;17:149.

91. Ekbom KA. Restless legs syndrome. Neurology 1960;10:868–873.

92. Coccagna G. Restless legs syndrome/periodic leg movements in sleep. In: Thorpy MJ, ed. Handbook of Sleep Disorders. New York: Marcel Dekker, 1990; 457–478.

93. Montagna P, Coccagna G, Cirignotta F, et al. Familial restless legs syndrome: Long-term follow-up. In: Guilleminault C, Lugaresi E, eds. Sleep/Wake Disorders: Natural History, Epidemiology and Long-Term Evolution. New York: Raven Press, 1983;231–235.

94. Montplaisir J, Godbout R, Boghen D, et al. Familial restless legs with periodic movements in sleep: Electrophysiologic, biochemical and pharmacologic study. Neurology 1985;35:130–134.

95. Akpinar S. Treatment of restless legs syndrome with levodopa plus benserazide. [letter] Arch Neurol 1982;39:739.

96. Von Scheele C, Kempi V. Long-term effect of dopaminergic drugs in restless legs. A 2-year followup. Arch Neurol 1990;47:1223–1224.

97. Buysse DJ, Reynolds CF: Insomnia. In: Thorpy MJ, ed. Handbook of Sleep Disorders. New York: Marcel Dekker, 1990;375–433.

98. Kales A, Bixler EO, Soldatos CR, et al. Quazepam and flurazepam: Long-term use and extended withdrawal. Clin Pharmacol Ther 1982;32:781–788.

99. Mitler MM, Carskadon MA, Phillips RL, et al. Hypnotic efficacy of temazepam: A long-term sleep laboratory evaluation. Br J Clin Pharmacol, 1979;8:63s–68s.

100. Kales A, Soldatos CR, Bixler EO, et al. Rebound insomnia and rebound anxiety: A review. Pharmacology 1983;26:121–137.

101. Gillin JC, Spinweber CL, Johnson LC. Rebound insomnia: A critical review. J Clin Psychopharmacol 1989;9:161–172.

102. Kay DC, Samiuddin Z. Sleep disorders associated with drug abuse and drugs of abuse. In: Williams RL, Karacan I, Moore CA, eds. Sleep Disorders: Diagnosis and Treatment, ed 2. New York: John Wiley & Sons, 1988;315–372.

103. Weil JV. Sleep at high altitude. In: Kryger M, Roth T, Dement WC, eds. Principles and Practice of Sleep Disorders Medicine. Philadelphia: WB Saunders, 1989;269–275.

104. Weitzman ED, Czeisler CA, Coleman RM, et al. Delayed sleep phase syndrome: A chronobiological disorder with sleep onset insomnia. Arch Gen Psychiatry 1981;38:737–746.

105. Rosenthal NE, Joseph-Vanderpool JR, Levendosky AA, et al. Phase-shifting effects of bright morning light as treatment for delayed sleep phase syndrome. Sleep 1990;13:354–361.

106. Czeisler CA, Richardson GS, Coleman RM, et al. Chronotherapy: Resetting the circadian clocks of patients with delayed sleep phase insomnia. Sleep 1981;4:1–21.

107. Allen RP. Early morning awakening insomnia: Bright-light treatment. In: Hauri PJ, ed. Case Studies in Insomnia. New York: Plenum, 1991:207–220.

108. Moldofsky H, Musisi S, Phillipson EA. Treatment of advanced sleep phase syndrome by phase advance chronotherapy. Sleep 1986;9:61–65.

109. Walsh JK, Sugerman JL. Disorders of initiating and maintaining sleep associated with adult psychiatric disorders. In: Kryger M, Roth T, Dement W, eds.

Principles and Practice of Sleep Medicine. Philadelphia: WB Saunders, 1989:448–455.

110. Kupfer DJ. REM latency: A psychobiological marker for primary depressive disease. Biol Psychiatry 1976;11:159–174.

111. American Psychiatric Association. Diagnostic and Statistical Manual of Mental Disorders, ed 3, revised. Washington, DC, American Psychiatric Association, 1987.

112. Roth T, Roehrs T, Zorick F. Pharmacological treatment of sleep disorders. In: Williams RL, Karacan IU, Moore CA, eds. Sleep Disorders: Diagnosis and Treatment, ed 2. New York: John Wiley & Sons, 1988;373–395.

113. Walsh JK, Mahowald MW. Avoiding the blanket approach to insomnia. Targeted therapy for specific causes. Postgrad Med 1991;90:211–224.

114. Jacobs EA, Reynolds CF, Kupfer DJ, et al. The role of polysomnography in the differential diagnosis of chronic insomnia. Am J Psychiatry 1988;145:346–349.

115. Edinger JD, Hoelscher TJ, Webb MD, et al. Polysomnographic assessment of DIMS: Empirical evaluation of its diagnostic value. Sleep 1989;12:315–322.

116. Bootzin RR, Epstein D, Wood JM. Stimulus control instructions. In: Hauri PJ, ed. Case Studies in Insomnia. New York: Plenum, 1991;19–28.

117. Spielman AJ, Saskin P, Thorpy MJ. Treatment of chronic insomnia by restriction of time in bed. Sleep 1987;10:45–56.

118. Hauri PJ ed. Case Studies in Insomnia. New York: Plenum, 1991.

119. National Institute of Mental Health, Consensus Development Conference. Drugs and insomnia: The use of medications to promote sleep. JAMA 1984; 251(8):2410–2414.

120. Balter MB, Uhlenhuth EH. The beneficial and adverse effects of hypnotics. J Clin Psychiatry 1991;52 Suppl:16–23.

121. Task Force of the American Psychiatric Association. Benzodiazepine Dependence, Toxicity, and Abuse. Washington, DC: American Psychiatric Association, 1990.

122. Roehrs T, Merlotti L, Zorick F, et al. Rebound insomnia and hypnotic self-administration. Psychopharmacology 1992;107:480–484.

123. Roehrs TA, Merlotti L, Beare D, et al. Benzodiazepine hypnotic self-administration and dose escalation. Sleep Res 1991;20:78.

124. Greenblatt DJ, Harmatz JS, Shapiro L, et al. Sensitivity to triazolam in the elderly. N Engl J Med 1991;324:1691–1698.

125. Greenblatt DJ, Harmatz JS, Zinny MA, et al. Effect of gradual withdrawal on the rebound sleep disorder after discontinuation of triazolam. N Engl J Med 1987;317:722–728.

126. Walsh JK, Fillingim JM. The role of hypnotics in general practice. Am J Med 1990;88(A):34S–38S.

127. Greenblatt DJ, Shader RI, Divoll M, et al. Adverse reactions to triazolam, flurazepam, and placebo in controlled clinical trials. J Clin Psychiatry 1984; 45:192–195.

128. Divoll M, Greenblat DJ, Harmatz JS, et al. Effect of age and gender on disposition of temazepam. J Pharm Sci 1981;70(0):11104–1107.

129. Bixler EO, Kales A, Manfredi RL, et al. Next-day memory impairment with triazolam use. Lancet 1991;337:827–831.

130. Scharf MB, Saskin P, Fletcher K. Benzodiazepine induced amnesia: Clinical laboratory findings. J Clin Psychiatry Monogr 1987;5:14–17.

131. Roth T, Roehrs TA, Stepanski EJ, et al. Hypnotics and behavior. Am J Med 1990;88(3A suppl):43S–46S.

132. Ankier SI, Goa KL. Quazepam. Drugs 1988;35:42–62.

133. Pierce MW, Shu VS, Groves LJ. Safety of estazolam. The United States clinical experience. Am J Med 1990;88(3A suppl):12–17S.

18

Narcolepsy

Christian Guilleminault

The word *narcolepsy* was first coined by Gelineau[1] in 1880 to designate a pathologic condition characterized by irresistible episodes of sleep of short duration that recur at close intervals. In the same report, he wrote that attacks were sometimes accompanied by falls or "astasias," a condition later referred to as cataplexy.[2] In the 1930s, Daniels[3] emphasized the association of daytime sleepiness, cataplexy, sleep paralysis, and hypnagogic hallucination. Calling these symptoms the clinical tetrad, Yoss and Daly[4] and Vogel[5] reported a nocturnal sleep-onset rapid eye movement (REM) period in narcoleptic patients, a finding confirmed in the following years.[6-9]

In 1975, participants in the First International Symposium on Narcolepsy defined the syndrome as follows: "The word *narcolepsy* refers to a syndrome of unknown origin that is characterized by abnormal sleep tendencies, including excessive daytime sleepiness (EDS) and, often, disturbed nocturnal sleep and pathologic manifestations of REM sleep. The REM sleep abnormalities include sleep-onset REM periods and the dissociated REM sleep inhibitory processes cataplexy and sleep paralysis. EDS, cataplexy, and, less often, sleep paralysis and hypnagogic hallucinations, are the major symptoms of the disease."[10] This definition highlighted the need for further research, for clearly, many unanswered questions remained about the causes of narcolepsy. It was agreed that the syndrome involved a dysfunction of REM sleep.

Recently, Honda and Juji criticized this definition[11] for being too broad and for overemphasizing the importance of polygraphic studies. He proposed the following diagnostic criteria:

A. Recurrent daytime naps and lapses into sleep occurring almost every day for a period of at least 6 months.
B. Concurrent with the history of napping, clinical confirmation of cataplexy in the patient's history.

These two criteria are based on strict findings:

A. Daytime sleep
The duration of each episode of daytime sleep is usually less than an hour. Sleep can be easily terminated by external stimulation.
The patient usually feels refreshed after sleeping.
Central nervous system (CNS) stimulants such as methylphenidate, pemoline, and amphetamine are effective against the somnolence.
The condition usually lasts over many years, 6 months at the very least.
B. Cataplexy
Consciousness and memory are not impaired during cataplexy.
The duration of cataplexy is usually short, from seconds to a few minutes.
Clomipramine and imipramine are effective in markedly reducing cataplexy.

With these clinical criteria, presence of human leukocyte antigen (HLA) DR2 and sleep-onset REM periods on polysomnography (PSG) confirms the diagnosis.[11]

At present there is controversy over this definition. Most controversial is the need for HLA-DR2 (or, by new World Health Organization nomenclature, DRw15) antigen to be present, and we do not subscribe to this notion. The requirement for clear investigation of clinical findings has the advantage of avoiding vagueness and of obtaining a good sleep history from patients.

CLINICAL FEATURES

Narcolepsy is characterized by a set of clinical symptoms, including abnormal sleep features, overwhelming episodes of sleep, EDS, hypnagogic hallucinations, disturbed nocturnal sleep, and manifestations of paroxysmal muscle weakness, cataplexy, and sleep paralysis.

Daytime Naps and Daytime Sleepiness

Unwanted episodes of sleep recur several times a day, not only under favorable circumstances such as monotonous sedentary activity or a heavy meal but also in situations when the subject is fully involved in a task. The duration of the episode may vary from a few minutes if the subject is in an uncomfortable position to more than an hour if the subject is reclining. Narcoleptics characteristically wake up refreshed, and there is a refractory period of one to several hours before the next episode occurs.

Apart from sleep episodes, patients may feel abnormally drowsy, spending the day in an unpleasantly low level of alertness that is responsible for poor performance at work, memory lapses, and even gestural, deambulatory, or speech automatisms.

Cataplexy

Cataplexy is an abrupt and reversible decrease or loss of muscle tone most frequently elicited by emotion. It may involve certain muscles or the entire voluntary musculature. Most typically, the jaw sags, the head falls forward, the arms drop to the side, and the knees unlock. The duration of a cataplectic attack, partial or total, is highly variable: from a few seconds to 30 minutes. Attacks can be elicited by emotion, stress, fatigue, or heavy meals. Laughter and anger seem to be the most common triggers, but the attacks can also be induced by feeling elation while listening to music, reading a book, or watching a movie. Cataplexy can also occur without clear precipitating acts or emotions.

The severity and extent of a cataplexy attack can vary from a state of absolute powerlessness that seems to involve the entire voluntary musculature to limited involvement of certain muscle groups, to no more than a fleeting sensation of weakness throughout the body. Though the extraocular muscles are probably not involved, weakness can occur, and the patient may complain of blurred vision. While complete paralysis of extraocular muscles has never been reported, the palpebral muscle may be affected. Speech may be impaired, and respiration may become irregular during an attack; this may be related to weakness of the abdominal muscles. Long diaphragmatic pauses have never been recorded, but short diaphragmatic pauses similar to those seen during nocturnal REM sleep can be noted. Complete loss of muscle tone may be experienced during a cataplectic attack. This causes total collapse with risk of serious injuries, including skull and other fractures. Commonly, however, the attacks are not so dramatic, and they may even be ignored by persons nearby. An attack may consist only of a slight buckling of the knees. Patients may perceive this abrupt and very short-lived weakness and may simply stop or stand against a wall. The condition may be slightly more obvious when there is a combination of sagging jaw and inclined head. Speech may be broken because of intermittent weakness affecting the arytenoid muscles. As seen during nocturnal REM sleep, the abrupt muscle inhibition is interrupted by sudden bursts of returning muscle tone, which at times even seems enhanced. If the weakness involves only the jaw or speech, the subject may exhibit masticatory movement or an attack of stuttering. If it involves the upper limbs, the patient complains of clumsiness, reporting activity such as dropping cups or spilling liquids when surprised, laughing, and so forth.

As these attacks are short and do not resemble a classic full-blown attack of cataplexy, they are often ignored by physicians, even though they are by far the most common. Without an electromyographic (EMG) recording, their transience may make them easy to miss, even by a skilled experimenter.

Cataplexy is associated with inhibition of the monysynaptic H and muscle stretch reflexes. Physiologically, H-reflex activity is fully suppressed only during REM sleep, which points to the relationship between the motor inhibitory components of REM sleep and the sudden atonia and areflexia seen during a cataplectic attack.

Sleep Paralysis and Hypnagogic Hallucinations

Sleep paralysis is a terrifying experience that occurs when a narcoleptic falls asleep or awakens. Patients find themselves suddenly unable to move the limbs, to speak, or even breathe deeply. The paralysis is frequently accompanied by hallucinations. During an episode of sleep paralysis, patients are powerless to move the extremities, to speak, or to open the eyes, though they are fully aware of the condition and are able to recall it completely afterward. In many episodes of sleep paralysis, especially the first occurrence, the patient may be prey to extreme anxiety associated with the fear of dying. This anxiety is often much intensified by the terrifying hallucinations that may accompany the sleep paralysis. With more experience of the phenomenon, however, the patient usually learns that episodes are brief and benign, rarely lasting longer than 10 minutes and always ending spontaneously. The narcoleptic's hypnagogic hallucinations often involve vision, and the manifestations usually consist of simple forms (colored circles, parts of objects) that may be constant in size or changing. The image of an animal or a person may present itself abruptly, in black and white, or, more often, in color. Auditory hallucinations are also common, but other senses are seldom involved. The auditory hallucinations can range from a collection of sounds to an elaborate melody. The patient may also be menaced by threatening sentences or harsh invective.

Sleep onset, either during daytime sleep episodes or at night, may be unpleasant, with vivid auditory or hypnagogic hallucinations. Another common and interesting type of hallucination reported at sleep onset involves elementary cenesthopathic (abnormal) feelings (i.e., picking, rubbing, light touching), changes in location of body parts (arm, leg), or feelings of levitation or extracorporeal experiences (moving the body in space, floating above the bed) which may be quite elaborate. For example, the patient may say, "I am above my bed and I can also see my body below," or, "I am a few feet up and people jump over my body." The association of sleep paralysis has led researchers to postulate gamma loop involvement in some of these hallucinations. The abrupt motor inhibition that involves the spinal cord motor neurons may lead to a significant decrease in feedback of information normally used by the CNS to gauge the position of the body and relation of the limb segments to each other. Night sleep is often interrupted by repeated awakenings and is sometimes interspersed with terrifying dreams.

ONSET OF CLINICAL SYMPTOMS

The first symptoms often develop near puberty. The peak age of reported symptoms is between 15 and 25 years in women, but narcolepsy and other symptoms have been noted at 5 or 6 years and a second, smaller peak of onset between 35 and 45 years, near menopause.

EDS and irresistible sleep episodes usually occur as the first symptoms, either independently or associated with one or more other symptoms. They are enhanced by high temperature, indoor activity, and idleness. Symptoms may abate with time but they never phase out completely. Attacks of cataplexy generally appear in conjunction with abnormal episodes of sleep, but they may occur as much as 20 years later. Occasionally, but seldom, they occur before the abnormal sleep episodes, in which case they are a major source of difficulty in diagnosis. They can vary in frequency from a few episodes during the subject's entire lifetime to one or several episodes per day.

Hypnagogic hallucinations and sleep paralysis do not affect all subjects and often are transitory. Disturbed nocturnal sleep seldom occurs in the first stages and generally builds with age.[12]

DIAGNOSTIC PROCEDURES: EVALUATION OF SLEEPINESS

The Stanford Sleepiness Scale (SSS),[13] a 6-point scale, was developed to quantify the subjective sleepiness of patients, but its reliability for chronically sleepy patients is questionable. Several tests have been designed to evaluate sleepiness objectively. Yoss and coworkers[14] described the electronic pupillogram (EPG) as a method of measuring increased levels of sleepiness. Recently, Schmidt

and Fortin[15] reviewed the advantages and limitations of EPG in arousal disorders. The use of EPG as a test is based on the facts that peripheral autonomic manifestations are associated with states of arousal or excitation as well as sleep and that the pupil is an index of autonomic (vagal) activity. Berlucchi and colleagues[16] clearly demonstrated the pupil's constriction during sleep. A normal, alert person sitting quietly in total darkness can maintain a stable pupil diameter, usually well above 7 mm, for at least 10 minutes, without subjective difficulty or pupillary oscillation.[15] The pupillary diameter in excessively sleepy patients, however, is unstable when they are adapting to the dark. The EPG technique is often performed with a series of light stimuli. (Schmidt and Fortin[15] recommend 15–foot candle intensity attenuated by a 4.0 log neutral-density filter.)

There are problems and limitations with this technique.[15] Patients with ocular problems or autonomic (CNS) lesions must be identified and excluded. A patient's ability and willingness to cooperate are critical. Excessively sleepy subjects have trouble avoiding lid drooping or closure. Small initial pupil diameter, dark irises, and excessive eye makeup all pose problems. Finally, the data may be difficult to interpret, particularly if recording conditions are not standardized. Though at one time experts did attempt to use EPG to diagnose narcolepsy, it essentially diagnoses only sleepiness. The test does not indicate the underlying causes of EDS.

The Multiple Sleep Latency Test (MSLT) was designed by Carskadon and Dement[17] to measure physiologic sleep tendencies in the absence of alerting factors. It consists of four or five scheduled naps, usually at 10:00, 12:00, 14:00, 16:00 and 18:00 hours, during which the subject is polygraphically monitored in a comfortable, soundproof, dark bedroom. The latency between lights out time and sleep onset is calculated for each nap. The criteria for sleep onset are those outlined in Rechtschaffen and Kales' international manual.[18] The type of sleep, REM or non-REM (NREM), is also noted. After each 20-minute monitoring period, patients stay awake until the following scheduled nap. The MSLT records the latency for each nap, the mean sleep latency, and the presence or absence of REM sleep in any of the naps. Based on polygraphic recording, REM sleep that occurs within 15 minutes of sleep onset is considered a sleep-onset REM period.[19] Guidelines for performance of the MSLT have been published by the American Sleep Disorders Association.[19]

In normal populations, MSLT scores vary with age. Puberty is the critical landmark; prepubertal children between age 6 and 11 years appear to be hyperalert. Mean MSLT scores under 8 minutes are generally considered to be in the pathologic range, whereas those over 10 minutes are considered normal.

When the range is between 8 and 10 minutes, age factors interact, so the test may be interpreted with greater care; mean scores of 9 to 10 minutes are in the gray zone.[20]

An MSLT performed alone has the same drawbacks as EPG (i.e., it measures sleepiness regardless of its cause, which may represent simply sleep deprivation). The MSLT also ignores repetitive microsleeps that can lead, in borderline cases, to daytime impairment not scored by conventional analysis. To be clinically relevant, it must be conducted under specific conditions. Subjects must be off medication for a sufficient period to avoid drug interaction (usually 15 days). On the basis of a sleep diary, their sleep-wake schedule must be stabilized. The night preceding the MSLT they must undergo nocturnal PSG i.e. polygraphic recording of variables defining wakefulness and sleep states and stages—electroencephalography [EEG], electrooculogram [EOG], chin EMG and other biologic variables (cardiac, pulmonary, gastrointestinal). Throughout the total nocturnal sleep period, any sleep-related biologic abnormalities responsible for sleep fragmentation and sleep deprivation should be recorded.

The nocturnal PSG indicates the underlying cause for the complaint of sleepiness; the MSLT indicates the severity of the problem. Once the nocturnal sleep recording has eliminated specific diseases and demonstrated that a patient is sleeping normally during the night, the MSLT confirms the presence of narcolepsy if there are two or more sleep-onset REM periods.

Recently Browman and associates[21] proposed adding a test for the maintenance of wakefulness to the MSLT. The patient is to remain awake in a comfortable sitting position in a dark room for five 20-minute trials given at 10:00, 12:00, 14:00, 16:00, and 18:00 hours. The test may be helpful in specific pharmacologic trials, but it has proven unsatisfactory as a diagnostic procedure.[21]

Another procedure is a continuous 24- or 36-hour PSG monitoring that provides information about the actual number, duration, times, and types of daytime sleep episodes and about disrupted nighttime sleep. In addition, this long polygraphic recording may identify the dissociated REM sleep inhibitory process that characterizes cataplexy. This dissociated REM process combines an awake EEG and EOG recording, associated with complete absence of chin EMG recording and bursts of muscle twitches also typical of REM sleep. This may allow monitoring of "microsleeps" and "microwakes." Microwakes, or, more aptly, microarousals or transient alpha arousals, are short bursts of alpha EEG activity lasting 3 to 14 seconds (usually 5 to 10) which interrupt any sleep stage or state. They may be (but do not have to be) associated with an increase in chin EMG activity,

eye movements, or both. The American Sleep Disorders Association (ASDA) Task Force[21a] on Terminology, Techniques, and Scoring System preliminary report indicates that a sleep EEG must last at least 10 seconds to be called a transient alpha arousal. Microsleeps, by analogy with transient alpha arousals, are changes in EEG to stage 1 NREM or a REM sleep pattern lasting 3 to 14 seconds.

Finally, Broughton and colleagues[22] recently proposed using auditorily evoked potentials to evaluate sleepiness, but, once again, this test, which may be very helpful in evaluating pharmacologic agents, has not been sufficiently discriminatory to be used as a diagnostic tool. All of these tests must be performed in association with a urine drug test to ascertain the presence or absence of stimulants or drugs that have an impact on the sleep-wake cycle.

The positive diagnosis of narcolepsy requires a minimum of two major symptoms: EDS and sleep attacks or attacks of cataplexy associated with objectively documented sleep-onset REM episodes. The clinical association of daytime sleepiness and cataplexy, when observed by a physician, is pathognomonic of the narcolepsy syndrome.

If EDS and cataplectic attacks are sufficient to confirm narcolepsy, why require PSG in other cases? The history of cataplexy may, at times, be difficult to affirm. Absolute cataplexy, which causes the patient to collapse on the floor, is uncommon. Often, subjects have time to reach a chair or wall to prevent a complete collapse. Most commonly, cataplexy is only partial, involving the head and neck, upper limbs, mandibular and upper airway muscles, or "weak knees." This partial cataplexy is often difficult to interpret, especially in cases when the subject has only a positive history of cataplexy without current symptoms. It is in these cases that polygraphic monitoring with positive MSLT findings can confirm the diagnosis.

Can a subject with EDS and a history of cataplexy have a negative MSLT (fewer than two sleep-onset REM periods)? Van den Hoed and coworkers[20] and Moscovitch and colleagues[23] reviewed this issue. Both groups analzyed patients seen at the Stanford University Sleep Disorders Clinic. Moscovitch's group had a larger population (306 narcoleptics). Seventy-seven percent of these patients had been seen by the same physician, who had much experience with narcolepsy. All were believed, based on clinical data, to have cataplexy, but only 84% of them presented with two or more sleep-onset REM periods at one PSG-MSLT period. Four successive days of MSLTs were necessary to observe two or more sleep-onset REM periods in every subject in the population.

Can someone be diagnosed as narcoleptic who has no cataplexy but has sleep-onset REM periods?
Considering the need to have strict criteria for epidemiologic studies and the gloomy prognosis linked to the diagnosis of narcolepsy (a lifelong illness), it is strongly recommended that physicians avoid using the term *narcolepsy* and, rather, describe the findings (i.e., excessive daytime somnolence with *x* sleep-onset REM periods). The subject may be developing narcolepsy and may not yet have developed cataplexy. Seven young persons followed by the Stanford Sleep Clinic had EDS and two or more sleep-onset REM periods at MSLT some 5 to 24 months before they exhibited cataplexy. (Some other teenagers exhibited cataplexy before they had two or more sleep-onset REM periods at 1-day MSLT). Thus, a subject with two or more sleep-onset REM periods may be narcoleptic. Also, family members of definite narcoleptics have presented with EDS and two sleep-onset REM periods (five subjects older than 30 years in the Stanford Sleep Clinic data base). However, 54 of 306 EDS subjects in the Stanford data base aged 32 years and older presented no cataplexy and two or more sleep-onset REM periods and had no family history of narcolepsy.

Can HLA aid in diagnosis? As indicated by Guilleminault and colleagues,[24] the DR2 DQwl haplotype is neither sufficient nor necessary for narcolepsy. The new World Health Organization nomenclature[25] labels the HLA haplotype most commonly associated with narcolepsy DRw15 Dw2 Dw6 (not DR2 DQw1), but, once again, though it is frequently noted, this haplotype may not be associated with independent and familial cases of narcolepsy.

Finally, can MSLT scores for EDS be outside the range usually reported? Once again, considering the Stanford University data base, out of 500 narcoleptics with clear cataplexy and complaints of mild sleepiness, two presented a mean MSLT score of 11 at two repeated investigations. Each of them had two sleep-onset REM periods at the MSLT; however, 85% of the narcoleptics with van den Hoed's[20] and Moscovitch's[23] groups had a mean sleep latency on MSLT of less than 5 minutes.

In summary, cataplexy is a key feature for the diagnosis of narcolepsy. A PSG evaluation followed by an MSLT the following day demonstrates two or more sleep-onset REM periods in 84% of the cases. Descriptive language is recommended in questionable cases.

EPIDEMIOLOGY AND GENETICS

Narcolepsy is not a rare condition. Its prevalence has been calculated at 0.05% in the San Francisco Bay area[26] and 0.067% in the Los Angeles area.[27] Males are affected somewhat more often than females. Age at onset varies from childhood to the fifth decade and peaks in the second decade. A special circumstance such as an abrupt change of sleep-wake schedule or a severe psychological stress—death of a relative, divorce—precedes the occurrence of the first symptom in half of the cases.[12]

The genetic aspect of narcolepsy has been investigated by several groups. Among the first-degree relatives of 50 narcoleptic probands, Kessler and coworkers[28] found 9 narcoleptic patients (18%) and 17 subjects with EDS (34%). Among the parents and siblings of 232 narcoleptic probands, Honda and associates[29] found 14 narcoleptic patients (6%) and 56 subjects with EDS (24%). This led these two groups of authors to suggest a two-threshold, multifactorial model of inheritance, EDS being the more prevalent and less severe manifestation and narcolepsy the less prevalent and more severe manifestation of the same genetic predisposition.

The discovery by Japanese researchers of a link between a class II antigen of the major histocompatibility complex (MHC) known as DR2 and narcolepsy led to a new investigation of the genetic basis of this disorder.[30] Honda and his team have discovered that 100% of the Japanese narcoleptic patients studied to date express DR2. British, French, Canadian, and U.S. investigators have confirmed the findings that, with few initial exceptions,[31–39] the great majority of Caucasian and black narcoleptics studied also express HLA-DR2 DQW1 (now called DQw15). This near-perfect association strongly supports a genetic basis for the susceptibility to the illness, which would involve a gene on the short arm of the sixth chromosome at the locus of HLA-DR2. However, recent family studies of narcoleptic index cases performed by our team and others have provided challenging data.

Montplaisir and Poirier,[40] in a recent survey (interviews and questionnaires) found that 23% of index cases had a family history of the disease and that 44% of them had at least one other relative who suffered from daytime sleepiness. In 1988, we pooled 334 probands who exhibited sleep attacks and cataplexy and abnormal sleep-onset REM periods at polygraphic recordings.[24] All of these patients would have met the strictest criteria for the definition of narcolepsy, including those of Honda. Direct patient interviews, rather than questionnaires sent to patients, assured us that questions were well understood. It became clear that the family history was often inaccurate and more vague than had been suspected. Deceased subjects were reported to have presented a higher rate of symptoms of daytime sleepiness or sleep attacks and cataplexy than living subjects, which obviously could not be verified.

After interviewing these well-documented probands, we obtained the following results: 176 patients (53%) had no known family history of sleep attacks and cataplexy; 18 patients (5%) reported a history of sleep attacks and cataplexy in a family member; and 132 patients (40%) reported EDS in another family member.[24]

We compared our results with our previous investigation[28] in 1972 and 1973. The 1972 study involved only 50 probands; at that time we had already found a low rate of narcolepsy and cataplexy (5.5%) in the surveyed population but a family history of EDS in 34%. To complete our new study, we asked 20 "sleepy" family members to be monitored for 24 hours (by nocturnal PSG and MSLT). These subjects were selected not randomly but according to location: they lived within a reasonable distance of the sleep center. Twelve presented obstructive sleep apnea, three had periodic leg movements during sleep and sleep fragmentation, two did not respond to objective criteria for sleepiness, one had an abnormal sleep-wake schedule, and only two would have qualified for the diagnosis of isolated idiopathic sleepiness. Though it is undoubtedly difficult to generalize from these findings, we believe that the published number of isolated EDS cases that can appropriately be related to narcolepsy (in questionnaire studies covering family members of narcoleptics) has been inflated. Determining the relationship between narcolepsy syndrome and isolated reports of EDS in a family member would require systematic monitoring of all suspected subjects. This could be very expensive and difficult; in our population, most relatives lived outside the Bay Area, or even out of state.

Thus, the first finding from these new data was that a relationship did not necessarily exist between narcolepsy and EDS in other family members.

Our second finding, echoed by the Japanese, Canadian, French, and German researchers, was that familial occurrence of narcolepsy is not a very frequent phenomenon.[41] Also, the implication of HLA-DR2 DQw6 (DQw15) in narcolepsy is now more complicated than was initially thought. The Japanese researchers still doubt the existence of non–HLA-DRw15 DQw6 narcolepsy cases.[41] However, the documentation of non–HLA-DR2 DQw1 cases is now fairly convincing, at least in Caucasians and in blacks as far as DRw15 is concerned.[24,32,38] Even if the percentage is estimated at 93% for HLA-DR2–positive narcoleptics, the present well-documented cases of non–HLA-DR2 narcoleptics prove that it is not necessary to be HLA-DR2 positive to be narcoleptic. Moreover, family studies throughout the world have shown that many family members have shared the HLA antigen haplotype for disease susceptibility with the proband and have never developed narcolepsy. For example, in one Japanese investigation of 17 families, 22 subjects had the same haplotype for disease susceptibility as the proband, but 13 subjects had no symptoms whatsoever, eight presented EDS in non-PSG studies, and only one suffered from narcolepsy.[39,40] Our investigation showed similar results in the 18 families studied.[24] We conclude that an association frequently exists between narcolepsy and the presence of HLA-DRw15 DQw6 (DR2 DQw1) but that the association is neither sufficient nor necessary for the development of narcolepsy, which indicates that other factors may be involved.

Investigation of published pedigrees of families with several affected members has further complicated the issue. It must be emphasized that families with at least three living narcoleptic members who also had HLA typing, are rare in the literature. We were able to review six families: three Canadians (J. Montplaisir, personal communication), one German, one French, and one Japanese.[41] In two of these six families, one proband was HLA DR2 homozygous. In the German family studied by Mueller-Eckhardt and associates,[39] three siblings and one of the parents presented narcolepsy. One affected sibling did not share the same HLA haplotype (coming from the affected parent) with the two other affected siblings. This rendered interpretation of the genetic transmission of the illness through HLA-DR2 very difficult. To explain the discrepancy, the authors suggested a recombinant haplotype.[39–41] This notion is credible, but at best it is only one of many possibilities. Probably the most damaging evidence against the genetic transmission of narcolepsy through DR2 or a closely located gene is our recent finding of a family in which six members presented all the clinical symptoms of narcolepsy and PSG documented sleep-onset REM periods but had negative tests for HLA-DR2 DQw1 (DQw6). Not only were all family members DR2 negative, but three-fourths of the patients with cataplexy did not share similar haplotypes. There was, however, a high familial incidence of both daytime sleepiness and cataplexy through several generations. The existence of a genetic element was thus once again strongly supported. The number 1 proband also had two affected daughters who had two different fathers, which eliminated, in that family, a recessive gene hypothesis. The transmission of narcolepsy in this family can, in some respects, be compared to the canine model of narcolepsy, in which the genetic transmission has been shown to be different from the dog leukocyte antigen (DLA) complex. A similar family was reported by Singh and colleagues.[42]

A final critical observation has been made by Montplaisir and Poirier[40] and our group at Stanford: we have observed monozygotic twin pairs who are discordant for narcolepsy. Twin studies are always important in genetic investigations, and cases of monozygotic twins in which narcolepsy was diagnosed are often cited as evidence for a genetic etiology of the disease. Many of the older cases, however, are unconvincing when judged by present-day standards. Before 1985, HLA typing was not widespread, and MSLTs often were not performed in the course of clinical evaluations of narcolepsy. Montplaisir and Poirier[40] (two pairs) and our team[24] (one pair) have now investigated in depth three pairs of monozygotic twins discordant for narcolepsy. The Canadian twins are over 50 years of age, and their monozygocity was established by HLA typing. Our own pair are 42 years old, and monozygocity was established by HLA typing and DNA fingerprinting. In each case, the affected twin developed symptoms during the teenage years. All express DR2 DQw1. The existence of discordant monozygotic twins indicates that non-genetic factors participate in the development of narcolepsy, but we reiterate that the genetic factor in narcolepsy, specifically the major association between HLA-DR2 (DRw15) and narcolepsy, cannot be dismissed, even though up to 4% of patients may not express HLA DR2.

The association between DRw15 DQw6 and narcolepsy is of particular interest because of the link between the human leukocyte antigen and autoimmune disease. Though there is very little evidence at this date to implicate the immune system in the pathogenesis of narcolepsy, the very strong associatiohn between DRw15 and the disease makes a compelling argument for immune system involvement. Investigations in Doberman pinschers have shown that, in this dog breed, narcolepsy is transmitted through a single autosomal recessive gene called CANARC 1. Gene markers for CANARC 1 have indicated that it is not linked to the canine major histocompatibility complex but is tightly linked to an S-like gene. SM is the switch region of the immunoglobulin heavy chain gene. This last finding also suggests also involvement of the immune system in the pathophysiology of the disease. One could propose a model in which a combination of several different factors would be necessary for the development of narcolepsy in most cases: (1) a genetic factor not linked to the HLA system, which would be a susceptibility gene, (2) the presence of HLA-DRw15 DQw6 (the key element being DQw6) and (3) the involvement of an environmental factor, possibly a viral infection. The hypothesis would not explain the non-DQw6 cases, which are much less common than the non-DRw15 cases, but until the susceptibility gene is identified such cases cannot be clearly explained.

Is there any support for possible immune system or viral involvement in the development of narcolepsy? Billiard and coworkers[43] have reported that in a study involving 52 narcoleptics, elevated antibody to streptolysin O (ABO titers) was found in 22 patients (compared with one in 49 controls), and elevated antibody to DNase B titers was observed in 13 patients and none of the controls. However, Montplaisir (personal communication) was unable to replicate the ABO findings in his patient population.

Clearly, at this time, one must conclude that some combination of genetic and environmental factors is probably involved in the development of human narcolepsy. The sequencing of DR in two narcoleptic patients (in England and USA) has not shown any difference between these patients and an unaffected subject. Further investigation of canine narcolepsy, which allows one to obtain back-crosses and several affected litters, may be of further help.

ETIOLOGIC AND PHARMACOLOGIC STUDIES AND THE ANIMAL MODEL

Over the past 10 years, an animal model of the narcolepsy-cataplexy syndrome has been developed at Stanford University. Several breeds of dogs have been collected that exhibit symptoms that closely resemble those of human narcolepsy. The usefulness of studying a naturally occurring disorder in an animal model depends on its similarity to the human form of the disorder. Of the four major symptoms of human narcolepsy, two, EDS and cataplexy, are present in most human patients and in dogs afflicted with narcolepsy.

Cataplexy is a brief episode of generalized nonreciprocal motor inhibition that is entirely reversible. It is essentially identical in humans and in dogs.[44,45] In canine cataplexy, the episode is often induced by a clear emotional component such as feeding, chewing, playing, or appetitive behaviors such as gnawing on a package of food or attempting sexual intercourse. As in humans, there is no loss of alertness during the briefer cataplectic attacks or during the initial stage of longer attacks in dogs. The waking-state sensorium remains intact, and the dog visually tracks objects if its eyes are open. Tendon reflexes are inactive during a cataplectic attack, but they return once cataplexy is terminated, and there are no residual neurologic abnormalities. Electrographic variables resemble those of wakefulness during the initial stage of cataplexy, whereas the later stage is indistinguishable from REM sleep. Finally, cataplexy in dogs is suppressed by the same REM-suppressant drugs that are used to treat human cataplexy.[46-50] Also, narcoleptic dogs consistently have short sleep latency, typically less than 5 minutes, on all tests, whereas normal dogs show much longer latencies.[48]

Investigations in Dobermans and Labrador retrievers have shown transmission via an identical autosomal recessive mode[49,50]; the recessive gene has full penetrance. Not all dog breeds exhibit genetic transmission of narcolepsy, as evidenced by unsuccessful efforts to breed affected poodles and beagles.[49] These findings suggest that there may be different causes for the canine narcolepsy syndrome: (1) inheritance via a single autosomal recessive gene with complete penetrance; (2) nongenetic mechanisms such as developmental accidents or CNS trauma, or (3) more complex polygenic mechanisms that produce unaffected offspring from narcoleptic parents. The Doberman and Labrador models have allowed the performance of pharmacologic studies searching for specific receptor defects.

CURRENT TREATMENT

The drugs most widely used against EDS are the CNS stimulants. Amphetamines were first proposed by Prinzmetal and Bloomberg[51] in 1935. The alerting effect of a single oral dose of amphetamine is at its maximum 2 to 4 hours after administration, and many patients require daily or twice-daily dosing. A number of side effects, including irritability, tachycardia, nocturnal sleep disturbances, and sometimes tolerance and drug dependence may arise. The use of methylphenidate was later encouraged,[52] because of faster action and lower incidence of side effects. Pemoline, an oxazolidine derivative with a longer half-life and slower onset of action, is less efficient but well tolerated.[53] CRL-40476 (Modanfinil), an alpha-stimulant medication currently under investigation in Europe, was recently reported, in France, to bring substantial improvement.[54] The new (MAOIB) selegiline has none of the tyramine-related side effects and appears to be helpful in the treatment of EDS.[55] The pharmacologic activity of the drug on sleepiness may be related to a levo-amphetamine metabolite.

Mazindol, an imidazoline derivative, has been shown to reduce the number of daytime sleep episodes in narcoleptics in a dose range of 3 to 8 mg. Side effects are minor.[56] γ-Hydroxybutyrate (GHB), a drug available in France and Canada and investigational in the United States, which is given orally at bedtime and at the time of a night awakening, has definite value even though its efficiency varies between patients.[57]

The treatment of cataplexy, sleep paralysis, and hypnagogic hallucinations calls for tricyclic medications. Both protriptyline in North America and clomipramine in Europe have been widely used, often with good responses. Other tricyclic medications such as imipramine and norpramine are also effective; however, the atropine-like side effects, particularly impotence in men, have prompted a search for new compounds. Viloxazine hydrochloride, a norepinephrine reuptake blocker that seems well-tolerated by patients, including elderly ones, is one of these new compounds. Incremental dose increases of viloxazine hydrochloride, from 100 to 200 or 300 mg daily, may completely prevent the rare appearance of headaches or nausea in elderly subjects.[58] Clonidine,[59] also a potent REM sleep suppressant, has too many side effects. Fluoxetine has been reported to be helpful against cataplexy.[60] MAOIs such as phenelzine[61] have been used to treat intractable narcolepsy-cataplexy, but the frequently dangerous side effects have severely limited its use, in comparison to selegiline.

Nocturnal sleep disturbances seem to be better controlled by GHB[62] than by the benzodiazepines. The advantage of improving nocturnal sleep is significant not only for daytime sleepiness but also for cataplexy, though stimulant medications are often necessary with GHB. Patients who present the full clinical tetrad frequently need a combination of drugs, particularly stimulants and tricyclics; GHB or a benzodiazepine may be needed at night.

Very recently Mouret and coworkers[63] reported a beneficial response with L-tyrosine in eight narcoleptic patients. They were treated over 6 months with daily doses ranging from 64 to 120 mg/kg (average 100 mg/kg) given orally in three doses (L-tyrosine 99.3% pure from Rexel Laboratories–Degussa Chemical Corporation, France). Despite the interest of this report and the fact that the beneficial effect of L-tyrosine could be related to some of the known pharmacologic abnormalities seen in canine narcolepsy, the results should be viewed with caution. This study was an open study with few patients, and the reported polygraphic data do not cover daytime. Our own investigation of L-tyrosine brought negative results, as did one performed by Parkes in England.

To better understand the efficacy of the different available drugs, Mitler and Hajdukovic[64] compared the efficacy of putative therapeutic agents on daytime sleepiness results from MSLT and maintenance of wakefulness test (MWT) published in the literature (Figure 18-1) The authors normalized the data, obtained on 179 narcoleptics, and reported the results as percentages of normal values obtained on a control group. The drugs tested were dextroamphetamine, methylphenidate, pemoline, modafinil (CRL-40476), protriptyline, viloxazine, ritanserin, codeine, and GHB.

The study shows that even with the largest recommended doses no drug brings narcoleptics to normal alertness. Dexedrine (dextroamphetamine) and methylphenidate most improved patients' alertness. GHB, protriptyline, and ritanserin had an insignificant impact. Viloxazine, modafinil, and pemoline had mild to moderate effect. Codeine is the least investigated of

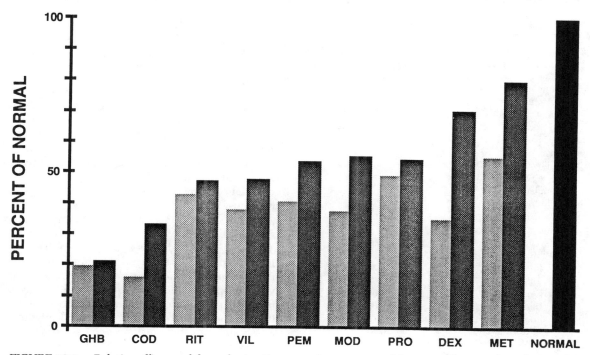

FIGURE 18-1. *Relative efficacy of drugs for treating narcolepsy presented in terms of percentage of normal levels of sleepiness. The lightest shading denotes baseline values; the intermediate shading treatment values. The darkest shading is used only for normal values. Key: GHB, γ-hydroxybutyrate; COD, codeine; RIT, ritanserin; VIL, viloxazine; PEM, pemoline; MOD, modafinil; PRO, protriptyline; DEX, dextroamphetamine; MET, methylphenidate. (From Miller M, Hajdukovic R. Relative efficacy of drugs for the treatment of sleepiness in narcolepsy. Sleep 1991;14:218–220, with permission.)*

these drugs, but it actually shows more promise than viloxazine, modafinil, or pemoline.

The drugs that stimulate norepinephrine release (amphetamines and methylphenidate) seem to have the greatest impact on sleepiness. This seems to be true also in the dog model of narcolepsy. As α-lb agonists appear to significantly improve canine narcolepsy, it is possible that such agents will prove beneficial to humans. Modafinil (CRL-40476) does not have a direct effect on the α-lb, which may explain its limited activity. More specific compounds may give better results.

Two other therapeutic approaches must be emphasized: short daytime naps and support groups. A 15- to 20-minute nap taken three times daily helps maintain a satisfactory level of vigilance. It has never been demonstrated that stimulant medications improve alertness more effectively. Naps have to be repeated throughout the day, as the "refractory" sleep period following a nap varies between 90 and 120 minutes. Undoubtedly, narcolepsy is a disabling disorder, leading in many instances to loss of gainful employment because of daytime sleepiness and automatic behavior. It is also often ill-understood by patients, family members, and peers. It can result in rejection from family and other social groups, in

divorce, loss of self-esteem, and depressive reactions. For these reasons, also, considering the young age at onset of the syndrome, it is important to put narcolepsy patients in contact with support groups and to help create regional narcolepsy associations and patient groups. Tables 18-1 and 18-2 summarize the drugs currently available and the treatment for narcolepsy.

CLINICAL VARIANTS AND ASSOCIATED ILLNESSES

The issue of "symptomatic" narcolepsy is difficult to resolve. There are, however, some rare but clearly documented forms of posttraumatic narcolepsy with EDS and cataplexy. The issue of narcolepsy (with or without cataplexy) and multiple sclerosis (MS) is conceptually interesting. Both have been postulated to be disorders of immunoreactivity, and the frequency of HLA-DR2 is also increased among MS patients, but a preliminary study has not demonstrated a significant difference in sleepiness complaints between MS patients who express DR2 and those who do not. Similarly, if rheumatoid arthritis, another DR2-linked disorder, may occur with narcolepsy

TABLE 18-1.   Currently Available Narcolepsy Drugs

Drugs	Maximum Dosage* (mg/day)
Treatment of EDS	
Stimulants	
Amphetamine	40
Methylphenidate	60 (in divided doses)
Mazindol	5
Pemoline	150
Adjunctive effect Drugs (i.e., improve EDS if associated with stimulant)	
Protriptyline	10
Viloxazine	200
Treatment of auxiliary effects	
Tricyclic antidepressants	
With atropine-like side effects:	
Protriptyline	20
Imipramine	200
Clomipramine	200
Desipramine	200
Without atropine side effects:	
Viloxazine	200
Experimental drugs or drugs available in very few countries	
Stimulant	
CRL 40476	
Codeine (given as stimulant)	
Cataplexy antagonist and mild stimulant: (γ-hydroxybutyrate)	

*All drugs are taken by mouth.

(personal observation), the association is far from frequent. As DQw6 may be more important than DRw15, the lack of association may not be surprising.

Sleep apnea may be seen more frequently with narcolepsy. As obstructive sleep apnea may lead to significant sleep fragmentation, the association of sleep-onset REM periods and daytime sleepiness at MSLT is insufficient to consider a disorder's association. A recent study on 100 sleep apnea patients found that 24% of them had two or more sleep-onset REM periods at MSLT (personal observation). However, the association of daytime sleepiness, cataplexy, and sleep apnea can undoubtedly be noted, with cataplexy affirming the presence of the narcolepsy syndrome.[65] The association of these two disorders enhances the disability linked to daytime sleepiness. The association between periodic leg movement syndrome (PLMS) and narcolepsy has been mentioned, though one must remember that imipramine, clomipramine, and protriptyline increase the number of PLMs during sleep, an increase that also is associated with aging. PLMS seem to be more frequent in narcoleptic patients than in the general population,[66] though Montplaisir and Godbout[67] do not believe, from their own analysis, that PMLS is an important factor in nocturnal sleep disturbance in narcolepsy.

The major items in the differential diagnosis are CNS hypersomnia syndrome and the syndromes associating EDS with the presence of one or several sleep-onset REM periods, as discussed in the Positive Diagnosis section. Idiopathic CNS hypersomnia syndrome, which is characterized by EDS, should be considered a possible diagnostic only when obstructive sleep apnea syndrome and upper airway resistance syndrome have been ruled out. The daytime somnolence is rarely relieved by short naps as in narcolepsy. In fact, naps may lead to sleep drunkenness and complaints of increased tiredness. Frequently reported with this syndrome are mild symptoms of autonomic nervous system dysfunction such as cold hands, cold feet (Raynaud's-type phenomena), lightheadedness (rarely associated with a drop in systolic blood pressure sufficient to be called orthostatic hypotension), and frequent dull headaches that may have a typical migraine presentation. In some instances the syndrome develops immediately following mononucleosis, Guillain-Barré syndrome, viral hepatitis, or atypical pneumonia, particularly that involving echoviruses, which suggests that a virus might participate in the appearance of idiopathic CNS hypersomnia. PSG and MSLT show lack of sleep-onset REM periods and a mean sleep latency of about 6 minutes. Tables 18-3 and 18-4 summarize the pertinent features for diagnosis and differential diagnosis of narcolepsy.

In conclusion, despite the many studies and publications on narcolepsy during the past 90 years, a complete understanding of the narcolepsy syndrome still eludes us. Narcolepsy remains a very disabling neurologic illness that is poorly or incompletely controlled by treatment. It leads to a variety of complications when it goes undiagnosed, such as traffic and industrial accidents. Narcolepsy is a major employment problem for its victims owing to many employers' unwillingness to allow short (15-minute) naps two or three times during the day. It is often responsible for job discrimination, job dismissal, early retirement, and depression secondary to these circumstances.[68]

The question of whether EDS slowly worsens with age is unresolved at this time. As aging is often associated with more disturbed nocturnal sleep, it is possible that the nocturnal sleep disturbances noted with aging worsen the EDS of narcoleptics. A survey performed on the Stanford Sleep Disorders Clinic narcoleptic population showed that 62% of narcoleptics older than 47 years of age had no recourse other than to apply for Social Security disability benefits.

TABLE 18-2. Treatment for Narcolepsy

I. Treatment for cataplexy and sleep paralysis, with or without hypnagogic hallucinations or panic reaction to sleep paralysis, is tricyclic antidepressants. Best medications are nonatropinic tricyclics, as they have fewer side effects.

    Viloxazine HCl (50-mg tablets) PO. Normal dose 150–200 mg daily.

    Fluoxetine HCl (20-mg tablets) PO. Normal dose (in the morning).

    Clomipramine (25 or 50-mg tablets) PO. Normal dose 75–125 mg daily (at bedtime).

  Other tricyclics with atropine-like side effects:

    Protriptyline (5-mg tablets) PO. Normal dose 10–15 mg (in the morning or divided) Impotence is common with 15–20 mg.

    Imipramine (25- or 30-mg tables) PO. Normal dose 75–125 mg daily (divided or in the evening).

II. Treatment for sleepiness

    Behavioral treatment

      Scheduled short 15-minute daytime naps

      Best time; 10:30 A.M., 1:00 P.M., 4:00 P.M.

      Schedules most frequently used by patients: 1:00 to 2:00 P.M., and 4:30 to 6:00 P.M.

    Nutrition

      Avoid heavy lunches, avoid alcohol and foods or beverages that have paradoxical effects, such as chocolate.

    Medication

      No medication completely alleviates daytime sleepiness, but will help to improve performance.

    Best medications:

      For children and adolescents:

      Pemoline (18.75- and 37.5-mg tablets).

      Efficacy increases progressively over 1 week. Dosage varies with age (weight), between 37 and 150 mg/day.

      For adults:

      1. Methylphenidate (5-mg tablets) PO, taken at least 30 to 45 minutes before or after a meal. Repeat doses throughout the day and avoid one large dose (short half-life)

          Advantages: can be taken when needed; rapid action

          Usual dosage: 20 to 40 mg/day.   Avoid more than 50 mg/day—no clinical gain.

      The slow-release form of this drug is available and may be used in the morning by U.S. Medicaid patients, whose only authorized dose is 20-mg tablets.

      2. Pemoline (37.5 mg tablets) PO. One or two daily doses (morning, noon). Normal dosage is 100 to 150 mg/day.

      3. Dexedrine (5-mg tablets) PO. Normal dosage 10 to 40 mg/day. Divided doses or slow-release formula recommended to avoid side effects. New patients should first be treated with other drugs.

      4. Mazindol (2-mg tablets) PO. Normal dosage 4 to 8 mg/day in two doses.

      5. Modafinil is available in several European countries on a restricted basis, presented as a nonamphetamine stimulant.

III. Examples of treatment packages

    Prepubertal children

      For sleepiness

        Contact school to alert teachers

        Nap at lunch time

        Nap at 4:00 to 5:00 P.M.

        Medication: Pemoline, one to three 18.75-mg tablets daily

      For cataplexy

        Clomipramine 25 to 50 mg at bedtime

    Pubertal children

      For sleepiness

        Contact school to alert teachers

        Emphasize need for regular nocturnal sleep schedule

        Try to obtain 9 hours' nocturnal sleep

        Nap at lunch time and 4:00 or 5:00 P.M.

        Medication: pemoline, one to three 37.5-mg tablets daily

    Adults

      Avoid shifting sleep schedule

      Avoid heavy meals and alcohol

      Regular timing of nocturnal sleep: 10:30 P.M. to 7:00 A.M.

      Naps: 15 minutes at lunch time and at 5:30 P.M.

      Medications:

        For daytime sleepiness

          Methylphenidate, 5 mg × ¾ or 20 mg SR morning, on empty stomach

          If difficulties persist:

            Methylphenidate (SR):   20 mg in the morning

                                   5 mg after noon nap

                                   5 mg at 4:00 P.M.

         If no response:

          Dexedrine spansule (SR): 15 mg at awakening

                                  5 mg after noon nap

                                  5 mg at 3:30 or 4:00 P.M.

                                15 mg at awakening

                                15 mg after noon nap

      For cataplexy:

        Clomipramine 75 to 125 mg *or*

        vivactil 150 to 200 mg *or*

        imipramine 75 to 125 mg

TABLE 18-3.   How to Diagnose Narcolepsy

A. Patient reports partial or complete cataplectic attacks, daytime sleepiness and napping. B. Patient reports a history of partial or complete cataplectic attacks and current daytime sleepiness and napping. C. Patient reports partial or complete cataplectic attacks and intermittent daytime drowsiness several times per week.	Patient is narcoleptic.	Confirm by nocturnal PSG and MSLT on the following day. MSLT shows short sleep latencies. PSG shows presence or absence of sleep apnea, presence or absence of PLMs. Risk of MSLT being negative with 1-day test is 3%.
D. Patient reports isolated cataplexy. No reports of EDS or napping. E. Patient reports isolated EDS and daytime napping. F. Patient reports EDS, daytime napping, hypnagogic hallucinations, sleep paralysis.	Patient has isolated cataplexy, is not narcoleptic, but . . . Patient is not narcoleptic. See Table 18-4.	1. Confirm absence of EDS by PSG and MSLT. 2. Investigate family history for narcolepsy. 3. Perform HLA typing to search for DR2 DQw6. Patient may be developing narcolepsy. Follow patient.

TABLE 18-4.   What To Do When Patient Is Not a Bona Fide Narcoleptic*

If patient presents with EDS, daytime napping, hypnagogic hallucinations, sleep paralysis,	(1) perform polygraphic recording and daytime MSLT; (2) investigate first-degree relatives for narcolepsy, and (3) consider patient's age.
If (1) patient is young, (2) Sleep latencies in MSLT are short, (3) there is more than one sleep-onset REM period, (4) PSG shows no cause for EDS, *and* (5) there is family history (first-degree relative) of narcolepsy,	patient is probably developing narcolepsy. Follow and treat as a narcoleptic. Do HLA typing and appreciate whether DR2 DQw6 is expressed.
If patient presents with isolated EDS and daytime napping,	(1) Obtain good sleep disorders history; (2) perform nocturnal PSG and daytime MSLT; (3) investigate family history for causes of EDS, and (4) consider patient's age.
If (1) patient has no clinical symptoms for other causes of EDS; (2) tests produce a good, undisrupted nocturnal PSG without evidence of sleep-related problems; (3) MSLT produces short latencies but ≤ 1 sleep-onset REM period; (4) the family history includes narcolepsy; *and* (5) patient is young,	patient may be developing narcolepsy. Follow and treat as a narcoleptic. Perform HLA typing.
If (1) Findings are identical to 1 through 4 directly above, and (2) patient is middle aged or older, with several years' history of sleepiness,	patient is considered to have a disorder of daytime sleepiness (probably related to narcolepsy but unproven to date). HLA typing is of scientific interest for better definition of the syndrome. Treat as a narcoleptic.

TABLE 18-4. *(Continued)*

If (1) patient has no clinical symptoms for other causes of EDS;

(2) tests produce good, undisrupted nocturnal PSG without evidence of sleep-related problems;

(3) MSLT produces short sleep latencies and ≥ 2 sleep-onset REM periods;

(4) there is no family history of narcolepsy; *and*

(5) Patient is young, middle-aged, or older with several years' history of sleepiness,

patient may be developing narcolepsy (i), and must be followed. Condition is considered a disorder of isolated sleepiness (possibly a disorder of REM sleep; the relation to narcolepsy is unknown). HLA typing is of scientific interest for better understanding of the syndrome. Treat with stimulants.

If (1) patient has no clinical symptoms for other causes of EDS;

(2) tests produce good, undisrupted nocturnal PSG without evidence of sleep-related problems;

(3) MSLT produces short sleep latencies with ≤ 1 sleep-onset REM periods,

(4) *and* there is no family history of narcolepsy,

patient of any age is considered to have CNS hypersomnia (relation to narcolepsy unknown). Investigate for viral infection concomitant with syndrome onset, and possibly perform serologic studies for positive history. Investigate family for history of isolated daytime sleepiness. HLA typing is of scientific interest for better definition of the syndrome (most commonly subjects express HLA-DR2 DQw6). Treat with stimulants.

* That is, if cataplexy is not currently and never has been, present.

REFERENCES

1. Gelineau J. De la narcolepsie. Gaz Hop (Paris) 1880;53:626–628; 54:635–737.
2. Henneberg R. Uber genuine Narkolepsie. Neurol Zb1 1916;30:282–290.
3. Daniels L. Narcolepsy. Medicine 1934;13:1–122.
4. Yoss RE, Daly DD. Criteria for the diagnosis of the narcoleptic syndrome. Proc Staff Meet Mayo Clin 1957;32:320–328.
5. Vogel G. Studies in the psychophysiology of dreams III. The dream of narcolepsy. Arch Gen Psychiatry 1960;3:421–425.
6. Rechtschaffen A, Wolpert E, Dement WC, et al. Nocturnal sleep of narcoleptics. Electroencephalogr Clin Neurophysiol 1963;15:599–609.
7. Takahashi Y, Jimbo M. Polygraphic study of narcoleptic syndrome with special reference to hypnagogic hallucinations and cataplexy. Folia Psychiatr Neurol Jap 1963;suppl 7:343–347.
8. Passouant P, Schwab RS, Cadilhac J, et al. Narcolepsie-cataplexie. Etude du sommeil de nuit et du sommeil de jour. Rev Neurol (Paris) 1964;3:415–426.
9. Hishikawa Y, Kaneko Z. Electroencephalographic study on narcolepsy. Electroencephalogr Clin Neurophysiol 1965;18:249–258.
10. Guilleminault C, Dement WC, Passouant P, eds. Narcolepsy. New York: Spectrum Publications, 1975;1–689.
11. Honda Y, Juji T, eds. HLA in Narcolepsy. Berlin: Springer-Verlag, 1988;208.
12. Billiard M, Besset A, Cadilhac J. The clinical and polygraphic development of narcolepsy. In: Guilleminault C, Lugaresi E, eds. Sleep/Wake Disorders: Natural History, Epidemiology, and Long-Term Evolution. New York: Raven Press, 1983;187–199.
13. Hoddes E, Dement WC, Zarcone V. The development and use of the Stanford Sleepiness Scale (SSS). Psychophysiology 1972;9:150.
14. Yoss RE, Mayer NJ, Ogle KN. The pupillogram and narcolepsy. Neurology 1969;19:921–928.
15. Schmidt HS, Fortin LD. Electronic pupillography in disorders of arousal. In: Guilleminault C, ed. Sleep and waking disorders: Indications and techniques. Menlo Park, Calif.: Addison Wesley, 1981;127–141.
16. Berlucchi G, Moruzzi G, Salva G, et al. Pupil behavior and ocular movements during synchronized and de-synchronized sleep. Arch Ital Biol 1964;102:230.
17. Carskadon MA, Dement WC. The multiple sleep latency test: What does it measure? Sleep 1982;5:67–72.
18. Rechtschaffen A, Kales AD. A Manual of Standardized Terminology, Techniques and Scoring System for Sleep Stages of Human Subjects. Los Angeles: Brain Information Service/Brain Research Institute, UCLA, 1968.
19. Association of Professional Sleep Societies Guidelines Committee. Guidelines for the Multiple Sleep Latency Test (MSLT): A standard measure of sleepiness. Sleep 1986;9:519–524.
20. Van den Hoed J, Kraemer H, Guilleminault C, et al. Disorders of excessive daytime somnolence: Polygraphic and clinical data for 100 patients. Sleep 1981;4:23–38.
21. Browman CP, Gujavarty KS, Sampson MG, et al. REM sleep episodes during the maintenance of wakefulness tests in patients with sleep apnea syndrome and patients with narcolepsy. Sleep 1983;6:23–28.
21a. EEG Arousals: Scoring Rules and Examples, A preliminary report from the Sleep Disorders Atlas Task Force of the American Sleep Disorders Association. Sleep 1992;15:174–184.
22. Broughton R, Low R, Valley V, et al. Auditory evoked potentials compared to EEG and performance measures of impaired vigilance in narcolepsy-cataplexy. Sleep Res 1981;10:184.
23. Moscovitch A, Partinen M, Patterson-Rhoads N, et al. Cataplexy in differentiation of excessive daytime somnolence. Sleep Res 1991;20:303.
24. Guilleminault C, Mignot E, Grumet C. Family study of narcolepsy. Lancet 1989;11:1376–1380.
25. World Health Organization (WHO) Nomenclature Committee for Factors of the HLA System. Nomenclature

for factors of the HLA system, 1989. Immunogenetics 1990;31:131–140.

26. Dement WC, Zarcone V, Varner V, et al. The prevalence of narcolepsy. Sleep 1972;1:148.

27. Dement WC, Carskadon MA, Ley R. The prevalence of narcolepsy. Sleep Res 1973;2:147.

28. Kessler S, Guilleminault C, Dement WC. A family study of 50 REM narcoleptics. Arch Neurol Scand 1974;50:503–512.

29. Honda Y, Asaka A, Tanimura M, et al. A genetic study of narcolepsy and excessive daytime sleepiness in 308 families with a narcolepsy of hypersomnia proband. In: Guilleminault C, Lugaresi E, eds, Sleep/Wake Disorders: Natural History, Epidemiology and Long-Term Evolution. New York: Raven Press, 1983;187–199.

30. Honda Y, Asaka A, Tanaka Y, et al. Discrimination of narcoleptic patients by using genetic markers and HLA [Abstr]. Sleep Res 1983;12:254.

31. Langdon N, Welch KI, Dam MV, et al. Genetic markers in narcolepsy. Lancet 1984;2:1178–1180.

32. Guilleminault C, Grumet C. HLA-DR2 and narcolepsy: Not all narcoleptic cataplectic patients are DR2. Hum Immuno 1986;17:1–2.

33. Juji T, Satake M, Honda Y, et al. HLA antigens in Japanese patients with narcolepsy—all the patients were DR2 positive. Tissue Antigens 1984;24:316–319.

34. Seignalet J, Billiard M. Possible associations between HLA-B7 and narcolepsy. Tissue Antigens 1984;23: 188–189.

35. Billiard M, Seignalet J. Extraordinary association between HLA-DR2 and narcolepsy. Lancet 1985;2:226–227.

36. Poirier G, Montplaisir J, Decary F, et al. HLA antigens in narcolepsy and idiopathic central nervous system hypersomnolence. Sleep 1986;9:153–158.

37. Langdon N, Lock C, Welsh K, et al. Immune factors in narcolepsy. Sleep 1986;9:143–148.

38. Neely SE, Rosenberg AS, Spire JP, et al. HLA antigens in narcolepsy. Neurology 1987;37:1858–1860.

39. Mueller-Eckhardt G, Meier-Ewert K, Schendel DJ, et al. HLA and narcolepsy in a German population. Tissue Antigens 1986;28:163–169.

40. Montplaisir J, Poirier G. HLA in narcolepsy in Canada. In: Honda Y, Juji T, eds. HLA in Narcolepsy. Berlin: Springer-Verlag, 1988;97–107.

41. Matsuki K, Honda Y, Satake M, et al. HLA in narcolepsy in Japan. In: Honda Y, Juji T, eds. HLA in Narcolepsy. Berlin: Springer-Verlag, 1988;58–76.

42. Singh S, George CFP, Kryger MH, et al. Genetic heterogeneity in narcolepsy. Lancet 1990;11:726–727.

43. Billiard M, Laaberki MF, Reygrobillet C, et al. Elevated antibody to streptolysin O and antibody to DNase B titers in narcoleptic subjects. Sleep Res 1989;18:201.

44. Mitler MM, Boysen BG, Campbell L, et al. Narcolepsy-cataplexy in a female dog. Exp Neurol 1974;45:332–340.

45. Mitler MM, Dement WC. Sleep studies on canine narcolepsy: Pattern and cycle comparisons between affected and normal dogs. Electroencephalogr Clin Neurophysiol 1977;43:691–699.

46. Delashaw J, Foutz Z, Guilleminault C, et al. Cholinergic mechanisms and cataplexy in dogs. Exp Neurol 1978;66:745–757.

47. Foutz AS, Delashaw JB Jr, Guilleminault C, et al. Monoaminergic mechanisms and experimental cataplexy. Neurology 1981;10:369–376.

48. Lucas EA. A study of the daily sleep and waking patterns of the laboratory cat and dog. Sleep Res 1978;7:142.

49. Foutz AS, Mitler MM, Cavalli-Sforza LL, et al. Genetic factors in canine narcolepsy. Sleep 1979;1:413–422.

50. Baker TL, Narver EL, Dement WC, et al. Effects of imipramine, chlorimipramine, and fluoxetine on cataplexy in dogs. Pharmacol Biochem Behav 1976;5:599–602.

51. Prinzmetal M, Bloomberg W. The use of benzedrine for treatment of narcolepsy. JAMA 1935;105:2051–2054.

52. Yoss RE, Daly DD. Treatment of narcolepsy with Ritalin. Neurology 1959;9:171–173.

53. Honda Y, Hishikawa Y. Effectiveness of pemoline in narcolepsy. Sleep Res 1970;8:192.

54. Farma L, Galland Y. Treatment of Narcoleptics with CRL-40476, an Alpha Stimulant Medication [Abstr]. 7th European Sleep Congress, abstract manual Munich, FRG, 1984.

55. Roselaar SE, Langdon N, Lock CB, et al. Selegiline in narcolepsy. Sleep 1987;10 491–495.

56. Parkes JD, Schacter M. Mazindol in the treatment of narcolepsy. Acta Neurol Scand 1979;60:250–254.

57. Broughton R, Mamelak M. Effects of nocturnal gamma-hydroxybutyrate on sleep/waking patterns in narcolepsy-cataplexy. Can J Neurol Sci 1980;7:23–31.

58. Guilleminault C, Mancuso J, Quera Salva MA, et al. Viloxazine hydrochloride in narcolepsy: A preliminary report. Sleep 1986;9:275–279.

59. Putkonen PT, Bergstrom L. Clonidine alleviated cataplectic symptoms in narcolepsy. In: Koella WP, ed, Sleep 1980. Basel: S Karger, 1981; 414–416.

60. Langdon N, Bandak S, Shindler J, et al. Fluoxetine in the treatment of cataplexy. Sleep 1986;9–371.

61. Wyatt R, Fram D, Buchbinder R, et al. Treatment of intractable narcolepsy with a monoamine oxidase inhibitor. Engl J Med 1971;285:987–999.

62. Mamelak M, Scharf MB, Woods M. Treatment of narcolepsy with γ-hydroxybutyrate. A review of clinical and sleep laboratory findings. Sleep 1986;9:285–289.

63. Mouret J, Sanchez P, Taillard J, et al. Treatment of narcolepsy with L-tyrosine. Lancet 1988;ii:1458–1459.

64. Mitler M, Hajdukovic R. Relative efficacy of drugs for the treatment of sleepiness in narcolepsy. Sleep 1991;14:218–220.

65. Guilleminault C, Van den Hoed J, Mitler MM. Clinical overview of the sleep apnea syndromes. In: Guilleminault C, Dement WC, eds. Sleep Apnea Syndromes. New York: Alan R. Liss, 1978;1–12.

66. Baker TL, Guilleminault C, Nino-Murcia G, et al. Comparative polysomnographic study of narcolepsy and idiopathic central nervous system hypersomnia. Sleep 1986;9:232–242.

67. Montplaisir J, Godbout R. Nocturnal sleep of narcoleptic patients: Revisited. Sleep 1986;9:159–161.

68. Broughton R, Ghanem Q, Hishikawa Y, et al. Life effects of narcolepsy in 180 patients from North America, Asia, and Europe compared to matched controls. Can J Sci 1981;8:299–304.

19

Motor Functions and Dysfunctions of Sleep

Wayne A. Hening
Arthur S. Walters
Sudhansu Chokroverty

The motor system is strongly modulated by the changes in state from wake to drowsiness to slow-wave sleep (SWS) and then to rapid eye movement (REM) sleep. Indeed, so significant are the changes in motor activity depending on state that various researchers have used quantitative recordings of motor activity, such as actigraphy, as a basis for determining sleep and wake states.[1] In this chapter, we will first briefly review normal motor activity and its changes during sleep, then examine motor disturbances associated with sleep.

Motor disturbances associated with sleep can be loosely sorted into two categories. First, there are motor disturbances (diurnal movement disorders) present during the daytime that may have an impact on sleep, either directly through their motor effects or indirectly through a variety of other mechanisms. These are the typical movement disorders that are seen by a movement disorder specialist. Second, there are motor disturbances that are predominantly associated with sleep. They may be motor activity similar to what is normally found during waking hours that intrudes upon sleep (some parasomnias, such as sleep walking, are of this type) or abnormal motor activity that does not occur during the wake state but is aroused by sleep. These are generally classified as sleep disorders and primarily are treated by a sleep disorder specialist. These two main categories are by no means completely unique, and it is not unusual for a patient with a disorder in one category to be seen by a specialist in the other category. For example, the waking involuntary movements of the restless legs syndrome (RLS) may bring such a patient to a movement disorder specialist. It is, therefore, useful to consider these two categories of sleep disturbances together in this chapter.

In line with the dual nature of motor disturbances of sleep, this chapter has two major purposes. First, it aims to provide both the movement disorder specialist and the sleep medicine specialist with a summary of sleep-related problems that might be expected to arise in connection with a patient who has

a diurnal movement disorder. Second, the chapter hopes to show how to approach the diagnosis and treatment of motor disturbances of sleep, in general, both those considered to be movement disorders and those considered to be primarily sleep disorders. While this chapter touches quite briefly on the distinctions between the various movement disorders, it does not pretend to be a general review of movement disorders. Those in the sleep field who wish a general review of movement disorders can find a number of recent treatises that deal extensively with a wide spectrum of movement disorders.[2-5] There are also a number of excellent, more abbreviated, treatments of this field in medical and neurologic textbooks.[6,7] Because this chapter is a volume that deals specifically with sleep medicine, the other chapters provide a suitable background for sleep-related issues for the neurologist or other persons whose primary field is movement disorders. Where issues have overlapped—such as the parasomnias that cause motor disturbances—other chapters in this volume are cited, so as not to unnecessarily increase the length of the entire volume.

THE MOTOR SYSTEM IN RELATION TO SLEEP

Before specific motor disturbances of sleep are discussed, we review the normal physiology of the motor system during sleep and the patterns of normal motor activity that vary with the circadian rhythm, different sleep stages, and human development and aging. Abnormal activity, in different cases, may follow this same background activity pattern or may deviate from it in striking ways.

Physiology of the Motor System in Relation to Sleep

The motor system can be considered very roughly to have three main units or levels: higher centers, segmental centers, and the motor unit (motor neuron and related muscle fibers). The higher centers are located in the brain and brain stem, where they receive diverse information from other brain regions, including those involved with the senses. These centers include the motor, premotor, and supplementary motor cortices, the basal ganglia and cerebellum, and various brain stem nuclei, including the reticular nuclei of the pons and the medulla. They provide descending control to segmental motor centers at the brain stem and spinal cord level, as well as some direct connections in humans to motor neurons. The segmental centers, in turn, channel and moderate descending and afferent inputs from somatosensory organs, so as to control the "final common path," the motor neuron. In addition to serving as way-stations or integrating stations, the segmental centers may also generate their own activity. Many studies have shown that the brain stem and spinal cord, even in complete isolation, can produce patterned motor activity such as locomotion.[8] This indicates that they have endogenous oscillators and other organized neural networks. The motor neuron, with its associated set of muscle fibers within a specific muscle, collectively known as the motor unit, is the ultimate effector responsible for motor activity. Between each of the levels, but especially between the segmental centers and higher centers, there is continuous two-way communication. Also, of course, the motor system is receiving a continuous flow of inputs from the various afferent systems, including the different sensory systems. In later sections of this chapter, as different normal and abnormal sleep-related motor activity is discussed, this model of the motor system is referred to, to suggest what levels are likely to be involved or disturbed in a particular condition.

A number of techniques have been used to study the physiology of the motor system. In this chapter, two important techniques are reviewed: neuronal recording, which has been used to examine, in animals, both the higher motor centers and the motor unit, and studies of reflexes, which examine the response of the motor system to defined afferent, often sensory, input.

Studies of activity in individual neurons

Two major kinds of studies have been done on individual neurons. First, patterns of activity in various brain centers have been studied, usually without clear knowledge of the function of the recorded neurons. These studies have indicated overall patterns of activity during different sleep stages. Second, extracellular and intracellular studies have been performed on identified motor neurons located in the brain stem and spinal cord. These studies have been able to identify some of the specific mechanisms of altered motor neuron function during sleep.

During waking, most brain cells tend to fire irregularly, at different frequencies in different brain regions. The general change during non-REM (NREM) sleep, and especially slow-wave sleep (SWS), is for cells to fire more slowly (lower frequency) but with more of a tendency to fire bursts.[9] During SWS, for example, thalamic cells fire slowly and are less responsive to afferent activity. These changes are related to the greater synchronization of surface electrical activity (electroencephalogram or EEG) during sleep. In REM sleep, by contrast, cellular activity is increased in many regions. Motor areas of the brain often show this activity increases, such as the primary motor cortex,[10] motor thalamus, red nucleus, and cerebellum.[9] This increased firing in the motor centers of the brain is thought to be related to the increased descending drive that occurs during REM sleep; however, since single unit studies have, in the main, merely examined rates of firing, it is not possible to say whether the neuronal activity in brain centers during REM sleep has the same pattern and organization as in the waking state. Studies of cerebral blood flow have largely paralleled those of cellular activity. Blood flow may be greater during REM than during wakefulness, but is widely depressed during NREM sleep, especially SWS.[11]

At the level of the motor unit, the motor neurons are less active during sleep. In relaxation and NREM sleep, they are slightly hyperpolarized (moved electrically away from their firing threshold) and less excitable.[12,13] This is due to inhibitory input inhibitory postsynaptic potentials (IPSPs). In REM sleep, the motor neurons are further hyperpolarized owing to the increased frequency of small IPSPs as well as large IPSPs that occur only during phasic REMs.[14] At least the larger, and perhaps both classes of, IPSPs can be suppressed by perfusion of strychnine, suggesting that they are mediated by the neurotransmitter glycine.[13] While both the pontine and medullary reticular formation, through centers located near the nucleus pontis oralis and the nucleus reticularis gigantocellularis, respectively,[13] are believed to play a role in producing this inhibition, the actual neuronal source of these different IPSPs is not yet known. As a result of this inhibition of the motor neurons, the increased activity of the central motor system in REM sleep is generally not reflected in increased motor activity. Rather, muscles, such as the mentalis, show atonia, while limb movements, generated either centrally or reflexly, are rare. The bursts of myoclonic movements that sometimes accompany REMs apparently arise from a superimposed phasic excitation via excitatory postsynaptic potentials (EPSPs). This excitations does not depend on the major voluntary motor pathways, such as the corticospinal or rubrospinal tract, but presumably originates in the brain stem.[15] Pharmacologic studies suggest that these EPSPs are mediated by non–NMDA (N-methyl-D-aspartate) excitatory synapses.[13]

Studies of reflex activity

Because much of motor behavior is reflexively generated, at least in part, it is also important to consider what happens to reflexes during sleep. The most commonly studied reflex has been the tendon reflex or its electrical counterpart the H reflex. Constant stimuli are applied and the resulting motor response, monitored as force, movement, or electromyographic (EMG) activity, is measured to determine the reflex gain (output per unit input). The tendon reflex is a monosynaptic reflex, so called because it is driven primarily by action across a single synapse, the excitatory connection from the afferent Ia muscle tendon fiber to the alpha motor neuron. This reflex is diminished in NREM sleep, especially SWS, and is then almost completely abolished in REM sleep, especially during REMs.[15,16] Polysynaptic spinal reflexes, which cross many synapses (e.g., cutaneous reflexes), are similarly depressed in NREM and REM sleep.[15] In contrast, it has been noted that brain stem reflexes such as vestibular reflexes and the blink reflex show decreased gain in NREM sleep but may then recover partially in REM sleep.[17,18] This recovery of brain stem reflexes during REM sleep parallels the relatively greater activity of the eye muscles, compared to trunk and limb muscles at that time.

While the basis for the reduced reflex gain during sleep is most likely inhibition of the motor output, even sensory transmission may be altered by sleep. Sensory transmission can be studied experimentally by evoked responses, synchronized electrical activity that arises as a result of sensory input (or electrical shocks to selected nerves) and that indicates the nervous systems response to the input.[19] Responses are labeled as short, medium, and long, latency depending on how long after the sensory stimulus they occur: earlier responses travel faster pathways, with fewer synaptic relays, than do later responses and are, thus, more purely "sensory" in nature. The general rule has been that medium- and long-latency components of evoked responses may be altered by NREM sleep whereas the short-latency components remain relatively stable,[20] however, even short-latency somatosensory evoked potentials (SEPs) may show diminished responsiveness with increased latency in stage 2 sleep.[21] Visual evoked responses, of course, are profoundly altered, even by drowsiness. During REM sleep, some later responses make at least a partial recovery: for example, the midlatency P1 potential of the brain stem auditory evoked response (BAER) returns to its waking configuration.[20]

Motor evoked potentials (MEPs) are muscle responses, usually measured by surface EMG, that are elicited by stimulating over motor nerves or the central nervous system. In one study of MEPs evoked by stimulating the motor cortex with a strong magnetic stimulus during sleep, it was noted that the MEPs decreased during NREM sleep.[22] Results during REM sleep have shown much greater variability in amplitude of evoked responses. Hess and colleagues[22] found that responses were of normal or increased amplitude, whereas Fish and coworkers[23] found that average amplitude was decreased in three normal subjects, despite some responses of higher amplitude than normal relaxed waking responses. The latter group also noted prolonged latencies of the MEPs, consistent with inhibitory processes. While these results remain to be harmonized, the variability is consistent with the fluctuating balance between inhibitory and excitatory processes in REM. A finding of decreased mean amplitude, however, is more consistent with the general inhibitory balance of REM sleep in normals.

It should be noted that sleep, though it dulls higher coordinated motor activity, does not abolish it. Complex responses such as scratching can occur during sleep, and human subjects can respond selectively to different sounds.[24] Such complex responses are most active in stage 1 sleep, least active in SWS, with responsiveness in REM being intermediate in level. Reflexes can also change their characteristic motor output in sleep,[25] indicating that sleep is not merely a general change in activity levels but a rearranged organization of responsiveness. In addition, certain reflexes that would be abnormal during waking, such as Babinski's sign, may be elicited during sleep[26,27] as discussed on pages 16 through 18 of the treatise by Kleitman[26] and later studied by Ryiki and colleagues.[27]

Summary of physiologic studies

The relatively consistent picture that has developed is that NREM sleep is a quiescent period marked by decreased activity and reduced responsiveness at all levels of the motor system in comparison to the waking state. REM sleep, in contrast, is a more unstable state in which excitatory and inhibitory influences are balanced. While the brain centers show increased activity, the motor unit is bombarded with both excitation and inhibition with, in the normal state, a functional preponderance of inhibitory tone. However, this result is precarious, and in some cases, such as reflexes, there may be increased activity during REM sleep.

The Normal Motor System and Sleep

The normal motor system shows marked variations in activity and responsiveness as a function both of time of day (based on circadian rhythm, as well as sleep history) and of sleep-wake state. Age is also an important factor, as the relation of the motor system to sleep changes throughout the life span.

Circadian activity cycles

In many, if not most, animal species, the motor system's level of activity depends on the time of day. Even in the absence of a day-night light cycle (constant conditions), such activity cycling persists in a "free-running state" that has circadian periodicity. As described in Chapter 23 on chronobiology, many of the important physiologic variables, such as temperature, also show circadian periods. While there are currently believed to be at least two important circadian "clocks" generating these rhythms,[28] the suprachiasmatic nucleus is thought to be the center responsible for the circadian variation of motor activity. Humans, of course, usually sleep at night, so that activity is concentrated during the daytime hours. This basic pattern, however, can be disturbed in a number of different settings: among shift workers or those with unusual schedules or in patients who have a variety of sleep disorders or degenerative neurologic conditions.

The motor system and sleep stages

During the night, a major change in motor activity depends on the sleep state (wakeful, REM, NREM). For example, one frequently used monitor of sleep-wake state, the chin EMG, is an indicator of brachial (brain stem) muscle tone. As discussed elsewhere under sleep staging, during wake, chin muscle tone is high and a tonically active chin EMG is interrupted by phasic contractions (e.g., facial expressions, tension, chewing). With relaxation and drowsiness the level of EMG activity decreases. It further decreases as NREM sleep is achieved and deepens to slow-wave sleep levels. Then, during REM sleep, EMG activity becomes minimal or even unapparent, though occasionally it may be interrupted with brief, irregular bursts of activity. These changes mirror, to a fair degree, the changes undergone by much of the motor system during sleep. Much of this variability can be understood on the basis of the altered activity of different levels of the motor system, as well as their interaction during different sleep stages.

While noting that motor activities are related to sleep stages, it is also important to remember that this relationship may need to be qualified in various contexts. First, at a technical level, sleep scoring may not adequately reflect the underlying brain processes

at the time of a given event, such as a movement. Sleep is generally scored as arbitrary epochs of fixed length, usually 30 seconds, whereas physiologic processes may occur on a whole variety of time scales. This has led some investigators to examine microepochs of a few seconds for momentary state.[29] Second, some sleep may not be adequately scorable according to the current rules. This has led to various proposals to revise the scoring system, or even to use very different methods of scoring. McGregor and colleagues, for example, have proposed the use of transitional or T sleep epochs, in which, because of disruptive events such as sleep apnea, there is an alternation of some sleep stage with arousal.[30] Third, the sleep stages themselves are not fully discrete. Fragments of a stage, such as REM-related atonia, may occur during other states such as wake, even in fully normal persons. Recently, Mahowald and Schenck[31] reported on six patients with marked admixtures of features from the different sleep-wake states (wake, NREM sleep, REM sleep). These patients showed abnormal distribution of motor activity with relation to sleep features. Fourth, motor events, while they are typical of one sleep stage or state, may less commonly occur in other stages. Though periodic limb movements in sleep (PLMS) occur primarily in NREM sleep, they may occur in REM sleep.[32] In our experience, similar movements may occur during arousals or wake periods after sleep onset, usually as part of a periodic sequence of movements that span the sleep-wake divide. Fifth, many conditions are not completely pure but contain a combination of disorders related to different sleep stages. For example, narcolepsy is closely associated with PLMS,[33] and patients with somnambulism, which typically occurs during NREM sleep, may show REM sleep motor abnormalities suggestive of the REM sleep behavior disorder (RBD).[34] Table 19-1 indicates our summary of the frequency of normal and abnormal motor activities that occur during the various phases of sleep and waking. Because many of these movements have not been fully and exhaustively studied, this table is a preliminary guide rather than a definitive pronouncement.

Drowsiness, sleep onset, and arousals. In the period before sleep begins, humans and other animals enter a period of relative repose. The transition to sleep is itself signalled by a variety of behavioral and EEG features.[35] Even before actual sleep onset, the motor system reduces its level of activity. It is during this period that the symptoms of RLS become prominent. RLS is relatively distinctive in that, unlike almost all other movement disorders, it is activated by relaxation.

The transition to sleep features a very common sleep-related movement, the sleep start or hypnic

TABLE 19-1. Persistence of Motor Activity in Sleep

Motor Activity	Awake/Active	Drowsiness/Sleep Onset	Arousal/Awakening	Stage 1NREM	Stage 2NREM	Stage 3 & 4NREM	REM Sleep
Normal Motor Activity							
Postural shifts	Very frequent	Frequent	Frequent	Common	Occasional	Rare	Occasional
Sleep myoclonus	Unreported	Rare	Rare	Common	Occasional	Rare	Frequent
Hypnic jerk	Unreported	Frequent	Occasional	Occasional	Rare	Rare	Unreported
Sleep paralysis*	N.A.	Common	Common	Rare	Unreported	Unreported	Frequent
Movement disorders							
Chorea	Very frequent	Frequent	Common	Occasional	Rare	Very rare	Rare
Dystonia	Very frequent	Common	Common	Occasional	Rare	Very rare	Rare
Hemiballismus	Very frequent	Common	Common	Occasional?	Occasional?	Very rare	Occasional?
Hemifacial spasm	Very frequent	Common	Common	Common	Common	Occasional?	Common
Myoclonus: cortical/subcortical	Very frequent	Common	Occasional?	Occasional?	Occasional?	Rare	Rare
Myoclonus: spinal	Very frequent	Frequent	Common	Common	Common?	Occasional	Common?
Palatal tremor	Constant	Frequent	Frequent	Frequent	Frequent	Common?	Common?
Parkinsonian tremor	Very frequent	Common	Common	Occasional	Rare	Very rare	Occasional
Tics	Very frequent	Common	Common	Occasional	Occasional	Rare	Common
Sleep disorders							
Benign infantile myoclonus	N.A.	Unreported	Unreported	Common	Common	Common	Common
Bruxism	Common	Occasional?	Occasional	Frequent	Frequent	Occasional	Frequent
Fragmentary myoclonus	Unreported	Unreported	Unreported	Frequent	Frequent	Common	Occasional
NPD	N.A.	Unreported	Common	Frequent	Frequent	Occasional	Rare
PLMS: Isolated or with RLS	N.A.	Occasional	Occasional	Frequent	Common	Rare	Rare
PLMS: Narcolepsy, RBD	N.A.	Occasional?	Occasional?	Frequent	Common	Rare	Common
RBD	N.A.	Unreported	Occasional?	Rare	Rare	Rare	Frequent
Rhythmic movement disorder	Common	Very frequent	Common	Common	Common	Rare	Occasional?
RLS: Restlessness	Rare	Very frequent	Frequent	Occasional	N.A.	N.A.	N.A.
Somnambulism	N.A.	Unreported	Common	Occasional	Common	Frequent	Occasional

Key: N.A., Not applicable; ?, Limited information.
*In narcolepsy, presents as cataplexy in wakeful state.

jerk.[36] This is an abrupt, myoclonic flexion movement, generalized or partial, often asymmetric, that may be accompanied by a sensation. There is often an illusion of falling. Unless it is very frequent (as it rarely is[37]), this is a benign movement that has little effect on sleep and carries no negative prognosis. It probably occurs in the majority of people. When it occurs, it is usually a single event that causes brief arousal. EMG records show relatively brief EMG complexes (less than 250 msec) that may be simultaneous or sequential in various muscles.

Arousals, brief periods of interrupted, lighter sleep that may lead to full awakening, are often associated with movements. Arousals may both follow and lead movements such as body shifts. Abnormal movements, such as parkinsonian tremor, may recur during arousals. Sleep-related movements, such as PLMS, may provoke frequent arousals or even awakenings and may also continue during periods of a waking from sleep.

Transitions into and out of sleep may also be associated with *sleep paralysis*, a condition that renders a person unable to move though awake. Breathing and eye movements are usually preserved. This condition is thought to represent a variety of REM sleep tonic motor inhibition. The state transition may be associated with arousal from a REM period or, less commonly except in narcolepsy, may progress into REM sleep from wake. Although it is most frequently associated with narcolepsy, sleep paralysis also occurs in many nonnarcoleptic persons, sometimes clustering in families. Recent studies suggest that, at least in some populations, sleep paralysis may be quite common.[38,39] It has been suggested that sleep paralysis may occur when there is an early-onset REM period, for example after a awakening from NREM.[40] In normal persons, it is generally infrequent, but it can cause significant anxiety, especially the first time it occurs. In the absence of other narcoleptic phenomena or abnormal neurologic findings, someone with occasional sleep paralysis may be reassured that it is almost certainly benign.

NREM sleep. Postural shifts, which may signal changes (into or out of wake or REM), occur. Motor activity is less in NREM sleep than in the waking or resting state. There are also small flickering movements, called *sleep myoclonus*, which may cause no apparent movement and are associated with very brief, highly localized EMG potentials.[41,42] In some cases, these movements may have a greater amplitude and increased frequency, at which point they are called *fragmentary myoclonus*, a possible sleep disorder.[43] The frequency of all movements decreases with depth of sleep, and they are least frequent in SWS sleep (NREM stages 3 and 4).[44,45]

Postural shifts rarely occur before SWS. This reduced activity is consistent with the quiescent stage of the nervous system documented by physiologic studies.

A number of abnormal motor activities, such as somnambulism or PLMS, occur predominantly during NREM sleep.

REM sleep. REM sleep is dramatically different from NREM. The motor system is dominated by central activation and peripheral inhibition, so muscle tone is reduced, even below the level of SWS, but bursts of small movements (sleep myoclonus), similar to those seen in NREM sleep but more clustered, occur phasically in association with REMs.

During REM there is increased nervous system activity and a close balance between strong upper motor center excitation and inhibition at the level of the motor effector. When the inhibitory influences break down, significant motor activity may be released. This can be achieved by lesioning the brain stem of animals, which destroy the inhibitory centers,[46] or can occur, it is believed, in human sleep disorders such as RBD. The resulting movements may represent "acting out" of dreams, which characteristically have a motor component.[47]

Ontogeny of the Motor System During Sleep

Normal sleep movements are affected by age as well as by sleep stage: the number of movements during sleep is greatest in infants and decreases with age.[44] For example, De Koninck and colleagues found that position shifts during sleep decreased from 4.7 per hour in 8- to 12-year-old sleepers to 2.1 per hour in persons aged 65 to 80 years.[48] Children are also thought to lack a fully mature sleep regulatory system, as a result of which they may be especially subject to a number of sleep motor disorders. Parasomnias such as bruxism, somnambulism, or soliloquy are present with greater prevalence during childhood and tend to become less and less frequent with age from early childhood on. Similarly, toward the end of life, as neural and other body systems begin to deteriorate, some forms of excessive motor activity may emerge again, including parasomnias such as bruxism, PLMS, and RBD.

MOVEMENT DISORDERS IN RELATION TO SLEEP

The relation between the diurnal movement disorders and sleep has become better known over the past several decades, in large part because of the major increase in the study of sleep. In this period of time, it has become more evident that movement disorders also have significant impact on sleep, even if most of their symptoms are appreciated during the daytime. It has also become clear that many movement disorders do persist to some extent during sleep. In some condition the level of symptoms may vary systematically with the sleep-wake cycle. For example, in dopa-responsive dystonia (DRD) patients feel best in the early morning, after sleeping and their well-being deteriorates as the day passes. Furthermore, movement disorder specialists have become more aware of certain conditions categorized primarily as sleep disorders, such as the RLS and nocturnal paroxysmal dystonia (NPD), which cause more activity during the night or during sleep.

Diurnal Movement Disorders

Most diurnal movement disorders are present during the daytime, and it is their impairment of function during the daytime that leads patients to seek medical care. It has become increasingly apparent, however, that movement disorders are not absent during sleep and that they may cause or be associated with a variety of sleep disturbances. Surveys of patients with Parkinson's disease have shown that the majority feel they have some difficulty with sleep.[49] In surveys performed by the first author at Parkinson's support groups, large numbers of patients (more than 30% in each category) complained of difficulty getting to sleep, inadequate time asleep, disrupted sleep, and daytime sleepiness. It has therefore become important for clinicians involved with movement disorders to be aware of the impact of these conditions on sleep and be ready to help patients with sleep problems. Sleep disorder specialists should also be sensitive to the increased sleep dysfunction of patients with movement disorders.

Persistence of movement disorders during Sleep

Different diurnal movement disorders show various degrees of persistence during sleep (see Table 19-1). Until fairly recently, it was almost universally believed that most movement disorders are abolished by sleep, such as the increased tonic spasms of dystonia or essential or parkinsonian tremor. However, careful studies generally find that there are remnants of abnormal activity that persist during sleep or occur during brief transitions to light sleep or wakefulness. As a rule, movement disorders are most likely to be present at transitions into and out of sleep or during the lighter stages of NREM sleep. Occasionally, they are reactivated during REM sleep as well.

Some movement disorders, though they subside, have been reported to occur fairly commonly during sleep. Tics, especially in children, have been noted to occur during sleep. In children, this may reflect a relative immaturity of the mechanisms for suppressing unwanted movement during sleep.

In a thorough and careful study using EMG, accelerometry, and split-screen video recording, Fish and colleagues[29] examined the relation of motor activity not only to conventional sleep staging but also to epochs with transitions (to lighter or deeper sleep stages or wakefulness). They also monitored the 2-second periods before onset of dyskinesias in patients with Parkinson's disease, Huntington's disease, Tourette's syndrome, and torsion dystonia (both primary generalized and secondary) and scored them for arousals, REMs, sleep spindles and slow waves. They compared these dyskinesias to normal movements in both patients and normal subjects. Of 43 patients, 41 had characteristic movements that persisted during sleep. Both normal movements and dyskinesias for every disorder followed the same general plan: most common in awakening epochs followed by lightening, stage 1 sleep, REM sleep, then stage 2 sleep, with no movements in pure stages 3, 4, and deepening sleep. Only Tourette's patients had dyskinesias during transition from wake to sleep. The 2-second period before both normal and abnormal movements most often showed arousals, followed by REMs, with spindles and slow waves both extremely unlikely to occur. These results support speculation[50] that both dyskinesias and normal movements are likely to be modulated by sleep in a similar fashion. The authors suggest this may be due either to the general suppression of centers for both normal and dyskinetic movements or to suppression of some common descending path, such as the pyramidal tract. It should be noted that all of these abnormal motor activities are thought to be generated in what we have called the *higher motor centers*.

Movement disorders associated with abnormalities of the lower motor centers most commonly persist during sleep. Most typical are the palatal myoclonus or palatal tremor family, in which there is low-frequency (typically, 1.5-Hz to 2.5-Hz) oscillatory activity associated with brain stem damage within Mollaret's triangle (dentatorubroolivary triangle, with damage most common in the central tegmental tract, which runs from the region of the red nucleus to the ipsilateral olive).[51] In addition, spinal myoclonus often persists during sleep. These can, in a general sense, be lumped together as segmental myoclonus. Similar persistence may be seen in hemifacial spasm, which is thought to involve damage either in the brain stem facial nucleus or in the peripheral nerve (cross-talk due to ephaptic transmission) or both. Also, fasciculations due to damaged lower motor neurons may persist during sleep.

It has been said that psychogenic movement disorders all subside during sleep or anesthesia, and, in general, they can be expected to do so. In some rare cases there are exceptions to this rule. These patients have not been studied systematically enough to reach a full conclusion but it can be expected that they would be most likely to show persistent abnormalities at sleep onset, during very light sleep stages, or in the course of arousals, and least likely in deep slow-wave sleep.

Sleep disorders associated with diurnal movement disorders

A basic problem occurs when movement disorders prevent sleep or arouse patients from sleep, but such direct effects of movement disorders are not the only effects on sleep. Additional problems arise because the movement disorder, or its treatment, may disturb sleep. Movement disorder patients may also be at risk for additional sleep disturbances, such as sleep apnea or parasomnias. Moreover, many movement disorder patients are elderly, some even demented, and they may have the impaired sleep often associated with aging or degenerative disease. Before discussing the sleep problems of individual movement disorders, we first review the general kinds of sleep problems that may occur in these patients.

Respiratory disturbances. A major problem for movement disorder patients is the prevalence of respiratory disturbances during sleep. Respiratory disturbances are common in the motor disorders that involve neuronal degeneration. Especially vulnerable are patients with degenerative diseases such as Parkinson's disease that involve brain stem loci. In the more widespread degenerative diseases such as olivopontocerebellar atrophy (OPCA) or multiple-system atrophy (MSA), there may be respiratory disturbances based on disturbed central regulation of breathing, problems with neuromuscular function leading to obstruction or laryngeal stridor, or impaired feedback control of respiration. These difficulties and the situation of patients with MSA are also discussed in Chapter 20 on neurologic disorders.

Sleep fragmentation. In many disorders, a primary concomitant of a degenerative movement disorder is disrupted sleep—more frequent awakenings, more stage transitions, partial and complete arousals. The result is usually sleep characterized by more time awake, less SWS, and, perhaps, less REM sleep. This has been reported as a complication of many different movement abnormalities. It should be remembered, however, that many of these movement disorders occur primarily in older patients and that sleep quality declines even in relatively healthy elderly persons. Sleep may improve once effective

therapy is found for the underlying condition.[52] Therapy for movement disorders may also interfere with sleep, and this must be considered in assessments of sleep problems. Because both the primary disease and its therapy may disrupt sleep, completely successful management may not be possible.

Dyssomnias and parasomnias. There are a number of movement disorders in which parasomnias or other motor disturbances of sleep are more likely to occur than in the general populations. Children with tics are reported to have an increased incidence of parasomnias such as somnambulism and somniloquy. Increased prevalence of PLMS or RLS has been reported with a variety of movement disorders, such as Huntington's disease (HD).[32] A number of movement disorders, especially MSA or OPCA, may be associated with RBD.[53]

The degree to which such additional motor abnormalities are seen in patients with diurnal movement disorders is not yet clear. Good epidemiologic studies have not been done; however, the frequency of associations reported does indicate that additional motor abnormalities during sleep must be considered when patients report a movement disorder.

Circadian rhythm disturbances. Circadian rhythm disturbances, especially changes in sleep phase or chaotic sleep rhythms, are especially common with the degenerative conditions. Many of these patients are elderly, severely incapacitated, or demented, all features that may weaken the circadian regulation of activity. Patients may have multiple factors that upset the circadian rhythm, including their medications. Nocturnal confusion or "sundowning" often occurs in this setting.

Circadian rhythm disturbances are difficult to treat, especially in patients whose cognition is compromised. Careful adjustment of medication, attempts to maintain wakefulness during the day, and good sleep hygiene may help. Sleeping medications may be counterproductive, leading to additional difficulties such as confusion. Because patients are often homebound and institutionalized, they may lack adequate exposure to bright light to reset their circadian rhythms. A trial of bright light therapy might be considered for selected patients.

Patients with Parkinson's disease are prone to endogenous and reactive depression.[54,55] They may show a classic pattern of sleep phase advance with increased and early-onset REM periods. In this situation, they may respond to judicious use of antidepressants.

Excessive daytime somnolence. Because of the varied difficulties associated with movement disorders—inadequate sleep, sleep fragmentation, sleep apnea, circadian rhythm disturbances—excessive daytime somnolence (EDS) may be a major problem for patients. This problem can be aggravated by medications such as L-dopa, which can induce sleepiness at peak blood concentrations.

*Sleep and sleep disturbances
in specific movement disorders*

Movement disorders have traditionally been categorized according to their appearance or phenomenology. Two major categories of movement disorders have been identified; the *akinetic or hypokinetic disorders*, predominantly Parkinson's disease and related entities, the most salient feature of which is a paucity or deficiency in movement or an inability to perform normal movements, and the *hyperkinetic disorders*, such as chorea or myoclonus, in which the most salient features are excessive movements superimposed upon normal motor behavior.

These two classes are by no means exclusive, as akinetic syndromes exhibit hyperkinetic features, even without treatment (for example, dystonia in Parkinson's disease). Indeed, in juvenile-onset cases of dystonia-parkinsonism, it has been difficult to distinguish one from another or to decide which is the primary motor disorder.

These two classes are applied primarily to the more classical basal ganglia or extrapyramidal disorders. Other motor problems of central origin, such as cerebellar ataxia or paresis due to stroke, often are not categorized along with the basal ganglia disorders.

Akinetic or hypokinetic disorders. The paradigmatic akinetic or hypokinetic disorder is Parkinson's disease; however, many other conditions have some of the same symptoms as part of their clinical picture. Patients with these conditions may be said to exhibit parkinsonism.[56] When many other systems are involved, as in multisystem atrophy, the clinical picture can become far more complicated. Such syndromes are dealt with in the chapter on breathing and neurologic disorders (see Chapter 20). This chapter focuses primarily on Parkinson's disease, which has been investigated to a fair degree from the point of view of sleep.

As well as being a common movement disorder, parkinsonism is associated with a variety of sleep complaints. This association is sufficiently important that it has been recognized in the new international sleep disorders classification. Sleep problems of parkinsonism are given their own coding category as medical-psychiatric sleep disorders associated with neurologic disorders (see the International Classification of Sleep Disorders,[57] p. 240–245 and Chapter 15).

Parkinson's Disease. Parkinson's disease is defined by the tetrad of resting tremor, rigidity (resistance to passive movement of the limbs), poverty of movement (slow movement, bradykinesia, and reduced spontaneous movement, akinesia), and poor postural reflexes leading to falls.[56] Classically, Parkinson's disease has been associated with the presence of Lewy bodies in the brain stem nuclei and depigmentation of the substantia nigra, the major nucleus providing dopaminergic innervation to the basal ganglia. Recently, it has become clear that these Lewy bodies are not specific to Parkinson's disease but may present with other features, such as dementia. In most patients with Parkinson's disease, dementia is seen only late in the course of the disease or in old age. Although juvenile cases of Parkinson's disease have been reported, most patients present after age 40 years and the incidence increases at least through the ninth decade. A typical course is progressive, though many patients achieve plateaus that last for years, and recent developments in therapy have succeeded in maintaining some degree of function in many patients for decades.

Pathologically, Parkinson's disease affects not only the substantia nigra but also other brain stem nuclei, such as the locus ceruleus and raphe nuclei,[58,59] which directly affect sleep (see Chapters 3 and 5). It is, therefore, reasonable to expect patients with Parkinson's disease or pathologically related disorders to have sleep disturbances. One interesting physiologic observation has been that Parkinson patients have diminished amplitude and frequency of sleep spindles,[60] which may be reversed by therapy.[61] The explanation for this phenomenon is not yet clear, but some patients with hyperkinetic disorders such as dystonia have been found to have increased spindles. These alterations may derive from interaction between the basal ganglia and the thalamus, where spindles originate, since the thalamus is a major target for basal ganglia output.

The characteristic motor abnormalities of parkinsonism, tremor and rigidity, were once thought to disappear during sleep. This was first pointed out by Parkinson himself, who, however, noted exceptions in very severe cases. More recently, some authors have pointed out that tremor could persist during sleep, usually occurring during lighter sleep stages and often associated with arousals.[62–64] While April[63] found that tremor could also appear in undisturbed SWS, Fish and colleagues recently found that tremor is associated with awakenings or lightenings, rarely or never with deep SWS.[29] The latter group found that in two cases tremor was precipitated in Parkinson's disease patients by PLMS.[29] In summary, this work appears to show that tremor may occur during the night but that it is almost invariably associated with intermediate states between sleep and wake and rarely occurs either in REM sleep or SWS.

Other motor activity may be abnormal in Parkinson's disease. Askenasy[52,65] found complex, unusual activity in patients with Parkinson's disease, as well as other presumed basal ganglia disorders, but the nature of this motor activity remains to be elucidated, though some may have been PLMS. Askenasy also noted an increased incidence of PLMS in these patients, which may involve the arms as well as the legs. In his patients, successful therapy for the underlying Parkinson's disease led to parallel improvements in sleep and normalization of the unusual motor activity.[52] Other investigators, however, have found normal large body movements such as position shifts to be decreased in Parkinson's disease.[66,67] One distinct, unusual sleep motor phenomenon reported in Parkinson's disease is REM-onset blepharospasm.[68] Mouret also noted increased chin muscle tone during REM sleep, a component of the RBD in some patients.[68] More recently, Comella and colleagues[68A] reported that 4 of 8 moderate to severely affected Parkinson's disease patients met polysomnographic criteria for RBD. Patients with RBD had a longer duration of disease (16 versus 7 years). Silber and Ahlskog in another recent report[68B] found that RBD could occur early in the course of Parkinson's disease (3 of their 11 patients had RBD before Parkinson's disease). Unfortunately, most of these observations are based on small samples, and it is too soon to generalize about what, if any, movement abnormalities are seen during sleep in Parkinson's disease. It may well be that the motor phenomena of sleep may depend on duration or stage of the disease, response to therapy, kind of therapy and dose, and any dyskinetic complications of therapy.

Sleep difficulties have been found to be common in patients with Parkinson's disease.[49] Indeed, survey studies have found that patients have an increased number of sleep complaints, at least part of which may be explained by the age of the patients since age-matched controls may have almost as many general sleep complaints.[69] In a study by Lees and colleagues[49] of 220 patients contacted through support groups, at least 32% of the respondents complained about each of the following sleep-related problems: excessive nocturia, inability to turn over during the night or upon waking, inability to get out of bed unaided,

leg cramps and jerks, dystonic spasms of the limbs or face, and back pain during the night. In this population, 44% felt their sleep was good but 18% rated it as poor. Only 4% of the patients had no sleep-related complaint. In a study by Factor and colleagues,[69] parkinsonian subjects had more sleep problems, but the difference from controls was not significant except for spontaneous episodes of falling asleep during the daytime. Nocturnal vocalizations occurred only in the parkinsonians.

Polysomnographic studies, usually uncontrolled, have identified poor sleep as common in Parkinson's disease.[60,70-72] It usually worsens as the disease progresses.[73] The most frequently found abnormal features of sleep include decreased sleep efficiency and increased time awake (WASO),[67] following a basic pattern of sleep fragmentation. There is no single reason that patients with parkinsonism have poor sleep, rather a series of associated sleep problems may impair sleep.

First, patients may have a variety of abnormal movements such as persistent tremor, or dyskinesias or disease-related dystonia. Second, there may be awakening with reactivation of symptoms such as difficulty changing position or getting out of bed or inability to initiate movement.[74] Third, other abnormal movements such as increased REM chin EMG activity (suggestive of RBD), PLMS, or REM-onset blinking may disrupt sleep. These may occur with increased frequency in Parkinson's disease.

Fourth, there may be an increase in respiratory sleep-fragmenting disorders such as sleep apnea or upper airway resistance syndrome, which may be more common in Parkinson's disease also. While respiratory problems are not prominent in Parkinson's disease, a number do occur, and they can affect sleep.[75,76] Patients have been noted to have a restrictive type of lung defect, owing to an intrinsic defect in breathing control, impaired respiratory muscle function due to rigidity, and faulty autonomic control of the lungs.[77] Patients may also have an obstructive respiratory defect,[78] stridor or laryngeal spasm associated with off-states or dystonic episodes,[79] diaphragmatic dyskinesias,[75,80] and upper airway dysfunction with tremorlike oscillations.[81] The incidence of respiratory difficulties is likely to be greater in patients with additional autonomic dysfunction.[72]

As a result of these respiratory difficulties that may be detected when patients are awake, it is not surprising that the prevalence of respiratory dysfunction has been reported to be increased in the sleep of parkinsonian patients. Obstructive, central, and mixed apneas can occur,[75,82] though not all authors have observed them.[72] Some authors have speculated that respiration-related sleep disorders in parkinsonism may be responsible for the increased rate of early morning mortality noted in these patients.[83]

Fifth, patients with Parkinson's disease, like those with degenerative diseases generally, may suffer a loss of central nervous system sleep regulation, leading to weakened circadian rhythmicity and poor sleep maintenance. Sixth, patients with Parkinson's disease are prone to depression, which in itself may cause sleep abnormalities, such as reduced REM sleep latency.[84] Depression may also aggravate the response to the parkinsonian symptoms such as pain and magnify their impact on sleep.[54,55]

Finally, medication effects can cause sleep disruption through varied mechanisms, including myoclonus or vivid and frightening nightmares.[85] Klawans and his group[73,85] have studied parkinsonian patients treated over long periods with L-dopa who develop a progressive sleep disturbance that includes impaired sleep maintenance, EDS with frequent naps, sleep talking, sleepwalking, frightening dreams, and myoclonic jerks. The condition may progress to hallucinosis and frank psychosis. Because it is assumed to be due to L-dopa therapy, it may be alleviated by reducing the dose or switching, in part or entirely, to other agents. Like many of the late complications of treated Parkinson's disease, this may require careful balancing of medications.

Treatment of Parkinson's disease has not been found to consistently improve sleep. Some authors report parallel benefits to sleep and movement,[52,74] whereas others have shown persistent abnormalities in sleep.[70,72] A difficulty of interpreting these studies, however, has been the failure to fully examine the different sources of sleep abnormalities in parkinsonism. It may be that, in undermedicated patients sleep will improve in parallel with Parkinson's disease when medication is increased but that over the course of time the patient may be caught between the need for medication to maintain function and side effects of the medication that disturb sleep. In patients with reactivation of parkinsonian symptoms during the night, adjustments in the timing and choice of medication may help. Patients who are taking medications only early in the day may benefit from evening or bedtime doses. Longer-acting preparations of L-dopa, such as are now available, may also help when taken near bedtime, as well as dopamine agonists (bromocriptine, pergolide), which have sustained action. Anticholinergics may help some patients sleep but can also cause vivid nightmares and awakenings. Other patients may require judicious balancing of their medication schedule or switching to a different combination of agents. Antihistamines, such as diphenhydramine, may be the most reasonable sleep medications, particularly in light of their modest anti-Parkinson effect.

While typical Parkinson's disease may occur at least as early as young adult life, some patients with early-onset disease have distinct conditions.[86] Yamamura and colleagues[87] reported on group of such patients who showed marked diurnal fluctuations in their symptoms. On initial presentation, these patients' condition often overlaps clinically with dopa-responsive dystonia (DRD), the Segawa variant,[88,89] so there remains some controversy about the distinction between these patient groups.[86] The DRD patients generally maintain a good response to L-dopa for long periods,[90] whereas the juvenile Parkinson's patients, though dopa responsive, quickly exhibit dyskinetic side effects. Improvement after sleep has also been reported to be common in later-onset Parkinson's disease,[91] though not all patients have such a benefit. Factor found that roughly equal groups of patients reported improvement, worsening, and no change after sleeping. The group that reported improvement had relatively mild disease.[69]

Neurologic Disorders Related to Parkinson's Disease. A number of degenerative diseases are similar to Parkinson's disease but have different and usually additional features referable to other central nervous system features. The MSAs and OPCA are discussed in Chapter 20. Here are discussed two specific conditions whose relationship to sleep have been studied and a particular syndrome of Parkinsonism and hypoventilation that has been described.

Postencephalitic parkinsonism is a condition due to infectious damage to the central nervous system, typically derived from the encephalitis lethargica epidemics of the 1920s (see Kleitman,[26] pp. 243–250 for discussion of encephalitis lethargica). While this has not been studied extensively, respiratory problems appear to be more common with postencephalitic parkinsonism than with Parkinson's disease, perhaps owing to the more widespread brain stem lesions of these patients.[75] They have been found to have poor voluntary respiratory control[92] and hypoventilation,[93] even while awake, which has been linked to decreased sensitivity of central chemoreceptors that regulate breathing.[93,94] These patients may also have greater sleep problems than idiopathic Parkinson's disease patients, including greater respiratory compromise during sleep.[83]

Progressive supranuclear palsy (PSP) is a condition with parkinsonism characterized by early gait disturbance and dystonia, especially of the neck and face, and progressive, eventually marked, impairment of eye movements.[95–97] The condition involves cell loss and overgrowth of glial cells in a number of brain stem nuclei, including the locus ceruleus. It is not surprising, then, that sleep is quite affected in this condition. A number of studies have been made of sleep in this condition. Patients have been reported to experience severe sleep disruption and reduced total sleep, reduced REM sleep time with abnormal REMs, disordered sleep architecture, and frequent awakenings.[98,99,99a] Sleep disruption increases with the severity of motor abnormalities.[100]

Therapy for PSP generally follows that for Parkinson's disease, but it is often relatively unavailing. For daytime symptoms a combination of L-dopa (with carbidopa) and a dopamine agonist may work better than either medication alone. Little is known about treatment of the sleep dysfunctions in this condition.

Purdy and colleagues[101] have described a *familial syndrome of parkinsonism with alveolar hypoventilation.* Two identical twins had ataxia of breathing with episodes of apnea that were more severe during sleep. The patient sustained breathing only by voluntary efforts, so their condition could be described as Ondine's curse, the failure of automatic breathing resulting in severe apnea during sleep. On autopsy, the twins had extensive damage to brain stem regions related to control of breathing as well as findings typical of Parkinson's disease.

Hyperkinetic disorders.   A diverse group of disorders are characterized by excessive involuntary movement, often coupled with deficiency of voluntary movement such as bradykinesia. In some cases, the conditions are known to have a very specific cause, such as HD, which is presumed always to be due to a single genetic defect.

Chorea.   Chorea consists of movements that occur in a flowing or irregular pattern and appear to migrate from one part of the body to another.[102] They may be exacerbated with action and typically are seen in the face and distal limbs.

The best-known cause of chorea is Huntington's disease (HD), a genetically dominant disease with almost complete penetrance whose gene has been linked to the short arm of chromosome 4. Patients also have prominent psychological symptoms, including depression, psychosis, and character disorders. Onset is typically between age 25 and 50 years, though it may occur even in the first decade or in late adult life. Progression is slow but relentless, with eventual debility, dementia, and inanition occurring when onset of disease occurs before old age.

Sleep has been studied by a number of investigators in HD. They observe variable persistence of chorea during sleep, chorea being most pronounced in the lighter stages of NREM sleep (stage 1 and 2).[62,65,103] In their recent study, Fish and colleagues[29] found that most choreiform movements occurred during awakening, lightening of sleep stages, or in stage 1 sleep. This is similar to other dyskinesias. One study reported an increase in overall sleep movements in HD.[66] Alterations in sleep spindles in HD have been inconsistent. One study found them to be largely absent,[104] but another found that their frequency was increased.[60]

Sleep has been found to be variably impaired in Huntington's disease, though most studies have not used matched control groups. The general finding has been that sleep is disturbed, and especially fragmented, particularly in patients with more advanced disease. Deficits include prolonged sleep latency, excessive waking, decreased slow-wave and REM sleep, and decreased sleep efficiency.[103-105] Some studies have reported that many patients have essentially normal sleep architecture and stages.[60] Unlike patients with parkinsonism, HD patients have not been found to have a significant number of sleep apneas that contribute to impaired sleep.[105,106]

Sleep has not been much studied in other conditions with predominant chorea. Broughton reported that four patients with Sydenham's chorea, which follows a streptococcal infection, had reactivation of their movements during REM sleep.[107] Because sleep complaints are not prominent in HD, little is known about the response to therapy or the effects on sleep features of treatment for the motor manifestations of HD.

Dystonia.   Dystonia[108] is a condition characterized by sustained distorting or twisting postures, often mixed with a variety of more jerky or oscillatory movements.[109] Dystonia can be primary or secondary and can be of variable extent, either focal, segmental, or generalized, depending on the area of involvement. Primary dystonia has been found to be at least in part genetic. A locus on chromosome 9 accounts for inheritance in a number of families.[110,111] One problem of evaluating sleep studies in dystonia is that they have often examined a fairly heterogeneous collection of patients with different distributions of dystonia and different causes.

Though they usually subside significantly, dystonic movements may persist during sleep at a reduced frequency and amplitude. They are maximally reduced during SWS and may be partially reactivated during REM sleep episodes.[65,112] In Fish and coworkers' study of dyskinetic movements, both primary and secondary dystonic patients followed the general pattern of greater dyskinetic movements during awakening or lightening epochs, followed by stage 1 sleep, and then with reduced frequency in stage 2, REM, and SWS, with movements absent during epochs of deepening sleep.[29] In a recent study including focal and segmental dystonias, Silvestri and colleagues found that Meig's syndrome (oromandibular dystonia), blepharospasm, and the tonic foot syndrome all showed persistent abnormal activity during sleep, with reduced amplitude, duration, and frequency of EMG bursts.[113] The greatest suppression was in SWS and REM sleep.

A number of studies have reported the presence of exaggerated sleep spindles in dystonia;[65,112,114] however, one more recent study found that this was, at best, a variable finding in a carefully studied group with primary and secondary dystonia.[115]

It has been suggested that inhibitory mechanisms are defective in dystonia.[116] This prompted Fish and colleagues[23] to study whether REM inhibition is intact in both primary and secondary dystonias. They found that primary dystonics had normal chin EMG atonia, while secondary dystonics showed significantly decreased chin EMG activity. No patients had complex abnormal activity during REM sleep. In an attempt to analyze motor excitability, the authors successfully stimulated three normal and four dystonic subjects with a magnetic coil over the vertex to evoke a motor response in the fifth finger abductor, the abductor digiti minimi. While response amplitudes were highly variable, dystonics, like controls, showed a decrease in the mean response relative to responses obtained before and after the sleep study in relaxed wakefulness. Latencies were prolonged on average in all groups. These findings—decreased amplitude and prolonged latency—were consistent with REM motor inhibition. Occasional high-amplitude responses may have corresponded to periods of phasic excitation. These results indicate that, whatever the decreased inhibitory processes in dystonia, they do not involve the descending inhibitory pathways of REM sleep.

Studies of sleep in dystonia have not been systematic; studies have involved small numbers of patients taking diverse medications, some of whom had undergone thalamic surgery. In these studies, sleep has been found to be inconsistently disrupted[65,114]; fragmentation is more severe in more advanced cases.[117] The major therapeutic effort in these patients is the attempt to reduce the dystonic movements (for review of therapy, see reference 108 and 109). It can be expected that successful therapy of the movements will also improve sleep, as reported after thalamotomy.[118]

It is not known to what degree different forms of dystonia—early versus late-onset, focal versus generalized—have different relations to sleep, though one striking form of dystonia, variably called, hereditary progressive dystonia with marked diurnal fluctuations (HPD), dopa-responsive dystonia (DRD), or the Segawa variant, often shows distinct circadian variability.[88,119] Patients present at quite a young age, often in the middle of the first decade, with postural dystonia, usually affecting one leg and sparing the trunk and neck. Thereafter, the dystonia spreads and parkinsonian signs, which are present at onset in a minority of patients, become more prominent. Many of these patients have a clear family history and large kindreds with many affected members have been described.[120] Interestingly, significantly more females

than males appear to be affected.[119,121] These patients may obtain significant symptomatic relief from sleep and therefore are minimally impaired early in the day,[88] though this is not true of all patients (57 of 86 in one review[121]) and some dystonic patients unresponsive to L-dopa may have similar benefit from sleep.[89,122] Patients with Parkinson's disease may also show sleep benefit.[69,91] Whether only REM sleep,[88] or NREM sleep, or even rest, can improve symptoms remains somewhat controversial.[89]

The patients do show abnormal sleep motility. Segawa and colleagues obtained movement counts from polysomnography with multiple EMG channels (eight to 12 surface EMG electrodes on trunk and limbs) and found that in DRD there is a decrease in gross body movements in stage one sleep, an increase in stage two, and decrease in REM, whereas localized twitch movements were depressed in all sleep stages but followed the normal relative distribution between stages.[88,123]

Both the diurnal dystonia and the nighttime sleep abnormalities of DRD patients are responsive to small doses of L-dopa, often as little as 50 to 200 mg per day with decarboxylase inhibitor. Unlike parkinsonian patients, some DRD patients can obtain a therapeutic effect even if they take L-dopa only every other day. Patients with long-standing disease (24 to 45 years before treatment) may benefit as well as those with new-onset disease.[121,124,125] This unusual pharmacologic profile led some investigators to suggest this condition may be an early-onset form of parkinsonism with dystonic features.[86] Against this finding is the continued responsiveness of DSD patients to L-dopa without the development of dyskinetic side effects that are very prominent in juvenile parkinsonism.[89,90,125] A few patients may develop a "wearing-off" phenomenon—reemergence of symptoms several hours after an oral dose of L-dopa.[125] Older family members may present with a parkinsonian picture but still show the same persistent, excellent response to L-dopa,[89,90,126] which is consistent with the idea that a single underlying disease has different manifestations that vary with age, dystonia being prominent early whereas parkinsonism appears late.[126]

Recently, with fluorodopa positron emission tomographic scanning, it has been shown in a number of families that patients with DRD exhibit normal to modestly reduced striatal uptake of fluorodopa,[127] including those who present with parkinsonian features later in life.[126] Because of this finding, it can be concluded these patients have relatively intact dopamine uptake, decarboxylation, and storage systems in the striatum. However, somewhere in the path of dopamine synthesis and release, at some other step, there is a metabolic block. A plausible site for this defect lies with the activities of tyrosine hydroxylase (TH),[126] the rate-limiting enzyme for synthesis of catecholamine neurotransmitters, though that enzyme itself is not the locus of the genetic defect in DRD.[128] Some DRD patients have reduced cerebrospinal fluid biopterin, a cofactor needed for TH activity.[129] Some authors have speculated that the diurnal fluctuations of the condition may be due to the circadian variation in dopamine production, greater synthetic activity being possible at night.[124]

Therapy for the condition is straightforward: L-dopa, either alone or with decarboxylase inhibitor (carbidopa, benserazide), begun in small doses with response expected in a few days, or at most weeks. Some patients also respond to anticholinergics (e.g., trihexyphenidyl) or carbamazepine.[125]

Myoclonus.   The myoclonias, which were recently extensively reviewed,[130] are actually a fairly diverse group of conditions in which abnormal movements are generated at different levels of the neuraxis, from cortex (cortical reflex or epileptic myoclonus) to spinal cord (spinal or segmental myoclonus). The basic abnormal movement is a single, repeated, or periodic jerk, most typically of an abrupt, lightning-like character. The categorization of these disorders is in a state of flux, and some conditions, such as nocturnal myoclonus, now known as *periodic limb movement disorder* (PLMD), are likely to be removed from the overall myoclonus category, principally because they lack the lightning-like characteristic of true myoclonus.

Most of the studies of myoclonus and sleep have focused on the persistence of myoclonic movements during sleep. Some of these dyskinesias are very persistent. Lugaresi and colleagues[131] studied a range of patients with myoclonus and found that persistence of the movements during sleep depended on the source of the abnormal discharge: myoclonus with a cortical source showed suppressed movements during sleep, whereas, similar to epilepsy, cortical discharges persisted; myoclonus of presumed subcortical origin was rapidly suppressed during sleep; whereas myoclonus of lower level origins (spinal cord or secondary to peripheral damage) persisted during sleep. Myoclonic jerks associated with startle disease also persist during sleep, though they are less intense.[132]

Among persistent myoclonic conditions, palatal myoclonus, sometimes more recently called palatal tremor, has been held to persist in sleep, and even during anesthesia.[51] Electrophysiologic studies in a small number of patients with palatal and associated eye, and sometimes limb, movements[133,134] have demonstrated that palatal contractions persist during sleep, albeit with shifts in amplitude and frequency, or even altered rhythmicity. The associated eye or limb movements show a greater decrease than

the palatal movements during sleep. This finding of persistent rhythmicity suggests a relatively autonomous oscillator, which is consistent with the idea that these segmental myoclonias may represent releases of primitive rhythmic centers.[51] In contrast to other forms of myoclonus, these dyskinesias appear to arise at a segmental level and to be associated with decreased motor control from higher centers. This dissociation may explain their resistance to modulation by descending inhibitory influences during sleep. Of course, they are not completely removed from higher motor centers or the periphery, as they may disappear in sleep, change with state, and be influenced by attention.[135,136] Spinal myoclonus, another segmental myoclonus, though it is more likely to disappear during sleep[137] can also persist (see reference 138, p. 316). The variable persistence of these segmental myoclonias is consistent with Lugaresi's[131] suggestion that they should persist during sleep.

A conclusion to be drawn from these findings is that when the sleep system is intact dyskinesias arising from dysfunction of the higher motor centers are blocked from expression by the normal inhibitory controls of sleep. Dyskinesias from lower centers, segmental and effector level (such as fasciculations), may be associated with damage to descending control systems and would thus be less regulated by the sleep-wake cycle.

Little is known about sleep in the myoclonic conditions. When movements persist, they are likely to disrupt sleep to some extent, though the movements of palatal myoclonus are usually too modest and continuous to be a source of arousal. Standard therapy for myoclonus may improve any sleep disruption related to the movements themselves.

Tics.   Tics are typically brisk, stereotyped, complex, often repetitive movements.[139,140] Usually, any given patient has a somewhat limited repertoire of movements that may change over periods of months to years. The prototypical tic disorder is Gilles de la Tourette's syndrome, a condition that involves multiple motor tics with vocalizations and usually begins in childhood or adolescence. Tourette's patients also have a number of commonly associated behavioral abnormalities, especially obsessive compulsive disorder. Most sleep studies have examined Tourette's patients.

Typically, younger Tourette's patients, who in most cases are more severely affected, have been studied with polysomnography or sleep monitoring.[141-143] Tics in Tourette's syndrome have been found to persist during sleep in most cases, mostly in the stage 1 and 2 NREM sleep and to a lesser extent during SWS or REM sleep.[143] In addition, body movements in general may be increased in persons with tics: Hashimoto and colleagues found that both twitchlike and gross body movements were more numerous than in control subjects during all stages of sleep, and total movements in tic patients were markedly increased during REM sleep.[142] Those authors did not attempt to analyze such movements in detail, so it is not clear what fraction of them were actual tics.

Sleep has been reported to be impaired in persons with tics. Various investigators have reported increased sleep disruption, higher prevalence of parasomnias, and respiratory disturbances during sleep by patients and family reports.[141] One large study (57 subjects in each group) finding increased parasomnias used two control groups, one of children with learning disorders and another of children with seizures[144]: 17.5% of tic patients exhibited somnambulism significantly more than in either of the two control groups. In one study patients were monitored after successful treatment of their movements with tetrabenazine, and it was found that their sleep had also improved.[145]

Other movement disorders. There are scattered reports of sleep studies of patients with a variety of other motor conditions that can be considered movement disorders. These have been studied less than the conditions discussed above, and a systematic picture of their relation to sleep has not yet been drawn.

In persons with *athetoid cerebral palsy*, abnormalities of REM sleep have been noted. Hayashi and colleagues[146] reported on a group of severely affected adolescent and young adult patients. The significant motor abnormalities all were associated with REM sleep: three patients had decreased numbers of REMS, two had increased chin muscle tone, and seven had reduced numbers of muscle twitches. The authors suggest this may be related to brain stem disease in these birth-injured patients.

Neuroacanthocytosis is an often inherited movement disorder with tics, chorea, vocalizations, and self-mutilation together with frequent seizures, associated with elevated acanthocytes (spiked red cells) in blood smears.[147] Silvestri and colleagues reported that abnormal movements persisted during sleep, but with decreased amplitude, duration, and frequency.[113] Patients frequently vocalized during REM sleep.

In *hemiballism* there are proximal flinging movements of one side of the body, which may be violent, associated with damage to the contralateral subthalamic nucleus.[148] It was initially thought that the movements subsided totally during sleep; however, Askenasy reported on a patient whose movements persisted in sleep,[65] and Silvestri and colleagues found that the movements were present during stage 1 and 2 NREM sleep as well as during REM sleep, though less intense and frequent than in the awake state.[113] Puca and colleagues reported one case in

which spindle density and amplitude were greater ipsilateral to the damaged subthalamic nucleus.[149] There was also disrupted sleep, with prolonged latency and an absence of both SWS and REM sleep. Successful treatment with haloperidol improved the sleep and decreased the spindling. In most cases, hemiballism is a transient phenomenon that follows local injury to the subthalamus, usually ischemic, though it may be transformed into a chronic choreiform disorder.

Hemifacial spasm is a synchronous contraction of one side of the face that is usually repetitive and jerky, but can be sustained.[150,151] It is thought to arise from damage to the facial nerve or nucleus. EMG recording shows highly synchronous discharges in upper and lower facial muscles. Montagna and colleagues[152] studied 16 patients, recording from upper and lower facial muscles during sleep studies. In most patients, the dyskinesias decreased during sleep, being approximately 80% less frequent in SWS and REM sleep. One patient showed almost no change in the prevalence of spasms. Current therapy for hemifacial spasm includes medications such as carbamazepine and botulinum toxin injection in the affected muscles. We are aware of no reports of sleep studies after successful therapy, but it seems likely that the dyskinesias are relieved.

A few final comments on therapy

Specific therapies for different sleep disturbances in the movement disorders have been discussed in the preceding text, but a number of specific suggestions can be made about how to proceed. The first step in tailoring therapy is to determine whether the sleep problem is a direct consequence of the movement disorder itself or is due to a coexisting sleep disorder, which may be primary (sleep apnea) or secondary (e.g., insomnia due to depression). Therapy should then be appropriately addressed to the movement disorder itself or to the coexisting sleep disorder or its underlying cause. Most sleep disorders that coexist with movement disorders would be treated in the usual fashion, continuous positive airway pressure for obstructive sleep apnea or antidepressants for insomnia due to depression.

A second consideration is whether behavioral measures, such as good sleep hygiene, can help the sleep problem. Even demented patients with highly disrupted circadian rhythms may benefit from some temporal order imposed on their daily activity.

Third is to begin therapy, especially in elderly persons or those with degenerative neurologic disease, with small doses and only gradually to build up to full dose schedules. This cautiousness may avoid many side effects. Of course, in some cases, slow buildup may be too discouraging to the patient, who may be looking for a more rapid effect. Then the process of building up to a therapeutic dose may need to be modified.

Fourth is to avoid regular, protracted use of hypnotic medications. In some cases, they may be used for a short time to regularize sleep or on an occasional basis to avid particularly difficult nights. Antihistamines such as diphenhydramine or anticholinergic antidepressants such as amitriptyline may substitute for benzodiazepines.

Movement Disorders Evoked by Sleep

Movement disorders evoked by sleep or rest fall into two primary categories in the International Classification of Sleep Disorders.[57] RLS and PLMS disorder are considered to be intrinsic sleep disorders, whereas other movement abnormalities are classified as parasomnias. At least one condition, fragmentary myoclonus, is categorized as a tentative disorder.

The motor parasomnias are reviewed extensively in the chapter in this volume on parasomnias (Chapter 24). Therefore, this discussion of these conditions is limited while RLS and PLMD are reviewed more

extensively. We also supplement the chapter on parasomnias (Chapter 24) with some additional commentary on two of the more important motor parasomnias, NPD and RBD.

The restless legs syndrome and periodic limb movements in sleep

The RLS, first described in a comprehensive manner by Ekbom[153] and reviewed a number of times since,[32,154-159] is an intrinsic sleep disorder in which leg symptoms lead to difficulties with sleep initiation and may disrupt sleep. The cardinal symptoms are leg paresthesias, provoked by rest, that are associated with an urge to move and relieved by movement such as walking. Most patients with RLS (approximately 70% to 80%[32,160,161]) studied by polysomnography have PLMS, repetitive, nearly periodic movements that occur predominantly during the lighter stages of sleep (Figure 19-1). PLMS, however, are common in patients without RLS, and they constitute a separate intrinsic sleep disorder, periodic limb movement disorder (PLMD). It has been estimated that approximately one-third of patients

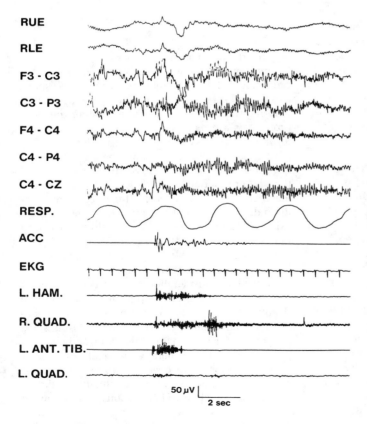

RUE	
RLE	
F3 - C3	
C3 - P3	
F4 - C4	
C4 - P4	
C4 - CZ	
RESP.	
ACC	
EKG	
L. HAM.	
R. QUAD.	
L. ANT. TIB.	
L. QUAD.	

50 µV
2 sec

FIGURE 19-1.   *Polysomnographic recording of PLMS. This movement occurred in stage 2 sleep and led to an arousal, as shown in the EEG traces (bipolar derivations as indicated in third through seventh traces). EMG recordings from left hamstring (HAM), anterior tibial (ANT TIB), and quadriceps (QUAD) muscles and right quadriceps. EMG bursts last 1 to 2 seconds, with some early brief burst components (see especially the left hamstring muscle), reflected in brief transients of the accelerometer (ACC) corresponding to jerklike movements. Accelerometer was placed on dorsum of left foot. Key: RESP, respirometer; RUE, RLE, EOG leads above and below the right eye, referenced to the right ear. (Reprinted, with the permission of Raven Press, from Walters A, Hening W, Côte L, Fahn S. Dominantly inherited restless legs with myoclonus and periodic movements of sleep: A syndrome related to the endogenous opiates? In: Fahn S, Marsden CD, Van Woert M, eds. Myoclonus. New York: Raven Press, 1986;309–319.)*

with PLMS have RLS. In many older—and possibly some newer—studies, specific questions were not asked to determine if patients also had RLS, so that those studies often examined mixed groups of patients, some with RLS and some with PLMS alone. How important this distinction would be is unknown. While the response of the two conditions to medications is quite similar, some differences may exist. One study reported that carbamazepine benefited RLS but had no effect on PLMS, suggesting that they have distinguishable pathophysiologic mechanisms.[160] Because PLMS are almost a component of RLS they are described first.

Periodic limb movements in sleep. PLMS are repetitive, often stereotyped movements that typically recur at intervals of 15 to 40 seconds during NREM sleep. They usually involve the legs and may consist of extension of the great toe associated with flexion at the ankle, knee, and hip. Because of their occasional jerky character and the initial lumping together of several different motor disorders, these movements were first called nocturnal myoclonus[162] and may still be so labeled in some papers. Later, the term *periodic movements in sleep* was introduced, to emphasize their periodicity and deemphasize their myoclonic nature, since they are not usually myoclonic in speed.[163] Subsequently (when the abbreviation for the condition, PMS, was confused with premenstrual syndrome) the name began to shift to *periodic leg (or limb) movements in sleep.* The latter is preferable, because although less common, the arms or trunk may be involved. In the 1990 classification of sleep disorders, the condition is known as periodic limb movement disorder (PLMD).[57]

A typical leg movement has been described as resembling a Babinski's reflex (extension of the great toe with fanning of the other toes)[164] or a triple flexion reflex.[165] A fairly large variety of movements have been described, and the arms or trunk are less often involved.[166] Most movements are not so rapid as to be called myoclonus, and they typically last a few seconds. However, in some cases, each movement may begin with one or more brief, myoclonic jerks, which then blend into a more tonic phase (see Figure 19-1),[32,138,159,165] or a more sustained movement may terminate in a jerk.[159] While most movements occur in the lighter stages of NREM sleep (stage 1 and 2), some movements may occur in SWS and REM sleep as well as during wakefulness, especially when it occurs in the middle of a sleep episode. Bouts of PLMS often end with a shift of body position, which may have occurred in response to the movements.[167]

In observing RBD, Lapierre and Montplaisir[168] found that PLMS occurred as often in REM as in NREM sleep. They concluded from this that the center driving these movements continues to be active during REM sleep but that in otherwise normal patients the movements are suppressed during REM sleep by the descending inhibition. Because the RBD patients lack the normal REM inhibition they have PLMS during REM sleep. Interestingly, patients with narcolepsy also have PLMS during REM sleep,[169] which may be consistent with their having a degree of decreased REM inhibition. It may not be surprising, then, that Schenck and Mahowald have recently reported that patients with narcolepsy have an increased incidence of REM atonia, including RBD,[33] further supporting the contention that deficient REM inhibitory control can disclose the continued operation of a PLMS pacemaker.

Patients with PLMS may be asymptomatic, but severely affected patients may complain of difficulty maintaining sleep or EDS. Bed partners may actually complain more about the movements than the patients and they are often an excellent source of information about the condition and its severity. The importance of PLMS has been questioned in the past,[163] though many sleep specialists now believe that severe cases may cause significant sleep disturbance and warrant therapy.

PLMS may begin at any age, but prevalence increases markedly in later life until more than 30% of persons older than 65 years may have a significant number of PLMS.[170] Indeed, because of night to night variability[170] it is possible that as many as 70% or 80% of elderly persons relatively frequently have more than 5 PLMS per hour. The importance of PLMS to sleep and wakefulness in the elderly is subject to question. Some studies have found no association between PLMS and either objective measures of sleep or symptomatic reports (or only very weak ones).[170] Other reports have not found that PLMS necessarily become more severe with time[171] though age is an important variable in their prevalence. In one large-scale and extensive study, Dickel and Mosko[172] examined 100 healthy, community-dwelling seniors with few sleep complaints (only 18% expressed complaints), and found that 71% had some PLMS on two nights of polysomnography (after one adaptation night); 58% had more than 5 per hour of sleep (a movement index, MI, greater than 5). But using a threshold MI of 5, 20, or 40 did not reveal significant associations with sleep complaints, although sleep was more disrupted in those with greater MIs. Interestingly, for the 71 subjects with PLMS, on average, only 25% of sleep time (PI or pervasiveness index) was dominated by epochs of PLMS. Because of these findings, elderly patients with PLMS on polysomnography or ambulatory recording should not be treated unless the PLMS can be linked to their sleep complaints.

PLMS is generally diagnosed by polysomnographic recording or ambulatory sleep monitoring.

TABLE 19-2.   Conditions associated with RLS and PLMS

Underlying Condition	Associated with RLS	Associated with PLMS
Sleep disorders		
OSA	×	×
Narcolepsy		×
RBD		×
Neurologic disorders		
Amyotropic lateral sclerosis		×
Huntington's disease		×
Isaac's syndrome		×
Multiple sclerosis	×	×
Myelopathies	×	×
Peripheral neuropathies	×	
Poliomyelitis	×	
Radiculopathies	×	
Spinal cord lesions		×
Startle disease		×
Stiff-man syndrome		×
Medical disorders		
Amyloidosis	×	
Anemia	×	
Cancer	×	
Chronic obstructive pulmonary disease	×	×
Diabetes	×	
Ferritin deficiency	×	
Fibrositis syndrome		×
Folate deficiency	×	
Gastrectomy	×	
Impotence		×
Iron deficiency	×	
Leukemia		×
Rheumatoid arthritis	×	
Telangiectasia	×	
Uremia	×	×
Vascular insufficiency	×	
Exogenous chemicals		
Caffeine	×	
L-Dopa		×
Lithium	×	×
Neuroleptics	×	
Tricyclic antidepressants		×
Withdrawal from sedative/ narcotic medications	×	

While the precise categorization of leg movement activity varies, most investigators use a definition that includes EMG burst duration, interval between movements, and number of movements in a series. A typical scheme counts movements if they occur in series of four or more during any sleep stage (wakefulness excluded) at intervals of 5 to 120 seconds. EMG bursts must last 0.5 to 5 seconds. The number of movements associated with arousals may also be counted.[173] Criteria for diagnosis or severity typically use an index determined by dividing the total number of movements (PLMS index) or movements associated with arousals (arousal index) by total sleep time. A PLMS index greater than 5 is considered abnormal. The International Classification defines severe PLMS as occurring with a PLMS index greater than 50 or an arousal index greater than 25.

One recent home study of disorders of initiating and maintaining sleep (DIMS) patients with previously documented PLMS found that their night to night variability, though significant in some individual cases, only rarely resulted in major changes in clinical classification.[174] Patients who were blindly rated as having severe PLMS by sleep clinicians based on home ambulatory sleep monitoring were usually (five of seven patients) rated as severe on each of the three night studies in which they participated. The initial night study was rated as severe in each of these patients.

PLMS may occur as an isolated condition or may be associated with a large number of other medical, neurologic, or sleep disorders or with medications and other pharmacologic agents (Table 19-2). Unfortunately, few studies are controlled and it is often not possible to say whether an association is more than a matter of chance. Now that it has become clear that large numbers of older persons have PLMS, the significance of a modest percentage of older patients with PLMS in association with some other condition must be more closely scrutinized. For instance, PLMS are common in patients with obstructive sleep apnea and RBD, but these patients are elderly. Some comparative studies have shown similar prevalence of PLMS among normal subjects and insomniacs.[175] Patients with sleep disorders may have a similar prevalence of PLMS.[163] Among sleep disorders, the more striking associations are with narcolepsy[33,176,177] and RLS, because PLMS are common in these patients even if they are relatively young. Obstructive sleep apnea patients may actually have more PLMS, sometimes with significant sleep fragmentation, after successful treatment of their apnea. Among medical conditions, the association with uremia is likely to be an important one. In some conditions, PLMS may be of great significance for sleep: in one actigraphic and polysomnographic study of 13 patients with rheumatoid arthritis, sleep efficiency was more highly negatively linked to PLMS than to measures of disease activity, suggesting that the PLMS were a major factor for sleep fragmentation in these patients.[178] In some cases, especially that of medications, it may be that PLMS are aggravated, rather than precipitated, by the condition or medication. In general, a full understanding of which conditions increase PLMS may have to await more sweeping epidemiologic studies. Until such studies are undertaken, however, it is probably worth keeping in mind the associations already suggested, with their general notion that altered nervous system function may often be expressed as PLMS, if patients with other disorders present with complaints of poor sleep maintenance or EDS.

Therapy for PLMS may be indicated when the movements seem to be the primary source of sleep disturbance. Benzodiazepines have been most commonly described as the first-line medications for PLMS and have been shown to improve sleep. Clonazepam, temazepam, and triazolam[179,180] have proven effective in blinded studies. Baclofen was reported to improve sleep with PLMS by decreasing movement intensity and arousals, but it did not decrease the number of movements.[181] Various medications effective for RLS have been reported to be active against PLMS as well.[182,183] It seems reasonable, in refractory cases, to try the range of medications that are useful for RLS, though, because carbamazepine had no effect on PLMS in patients with RLS treated successfully in one study,[160] this may be a medication to try only if a number of others have failed. Nonpharmacologic therapy for PLMS, such as muscle or nerve stimulation,[184] occasionally has been reported to be helpful and is, therefore, worth trying when patients prefer not to take medications or cannot tolerate them. Withdrawal of medications that likely aggravate PLMS may also be useful.

Because no clear pathologic mechanism has been demonstrated for isolated PLMS, its pathogenesis, like that of RLS, is unknown. It seems reasonable, given the periodic nature of the movements, to postulate that they are driven by an oscillator that is able to overcome the motor inhibition of NREM sleep. This oscillator is modulated by the sleep-wake alternation, and, in many persons is largely or completely suppressed throughout life. The very high prevalence of PLMS in elderly persons, and the increased prevalence among persons with neurologic conditions, argue that the balance of favor of the oscillator's suppression is a relatively slight one. Lugaresi and colleagues have suggested that the oscillation may be linked to autonomic periodicities generated primarily within the brain stem.[185] This would couple the oscillator to apparently normal rhythmicities in the central nervous system. Further support for this proposal is found in the shifts in heart rate and respiratory rate reported in some patients in phase with the PLMS.[186] Because PLMS are predominant in the legs, an oscillator located in the spinal cord is a definite possibility, though, for now, the location remains uncertain. One recent report[165] does support a spinal location, since two of ten patients with spinal cord lesions and PLMS were believed to have complete spinal cord transections at the cervical (C-7) and thoracic (T-6) levels, respectively. These patients without evidence for descending motor influences showed phenomenologically typical PLMS throughout all sleep stages. Unless the transection in these patients was not complete, the minimum con-clusion to be drawn from this finding is that the lower spinal cord can support movements like PLMS. Recent studies in RBD, which show persistent PLMS during REM sleep, suggest that the oscillator may be active throughout all sleep stages but that its manifestations, the leg movements, are suppressed selectively during REM sleep.[168] The same suppression may apply during SWS. Alternatively, the oscillator may itself be inhibited by the REM-generated mechanism in patients without RBD, whereas RBD patients have a parallel failure of atonia and suppression of the PLMS oscillator.

The restless legs syndrome. Table 19-3 indicates the features of the RLS. The most distinctive one is that the sensory and motor symptoms are evoked by rest, either quiet wakefulness or attempts to sleep. Patients typically report their symptoms are worst when they are lying down or sitting. They almost always describe uncomfortable sensations, most common in the legs, especially in the region of the calves, that may be variably described as tingling, burning, like water moving or insects crawling, aching, grabbing, or painful, though a wide variety of other descriptions may be offered and a significant number of patients cannot describe the sensations at all. These sensations are usually associated with an urge to move, though some patients report such an urge or inner feeling of restlessness independent of any clear precipitating sensation. In response to the urge to move, patients typically walk around, though a wide variety of movements such as rocking, shaking, stretching, marching in place, or bending may be tried for relief. These varied movements that patients select to reduce their symptoms are under voluntary control and can be suppressed by the patient on command. Suppression, however, may

TABLE 19-3. Clinical features of the idiopathic RLS

Uncomfortable sensations, primarily in the legs
Motor restlessness, relieved by activity
Dyskinesias while awake that occur almost exclusively at rest
PLMS
Exacerbation of sensorimotor features by repose
Sleep disturbance, especially difficulty in sleep initiation
Circadian variability with symptoms worst in the evening and early in the night
Suggestive family history consistent with dominant inheritance
Exclusion of potential underlying causes for RLS
Absence of associated abnormalities on neurologic examination
Onset at any age, typically with chronic and progressive course. Most severely affected persons are middle aged to older. Occasional remissions. Frequent onset of aggravation during pregnancy.

greatly increase the patient's discomfort and few severely affected patients are willing to suppress their restless movements for more than a brief period when they are symptomatic. Many patients report that they use also a variety of sensory stimuli such as massage, applying oils or other materials, hot baths, or cold showers to get at least temporary relief.

While awake, patients may also have involuntary movements that they cannot suppress by will alone. These are typically jerky movements that have an appearance and distribution similar to that of PLMS but are more intense and rapid (Figure 19-2), which we have termed *dyskinesias while awake* (DWA).[187] Although the movements may take a variable form they are most characteristically a flexion jerk, with flexion at hip, knee, and ankle. In the flexed leg, the movements may appear to be primarily extensions, consistent with our EMG observation (unpublished studies) that there is usually cocontraction in flexor and extensor muscles during the dyskinesias. Although they may have a wide range of speeds, DWAs are often myoclonic in speed. Because these jerks are influenced by ongoing voluntary movements or position (flexion may suppress the jerks), they are less periodic than PLMS and may appear to be either aperiodic or clustered in bursts. In some patients

these movements may merge with PLMS at sleep onset or termination. It has been noted that DWAs have a shorter period than PLMS (Figure 19-3).[138,188] A recent review of RLS with accompanying videotape illustrates the different voluntary and involuntary movements that patients experience.[187]

Most commonly, the various symptoms occur during the evening or early part of the night (between about 6:00 P.M. and 4:00 A.M.). Patients are less bothered by symptoms during the daytime and, even if severely affected, often obtain some relief near dawn. In general, patients experience the abnormal sensations, involuntary movements, and urge to move or restlessness under the same conditions. Indeed, these different symptoms tend to respond to the same medications.[189–191] They can be shown to be associated by tests that relatively immobilize patients as a means of provoking repose-dependent symptoms,[192,193] though it does not seem likely that they are invariably related as a single phenomenon, since some patients complain of either uncomfortable sensations or involuntary movements alone.

Patients with RLS have disturbed sleep because of their symptoms and their PLMS. They have a primary difficulty getting to sleep because lying down

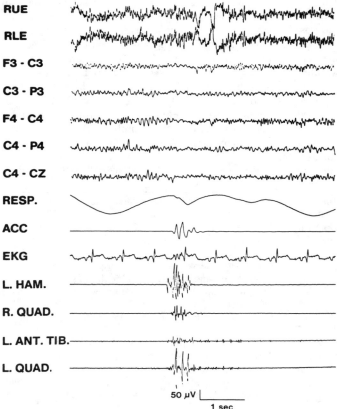

FIGURE 19-2. *Polysomnographic recording of dyskinesia while awake in patient with RLS. Labels as in Figure 19-1. EMG and accelerometer traces show a series of brief (less than 250 msec) jerking movements of myoclonic speed. EEG traces show waking state with desynchronization and lower-amplitude potentials during the movement. (Reprinted, with the permission of Raven Press, from Walters A, Hening W, Côte L, Fahn S. Dominantly inherited restless legs with myoclonus and periodic movements of sleep: A syndrome related to the endogenous opiates? In: Fahn S, Marsden CD, Van Woert M, eds. Myoclonus. New York: Raven Press, 1986;309–319.)*

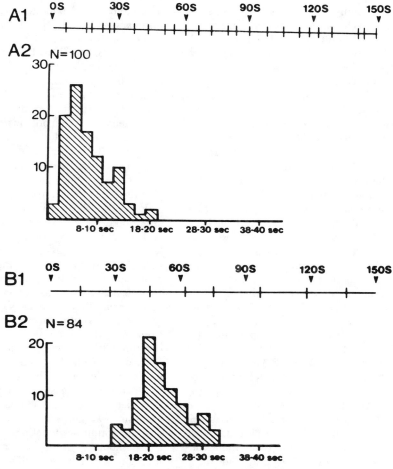

FIGURE 19-3.   *Periodicity of DWA (A) and PLMS (B) in RLS.* Data drawn from one subject in whom 100 consecutive DWA and 84 consecutive PLMS were timed during long epochs of constant activity. During DWA, the patient was awake holding legs extended. During PLMS, the patient was in stage 1 or 2 NREM sleep. (*A1, B1*) 150 second (2½-minute) time lines with each vertical mark indicating one movement. Cumulative time indicated by arrows. (*A2, B2*) Histograms show the distributions of intermovement intervals (periods of movements). The DWA have significantly shorter intervals (< 0.001) and a greater coefficient of variation (53.3% versus 20.2%) than PLMS, indicating a shorter periodicity and more irregular occurrence for the DWA. (Reprinted, with the permission of Raven Press, from Walters A, Hening W, Côte L, Fahn S. Dominantly inherited restless legs with myoclonus and periodic movements of sleep: a syndrome related to the endogenous opiates? In: Fahn S, Marsden CD, Van Woert M, eds. Myoclonus. New York: Raven Press, 1986;309–319.)

and trying to relax activates the symptoms, which may be relieved only by activity. In severe cases, patients may have frequent nights when sleep is delayed several hours because of their symptoms. In addition to prolonged sleep latency, patients may have difficulty maintaining sleep. An important con-tribution to this may be their PLMS, which can arouse and awaken them. Approximately 70% to 80% of patients with RLS have associated PLMS.[161] In severe cases this disturbance can be quite significant.[194] As a result of these difficulties in achieving sleep, patients may, in severe cases, have a total sleep time of only 3 or 4 hours a night. In such cases, excessive daytime sleepiness can occur that may be severe and significant. It has been noted, though not formally studied, that RLS patients are less likely to complain of EDS than patients with similarly sleep-disruptive obstructive sleep apnea, patients with equivalent sleep reduction, or patients with narcolepsy. While RLS is generally a condition that impairs the quality of life, it has not generally been thought to carry an adverse general prognosis. However, in one study, Pollak and colleagues found that in women RLS was a significant predictor of death during the study period.[195] The significance of that association remains to be further defined.

While our impression is that the majority of cases of RLS are idiopathic (though no studies have been done to establish this epidemiologic point), RLS has also been associated with a variety of other illnesses (see Table 19-2). One important condition in which RLS has been reported is uremia. RLS is only one of a spectrum of motor abnormalities that occur in uremia, and it may need to be distinguished from action myoclonus, asterixis, tremor, and akathisia. While it has not been satisfactorily documented (as by videotape study), it is our clinical impression and that of at least one other group (P Montagna, personal communication) that RLS in uremia may be phenomenologically identical to that in idiopathic cases. Uremic patients may have abnormal sensations, an urge to move, and abnormal jerks associated with rest. In one study, patients with RLS (40% of 55 dialysis patients) were more likely to be anemic, but they had no more neuropathy than those without RLS.[196] Correcting the anemia in an open-label long-term trial led to significantly decreased subjective complaints.

In secondary cases, it is important to distinguish RLS from akathisia, which, to be more confusing, has at times been called restless legs. Akathisia, most typically due to neuroleptic medications (neuroleptic-induced akathisia or NIA), is a similar motor restlessness that may have sleep abnormalities and associated PLMS.[197] However, Lipinski and colleagues in one study did not find PLMS, but rather a distinctive rhythmic activity at sleep onset and during arousals that may represent a rhythmic manifestation of the akathisia.[198] Akathisia can be distinguished from RLS by history and examination of the patient.[197,199] We have noted, based on patient interview and observation, that there are several telling historical distinctions between RLS and NIA[197]: (1) RLS patients complain most about uncomfortable sensations as a source of restlessness (19/20), while this is less common in NIA patients (5/20), who have a more primary sense of inner restlessness (15/20). (2) RLS patients more commonly complain about nighttime aggravation of their symptoms (18/20 com-

pared to 6/20 NIA patients); NIA patients have continuous symptoms or symptoms related to the timing of neuroleptic doses. (3) RLS patients more frequently report they feel worst when lying down (16/20 versus 3/20 NIA patients). (4) NIA patients tend to have persistent, repetitive, cyclic movements like body rocking and marching in place, whereas RLS patients less commonly have similar kinds of movements, and then only in association with nighttime symptoms and restlessness. Akathisia is associated with a number of disorders such as Parkinson's disease, as well as medications, but it is almost always secondary. Idiopathic or essential akathisia is at least rare.

Idiopathic RLS begins at any age, even in early childhood,[200,201] but prevalence increases with age and some persons become symptomatic only when elderly. Studies of prevalence suggest that there may be a significant fraction of older persons who have symptoms of RLS. In some surveys as many as 29% in some patient groups have reported symptoms consistent with RLS.[202] Because the features of RLS were only recently fully clarified, there have not been any full-scale studies that are truly adequate to determine the exact prevalence. Pregnancy is a known precipitant of the condition, which may subsequently remit. The course of the illness may fluctuate, but, at least in severe cases, it progresses over periods of years or decades. At least partial remissions are not rare, but in most cases RLS is a chronic condition, whether it is treated or not.[203] Since Ekbom,[153] it has been noted that RLS can be found in first-degree relatives, and efforts to find familial clusters have been quite successful.[200,203] This has led to the proposition that RLS may be a dominantly inherited condition. Genetic studies are now under way, in an attempt to find linkage for the putative RLS gene.[204] One factor that has made the familial clustering less obvious is that probands are often uninformed about the presence of the condition even in close relatives. In addition, since many individuals are not affected until late in life, full detection of those carrying the gene currently is not possible.

Evaluation of the RLS involves a general medical history and physical examination, to rule out possible secondary causes of the syndrome. In idiopathic RLS, findings of the neurologic examination are normal unless some additional neurological disorder is present. Blood tests should probably be performed to exclude anemia (including iron, ferritin, and folate levels) and uremia, if recent results are not available. In longstanding cases with no findings on history or examination that may end the work-up for cause. With sensory findings or a complaint suggestive of root damage, an EMG and nerve conduction study should be performed. Evaluation of RLS should include sleep logs, as part of the general evaluation of the sleep complaint, and specific questions about the RLS. We have rated subjective discomfort on a scale of 0 to 3, where 0 is asymptomatic and 1 through 3 represent mild, moderate, or severe symptoms. Patients assess their leg discomfort, restlessness, jerks while awake, difficulty getting to sleep, difficulty staying asleep, and daytime somnolence. The most profoundly affected patients would have an RLS score of 18. This scale has been helpful in assessing subjective response to therapy (Figure 19-4). Polysomnography is indicated to document the

degree of sleep disorder and establish whether PLMS are present.

Despite the suggestion that idiopathic RLS may have a genetic basis, no pathologic mechanism is known to be associated with the syndrome. The only exceptions to this observation are secondary cases, when lesions typical of the primary disorder may be present. Because of the caudal distribution of the symptoms, the activation of symptoms during periods of decreased voluntary activity, and the lack of signs of cortical lesions or irritation, it is generally believed that the primary generator for the condition

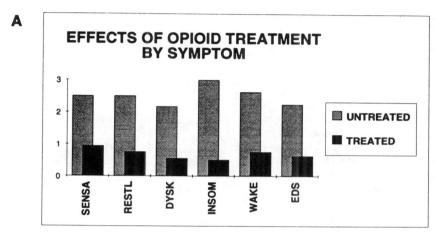

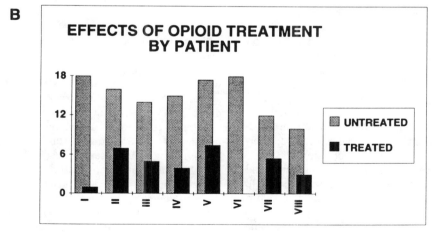

FIGURE 19-4. *Effects of opioid therapy on eight patients with RLS. Patients rated six symptoms on 0 to 3 scale before therapy (*untreated*) and on opioid therapy (*treated; for five patients, treatment included additional medications). Symptoms include SENSA, Uncomfortable sensations; RESTL, degree of motor restlessness or urge to move; DYSK, dyskinesias while awake; INSOM, difficulty in getting to sleep; WAKE, waking after sleep onset; and EDS, excessive daytime somnolence. (A) Mean rating per symptom across 8 patients (all differences significant, P < .05, paired t test). (B) Sum of the six ratings for each individual patient, I–VIII (sum ranges from 0 to 18).*

must be subcortical, lying somewhere between the basal ganglia and the spinal cord. Evidence of enhanced polysynaptic reflex excitability in some of these patients[205] suggests that they may have a generalized deficiency of inhibitory processes, but other manifestations of this deficiency are absent in most patients. Moreover, other reports have not found increased reflex excitability.[165,206] If increased excitability is present, it may point generally to some synaptic or related process that may be genetically abnormal in patients with idiopathic disorders. Impairment of a descending inhibitory system could explain the sensorimotor systems of RLS as lower level (presumably segmental) sensorimotor activity that is released by the impaired descending inhibition. The symptoms, then, would be somewhat similar to such release phenomena as hyperreflexia, clonus, and flexor spasms that occur in patients with damage to the descending pyramidal tract.

Cortical motor prepotentials may also help localize the source of an abnormal discharge leading to an involuntary movement. These prepotentials are EEG events time-locked to a movement, but occurring before it and indicating that associated activity is developing before the movement. Short latency cortical prepotentials are taken as evidence that there is a cortical source for a particular movement.[207] Some groups have failed to find a prepotential before PLMS or DWA,[32,207A] while we have found a cortical prepotential occurring before leg jerks in some patients that was unlike the prepotential before stimulated leg jerks.[206,208] However, because this is a long-lived, slowly rising potential, it cannot provide strong evidence for a cortical source for the leg jerks. Rather, the cortical potential may be a manifestation of some subcortical event projected upward to the cortex, perhaps an event related to the uncomfortable sensations of RLS that may accompany leg jerks.[193] A final clue to the pathophysiology of RLS may be the spectrum of medications to which the condition responds. These would indicate participation in some fashion of the opioidergic, dopaminergic, or GABA-ergic systems in producing RLS.

Therapy for RLS (Table 19-4) has been developed over the last 10 or 12 years, until it is now possible to treat most patients with a fair degree of success (for reviews, see references 157 to 159 and 161). The mainstays of therapy are the benzodiazepines, the dopaminergic drugs, and the opioids. A number of multipatient, controlled studies have provided support for the proposition that each of these classes of drugs ameliorates the symptoms of RLS. A successful strategy may be to start patients on a benzodiazepine in fairly small doses (0.5 to 2 mg clonazepam or 15 mg temazepam), gradually increase to moderate-sized doses (4 mg clonazepam or 30 mg temazepam nightly) as tolerated, and then add either

TABLE 19-4. Medications useful in RLS

Primary therapy
  Benzodiazepines
    Clonazepam
    Temazepam
    Nitrazepam
    Alprazolam
    Triazolam
    Diazepam
  Dopaminergic agents
    L-Dopa combined with carbidopa or benserazide
    Long-acting combined L-Dopa preparations
    Bromocriptine
    Selegiline
  Opioids
    Oxycodone
    Propoxyphene
    Codeine
    Methadone
    Pentazocine
Back-up Therapy
  Carbamzepine
  Clonidine
  Propranolol
Secondary or symptomatic therapy
  Baclofen
  Folate
  5-Hydroxytryptophan (5-HTP)
  Iron
  Orphenadrine citrate
  Phenoxybenzamine
  Vasodilators
  Vitamin B_{12}
  Vitamin E

a dopaminergic agent or an opioid, again beginning with small doses and titrating upward. Sinemet 25/100 (which can be split), Sinemet CR (beginning with a half pill), or 2.5 to 5 mg of bromocriptine would be a useful starting dose of a dopaminergic agent. For opioid agents, either propoxyphene at doses of 65 to 130 mg (or equivalent) or 30 mg codeine (which may be combined with acetaminophen) would be a useful starting dose. In both cases, it may be necessary to gradually increase the dose to achieve adequate control. Patients generally tolerate the opioid medications well, but most require incremental adjustment of doses over several years after adequate dosage is initially established. Severely affected patients may require two or even three classes of medications for adequate control. Those with a mild disturbance often obtain adequate relief by taking medication as needed. Some authors have suggested that rotating medications may be a useful strategy to prevent development of tolerance to any one.[158]

Each of the therapies has potential drawbacks. Benzodiazepines can cause drowsiness or depression and, in elderly persons, also confusion. Doses of long-acting agents such as diazepam may result in accumulating effects that last through the daytime. A possible drawback to dopaminergic therapy is the development of late night reemergence of symptoms or displacement of symptoms into the day after treatment with L-dopa.[161,183,189] Sinemet CR, a longer-acting medication, may obviate this problem to some extent, but definitive proof is so far lacking. Some patients have required around-the-clock treatment with L-dopa for control after they develop daytime symptoms. Others patients have also complained of insomnia while taking L-dopa.[146] Another worry is the long-term effects of dopaminergic agents, which are associated with dyskinesias and other abnormal motor phenomena in patients with Parkinson's disease. So far, this has not been a problem with RLS patients.[161] Von Scheele and Kempi reported a two-year period of therapy with levodopa (combined with benserazide) in 26 patients who remained without significant dyskinesias and continued to be responsive to the medications though 9 of them needed to increase their daily dose.[209] Opioids should obviously be avoided in persons with an addictive personality, but aside from such patients, for us the major drawback to using opioids has been the potential for criticism by reviewing authorities. We have found that some patients can be controlled on opioids at a stable dose for more than 10 years.[191] We recently studied oxycodone as a treatment for RLS and found, in a double-blind crossover placebo study that it alleviated PLMS and improved objective measures of sleep and subjective measures of RLS symptoms.[210] Most patients tolerate opioids well; constipation and a modest degree of sedation are the most significant complaints.

Despite these drawbacks, it is our impression that the majority of even severely affected RLS patients may experience significant amelioration of their condition with some medication or combination of medications from these groups. In our experience, severely affected patients rarely find the therapy intolerable and rarely decide to stop using the drugs.

A number of other medications have been tried in variably controlled studies and have shown promise for RLS. Carbamazepine, at anti-seizure doses with therapeutic drug levels, was effective for RLS in a large-scale double-blind clinical trial.[211] An open-label polysomnographic study on nine patients with RLS and PLMS found significant subjective improvement and significant improvement in some sleep measures (sleep efficiency, sleep latency) with a trend toward improvement in other measures (decreased WASO and percentage of stage 1 NREM sleep).[160] PLMS were unaffected in number, frequency, and tendency to cause arousals. β-blockers such as propranolol[212] and α-adrenergic blockers such as clonidine[213] have also been reported to be successful.

The secondary medications listed in Table 19-4 may be considered if, for some reason, the primary medications are not helpful or are limited by other problems of the patient. Experience with these is limited, but as a general rule, introducing a medication with small doses and gradually increasing the dose is probably a useful strategy.

Nocturnal paroxysmal dystonia and related conditions

NPD (see also Chapter 24) was first described by Lugaresi's group as a condition of uncertain cause that might be considered analogous to diurnal paroxysmal movement disorders.[214] More recently, Montagna[215] has linked the form of paroxysmal nocturnal dystonia with short-lived (seconds to minutes) attacks together with two other conditions, paroxysmal arousals[216] and episodic nocturnal wanderings,[217] and proposed that these three disorders represent a spectrum of related disorders. They share the main features of sudden arousals or awakenings from NREM sleep, dyskinetic or semipurposive movement and vocalizations, which can be quite forceful, and a link to epilepsy in some patients. This link consists of increased prevalence of seizures in patients, interictal EEG abnormalities, response of many patients to anticonvulsants, and the resemblance of the episodes to complex partial seizures, especially those of deep frontal lobe origin.[218] Though ictal records have not shown epileptic activity on the EEG, Montagna postulates this may be due to the deep-seated locus of the attacks, which prevents them from being seen at the cortical surface. Meierkord and colleagues recently further supported the epileptic nature of these attacks by showing that they overlap substantially in character with nocturnal attacks of patients who have an established diagnosis of nocturnal epilepsy.[219]

Lugaresi's group also recently described a form of NPD[220] that occurs periodically (every 30 seconds to 2 minutes) with usually quite brief attacks (2 to 13 seconds in duration) and arousals that they have called *atypical periodic movements in sleep*. While it "overlaps" with the short-lived NPD, this condition has been unresponsive to seizure medications, even though one patient had a vascular orbital frontal tumor on CT and spikes on depth recording.

Short-lived attacks of NPD begin with arousal, including an abrupt autonomic activation that can include substantial tachycardia, followed by dystonic movements and large-scale semipurposeful movements of all limbs. Vocalizations are common. The attacks are quite diverse if considered between patients but appear to be stereotyped in a single patient. Attacks last about a minute (typical range 15 seconds to 2 minutes) and may be vaguely remembered. Neither tongue biting nor urinary incontinence has so far been reported.

Paroxysmal arousals are brief attacks lasting several seconds in which patients awake abruptly from NREM sleep, perhaps with a start or cry, have fleeting dyskinetic movements, then fall back to sleep. Episodic nocturnal wanderings are attacks of sudden motor activity, including violent ambulation, loud vocalizations, and a variety of forceful gestures that can cause significant injury. The attacks commonly occur in stage 2 NREM sleep.

Other dystonic attacks, especially those of longer duration (2 to 50 minutes) have not been so clearly associated with epilepsy and may represent more primary movement disorders.[215] In one case, a patient afflicted with such attacks for 20 years developed HD; however, a full classification of these attacks cannot yet be made.

NPD events must be distinguished from nocturnal seizures with clear epileptic EEGs, which can look similar, from PLMS, if periodic, and from RBD. The main distinction between NPD and RBD is the clear association of the latter with REM sleep and the response of the two conditions to dissimilar medications.

The epilepsy-like attacks are treated with anticonvulsants, especially carbamazepine. Treatment of the nonepileptic attacks remains uncertain.

REM sleep behavior disorder

Patients with RBD (see also Chapter 24) typically present with a history of vivid dreams and excessive movements in sleep, sometimes violent ones that cause injury to the patient or bed partner.[221–223] The condition may begin insidiously and progress over many years. A so-called prodrome, consisting principally of vocalizations and limb jerks, was reported in 17 of 70 patients in a large series described by Schenck and Mahowald.[224] Violent behavior may be specifically related to dream content, which is often repetitive and stereotyped and commonly involves the patient's engaging with some form of threat. For example, the patient may dream that he is rescuing his wife from attackers, though at the time he is actually striking her.[223]

While RBD may occur at any age, including childhood, it is far more common in elderly persons. Men are more commonly afflicted than women, and there may be a familial tendency in some cases.[223] Although it can clearly occur in otherwise healthy and neurologically intact persons, RBD appears to have a significantly increased prevalence in those with neurodegenerative disorders, including Parkinson's disease.[68A, 68B, 224] It may be particularly common in OPCA and Shy-Drager syndrome.[53] In some cases it may herald the onset of such a condition.[225] The

condition has also been associated with brain stem insults, such as infarcts.[226] Similar transient conditions may occur in situations of drug toxicity or withdrawal as well as other conditions of acute brain stem insult.[223]

In contrast to the usual predilection for the elderly, Schenck and Mahowald have recently reported RBD to be common in narcolepsy (more than 10% of patients polysomnographically studied).[33] Narcolepsy, of course, involves various abnormalities of REM organization. This group is exceptional in the youthful age of onset of RBD (the mean age in Schenck and Mahowald's study was 28.4 years). These patients also had a high incidence of PLMS (10 of 17), another condition more typically associated with advanced years.

Patients with this condition show increased EMG tone in the mentalis on polysomnography during REM sleep, together with excessive phasic movement outbursts. Patients also have other sleep motor disturbances, and many have both PLMD and excessive fragmentary myoclonus in NREM sleep or other NREM periodic movements.[222,226] In a recent series reported by Schenck and Mahowald, 44 of 70 patients had PLMD and 28 of 70 had aperiodic NREM movements.[224] Lapierre and Montplaisir found in a small controlled series that the PLMS of RBD occurred as often in REM as in NREM sleep.[168] They conclude that this occurs because the RBD patients lack a normal atonia that would mask the PLMS.

Other than the motor disturbances, sleep architecture is usually normal in RBD patients, though they may have more SWS and REM sleep than expected for their age. In the Schenck and Mahowald series, 28 of 65 evaluable patients had increased REM percent (more than 25% of total sleep time), and 42 of 50 patients older than 57 years had increased SWS (more than 15% of total sleep time).[224] In another study of seven otherwise healthy elderly patients, Tachibana and colleagues[227] found normal sleep architecture. The patients had increases in both tonic REM sleep EMG and in phasic EMG, as measured in chin EMG. Their only other abnormality was increased REM density (number of REMs per minute of REM sleep).

Diagnosis relies on a mixture of clinical and polysomnographic features. On PSG, patients must have at least some tonic or phasic abnormality in muscle tone. (Usually they have both: Lapierre and Montplaisir have proposed that both be required.[168]) Violent, dream-related behaviors must be documented by excessive, complex, or violent behavior during polysomnographically recorded REM sleep or a significant history of abrupt, dangerous, or sleep-disrupting behaviors. In addition, seizures must be excluded by suitable EEG recording.[223] The differential diagnosis includes sleep disorders that cause disrupted movements and sleep, as well as awakenings—somnambulism, night terrors, NPD, as well as some cases of sleep apnea or PLMD. Dissociated states can also be confused with RBD. All of these can generally be distinguished by a combination of a careful sleep history, including interview of the bed partner, and adequate polysomnography (with video or observational monitoring, EMG leads on legs, and suitable EEG montage for seizure study).

Most patients respond well to clonazepam, which may be particularly effective in suppressing the dangerous, violent sleep behavior[223]; however, occasional breakthrough behavior may occur, so the patient's environment should be rendered safe even if treatment appears to be working. Other medications that may be effective include L-dopa (combined with carbidopa) and clonidine.[224]

Pathophysiologically, this condition appears to be a human analogue of REM sleep without atonia, a breakdown of the normal REM inhibition of the lower motor neuron with resulting translation of cortical impulses into motor behavior. It is, therefore, likely an abnormality of the higher regulatory centers. Animal models of this condition have been available for several decades. They are caused by specific lesions in the brain stem: different lesions may cause different forms of behavioral abnormality.[46] The disruption may be specific to atonia, with normal descending drive intact, since, in one controlled study, patients had the same number of REMs as normal subjects.[168]

Other sleep-related movement disorders

Benign neonatal myoclonus, also a parasomnia, is a transient, sometimes familial condition that begins soon after birth and resolves within months.[228] The myoclonic jerks are brief, asynchronous, and repetitive, involving primarily the distal limbs but also the trunk. The jerks occur during all stages of sleep, most in NREM sleep, and typically do not arouse or wake the infant.[229] The pathophysiology of this disorder is unknown. It is not typically associated with other nervous system disease, and the EEG is not epileptogenic, distinguishing this condition from a seizure disorder. It may be an exaggeration of the normally greater sleep-related movements of infants.[230]

Fragmentary myoclonus is considered a possible sleep disorder.[57] The abnormal movements of this condition are brief, asymmetric, focal jerks of the face and limbs that occur primarily during NREM sleep.[43] The associated EMG shows brief (less than 150 msec) bursts of variable amplitude, the larger bursts associated with visible movements. Fragmentary myoclonus may be associated with one of a variety of sleep disorders, or it can occur in isolation.[43] Because the myoclonus is similar to the jerks of sleep starts or hypnic myoclonus, it may represent an exaggeration of normal sleep movements. This condition may be another in which inadequate inhibitory drive fails to block descending activation from higher centers, or it may represent a condition of excessive activation of higher centers during NREM sleep.

Fatal familial insomnia (FFI)[231] is a recently described condition that involves progressive insomnia with derangement of sleep states, autonomic changes, and motor signs, especially ataxia (loss of coordination) and myoclonus. It is classified as a medical or psychiatric sleep disorder associated with a neurologic disorder in the current sleep classification.[57] In some patients the motor symptoms are noted first.[231] The condition appears to be inherited in an autosomal dominant pattern (transmitted from a parent to children of both sexes). Genetic linkage studies have established that the disease is related to a mutation in the prion protein that also causes Creutzfeld-Jakob disease (CJD), a rapidly progressive dementia often accompanied by myoclonus. Indeed, the mutation in FFI is identical to that of one familial form of CJD (asparagine substituted for aspartic acid at locus 178 of the prion protein).[232] Familial manifestations as either FFI or CJD apparently depends on which common polymorphism occurs in the mutant allele at locus 129: methionine results in FFI; valine yields CJD.

A number of the more classical parasomnias (see Chapter 24) such as rhythmic movement disorders (formerly known as head banging or jactatio capitis nocturna for the paradigmatic form of this disorder), bruxism, or somnambulism, contain a prominent motor component. Therefore, they may be part of the differential diagnosis for the other sleep-related motor disorders and, so, must be kept in mind by the investigator who is studying an unknown sleep-related motor disturbance.

Somnambulism, for instance, might be considered in the differential diagnosis of RBD or PND, conditions that may involve similar motor activity in sleep, or RLS, in which patients may wake up and seek relief in walking. Recently, it has been reported that somnambulism in adults may be characterized by bursts of hypersynchronous delta and SWS interruptions on a background of an increased amount of SWS.[233] Somnambulism is a frequent cause of injury to adults.[34] Like RBD, which it may resemble, somnambulism responds well to clonazepam.

Rhythmic movement disorder may need to be distinguished from tremor or segmental myoclonias, whereas *bruxism* may need to be distinguished from oromandibular dystonia. It must also be remembered that in some patients, such as children with tics, such parasomnias may be more common. This may also be true in patients with diurnal movement disorders, especially elderly patients suffering from a degenerative process. In evaluating the significance of parasomnias in a patient with another motor disturbance of sleep, however, it should be remembered that parasomnias are quite common in children, especially if they are only occasional, and also more prevalent in elderly persons. Therefore, their association with another motor disturbance of sleep may be a benign coincidence.

SOME REMARKS ABOUT SPECIAL CONSIDERATIONS FOR EVALUATING AND TREATING DISORDERS OF THE MOTOR SYSTEM IN SLEEP

History and Examination

As for all sleep disorders, a detailed sleep history is important in evaluating these patients. A sleep diary and specific questions about sleep symptoms are useful. Frequency and timing of the movements are also important to note, as these may provide diagnostic clues or indicate how likely studies are to uncover the nature of the movements. In women, the relation of the disorder to pregnancy or the menstrual cycle should be ascertained. The history should also include all associated medical conditions, whether neurologic or referable to other organ systems, as a motor sleep disturbance may be secondary to an antecedent medical condition. All medications should also be ascertained, as they may cause secondary motor and sleep disturbances, aggravate preexisting conditions, or even mask some sleep problems serendipitously (pain medications can ameliorate RLS).

In patients with movement disorders, it is important to elucidate the relation and timing of the sleep complaint relative to the motor disease and its treatment. It is important to consider whether the sleep problem is (1) due to the movement disorder itself (in which case management may be directed at the symptoms of the movement disorder as a first approach); (2) a secondary consequence of the movement disorder; (3) independent of the movement disorder (as a preexisting condition or one only coincidentally present, which may be then best addressed by the specific therapy for the sleep problem); or (4) a consequence of the treatment of the movement disorder (in which case therapy might be adjusted, if feasible). This categorization provides some guidance to which way therapy should be directed. The sleep specialist may need to become somewhat familiar, through reading or consultation, with the features of the movement disorder. Obtaining a clear picture from a referring neurologist or movement disorders specialist, through discussion or review of notes and summaries, of the evaluation and treatment of the patient's movement disorder may often be critical to rational advice and therapy. Ideally, there is active collaboration, when needed, between a sleep medicine specialist and a specialist capable of handling the movement disorder itself.

Because motor sleep disturbances are not generally evident in the physician's office, and may provide little that could assist diagnosis on physical examination, it is important to probe more deeply in the patient's symptoms than one usually does. The bed partner may provide a wealth of information about movements, their timing during the night, drowsiness during the daytime, the frequency of motor disturbances, noises, confusion, and hallucinations. As appropriate, all of these should be discussed, as the patient may be unaware of these phenomena or reluctant to discuss them. We have found it helpful to probe waking movements by asking the patient to reenact them in the office, discussing whether or not they can be suppressed, finding details of how the patient handles the movements or uncomfortable sensations (as in RLS), and eliciting provocative factors, such as time of day or night and position. When patients do not freely provide information on their own, we have sometimes modeled potential movements for them, to show them what might have occurred.

It is important to probe specific features of the patient's history when particular diagnoses are under consideration. For example, in considering whether epilepsy might figure in the clinical picture, it is important to ask about such sequelae of epileptic attacks as incontinence, tongue biting, or muscle soreness. In considering the possibility of RBD it is important to determine the character of the movements, whether they can injure the patient, and whether he or she actually leaves the bed in the course of the attack.

Some motor conditions, such as RLS, may cluster in families. It is important, therefore, to attempt to obtain a good family history. In cases of RLS this may require independent interviewing of other family members, since, we have found, the symptoms of RLS often are not communicated to other family members, even those who might be expected to be quite close. For example, we interviewed two sisters, both single and quite close who had weekly contact, each of whom was severely affected by RLS and was unaware that the other sister was also affected.

As a final consideration, in this day of the camcorder, may patients may own home videotaping equipment and may be willing to take some videos of their movements awake or asleep. These can provide invaluable insights into the patient's situation.

In sleep-related motor disturbances, as in sleep disturbances generally, a variety of paper instruments—symptom checklist, lists of sleep complaints, sleep log, or questionnaire aimed at specific sleep symptoms (e.g., EDS[234])—can be helpful in delineating the clinical picture. When using such instruments, it is important to review them with regard to relevant motor complaints. It is also important to utilize bed partners or others close to the patient as sources of additional information.

Sleep Studies

The value of standard sleep studies in evaluating motor disturbances of sleep is established.[235] A standard polysomnogram, with at least one EMG lead for the legs, provides a fair amount of information about motor disturbances. This should be supplemented by technician observations, wherever feasible, to explain motor events on the record. Where motor disturbances are the primary concern and seizures are part of the differential diagnosis, it is helpful to perform video-polysomnography. In an optimal setup, this may include multiple EEG channels, as for a regular EEG study (eight to 12 channels in a montage that can span the head and provide information about frontal and temporal activity), split-screen recording, and a facility for playing back the EEG record at the conventional daytime paper speed of 30 mm per second.

The following sections contain a number of suggestions about the use of different modalities for studying motor phenomena in sleep, then comment on alternate schemes from the regular polysomnogram for assessing sleep-related motor disturbances. Polysomnography, together with the Multiple Sleep Latency Test (MSLT), has been accepted as having established value for studies of PLMD as well as movements that can provoke violence in sleep (which includes RBD, seizures, somnambulism, and related conditions).[235]

Polysomnography

In selecting how to proceed with polysomnography, it is important to think about what conditions are being studied. Because the differential diagnosis of unknown motor disorders of sleep is relatively broad, it is usually important to monitor breathing as well as extensive EEG and EMG recordings. Accurate technician observation and videotaping may be extremely helpful in conducting studies that yield accurate diagnoses.

EEG montages. The standard sleep study may use only two EEG leads, a central lead (C_3-A_2 or C_4-A_1) together with an occipital lead (O_1, O_2, or O_z linked to an ear electrode). When seizures may be in the differential, as in unknown motor disorders of sleep, more elaborate montage may be necessary to adequately rule out seizure activity. Special electrodes may be required (see Chapters 27 and 6).

EMG recording. Standard sleep recording uses the chin EMG and leads on one or both legs for evaluation of possible PLMS. Where a specific motor complaint is noted that involves movement of other body parts—arms, trunk, abdomen, neck, face—additional leads can be applied. Most laboratories perform EMGs with a standard EEG filter setting (bandpass of 5 to 70 Hz), but we have found that a more artifact-free recording can be obtained if a higher bandpass (e.g., 50 to 150 Hz) is employed. We also set the amplitude before the study, so that a strong voluntary contraction is near or slightly above the full pen excursion for a polygraphic recorder.

Videotaping. Videotape studies can be extremely helpful in sorting out various abnormal movements or gaining some insight into their severity. This can permit correlation of paper records of movement or EMG potentials with actual movements and in some cases affords a better impression of the character of the movements. Split-screen studies, with polygraphic montages correlated directly with videotape of the associated behavior, are especially helpful in this regard. Patients may also have different categories of movements that may be distinguished by the videotape record but not the polysomnogram. To provide best natural conditions, infrared cameras are optimal, though many modern color video cameras can perform under relatively low light conditions. If possible, subjects should sleep with minimal covers, as this makes visualization of movements much easier. For this, carefully temperature-controlled rooms, especially warmer ones, are helpful. Time bases, including those added by special effects generators or an on-screen clock, can facilitate search and retrieval of movements.

In one study of the utility of video polysomnography, Aldrich and Jahnke[236] found that, in 86 patients without known epilepsy who had reported abnormal motor activity in sleep, these studies provided useful diagnostic information for 52 patients. Fully 69% of those with prominent motor activity received such information. Among 36 patients with known epilepsy, the studies provided useful diagnostic information about unclear motor phenomena in 28 (78%). For both groups of patients, the diagnostic outcomes included both seizure and nonseizure disorders. The authors emphasize that ability to play back the record at slower speed, afforded by some digital EEG systems, improves the ability to discriminate seizure activity from other motor phenomena. They also emphasize, as is generally true of polysomnography to evaluate motor abnormalities, that yield increases with the frequency of the disturbance. Conditions that are manifested every night can usually be usefully evaluated.

Accelerometers, activity meters, and related equipment.   Accelerometers, which now may be found in very miniaturized forms, can serve either as event markers or, if sufficiently accurate and calibrated, to quantify the degree of movement. Most accelerometers are linear and measure acceleration only along a single axis, but three-dimensional, triaxial models are also available. Accelerometers can discriminate actual movement from EMG potentials, which may occur without any significant displacement of a limb. While they are utilized for research purposes, they have not yet been established as standard for clinical studies.

Activity meters are now available in a number of forms.[1] They are usually self-contained devices that measure acceleration and digitize a measure of the number of accelerations, either those that exceed threshold in a given time period (sampling bin) or the number of smaller periods within a sampling bin during which threshold is exceeded. This provides a measure of movement. They can be set to sample over long or short periods: the longer the sampling period, the longer the overall period of time whose record can be stored by the device. As improvements are made in memory, it becomes possible to record with shorter sampling periods for longer overall periods of time. When the meter is removed from the subject, it is interfaced to a computer, usually a desktop IBM compatible type or MacIntosh, and the accumulated activity records are downloaded. Though theoretically such meters are capable of examining abnormal motor states, during either wakefulness (e.g., RLS) or sleep (e.g., PLMS or RBD), they have not yet been effectively utilized for this purpose. It seems likely that such systems will be developed in the future.

Other recording systems

The static charge–sensitive bed is a device[237] suitable for adult and pediatric[238] recordings, that is very sensitive to movements, including such physiologic movements as those associated with breathing or the heartbeat. Different kinds of movement, such as body movements or respiratory pauses, can be differentiated by selective filtration of the potentials transmitted by the bed.[239] This can allow for quantification of sleep states[240] or for counting movements. Because the bed itself is rather simple and not particularly expensive it may offer an alternative to some polysomnography in the future, though, like other simplified recording systems, it is not yet as accurate as polysomnography for detailing sleep states and associated movements.[241]

Ambulatory monitoring

A variety of systems are available for home or ambulatory monitoring of sleep, and capacity can be as great as 16 channels. Most of the customary sleep monitors can be used in the ambulatory setting. Generally, technicians prepare the patient for study either in the laboratory or at home. The various channels are recorded on tape for later display and analysis with computer systems. The advantage of these systems is that they reduce the personnel required and can reduce cost. This may permit analysis of less frequent phenomena than those that can profitably be studied under normal conditions in the more relevant home environment. Because these systems lack supervision, however, clear identification of abnormal events may not be feasible. Thus, for diagnostic purposes they may best be used as screening procedures. Once a clear question is available— How well is the patient sleeping? How many typical events occur?—they may provide more definitive answers to questions.

In an even more simplified system, activity meters have been used for long-term monitoring of sleepwake cycles and for sleep scoring. Typically, activity meters give a less clear picture of the motor activity than polysomnography with relevant EMG recording; however, given the ability of activity meters to make long-term recordings, especially with improved capacity, with little technician time, and ready computer analysis of the resulting data, it seems likely they will be used increasingly in future to study disorders of motor activity, including those associated with sleep.

Automatic scoring

One of the more interesting and challenging current developments in the sleep field is the development of technologies based on digitized polysomnograms that are processed by computer and stored on electronic media. This leads, in some cases, to "paperless" records. As a corollary of the computerized processing of studies, it becomes possible to perform automatic sleep analysis. This can offer the advantage of decreased scorer time, more consistent scoring criteria, and the ability to readily rescore records. Cost may decrease. All current digital systems are in a state of development: an experienced scorer may take more out of a record and can respond far more flexibly to altered recording conditions. The longterm prospect, nevertheless, is that digital systems with automatic scoring will increasingly play a role in sleep studies. We feel that within 10 years these systems may be the predominant ones used for sleep studies, whether in a sleep laboratory or in the ambulatory setting. In the ambulatory setting, some systems have utilized actigraphy as the basis for automatic sleep scoring. With current refinement, such sleep-scoring systems may achieve 88% agreement (sleep versus wake discrimination) with hand scoring.[242]

In the area of motor disturbances, the greatest promise for automatic scoring is the ability to score PLMS, whose stereotyped form allows relatively simple discrimination of PLMS from other phenomena. A number of systems for such scoring are currently available that have reasonable reliability with respect to human scorers. Kayed and colleagues reported one system that matched human performance but on occasion disregarded PLMS because they did not meet exact criteria though they were accepted as PLMS by human scorers.[243] In scoring PLMS, one distinct advantage of these systems is the ability to readily prepare graphic displays of the movements and to analyze them quantitatively. Other possible functions of automated scoring in the area of motor function may be the quantification of muscle activity (such as chin EMG), as by rectification and integration, and automatic scoring of movement time epochs. It should also be possible to relate various motor activities to other sleep events, such as arousals, awakenings, or K complexes. In the more distant future, the combination of expert systems with digital polysomnography may lead to scoring and record analysis that far exceeds the capacity of even the most experienced scorer.

Daytime and Evening Evaluation

Patients with sleep motor disturbances can be evaluated with MSLT for EDS, as can sleep patients generally. The American Academy of Neurology now accepts these studies as useful for patients with a variety of sleep disorders who complain of EDS.[235]

Daytime sleep studies, sometimes done with sleep deprivation the night before, can occasionally be useful in disclosing sleep motor disturbances such as RLS or PLMS or may assist in the evaluation of a possible case of epilepsy. Negative findings under these conditions are not helpful, however, and the limited yield of daytime studies makes full nighttime polysomnography far more desirable.

There is a great need for developing a test for the waking movements and discomfort of RLS. A number of investigators have proposed preliminary tests that allow for quantification of movements through EMG or videotapes, together with subjective indicators of abnormal sensations. In our studies, we asked patients to lie quietly for a half hour to an hour, asked patients to rate severity of uncomfortable sensations and involuntary jerks every 10 minutes, and counted abnormal movements with EMG and videotape (Figure 19-5).[192] Pelletier and group have developed a number of protocols, most recently the forced immobilization test (FIT),[193] in which patients' legs are restrained in bed in an extended

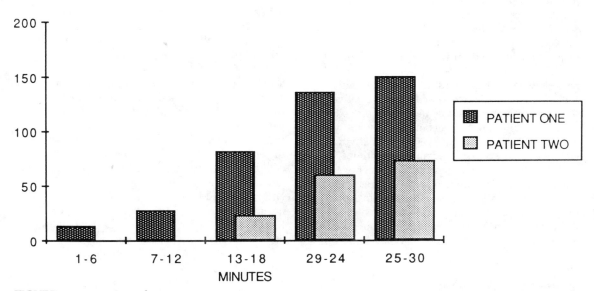

FIGURE 19-5. *RLS involuntary movements during instructed repose. During the test, the patients lay down with their legs held extended for a half hour. In these two patients, three studies were done at approximately 8-hour intervals around the clock and results combined for the figure. Movements are recorded by videotape and EMG tracings. Number of movements is charted by 6-minute intervals beginning when the patient lay down. Note that, for both patients, the largest number of movements occurred in the final 6-minute interval.*

position for an hour. Patients press a button at the onset of every abnormal sensation, while movements are quantified by EMG. In the future, it should be possible to use activity meters, together with a patient diary, to quantify general movements, including both involuntary movements and voluntary movements of motor restlessness.

SUMMARY

The past two decades have witnessed a great increase in knowledge about the motor disorders and sleep. New disorders—such as RBD and PND—have been described and other disorders, such as RLS, have been clarified. The importance of sleep dysfunction in the diurnal movement disorders, especially Parkinson's disease and related conditions, has been established. From the viewpoint of treatment, new therapies, for both long-known and recently described disorders, have been developed.

In this decade of the brain (1990s), there is promise that an explosion of knowledge about brain function will also produce much better answers about why sleep is needed and how it is regulated. We may gain a better understanding of how motor disturbances of sleep intrude on normal function. These answers should help provide guides for more specific therapy. Advances in understanding the genetics of a number of conditions, both diurnal movement disorders and sleep disorders such as RLS, may provide specific clues to how the sleep-regulating system is disordered.

As of now, we are beginning to develop a sharper picture of how both normal and abnormal movements are controlled during sleep. In the normal or "ideal" case there are three discrete states: wakefulness, NREM sleep, and REM sleep.[31] Both sleep states act to provide two key functions: relative dissociation of higher sleep centers from the external world and from lower levels of the nervous system and partial suppression of overt motor activity. The waking state, in contrast, attempts to optimize association between higher centers, lower centers, and the world, and to facilitate motor expression. The two sleep states differ in the autonomous activity of higher centers, which appears to be much greater in REM sleep. Both normal movements and most abnormal movements due to diurnal movement disorders show a characteristic pattern in sleep. They are most likely to occur during the lightest stages of sleep (stage 1 NREM), often in association with lightenings of sleep or arousal. They are less likely to occur in stage 2 NREM or REM sleep and least likely to occur in SWS or during deepening sleep. This pattern seems to be followed by movement disorders whose presumed generator is in a higher motor cen-

ter, either cortical or subcortical. In contrast, movements generated at the segmental level or at the level of the motor neuron are relatively resistant to modulation by sleep, perhaps because their mere presence is evidence for a reduced degree of higher control.

NREM and REM sleep disorders involve separate but interrelated motor dysfunctions. NREM disorders, such as many parasomnias, RLS, and PLMD, are activated by repose and sleep. In the case of RLS, the activation may begin in the predormital phase, as relaxation and drowsiness overshadow wakeful alertness. Presumably, these conditions arise, especially RLS and PLMD, because of some changing control from higher centers that allows the expression of a more primitive motor rhythmicity. In case of parasomnias that are similar to normal motor behavior, such as somnambulism or somniloquy, the major defect may be excessive activity of higher centers or relative failure of the NREM motor inhibitory system. NREM disorders probably would occur during REM sleep as well, as is observed with PLMD in the RBD[168] and narcolepsy,[169] but the additional inhibition that occurs during REM sleep suppresses them. REM disorders, by contrast, involve some shift in the critical REM sleep balance between excitation and inhibition. Though the exact changes are not clear, it seems likely that this is a change in higher influence and most likely a deficiency in inhibitory systems in the brain stem, analogous to the animal lesion models of REM sleep without atonia.[46] A unifying thesis for both NREM and REM disorders is that they can involve a failure of descending inhibition. The different conditions are likely to involve partially distinct but related inhibitory processes.

NREM and REM disorders, then, are likely to be activated by processes that impinge on the inhibitory systems of the brain stem. Because the balance between excitation and inhibition is fairly exacting, a variety of different influences, such as neurodegenerative disorders or even normal aging, may result in the emergence of disorders. Conditions such as narcolepsy, which are associated with poor state regulation, are very likely to be associated with additional NREM and REM disorders; thus the report that narcoleptics may at a young age have both PLMD and RBD.[33] The overall interrelatedness of failures of sleep inhibitory control can be appreciated in two other facts. First, REM and NREM disorders often overlap. For example, there is a high incidence of PLMD and fragmentary myoclonus in RBD.[224] Second, certain medications, such as the benzodiazepines and dopaminergic agents, may be useful for a number of the NREM and REM motor disturbances, as well as for state dyscontrol conditions such as narcolepsy.

The further resolution of the pathophysiology of motor disturbances of sleep now awaits a more exact understanding of the sleep regulatory systems of the brain, especially those responsible for the descending inhibition of the segmental and effector levels of the motor system.

REFERENCES

1. Tyron WW. Activity Measurement in Psychology and Medicine. New York: Plenum Press, 1991.
2. Marsden CD, Fahn S. Movement Disorders 2. Boston: Butterworths, 1987.
3. Quinn, NP, Jenner, PG. Disorders of Movement: Clinical, Pharmacological, and Physiological Aspects. New York: Academic Press, 1989.
4. Weiner WJ, Lang AE. Movement disorders: A Comprehensive Survey. Mount Kisco, NY: Futura, 1989.
5. Chokroverty S. Movement Disorders. Costa Mesa, CA: PMA, 1990.
6. Wilson JD, Braunwald E, Isselbacher KJ, et al. Harrison's Principles of Internal Medicine, ed 12. New York: McGraw-Hill, 1991.
7. Rowland LP, ed. Merritt's Textbook of Neurology. Philadelphia: Lea & Febiger, 1989.
8. Grillner S. Neurobiological bases of rhythmic motor acts in vertebrates. Science 1985; 228:143–149.
9. Steriade M, Hobson JA. Neuronal activity during the sleep-waking cycle. Prog Neurobiol 1976;6:155–376.
10. Evarts EV. Temporal patterns of discharge of pyramidal tract neurons during sleep and waking in the monkey. J Neurophysiol 1964;27:152–171.
11. Balkin TJ, Wesensten NJ, Brain AR, et al. Sleep-mediated changes in regional cerebral blood flow in humans. J Sleep Res 1992;1(suppl):14.
12. Chase MH, Morales FR. The control of motoneurons during sleep. In: Kryger MH, Roth T, Dement WC, ed. Principles and Practice of sleep medicine. Philadelphia: WB Saunders 1989;74–85.
13. Chase MH, Morales FR. The atonia and myoclonia of active (REM) sleep. Ann Rev Psychol 1990;41:557–584.
14. Morales FR, Boxer P, Chase MH. Behavioral state-specific inhibitory postsynaptic potentials impinge on cat lumbar motoneurons during active sleep. Exp Neurol 1987;98:418–435.
15. Pompeiano O. The neurophysiological mechanisms of the postural and motor events during desynchronized sleep. In: Kety SS, Evarts EV, Williams HL, ed. Sleep and Altered States of Consciousness. Baltimore: Williams & Wilkins, 1967;351–423.
16. Hodes R, Dement WC. Depression of electrically induced reflexes ("H-reflexes") in man during low voltage EEG "sleep." Electroencephalogr Clin Neurophysiol 1964;17:617–629.
17. Kimura J, Harada O. Excitability of the orbicularis oculi reflex in all night sleep: Its suppression in non-rapid eye movement and recovery in rapid eye movement sleep. Electroencephalogr Clin Neurophysiol 1972;33:369–377.
18. Redeng GR, Fernandez C. Effects of vestibular stimulation during sleep. Electroencephalogr Clin Neurophysiol 1968;24:75–79.
19. Chiappa KH, ed. Evoked Potentials in Clinical Medicine, ed. 2. New York City: Raven Press, 1990.
20. Erwin R, Buchwald JS. Midlatency auditory evoked responses: Differential effects of sleep in humans. Electroencephalogr Clin Neurophysiol 1986;65:383–392.
21. Emerson RG, Sgro JA, Pedley TA, et al. State-dependent changes in the N2O component of the median nerve somatosensory evoked potential. Neurology 1988;38:64–68.
22. Hess CW, Mills KR, Murray NMF, et a. Excitability of the human cortex is enhanced during REM sleep. Neurosci Let 1987;82:47–52.
23. Fish DR, Sawyers D, Smith SJM, et al. Motor inhibition from the brainstem is normal in torsion dystonia during REM sleep. J Neurol Neurosurg Psychiatry 1991;54:140–144.
24. Williams HL, Morlock HC Jr, Morlock JV. Instrumental behavior during sleep. Psychophysiology 1966;2:208–216.
25. Cirignotta F, Montagna P, Lugaresi E. Reversal of motor excitation to motor inhibition induced by sleep in man. In: Chase M, Weitzman ED, ed. Sleep Disorders: Basic and Clinical Research. New York: Spectrum Publications, 1983;129–135.
26. Kleitman N. Sleep and Wakefulness, ed 2. Chicago: University of Chicago Press, 1963.
27. Fujiki A, Shimizu A, Yamada Y, et al. The Babinski reflex during sleep and wakefulness. Electroencephalogr Clin Neurophysiol 1971;31:610–613.
28. Minors DS, Waterhouse JM. Circadian rhythms and their mechanisms. Experientia 1986;42:1–13.
29. Fish DR, Sawyers D, Allen PJ, et al. The effect of sleep on the dyskinetic movements of Parkinson's disease, Gilles de la Tourette syndrome, Huntington's disease, and torsion dystonia. Arch Neurol 1991;48:210–214.
30. McGregor P, Thorpy MJ, Schmidt-Nowara WW, et al. An improved method for scoring breathing-disordered sleep. Sleep 1992;15:359–363.
31. Mahowald MW, Schenck CH. Status dissociatus—a perspective on states of being. Sleep 1991;14:69–79.
32. Lugaresi E, Cirignotta F, Coccagna G, et al. Nocturnal myoclonus and restless legs syndrome. In: Fahn S, Marsden CD, Van Woert M, eds. Myoclonus. New York: Raven Press, 1986;295–307.
33. Schenck CH, Mahowald MW. Motor dyscontrol in narcolepsy: Rapid eye movement (REM) sleep without atonia and REM sleep behavior disorder. Ann Neurol 1992;32:3–10.
34. Schenck CH, Milner DM, Hurwitz TD, et al. A polysomnographic and clinical report on sleep-related injury in 100 adult patients. Am J Psychiatry 1989;146:1166–1173.

WAH supported by the Department of Veterans Affairs Medical Research Service Career Development Program. WAH and ASWQ supported by the Department of Veterans Affairs Medical Research Service Merit Review Program.

35. Santamaria J, Chiappa KH. The EEG of drowsiness in normal adults. J Clin Neurophysiol 1987;4:327–382.
36. Oswald I. Sudden bodily jerks on falling asleep. Brain 1959;82:92–103.
37. Broughton R. Pathological fragmentary myoclonus, intensified sleep starts and hypnagogic foot tremor: Three unusual sleep related disorders. In: Koella WP, ed. Sleep 1986. New York: Fischer-Verlag, 1988;240–243.
38. Bell CC, Dixie-Bell DD, Thompson B. Further studies on the prevalence of isolated sleep paralysis in black subjects. J Natl Med Assoc 1986;78:649–659.
39. Fukuda K, Miyasita A, Inugami M, et al. High prevalence of isolated sleep paralysis: *Kanashibari* phenomenon in Japan. Sleep 1987;10:279–286.
40. Takeuchi T, Miyasita A, Sasaki Y, et al. Isolated sleep paralysis elicited by sleep interruption. Sleep 1992;15:217–225.
41. Dagnino N, Loeb C, Massazza G, et al. Hypnic physiological myoclonus in man: An EEG-EMG study in normals and neurological patients. Eur Neurol 1969;2:47–58.
42. Montagna P, Liguori R, Zucconi M, et al. Physiological hypnic myoclonus. Electroencephalogr Clin Neurophysiol 1988;70:172–176.
43. Broughton R, Tolentino MA, Krelina M. Excessive fragmentary myoclonus in NREM sleep: A report of 38 cases. Electroencephalogr Clin Neurophysiol 1985;61:121–133.
44. Gardner R Jr., Grossman WI. Normal motor patterns in sleep in man. In: Weitzman E, ed. Advances in Sleep Research. New York: Spectrum, 1975;2:67–107.
45. Wilde-Frenz J, Schulz H. Rate and distribution of body movements during sleep in humans. Percept Mot Skills 1983;56:275–283.
46. Hendricks JC, Morrison AR, Mann GL. Different behaviors during paradoxical sleep without atonia depend on pontine lesion site. Brain Res 1982;239:81–105.
47. McCarley RW. The biology of dreaming sleep. In: Kryger MH, Roth T, Dement WC, ed. Principles and Practice of Sleep Medicine. Philadelphia: WB Saunders, 1989;173–183.
48. DeKoninck J, Lorrain D, Gagnon P. Sleep positions and position shifts in five age groups: An ontogenetic picture. Sleep 1992;15:143–149.
49. Lees AJ, Blackburn NA, Campbell VL. The nighttime problems of Parkinson's disease. Clin Neuropharmacol 1988;11:512–519.
50. Hening WA, Walters AS, Chokroverty S. Movement disorders and sleep. In: Chokroverty S, ed. Movement Disorders. Costa Mesa, CA: PMA, 1990;127–157.
51. Lapresle J. Palatal myoclonus. In: Fahn S, Marsden CD, Van Woert MH, eds. Myoclonus. New York: Raven Press, 1986;265–273.
52. Askenasy JJM, Yahr MD. Reversal of sleep disturbance in Parkinson's disease by antiparkinsonian therapy: A preliminary study. Neurology 1986;35:527–532.
53. Shimizu T, Inami Y, Sugita Y, et al. REM sleep without muscle atonia (stage 1–REM) and its relation to delirious behavior during sleep in patients with degenerative diseases involving the brainstem. Jpn J Psychiatr Neurol 1990;44:681–692.
54. Goetz CG, Wilson RS, Tanner CM, et al. Relationships among pain, depression, and sleep alteration in Parkinson's disease. In: Yahr MD, Bergmann KJ, eds. Parkinson's Disease. New York: Raven Press, 1986;345–347.
55. Starkstein SE, Preziosi TJ, Robinson RG. Sleep disorders, pain, and depression in Parkinson's disease. Eur Neurol 1991;31.
56. Duvoisin RC, Sage JI. The spectrum of parkinsonism. In: Chokroverty S, ed. Movement Disorders. Costa Mesa, CA: PMA, 1990;159–177.
57. Diagnostic Classification Steering Committee of the American Sleep Disorders Association. The International Classification of Sleep Disorders: Diagnostic and Coding Manual. Rochester, Minn.: American Sleep Disorders Association, 1990.
58. Jellinger K. Overview of morphological changes in Parkinson's disease. In: Yahr MD, Bergmann KJ, eds. Parkinson's Disease. New York: Raven Press, 1987;1–18.
59. German DC, Manaye KF, White CL III, et al. Disease-specific patterns of locus coeruleus cell loss. Ann Neurol 1992;32:667–676.
60. Emser W, Brenner M, Stober T, et al. Changes in nocturnal sleep in Huntington's and Parkinson's disease. J Neurol 1988;235:177–179.
61. Puca FM, Bricolo A, Turella G. Effect of L-dopa on amantadine therapy on sleep spindles in parkinsonism. Electroencephalogr Clin Neurophysiol 1973;35:327–330.
62. Tassinari CA, Broughton R, Poire R, et al. Sur l'évolution des mouvements anormaux au cours du sommeil. In: Fischgold H, ed. Le Sommeil de Nuit Normal et Pathologique. Paris: Masson, 1965;314–333.
63. April R. Observations on parkinsonian tremor in all-night sleep. Neurology 1966;16:720–724.
64. Stern M, Roffwarg H, Duvoisin R. The parkinsonian tremor in sleep. J Nerv Ment Dis 1968;147:202–210.
65. Askenasy JJM. Sleep patterns in extrapyramidal disorders. Int J Neurol 1981;15:62–76.
66. Shima F, Imai H, Segawa M. Polygraphic study on body movements during sleep in cases with involuntary movement. Clin Electroencephalogr 1974;16:229–235.
67. Laihinen A, Alihanka J, Raitasuo S, et al. Sleep movements and associated autonomic nervous activities in patients with Parkinson's disease. Acta Neurol Scand 1987;76:64–68.
68. Mouret J. Differences in sleep in patients with Parkinson's disease. Electroencephalogr Clin Neurophysiol 1975;38:653–657.
68a. Comella CL, Ristanovic R, Goetz CG. Parkinson's disease patients with and without REM behavior disorder (RBD): A polysomnographic and clinical comparison. Neurology 1993;43(Supp 2):A301.
68b. Silber MH, Ahlskog JE. REM sleep behavior disorder and Parkinson's disease. Neurology 1993;43(Supp 2):A338.
69. Factor SA, McAlarney T, Sanchez-Ramos JR, et al. Sleep disorders and sleep effect in Parkinson's disease. Mov Disord 1990;5:280–285.
70. Kales A, Ansel RD, Markham CH et al. Sleep in patients with Parkinson's disease and normal subjects

prior to and following levodopa administration. Clin Pharmacol Ther 1971;12:397–406.

71. Bergonzi P, Chiurulla C, Cianchetti C, et al. Clinical pharmacology as an approach to the study of biochemical sleep mechanisms: The action of L-dopa. Confin Neurol 1974;36:5–22.

72. Apps MCP, Sheaff PC, Ingram DA, et al. Respiration and sleep in Parkinson's disease. J Neurol Neurosurg Psychiatry 1985;48:1240–1245.

73. Nausieda PA, Weiner WJ, Kaplan LR, et al. Sleep disruption in the course of chronic levodopa therapy: An early feature of the levodopa psychosis. Clin Neuropharmacol 1982;5:183–194.

74. Bergonzi P, Chiurulla C, Gambi D, et al. L-dopa plus decarboxylase inhibitor: Sleep organization in Parkinson's syndrome before and after treatment. Acta Neurol Belg 1975;75:5–10.

75. Chokroverty S. The spectrum of ventilatory disturbances in movement disorders. In: Chokroverty S, ed. Movement Disorders. Costa Mesa, CA: PMA, 1990;365–392.

76. Hovestadt A, Bogaard JM, Meerwaldt JD, et al. Pulmonary function in Parkinson's disease. J Neurol Neurosurg Psychiatr 1989;52:329–333.

77. Lilker ES, Woolf CR. Pulmonary functions in Parkinson syndrome. Can Med Assoc J 1968;99:752–757.

78. Obenour WH, Stevens PM, Cohen AA, et al. The causes of abnormal pulmonary function in Parkinson's disease. Am Rev Respir Dis 1972;105:382–387.

79. Vas CJ, Parsonage M, Lord OC. Parkinsonism associated with laryngeal spasm. J Neurol Neurosurg Psychiatry 1965;28:401–403.

80. Weiner WJ, Goetz G, Nausieda PA, et al. Respiratory dyskinesias: Extrapyramidal dysfunction and dyspnea. Ann Intern Med 1978;88:327–331.

81. Vincken WG, Gauthier SG, Dollfuss RE, et al. Involvement of upper airway muscles in extrapyramidal disorders. N Engl J Med 1984;311:438–442.

82. Hardie RJ, Efthimiou J, Stern GM. Respiration and sleep in Parkinson's disease. J Neurol Neurosurg Psychiatry 1986;50:1326.

83. Efthimiou J, Ellis SJ, Hardie RJ, et al. Sleep apnea in idiopathic and postencephalitic parkinsonism. In: Yahr MD, Bergmann KJ, eds. Parkinson's Disease. New York: Raven Press, 1986;275–276.

84. Kostic VS, Susic V, Covickovic-Sternic N, et al. Reduced rapid eye movement sleep latency in patients with Parkinson's disease. J Neurol 1989;236:421–423.

85. Sharf B, Moskovitz C, Lupton MD, et al. Dream phenomena induced by chronic levodopa therapy. J Neural Transm 1978;43:143–151.

86. Quinn N, Critchley P, Marsden CD. Young onset Parkinson's disease. Mov Dis 1987;2:73–91.

87. Yamamura Y, Sobue I, Ando K, et al. Paralysis agitans of early onset with marked diurnal fluctuations of symptoms. Neurology 1973;23:239–244.

88. Segawa M, Hosaka A, Miyagawa F, et al. Hereditary progressive dystonia with marked diurnal fluctuations. Adv Neurol 1976;14:215–233.

89. Nygaard TG. Dopa-responsive dystonia: 20 years into the L-dopa era. In: Quinn NP, Jenner PG, eds. Disorders of Movement: Clinical, Pharmacological, and

Physiological Aspects. New York: Academic Press, 1989;323–337.

90. Segawa M, Nomura Y, Yamashita S, et al. Long-term effects of L-dopa on hereditary progressive dystonia with marked diurnal fluctuation. In: Berardelli A, Benecke R, Manfredi M, et al. eds. Motor disturbances II. New York: Academic Press, 1990;305–318.

91. Marsden CD, Parkes JD, Quinn N. Fluctuations of disability in Parkinson's disease—clinical aspects. In: Marsden CD, Fahn S, eds. Movement Disorders. Boston: Butterworth, 1982;96–122.

92. Kim R. The chronic residual respiratory disorder in post-encephalitic Parkinsonism. J Neurol Neurosurg Psychiatry 1968;31:393–398.

93. Garland T, Linderholm H. Hypoventilation syndrome in a case of chronic epidemic encephalitis. Acta Med Scand 1958;162:333–349.

94. DaCosta JL. Chronic hypoventilation due to diminished sensitivity of the respiratory centre associated with Parkinsonism. Med J Aust 1972;1:373–376.

95. Steele JC, Richardson JC, Olszewski J. Progressive supranuclear palsy. Arch Neurol 1964;10:333–359.

96. Golbe LI, Davis PH, Schoenberg BS, et al. Prevalence and natural history of progressive supranuclear palsy. Neurology 1988;38:1031–1034.

97. Jankovic J, Van der Linden C. Progressive supranuclear palsy (Steel-Richardson-Olszewski syndrome). In: Chokroverty S, ed. Movement Disorders. Costa Mesa, CA: PMA, 1990;267–286.

98. Gross RA, Spehlmann R, Daniels JC. Sleep disturbances in progressive supranuclear palsy. Electroencephalogr Clin Neurophysiol 1978;45:16–25.

99. Laffont F, Autret A, Minz M, et al. Étude polygraphique du sommeil dans 9 cas de maladie de Steele-Richardson. Rev Neurol 1979;135:127–142.

99a. Aldrich M, Foster NL, White RF, et al. Sleep abnormalities in progressive supranuclear palsy. Ann Neurol 1989;25:577–581.

100. Perret JL, Jouvet M. Étude du sommeil dans la paralyse supra-nucléaire progressive. Elecroencephalogr Clin Neurophysiol 1980;49:323–329.

101. Purdy A, Hahn A, Barnett JM, et al. Familial fatal Parkinsonism with alveolar hypoventilation and mental depression. Ann Neurol 1979;6:523–531.

102. Thompson PD. Chorea. In: Quinn NP, Jenner PG, eds. Disorders of Movement: Clinical, Pharmacological and Physiological Aspects. New York: Academic Press, 1989;455–468.

103. Spire JP, Bliwise DL, Noronha ABC, et al. Sleep profiles in Huntington disease. Neurology 1981;31:151–152.

104. Sishta SK, Troupe A, Marszalek KS, et al. Huntington's chorea: An electroencephalographic and psychometric study. Electroencephalogr Clin Neurophysiol 1974;36:387–393.

105. Hansotia P, Wall R, Berendes J. Sleep disturbances and severity of Huntington's disease. Neurology 1985;35:1672–1674.

106. Bollen EL, Den Heijer JC, Ponsioen C, et al. Respiration during sleep in Huntington's chorea. J Neurol Sci 1988;84:63–68.

107. Broughton R, Tassinari CA, Gastaut JR, et al. A polygraphic study of abnormal movements during different stages of sleep. Can Med Assoc J 1967;97:243–244.

108. Fahn S. Recent concepts in the diagnosis and treatment of dystonias. In: Chokroverty S, ed. Movement Disorders. Costa Mesa, CA: Raven Press, 1990;237–258.

109. Fahn S, Marsden CD, Calne DB, eds. Dystonia 2. New York: Raven Press, 1988.

110. Ozelius L, Kramer PL, Moskowitz C. Human gene for torsion dystonia located on chromosome 9q32-34. Neuron 1989;2:1427–1434.

111. Kramer PL, de Leon D, Ozelius L, et al. Dystonia gene in Ashkenazi jewish population is located on chromosome 9q32-34. Ann Neurol 1990;27:114–120.

112. Shiozawa Z, Mano T, Sobue I. Polygraphic studies on involuntary movements during sleep in cases of dystonia, choreo-athetosis, and ballism. Rinsho Shinkeigaku 1978;18:547–556.

113. Silvestri R, De Domenico P, Di Rosa AE, et al. The effect of nocturnal physiological sleep on various movement disorders. Mov Disord 1990;5:8–14.

114. Jankel WR, Allen RP, Niedermeyer E, et al. Polysomnographic findings in dystonia musculorum deformans. Sleep 1983;6:281–285.

115. Fish DR, Allen PJ, Sawyers D, et al. Sleep spindles in torsion dystonia. Arch Neurol 1990;47:216–218.

116. Berardelli A. The pathophysiology of dystonia. In: Quinn NP, Jenner PG, ed. Disorders of Movement: Clinical, Pharmacological, and Physiological Aspects. New York: Academic Press, 1989;251–261.

117. Wein A, Golubev V. Polygraphic analysis of sleep in dystonia musculorum deformans. Waking Sleeping 1979;3:41–50.

118. Jankel WR, Niedermeyer E, Graf M, et al. Case report: Polysomnographic effects of thalamotomy for torsion dystonia. Neurosurgery 1984;14:495–498.

119. Segawa M, Nomura Y. Hereditary progressive dystonia with marked diurnal fluctuations. In: Nagatsu T, Narabayashi H, Yoshida M, eds. Parkinson's Disease From Clinical Aspects to Molecular Basis. New York: Springer-Verlag, 1991;167–177.

120. Nygaard TG, Trugman JM, de Yebenes JG, et al. Dopa-responsive dystonia: The spectrum of clinical manifestations in a large North American family. Neurology 1990;40:66–69.

121. Nygaard TG, Marsden CD, Duvoisin RC. Dopa-responsive dystonia. In: Fahn S, Marsden CD, Calne DB, eds. Dystonia 2. New York: Raven Press, 1988;377–384.

122. Montagna P, Procaccianti G, Lugaresi A, et al. Diurnal variability in cranial dystonia. Mov Disord 1990;5:44–46.

123. Segawa M, Nomura Y, Tanaka S, et al. Hereditary progressive dystonia with marked diurnal fluctuations—consideration on its pathophysiology based on the characteristics of clinical and polysomnographical findings. In: Fahn S, Marsden CD, Calne DB, eds. Dystonia 2. New York: Raven Press, 1988;367–376.

124. de Yebenes JG, Moskowitz C, Fahn S, et al. Long-term treatment with levodopa in a family with autosomal dominant torsion dystonia. In: Fahn S, Marsden CD, Calne DB, eds. Dystonia 2. 1 New York: Raven Press, 1988;101–111.

125. Nygaard TG, Marsden CD, Fahn S. Dopa-responsive dystonia: Long-term treatment response and prognosis. Neurology 1991;41:174–181.

126. Nygaard TG, Takahashi H, Heiman GA, et al. Long-term treatment response and flurodopa positron emission tomographic scanning of parkinsonism in a family with dopa-responsive dystonia. Ann Neurol 1992;32:603–608.

127. Sawle GV, Leenders KL, Brooks DJ, et al. Dopa-responsive dystonia: [^{18}F]Dopa positron emission tomography. Ann Neurol 1991;30:24–30.

128. Fletcher NA, Holt IJ, Harding AE, et al. Tyrosine hydroxylase and levodopa-responsive dystonia. J Neurol Neurosurg Psychiatry 1989;52:112–114.

129. Fink JK, Barton N, Cohen W, et al. Dystonia with marked diurnal variation associated with biopterin deficiency. Neurology 1988;38:707–711.

130. Fahn S, Marsden CD, Van Woert M, eds. Myoclonus. New York: Raven Press, 1986.

131. Lugaresi E, Coccagna G, Mantovani M, et al. The evolution of different types of myoclonus during sleep. A polygraphic study. Eur Neurol 1970;4:321–331.

132. Lugaresi E, Cirignotta F, Montagna P, et al. Myoclonus and related phenomena during sleep. In: Chase M, Weitzman ED, eds. Sleep Disorders: Basic and Clinical Research. New York: Spectrum, 1983;123–127.

133. Chokroverty S, Barron KD. Palatal myoclonus and rhythmic ocular movements: A polygraphic study. Neurology 1969;19:975–982.

134. Tahmoush AJ, Brooks JE, Keltner JL. Palatal myoclonus associated with abnormal ocular and extremity movements: A polygraphic study. Arch Neurol 1972;27:431–440.

135. Jacobs L, Newman RP, Bozian D. Disappearing palatal myoclonus. Neurology 1981;31:748–751.

136. Kayed K, Sjaastad O, Magnussen I, et al. Palatal myoclonus during sleep. Sleep 1983;6:130–136.

137. Hoehn MM, Cherington M. Spinal myoclonus. Neurology 1977;27:942–946.

138. Walters A, Hening W, Côte L et al. Dominantly inherited restless legs with myoclonus and periodic movements of sleep: A syndrome related to the endogenous opiates? In: Fahn S, Marsden CD, Van Woert M, eds. Myoclonus. New York: Raven Press, 1986; 309–319.

139. Jankovic J. The neurology of tics. In: Marsden CD, Fahn S, eds. Movement Disorders 2. Boston: Butterworth, 1987;383–405.

140. Van Woert MH. Gilles de la Tourette syndrome. In: Chokroverty S, ed. Movement Disorders. Costa Mesa, CA: PMA, 1990;309–317.

141. Nee LE, Caine ED, Polinsky RJ, et al. Gilles de la Tourette syndrome: Clinical and family study of 50 cases. Ann Neurol 1980;7:41–49.

142. Hashimoto T, Endo S, Fukuda K, et al. Increased body movements during sleep in Gilles de la Tourette syndrome. Brain Dev 1981;3:31–35.

143. Glaze DG, Frost JD Jr, Jankovic J. Sleep in Gilles de la Tourette syndrome: Disorder of arousal. Neurology 1983;33:586–592.

144. Barabas G, Matthews WS, Ferrari M. Somnambulism in children with Tourette syndrome. Dev Med Child Neurol 1984;26:457–460.

145. Jankovic J, Glaze DG, Frost JD Jr. Effect of tetrabenazine on tics and sleep of Gilles de la Tourette's syndrome. Neurology 1984;34:688–692.

146. Hayashi M, Inoue Y, Iwakawa Y, et al. REM sleep abnormalities in severe athetoid cerebral palsy. Brain Dev 1990;12:494–497.

147. Yamamoto T, Hirose G, Shimazaki K, et al. Movement disorders of familial neuroacanthocytosis syndrome. Arch Neurol 1982;39:298–301.

148. Shannon KM, Klawans HL. Hemiballismus. In: Chokroverty S, ed. Movement Disorders. Costa Mesa, CA: PMA, 1990;353–364.

149. Puca FM, Minervini MG, Savarese M, et al. Evoluzione del sonno in un caso di emiballismo. Boll Soc It Biol Sper 1984;60:981–987.

150. Auger RG. Hemifacial spasm: Clinical and electrophysiologic observations. Neurology 1979;29:1261–1272.

151. Digre KB, Corbett JJ. Hemifacial spasm: Differential diagnosis, mechanism and treatment. In: Jankovic J, Tolosa E, eds. Facial Dyskinesias. New York: Raven Press, 1988;151–175.

152. Montagna P, Imbriaco A, Zucconi M, et al. Hemifacial spasm is sleep. Neurology 1986;36:270–273.

153. Ekbom KA. Restless legs: A clinical study. Acta Med Scand Suppl 1945;158:1–122.

154. Ekbom KA. Restless legs syndrome. Neurology 1960;10:868–873.

155. Bornstein B. Restless legs. Psychiatr Neurol 1961;141:165–201.

156. Coleman RM. Periodic movements in sleep (nocturnal myoclonus) and restless legs syndrome. In: Guilleminault C, ed. Sleeping and Waking Disorders: Indications and Techniques. Menlo Park, Calif.: Addison Wesley, 1982;265–295.

157. Walters AS, Hening W. Review of the clinical presentation and neuropharmacology of restless legs syndrome. Clin Neuropharmacol 1987;10:225–237 (erratum 482).

158. Krueger BR. Restless legs syndrome and periodic movements of sleep. Mayo Clin Proc 1990;65:999–1006.

159. Coccagna G. Restless legs syndrome/periodic leg movements in sleep. In: Thorpy MJ, ed. Handbook of Sleep Disorders. New York: Marcel Dekker, 1990;457–478.

160. Zucconi M, Coccagna G, Petronelli R, et al. Nocturnal myoclonus in restless legs syndrome: Effect of carbamazepine treatment. Funct Neurol 1989;4:263–271.

161. Montplaisir J, Lapierre O, Warnes H, et al. The treatment of the restless legs syndrome with or without periodic leg movements in sleep. Sleep 1992;15:391–395.

162. Symonds CP. Nocturnal myoclonus. J Neurol Neurosurg Psychiatry 1953;16:166–171.

163. Coleman RM, Pollak CP, Weitzman ED. Periodic movements in sleep (nocturnal myoclonus): Relation to sleep disorders. Ann Neurol 1980;8:416–421.

164. Smith RC. Relationship of periodic movements in sleep (nocturnal myoclonus) and the Babinski sign. Sleep 1985;8:239–243.

165. Yokota T, Hirose K, Tanabe H, et al. Sleep-related periodic leg movements (nocturnal myoclonus) due to spinal cord lesion. J Neurol Sci 1991;104:13–18.

166. Walters A, Hening W, Kavey N, et al. Restless legs syndrome: A pleomorphic sensorimotor disorder. Neurology 1984;34 (suppl 1):129.

167. Dzvonik ML, Kripke DF, Klauber M, et al. Body position changes and periodic movements in sleep. Sleep 1986;9:484–491.

168. Lapierre O, Montplaisir J. Polysomnographic features of REM sleep behavior disorder: Development of a scoring method. Neurology 1992;42:1371–1374.

169. Godbout R, Montplaisir J, Poirier G, et al. Distinctive electrographic manifestations of periodic leg movements during sleep in narcoleptic vs insomniac patients. Sleep Res 1988;17:182.

170. Ancoli-Israel S, Kripke DF, Klauber MR, et al. Periodic limb movements in sleep in community-dwelling elderly. Sleep 1991;14:496–500.

171. Phoha RL, Dickel MJ, Mosko SS. Preliminary longitudinal assessment of sleep in the elderly. Sleep 1990;13:425–429.

172. Dickel MJ, Mosko SS. Morbidity cut-offs for sleep apnea and periodic leg movements in predicting subjective complaints in seniors. Sleep 1990;13:155–166.

173. Sleep Disorders Atlas Task Force of the American Sleep Disorders Association. EEG arousals: Scoring rules and examples. Sleep 1992;15:173–184.

174. Edinger JD, McCall WV, Marsh GR, et al. Periodic limb movement variability in older DIMS patients across consecutive nights of home monitoring. Sleep 1992;15:156–161.

175. Kales A, Bixler EO, Soldatos CR, et al. Biopsychobehavioral correlates of insomnia. Part 1: Role of sleep apnea and nocturnal myoclonus. Psychosomatics 1982;23:589–600.

176. Wittig R, Zorick F, Piccione P, et al. Narcolepsy and disturbed nocturnal sleep. Clin Electroencephalogr 1983;14:130–134.

177. Baker TL, Guilleminault C, Nino-Murcia G, et al. Comparative polysomnographic study of narcolepsy and idiopathic central nervous system hypersomnia. Sleep 1986;9:232–242.

178. Lavie P, Epstein R, Tzischinsky O, et al. Actigraphic measurements of sleep in rheumatoid arthritis: Comparison of patients with low back pain and healthy controls. J Rheumatol 1992;19:362–365.

179. Mitler MM, Browman CP, Menh SJ, et al. Nocturnal myoclonus: Treatment efficacy of clonazepam and temazepam. Sleep 1986;9:385–392.

180. Bonnet MH, Arand DL. The use of triazolam in older patients with periodic leg movements, fragmented sleep, and daytime sleepiness. J Gerontol 1990;45:M139-144.

181. Guilleminault C, Flagg W. Effect of baclofen on sleep-related periodic leg movements. Ann Neurol 1984;15:234–239.

182. Kavey N, Walters AS, Hening W, et al. Opioid treatment of periodic movements in sleep in patients without restless legs. Neuropeptides 1988;11:181–184.

183. Allen RP, Kaplan PW, Buchholz DW, et al. Double-blinded, placebo-controlled comparison of high dose propoxyphene and moderate dose carbidopa/levodopa for treatment of periodic limb movements in sleep. Sleep Res 1992;21:166.

184. Kovacevic-Ristanovic R, Cartwright RD, Lloyd S. Non-pharmacologic treatment of periodic leg movements in sleep. Arch Phys Med Rehab 1991;72:385–389.

185. Lugaresi E, Coccagna G, Montovani M, et al. Some periodic phenomena arising during drowsiness and sleep in man. Electroencephalogr Clin Neurophysiol 1972;32:701–705.

186. Ali NJ, Davies RJO, Fleetham JA, et al. Periodic movements of the legs during sleep associated with rises in systemic blood pressure. Sleep 1991;14:163–165.

187. Walters AS, Hening WA, Chokroverty S. Review and videotape recognition of the restless legs syndrome. Move Disord 1991;6:105–110.

188. Montplaisir J, Godbout R, Boghen D. Familial restless legs with periodic movements in sleep: Electrophysiologic, biochemical and pharmacologic study. Neurology 1985;35:130–134.

189. Montplaisir J, Godbout R, Poirier G, et al. Restless legs syndrome and periodic movements in sleep: Physiopathology and treatment with L-dopa. Clin Neuropharmacol 1986;9:456–463.

190. Walters A, Hening W, Kavey N, et al. A double-blind randomized crossover trial of bromocriptine and placebo in the restless legs syndrome. Ann Neurol 1988;24:455–458.

191. Hening WA, Walters AS. Successful long-term therapy of the restless legs syndrome with opioid medications. Sleep Res 1989;18:241.

192. Hening WA, Walters AS, Chokroverty S. A test for monitoring symptom severity in the restless legs syndrome. Neurosci Abstr 1988;14:908.

193. Pelletier G, Lorrain D, Montplaisir J. Sensory and motor components of the restless legs syndrome. Neurology 1992;42:1663–1666.

194. Kwan PC, Hening WA, Chokroverty S, et al. Periodic limb movements in sleep may cause significant sleep disruption in patients with the restless legs syndrome. Sleep Res 1992;21:222.

195. Pollak CP, Perlick D, Linsner JP, et al. Sleep problems in the community elderly as predictors of death and nursing home placement. J Community Health 1990; 15:123–135.

196. Roger SD, Harris DCH, Stewart, JH. Possible relation between restless legs and anaemia in renal dialysis patients. Lancet 1991;337:1551.

197. Walters AS, Hening W, Rubinstein M, et al. A clinical and polysomnographic comparison of neuroleptic-induced akathisia and the idiopathic restless legs syndrome. Sleep 1991;14:339–345.

198. Lipinski JF, Hudson JI, Cunningham SL, et al. Polysomnographic characteristics of neuroleptic-induced akathisia. Clin Neuropharmacol 1991;14:413–419.

199. Walters AS, Hening WA, Chokroverty S. Frequent occurrence of myoclonus while awake and at rest, body rocking and marching in place in a subpopulation of patients with restless legs syndrome. Acta Neurol Scand 1988;77:418–421.

200. Godbout R, Montplaisir J, Poirier G. Epidemiological data in familial restless legs syndrome. Sleep Res 1987;16:338.

201. Hickey K, Walters A, Hening W. Hyperactivity and "growing pains" as possible misdiagnosis in young-age onset restless legs syndrome. Sleep Res 1992; 21:209.

202. Oboler SK, Prochazka AV, Meyer TJ. Leg symptoms in outpatient veterans. West J Med. 1991;155:256–259.

203. Montagna P, Coccagna G, Cirignotta F, et al. Familial restless legs syndrome: Long-term follow-up. In: Guilleminault C, Lugaresi E, eds. Sleep/Wake Disorders: Natural History, Epidemiology, and Long-Term Evolution. New York: Raven Press, 1983;231–235.

204. Johnson W, Walters A, Lehner T, et al. Affecteds only linkage analysis of autosomal dominant restless legs syndrome. Sleep Res 1992;21:214.

205. Wechsler LR, Stakes JW, Shahani BT, et al. Periodic leg movements of sleep (nocturnal myoclonus): An electrophysiological study. Ann Neurol 1986;19:168–173.

206. Hening WA, Chokroverty S, Walters AS. Presence of a biphasic cortical potential before leg jerks in the restless legs syndrome. Sleep Res 1990;19:235.

207. Shibasaki H, Yamashita Y, Tobimatsu S, et al. Electroencephalographic correlates of myoclonus. In: Fahn S, Marsden CD, Van Woert MH, eds. Myoclonus. New York: Raven Press, 1986;357–372.

207a. Trenkwalder C, Bucher SF, Oertel WH, et al. Bereitschaftspotential in idiopathic and symptomatic restless legs syndrome. Electroencephalogr Clin Neurophysiol 1993;89:95–103.

208. Hening W, Chokroverty S, Rolleri M, et al. The cortical premovement potential of restless legs syndrome jerks: Differences in potentials before simulated versus symptomatic jerks. Sleep Res 1991;20:355.

209. Von Scheele C, Kempi V. Long-term effect of dopaminergic drugs in restless legs: A 2-year follow-up. Arch Neurol 1990;47:1223–1224.

210. Walters AS, Wagner M, Hening WA, et al. Successful treatment of the idiopathic restless legs syndrome in a randomized double-blind trial of oxycodone. Sleep 1993;16:327–332.

211. Telstad W, Sørenson O, Larsen S, et al. Treatment of the restless legs syndrome with carbamazepine: A double blind study. Br Med J 1984;288:444–446.

212. Strang RR. The symptoms of restless legs. Med J Aust 1967;1:1211–1213.

213. Handwerker JV, Palmer RF. Clonidine in the treatment of restless legs syndrome. N Engl J Med 1985;313:1228–1229.

214. Lugaresi E, Cirignotta F, Montagna P. Nocturnal paroxysmal dystonia. J Neurol Neurosurg Psychiatry 1986;49:375–380.

215. Montagna P. Nocturnal paroxysmal dystonia and nocturnal wandering. Neurology 1992;42:61–67.

216. Peled R, Lavie P. Paroxysmal awakenings from sleep associated with excessive daytime somnolence: A form of nocturnal epilepsy. Neurology 1986;36:95–98.

217. Pedley TA, Guilleminault C. Episodic nocturnal wanderings responsive to anticonvulsant drug therapy. Ann Neurol 1977;2:30–35.

218. Tinuper P, Cerullo A, Cirignotta F, et al. Nocturnal paroxysmal dystonia with short-lasting attacks. Three cases with evidence for an epileptic frontal lobe origin of seizures. Epilepsia 1990;31:549–556.

219. Meierkord H, Fish DR, Smith SJM, et al. Is nocturnal paroxysmal dystonia a form of frontal lobe epilepsy? Mov Disord 1992;7:38–42.

220. Lugaresi E, Montagna P, Sforza E. Nocturnal paroxysmal dystonia. In: Terzano MG, Halasz P, Declerck AC, eds. Phasic Events and Dynamic Organization of Sleep. New York: Raven Press, 1991;1–5.

221. Schenck CH, Bundlie SR, Ettinger MG, et al. Chronic behavioral disorders of human REM sleep: A new category of parasomnia. Sleep 1986;293–308.

222. Schenck CH, Bundlie SR, Patterson AL, et al. Rapid eye movement sleep behavior disorder. JAMA 1987;257:1786–1789.

223. Mahowald MW, Schenck CH. REM sleep behavior disorder. In: Kryger MH, Roth T, Dement WC, eds. Principles and Practice of Sleep Medicine. Philadelphia: WB Saunders, 1989;389–401.

224. Schenck CH, Mahowald MW. Polysomnographic, neurologic, psychiatric, and clinical outcome report on 70 consecutive cases with REM sleep behavior disorder (RBD): Sustained clonazepam efficacy in 89.5% of 57 cases. Cleve Clin J Med 1990;57 (Suppl: S9–S23.).

225. Wright BA, Rosen JR, Buysse DJ, et al. Shy-Drager syndrome presenting as a REM behavioral disorder. J Geriatr Psychiatry Neurol 1990;3:110–113.

226. Culebras A, Moore JT. Magnetic resonance findings in REM sleep behavior disorder. Neurology 1989;39:1519–1523.

227. Tachibana N, Sugita Y, Terashima K, et al. Polysomnographic characteristics of healthy elderly subjects with somnambulism-like behaviors. Biol Psychiatry 1991;30:4–14.

228. Coulter DL, Allen RJ, Benign neonatal sleep myoclonus. Arch Neurol 1982;39:191–192.

229. Resnick TJ, Moshe SL, Perotta L, et al. Benign neonatal sleep myoclonus. Relationship to sleep states. Arch Neurol 1986;43:266–268.

230. Fukimoto M, Mochizuki N, Takeishi M, et al. Studies of body movements during night sleep in infancy. Brain Dev 1981;3:37–43.

231. Manetto V, Medori R, Cortelli P, et al. Fatal familial insomnia: Clinical and pathological study of five new cases. Neurology 1992;42:312–319.

232. Goldfarb LG, Petersen RB, Tabaton M, et al. Fatal familia insomnia and familial Creutzfeld-Jakob disease: Disease phenotype determined by a DNA polymorphism. Science 1992;258:806–808.

233. Blatt I, Peled R, Gadoth N, et al. The value of sleep recording in evaluating somnambulism in young adults. Electroencephalogr Clin Neurophysiol 1991;78:407–412.

234. Johns MW, A new method for measuring daytime sleepiness: The Epworth Sleepiness scale. Sleep 1991;14:540–545.

235. Therapeutic and Technology Assessment Subcommittee of the American Academy of Neurology. Assessment: Techniques associated with the diagnosis and management of sleep disorders. Neurology 1992;42:269–275.

236. Aldrich MS, Jahnke B. Diagnostic value of video-EEG polysomnography. Neurology 1991;41:1060–1066.

237. Alihanka J, Vaahtoranta K, Saarikivi J. A new method of long-term monitoring of the ballistocardiogram, heart rate and respiration. Am J Physiol 1981;240:384–392.

238. Erkinjuntti M, Vaahtoranta K, Alihanka J, et al. Use of the SCSB method for monitoring of the respiration, body movements, and ballistocardiogram in infants. Early Hum Dev 1984;9:119–126.

239. Salmi T, Leinonen L. Automatic analysis of sleep records with static charge-sensitive bed. Electroencephalogr Clin Neurophysiol 1986;64:84–87.

240. Erkinjuntti M, Kero P, Halonen JP, et al. SCSB method compared to EEG-based polygraphy in sleep state scoring of newborn infants. Acta Pædiatr Scand 1990;79:274–279.

241. Salmi T, Telakivi T, Partinen M. Evaluation of automatic analysis of SCSB airflow and oxygen saturation signals in patients with sleep related apneas. Chest 1989;96:255–261.

242. Cole RJ, Kripke DF, Gruen W, et al. Automatic sleep/wake identification from wrist activity. Sleep 1992;15:461–469.

243. Kayed K, Roberts S, Davies WL. Computer detection and analysis of periodic movements in sleep. Sleep 1990;13:253–261.

20

Sleep, Breathing, and Neurological Disorders

Sudhansu Chokroverty

To understand the effects of neurologic lesions on sleep-wake cycles and sleep states, and to understand the normal interactions of sleep and breathing, it is important to have a clear understanding of the functional anatomy of sleep and breathing. In the first section of the chapter, therefore, a brief overview of the anatomy and physiology of sleep is presented. The section of the functional anatomy of sleep is followed by a short discussion of the control of breathing during sleep. For details readers are referred to some excellent reviews[1-10] and monographs and to Chapters 3 and 5 in this volume.

Most of the anatomic structures that control sleep and breathing are located in the central nervous system (CNS). These regions are influenced not only by other CNS structures but also by inputs from the peripheral neuromuscular system and other body systems. It is very common to encounter in practice a variety of neurologic disorders that affect sleep and breathing. It is important to understand not only that the neurologic illnesses may affect sleep and breathing but also that alterations of sleep and breathing may adversely affect the natural history of a neurologic disorder. A number of excellent sources provide systematic descriptions of the effects of neurologic lesions on the pattern and control of breathing.[11-21] The effect of acute and chronic neurologic disorders on the state of sleep and the resulting interaction on breathing have received scant attention. An understanding of such an interaction is essential for treatment and prognostic purposes in various neurologic disorders. In neurologic illnesses, breathing disorders may manifest as hypopnea, apnea, irregular or periodic breathing, or cessation of breathing. Similarly, sleep disturbances may manifest as hypersomnia, hyposomnia (insomnia), parasomnia, or circadian rhythm sleep disorders. The sections following those on functional anatomy and physiology of sleep and breathing deal with the clinical manifestations, laboratory assessment, and treatment of sleep and breathing disorders that accompany neurologic illnesses. The discussion is grouped into two major sections: (1) sleep and breathing disorders secondary to somatic neurologic illness and (2) sleep and breathing disorders secondary to autonomic failure. The somatic neurologic disorders are subdivided into CNS disorders and peripheral neuromuscular disorders.

FUNCTIONAL ANATOMY OF SLEEP (SEE CHAPTER 3)

Neurophysiologic studies of sleep really began after astute clinicopathologic observers examined patients with encephalitis lethargica at the beginning of this century.[22] It was noted that lesions of encephalitis lethargica, which severely affected the posterior hypothalamic and preoptic area, were associated with the clinical manifestation of extreme somnolence whereas morphologic alterations in the anterior hypothalamic region were associated with sleeplessness. These observations led scientists to believe in the existence of the so-called sleep-wake centers.[22-25]

Before the middle of the century the emphasis of sleep physiologists was on the passive[25-27] theories of sleep. Beginning in the late 1950s thought shifted toward active sleep theories.[3,5,28-37] The passive theory postulates that sleep results from withdrawal of both specific and nonspecific afferent stimuli to the brain stem and the cerebral hemispheres. Proponents of active sleep theories suggest that activity of sleep-promoting neurons or the fibers of these so-called centers determines the onset of sleep. Most likely, proponents of both active and passive theories are partially correct, as far as the physiology and anatomy of sleep are concerned. These conclusions are based on stimulation, ablation, or lesion experiments. Later on, these studies were extended to include extracellar as well as intracellar recordings, and pharmacologic injections of chemicals into discrete areas to induce different states of sleep or to inhibit sleep.[38]

The passive theory originated with two classic preparations in cats by Bremer,[26,39] *cerveau isolé* and *encéphale isolé*. Bremer found that midcollicular transection (cerveau isolé) produced somnolence in the acute stage and that transection at C-1 vertebral level, to disconnect the entire brain from the spinal cord (encéphale isolé), caused electroenceph-alographic recordings to fluctuate between wakeful-ness and sleep. From these experiments Bremer con-cluded that in cerveau isolé preparations all the specific sensory afferent stimuli were withdrawn and thus sleep was facilitated whereas such stimuli maintained the activation of the brain in encéphale isolé preparation. These conclusions, however, have been modified since the discovery by Moruzzi and Magoun in 1949[27] of the existence of nonspecific groups of neurons and fibers in the center of the brain stem called the reticular formation. Moruzzi and Magoun[27] stated that the ascending reticular activating brain stem system energized the forebrain and that withdrawal of this influence in cerveau isolé preparation resulted in somnolence or coma. The observations of Moruzzi and Magoun[27] that EEG desynchronization results from activation of the midbrain reticular neurons, which directly excite the thalamocortical projections, have been con-firmed by recent intracellular studies.[40,41] It was thought that wakefulness results from activation of the ascending reticular activating system and diffuse thalamocortical projections.[1] Following stimulation of these structures, EEG shows diffuse desynchroni-zation, whereas lesions in these structures produce EEG synchronization or the EEG non–rapid eye movement (NREM) sleep pattern. The origin of the sleep spindles was recently shown to be related to the reticular nucleus of the thalamus.[1] Stimulation of this nucleus produces spindle-like activity while destruction of it abolishes the spindles unilaterally and bilateral destruction abolishes the spindles on both sides.

The passive sleep theories were challenged by findings that came in the wake of midpontine pre-trigeminal brain stem transection in cats performed by Batini and coworkers.[29,30] This preparation is only a few millimeters below the section that pro-duces cerveau isolé preparation. In contrast to the somnolence produced by cerveau isolé preparation, the midpontine pretrigeminal section produced per-sistent EEG and behavioral signs of alertness. These observations imply that structures located in the brain stem regions between these two preparations (cerveau isolé and midpontine pretrigeminal prepa-rations) are responsible for wakefulness. Recent data demonstrate cholinergic neurons in the pedunculo-pontine tegmental nucleus (PPT) and in the latero-dorsal tegmental (LDT) nucleus in the region of the midbrain-pontine junction.[1] These groups of cholin-ergic neurons have been shown to have thalamic and basal forebrain projections as well as projections toward the medial pontine reticular formation. The neurons are likely responsible for activation and for generation of REM sleep (see Chapter 3). The fore-brain cholinergic neurons from the basal nucleus of

Meynert project to the cerebral hemisphere, partic-ularly to the sensory-motor cortex, and lesions in these neurons disrupt the EEG waves and elicit dif-fuse slow waves.[1] The finding of cholinergic neu-rons at the mesopontine junction confirms the con-clusions drawn by Batini[29,30] and colleagues after midpontine pretrigeminal transections. Transection experiments by Jouvet[42] through different regions of the midbrain, pons, and medulla of cats clearly show the existence of REM sleep–generating neurons in the pontine catbrain (see Chapter 3).

The active hypnogenic neurons for NREM sleep are thought to be located in two regions[1]: (1) the region of the nucleus tractus solitarius in the medulla, and (2) the preoptic area of the hypothalamus and the basal forebrain area. The evidence is based on stim-ulation, lesion, and ablation studies, and recently on extracellular and intercellular recordings.[1] The ac-tive inhibitory role of the lower brain stem hypno-genic neurons on the upper brain stem ascending reticular activating systems has been clearly demon-strated by Batini's[29,30] experiment of midpontine pretrigeminal section. Similarly, electrical[34] stimu-lation of the preoptic area, which produced EEG synchronization and behavioral state of sleep, sup-ported the idea of the existence of active hypnogenic neurons in the preoptic area.[1] Nauta's[25] experiments in 1946 that showed insomnia following lesion of the preoptic region also supported the hypothesis of active hypnogenic neurons in the forebrain preoptic area. Later experiments by McGinty and Sterman[36] in 1968 confirmed Nauta's observations. Recently, ibotenic[43] lesions in the preoptic region have been found to produce insomnia, and these results sup-port the active hypnogenic role of preoptic area.[1] Intracellular studies by Szymusiak and McGinty[44] again challenged the concept of active hypnogenic neurons in the preoptic area. In these experiments, only a small number of neurons showed discharge rates that were higher during EEG synchronization than in REM sleep or wakefulness; therefore, the majority of these forebrain neurons are found to be state indifferent or waking active.[1,44] On the other hand, experiments in cats by Detari[45] and Buzsaki[46] and their coworkers have clearly shown increased firing rates for basal forebrain neurons during EEG desynchronization associated with appropriate be-havioral state. Thus, Steriade and McCarley[1] con-cluded that the idea of an active hypnogenic center or group of neurons still awaits confirmation at the cellular level. They,[1] however, suggested that the search for the active hypnogenic neurons should be conducted in the region of the basal forebrain rather than any other brain region, because recently cholin-ergic[47] pathways were shown that descend from the basal forebrain[48] to the PPT nucleus in the mesopon-tine junction. In summary, the active and passive theories of sleep may be viewed as complimentary rather than mutually exclusive mechanisms.[1]

FUNCTIONAL ANATOMY OF RESPIRATION AND SLEEP IN WAKEFULNESS

The neuroanatomy of respiration, its control, and physiologic changes during sleep in healthy persons are described in detail in Chapter 5. Briefly, respiration is controlled by the automatic metabolic and behavioral systems.[11-14,49-52] The two systems are complemented by a third system known as the arousal system, which may also be called the *system for wakefulness stimulus*.[52,53] These respiratory systems work in concert with the various peripheral and central inputs to maintain acid-base regulation and respiratory homeostasis.[9] The location of the respiratory neurons makes them easily vulnerable to a variety of central and peripheral neurologic disorders, particularly central neurologic disorders involving the brain stem. Many acute and chronic neurologic illnesses may affect central or peripheral respiratory pathways, giving rise to acute respiratory failure in wakefulness and sleep. Some conditions may affect control of breathing only during sleep. Such a condition may cause undesirable, often catastrophic, results, including cardiorespiratory failure and even sudden death.

THE SPECTRUM OF SLEEP-RELATED RESPIRATORY DYSRHYTHMIAS IN NEUROLOGIC DISORDERS

Many different types of sleep-related respiratory dysrhythmias have been noted in association with neurologic illnesses[52,54,55] (Figure 20-1). The commonest type is sleep apnea or sleep hypopnea.

Sleep Apnea

Three types of sleep apnea have been noted[56]: central, upper airway obstructive, and mixed. Normal persons may experience a few episodes of sleep apnea, particularly central apnea, at the onset of NREM sleep and during REM sleep. To be of pathologic significance, the sleep apnea should last at least 10 seconds, apnea index (number of apneas per hour of sleep) should be at least 5, and the patient should have at least 30 periods of apneas during 7 hours of all-night sleep.[57]

Cessation of airflow with no respiratory effort constitutes central apnea. During this period there is no diaphragmatic and intercostal muscle activity or air exchange through the nose or mouth. Upper airway obstructive sleep apnea (OSA) is manifested by absence of air exchange through the nose or mouth but persistence of the diaphragmatic and intercostal muscle activity.

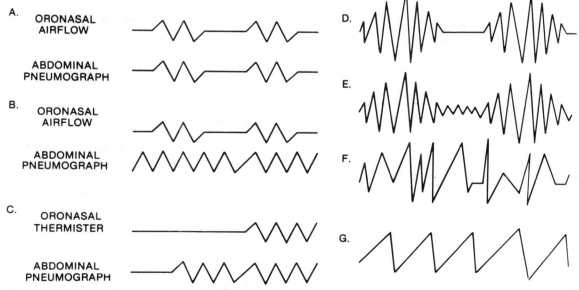

FIGURE 20-1.   *Schematic diagram to show different types of sleep-related breathing patterns in neurological illness. (A) Central apnea. (B) Upper airway obstructive apnea. (C) Mixed apnea (initial central followed by obstructive apnea). (D) Cheyne-Stokes respiration. (E) Cheyne-Stokes variant pattern. (F) Dysrhythmic breathing. (G) Apneustic breathing. (Reproduced with permission from Chokroverty S.) Sleep apnea and respiratory disturbances in multiple system atrophy with progressive autonomic failure (Shy-Drager syndrome). In: Bannister R, ed. Autonomic Failure, Ed 2. London: Oxford University Press, 1988;432–450.)*

During mixed apnea, initially airflow ceases, as does respiratory effort (central apnea); this is followed by a period of upper airway OSA. On rare occasions this pattern may be reversed: an initial period of OSA followed by central apnea (Figure 20-2).

Sleep-Related Hypopnea

Sleep-related hypopnea is manifested by a decrease in airflow at the mouth and nose and decreased chest movement, which causes a reduction in tidal volume and a reduction of the amplitude of the oronasal thermistor or the pneumographic signal to half the volume measured during the preceding or following respiratory cycles.[58] Respiratory disturbance index (RDI) or apnea-hypopnea indexed (AHI) is defined as the number of apneas plus hypopneas per hour of sleep, and again the index should be at least 5 to be significant.

Sleep-related apneas and hypopneas in neurologic diseases are secondary sleep apnea syndromes, in contrast to primary OSA syndrome, in which no cause is found to account for the appearance of

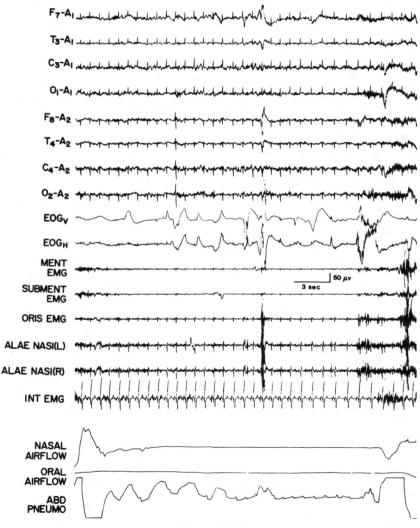

FIGURE 20-2.   *PSG recording in a patient with narcolepsy and sleep apnea showing EEG (top eight channels), vertical (EOG$_V$) and horizontal electrooculograms (EOG$_H$), submental (SUBMENT), orbicularis oris (ORIS), left (L) and right (R) alae nasi and intercostal (INT) muscles, nasal and oral airflow and abdominal pneumogram (ABD PNEUMO). Note unusual type of mixed apnea (initial period of 14 seconds' obstructive apnea followed by 8 seconds' central apnea) during REM sleep.*

apnea. The neurologic illness may be aggravated by the secondary sleep apnea because of the adverse effects of sleep-induced hypoxemia and hypercapnia and repeated sleep arousals with sleep fragmentation. In longstanding cases there may be pulmonary hypertension, congestive cardiac failure, and other manifestations of chronic sleep deprivation.

Cheyne-Stokes and Cheyne-Stokes Variant Pattern of Breathing[58–60]

Cheyne-Stokes breathing is a special type of central apnea manifested as cyclic changes in breathing with crescendo-decrescendo sequence separated by central apneas. The Cheyne-Stokes *variant pattern* of breathing is distinguished by the substitution of hypopneas for apneas.[19,21] In neurologic disorders, Cheyne-Stokes type of breathing is mostly noted in bilateral cerebral hemispheric lesions[12,13] and it worsens during sleep, whereas Cheyne-Stokes variant pattern of breathing may also be noted in brain stem lesions, in addition to bilateral cerebral hemisphere disease.

Dysrhythmic Breathing[58,61]

Dysrhythmic breathing is characterized by non-rhythmic respiration of irregular rate, rhythm, and amplitude during wakefulness that becomes worse during sleep. Dysrhythmic breathing may result from an abnormality in the automatic respiratory pattern generator in the brain stem.

Apneustic Breathing

Apneustic breathing is characterized by prolonged inspiration with an increase in the ratio of inspiratory to expiratory time.[59] This type of breathing may result from a neurologic lesion in the caudal pons that disconnects the so-called apneustic center in the lower pons from the pneumotaxic center (parabrachial and Kolliker-Fuse nuclei) in the upper pons in association with vagotomy.[62,63]

Inspiratory Gasp

Inspiratory gasp is characterized by a short inspiration time and a relatively prolonged expiration (reduced inspiratory-expiratory time ratio).[64] Gasping or irregular breathing has been noted after lesion in the medulla.[16,59]

In addition to these, the following abnormal breathing patterns are also noted in neurologic disorders, particularly in patients with Shy-Drager syndrome[52,55]:

Nocturnal stridor causing severe inspiratory breathing difficulty.

Periodic central apnea in the erect position accompanied by postural fall of blood pressure in the Shy-Drager syndrome.[65]

Prolonged periods of central apnea accompanied by mild oxygen desaturation *in relaxed wakefulness,* as if the respiratory centers "forgot" to breathe.[58,61]

Transient occlusion of the upper airway or transient uncoupling of intercostal and diaphragmatic muscle activity[61]

Transient sudden respiratory arrest.

MECHANISM OF RESPIRATORY DYSRHYTHMIAS IN NEUROLOGIC DISEASES

Several mechanisms may be responsible for the respiratory abnormalities in sleep associated with neurologic disorders.[52,58]

1. Direct involvement causing structural alterations of the medullary respiratory neurons (automatic or metabolic respiratory controlling system). This mechanism may result in apnea or hypopnea during NREM and REM sleep. During REM sleep this problem may be aggravated because of the additional complicating factor of oropharyngeal or other upper airway muscle hypotonia contributing to upper airway OSA.

2. Involvement of the voluntary respiratory control system would, of course, cause respiratory dysfunction during wakefulness and may give rise to respiratory apraxia.

3. Functional or neurochemical alteration of the respiratory neurons.

4. Interference with the afferent inputs to the medullary respiratory neurons (for example, compromise of the peripheral chemoreceptors located in the vagal and glossopharyngeal nerve endings), supramedullary pathways, and central chemoreceptors in the ventrolateral medulla.

5. Direct involvement of the efferent mechanism through respiratory muscle weakness may result from either direct involvement of the muscles, as in myopathies, or involvement of the lower motor neurons to the respiratory muscles. In such patients with weakness of the principal respiratory and the accessory respiratory muscles, the central respiratory neurons may increase their rate of firing or recruit additional respiratory neurons during wakefulness to maintain ventilation at a level adequate to drive the weak respiratory muscles in such patients. Because of the normal vulnerability of the respiratory neurons during sleep, ventilatory problems may be aggravated, causing more severe hypoventilation, and even apnea, during sleep. In addition, weakness of the upper airway muscles, which in fact are

respiratory muscles and receive phasic inspiratory drive from the respiratory neurons in the brain stem, may cause obstructive apnea.

CLINICAL MANIFESTATIONS

Sleep disorders in the neurologic illnesses may be divided broadly into two groups: (1) *dyssomnias*, which include insomnia, hypersomnia, and circadian rhythm sleep disorders, and (2) *parasomnias*, which are not primary disorders of sleep but disorders of arousal and sleep stage transition, associated with intrusion into sleep but not with alteration of the sleep architecture.

Insomnia may be manifested as difficulty in initiating or maintaining sleep, and hypersomnia as excessive daytime somnolence (EDS) and other symptoms. Most of the neurologic disorders cause hypersomnia, but sometimes insomnia is the presenting complaint. An important but rare example, fatal familial insomnia, is described later in this chapter.

Hypersomnia is generally noted in patients with sleep-related respiratory dysrhythmias. In acute neurologic disorders the clinical features of neurologic dysfunction may overshadow the sleep and sleep-related respiratory problems.[58] Furthermore, many patients with acute neurologic disorders are actually in stupor or coma. Neurologic lesions may disrupt the sleep architecture, for example, altering the percentage of different sleep stages, increasing awakenings, or causing sleep stage shifts. In addition, sleep apnea, which may occur in various neurologic diseases, intrusion of abnormal movements in sleep and repeated seizures may disrupt the morphology of sleep and sleep stages. Sleep disturbances may impair memory, cognition, or behavior or cause cardiopulmonary changes secondary to repeated hypoxemia. These effects secondary to sleep disturbance can aggravate the primary neurologic condition.

The clinical manifestations of sleep and breathing disorders in chronic neurologic illnesses may be divided into specific and general features.[52,58] The specific manifestations depend on the nature of the neurologic deficit. The general features that are relevant to the diagnosis of sleep-related hypoventilation and apnea include EDS, fatigue, early morning headache, disturbed nocturnal sleep, intellectual deterioration, personality changes, and in men, impotence. Breathlessness is generally not an important feature of CNS disorders except those illnesses that affect the lower motor neurons to the respiratory muscles. The general symptoms of daytime fatigue,

somnolence, and morning headache may be related to frequent arousals at night secondary to repeated apnea or hypopnea and carbon dioxide retention.[66] In patients with neurologic disorders it is very important to recognize alveolar hypoventilation during sleep because assisted ventilation at night improves the symptoms and protects patients from fatal apnea during sleep. Furthermore, such treatment may prevent the development of serious complications resulting from episodic or prolonged hypoxemia, hypercapnia, and respiratory acidosis in sleep, complications that may include pulmonary hypertension, cor pulmonale, congestive cardiac failure, and occasionally cardiac arrhythmias.

To make a clinical diagnosis of sleep disorder or sleep-related breathing disorders, a careful history—not only from the patient but also from the caregiver—and a physical examination are essential.

In summary, the sleep disturbances in neurologic disorders may result from any of the following mechanisms[52,58,67]:

1. Direct involvement of the hypnogenic neurons; for example, hypofunction of the hypothalamic preoptic nuclei or the lower brain stem hypnogenic neurons alters the balance between the waking and the sleeping brain, causing wakefulness or sleeplessness. Similarly an affection of the posterior hypothalamic, the ascending reticular activating system, or other brain regions responsible for waking and alertness cause hypersomnolence.

2. Indirect mechanisms are the associated manifestations, for example, pain, confusional episodes, changes in the sensorimotor system, and movement disorder that interfere with sleep.

3. Medications used to treat neurologic illnesses may have a direct effect on sleep and breathing (e.g., anticonvulsants, antidepressants, dopamine agonists, anticholinergics, hypnotics, sedatives).

4. Neurologic diseases may change the neurochemical environment of the sleep-generating and sleep-promoting neurons (e.g., hyperkinetic movement disorders, Rett syndrome).[68]

5. Associated depression or anxiety, which may be a secondary manifestation of neurologic disease can disrupt sleep.

6. Sleep-wake schedule disturbances.

7. Sleep-related respiratory dysrhythmias.

Neurologic disorders could be metabolic or structural (e.g., head injury, tumors, infection, toxic-metabolic brain dysfunction, vascular and degenerative CNS diseases, headache from any cause, painful peripheral neuropathy, or another neuromuscular disorder).

SLEEP AND BREATHING DYSFUNCTION

Cerebral Hemispheric and Diencephalic Diseases

Sleep disturbances in neurologic diseases affecting the cerebral hemispheres and the diencephalon have been noted in two groups of patients: those with sleep-related breathing disorders and those without sleep-disordered breathing. Plum and co-workers noted[11–13,17,69] that the major effects of cerebral hemispheric disease on respiration in sleep consisted of these: (1) Cheyne-Stokes respiration or long-cycle Cheyne-Stokes breathing associated with hypocapnia; this was associated with brain damage deep in both cerebral hemispheres. In unilateral cerebral infarction this may be due to the phenomenon of diaschisis.* 2. Posthyperventilation apnea was noted in 70% of patients with bilateral and 6% with unilateral cerebral dysfunction, and the apnea became more marked during sleep. On the other hand, Lee and coworkers[21] found Cheyne-Stokes and Cheyne-Stokes variant pattern breathing in patients with extensive bilateral pontine lesions. Plum and coworkers[11–13,69] rarely found Cheyne-Stokes respiration in lesions located as low as the upper pons but mostly noted it with bilateral cerebral hemispheric or diencephalic lesions. It must be remembered that many patients with cerebral hemispheric and diencephalic lesions remain in stupor and coma; these patients' sleep and respiration during sleep cannot be assessed.

Sleep disturbances in cerebral hemispheric and diencephalic diseases may result from cerebral vascular diseases, brain tumors, degenerative dementia (e.g., Alzheimer's disease [AD]), head trauma, encephalitis, or toxic-metabolic encephalopathy or any diffuse cerebral dysfunction that could directly or indirectly affect the diffuse thalamocortical projection system and thalamic-hypothalamic regions.

Sleep and Respiration in Alzheimer's Disease

AD, or senile dementia of the Alzheimer's type, is characterized by progressive intellectual deterioration occurring in middle or later life associated with characteristic neuropathologic findings, including cerebral cortical atrophy and neuronal loss in the nucleus basalis of Meynert. There is also evidence of alterations in the forebrain cholinergic, and in many cases also in the noradrenergic, system.[70] For the diagnosis of probable, possible, and definite AD readers are referred to the clinical criteria developed

---

Diaschisis implies physiologic dysfunction of the contralateral homologous area without anatomic disconnection.

by NINCDS-ADRDA work (Table 20-1).[71] Sleep disturbances in AD may be related partly to the severity of the loss of the cholinergic neurons in the basal forebrain regions, as well as to changes in the brain stem aminergic systems.

Sleep disorders in AD may increase cognitive and behavioral dysfunction. Such sleep disorders may arise directly from the disease itself, as a consequence of the degeneration of the brain stem and other centers that regulate sleep,[72] or indirectly from changes in sleep associated with aging (see Chapter 25). Sleep disorders can have a number of undesirable consequences: they can increase cardiovascular and even cerebral vascular morbidity and impair daytime alertness and functioning.[56,57,73]

A number of studies have now examined the differences between demented patients and normal elderly persons and have demonstrated higher prevalence for sleep apnea and for poorer sleep quality when patients are compared to age-matched controls.[72–74] Though the results vary somewhat from study to study, these investigations have shown deterioration of sleep parameters, including reduced total length of sleep, decreased REM and stage 4 NREM sleep, loss of phasic components (spindles and K complexes) of NREM sleep, and sleep-wake rhythm disturbances in demented patients.[74–78] This pattern of disorder is different from that of depressed elderly patients, who most clearly show poor sleep maintenance, often with increased REM sleep.[75] Most of the studies, however, have not used current diagnostic criteria for dementia and have lumped together patients with different forms of it. When more accurate diagnostic groupings were made, similar results were found for AD patients usually defined by clinical course. Some studies have shown a clear association between greater sleep disturbance and impaired mental functioning or severity of dementia.[72,79–81]

Sleep apnea has been observed in some 33% to 53% of demented patients with probable AD.[72,80–82] While sleep apnea may be associated with disease severity, no longitudinal studies have been conducted to determine whether sleep apnea increases the severity of disease in individual patients and whether sleep apnea may be associated with more rapid progression of the disease. Such a deleterious effect of sleep apnea is to be expected, as it is thought to increase the intellectual deficit of demented patients.[75,82] Because sleep apnea may be treated by a number of modalities, it is possible that therapy may improve behavior and cognitive function, though as yet there are no reports of the effects of treatment of sleep apnea in AD or dementia.

According to Smallwood and colleagues,[81] the incidence of sleep apnea in male AD patients is similar

TABLE 20-1. Criteria for Clinical Diagnosis of Alzheimer's Disease

---

I. The criteria for the clinical diagnosis of PROBABLE Alzheimer's disease include:
Dementia established by clinical examination and documented by the Mini-Mental Test, Blessed Dementia Scale, or some similar examination, and confirmed by neuropsychological tests
Deficits in two or more areas of cognition
Progressive worsening of memory and other cognitive functions
No disturbance of consciousness
Onset between ages 40 and 90, most often after age 65 *and*
Absence of systemic disorders or other brain diseases that, in and of themselves, could account for the progressive deficits in memory and cognition.

II. The diagnosis of PROBABLE Alzheimer's disease is supported by:
Progressive deterioration of specific cognitive functions such as language (aphasia), motor skills (apraxia), and perception (agnosia)
Impaired activities of daily living and altered patterns of behavior
Family history of similar disorders, particularly if confirmed neuropathologically
and
Laboratory results:
Normal lumbar puncture as evaluated by standard techniques
Normal pattern or nonspecific changes in EEG, such as increased slow-wave activity
and
Evidence of cerebral atrophy on CT with progression documented by serial observations

III. Other clinical features consistent with the diagnosis of PROBABLE Alzheimer's disease, after exclusion of causes of dementia other than Alzheimer's disease, include:
Plateaus in the course of progression of the illness
Associated symptoms of depression, insomnia, incontinence, delusions, illusions, hallucinations, catastrophic verbal, emotional, or physical outbursts, sexual disorders, and weight loss; other neurologic abnormalities in some patients, especially with more advance disease and including motor signs such as increased muscle tone, myoclonus, or gait disorder
Seizures in advanced disease
and
CT normal for age.

IV. Features that make the diagnosis of PROBABLE Alzheimer's diseases uncertain or unlikely include:
Sudden, apoplectic onset
Focal neurologic findings such as hemiparesis, sensory loss, visual field deficits, and incoordination early in the course of the illness
and
Seizures or gait disturbances at the onset or very early in the course of the illness.

V. Clinical diagnosis of POSSIBLE Alzheimer's disease:
May be made on the basis of the dementia syndrome, in the absence of other neurologic, psychiatric, or systemic disorders sufficient to cause dementia, and in the presence of variations in the onset, in the presentation, or in the clinical course;
May be made in the presence of a second systemic or brain disorder sufficient to produce dementia, which is not considered to be the cause of the dementia
and
Should be used in research studies when a single, gradually progressive severe cognitive deficit is identified in the absence of other identifiable cause.

VI. Criteria for diagnosis of DEFINITE Alzheimer's disease are:
The clinical criteria for probable Alzheimer's disease and histopathologic evidence obtained from a biopsy or autopsy.

VII. Classification of Alzheimer's disease for research purposes should specify features that may differentiate subtypes of the disorder, such as:
Familial occurrence;
Onset before age 65
Presence of trisomy 21
and
Coexistence of other relevant conditions, such as Parkinson's disease.

(Reprinted with permission from McKhann G, Drachman D, Folstein M, et al. Clinical diagnosis of Alzheimer's disease: Report of the NINCDS-ADRDA work under the auspices of Department of Health and Human Services Task Force on Alzheimer's Disease. Neurology 1984;34:939–944.)

to that of healthy elderly subjects. Reynolds and coworkers[83] reported a higher prevalence of sleep apnea in female AD patients during the later stage of the illness than in controls. These findings have been confirmed later by Vitiello[84] and Mant[85] and their associates. Periodic limb movements in sleep (PLMS) are common in elderly persons, and there is no significant difference in incidence between AD patients and healthy elderly subjects.[86] The incidence and severity of sleep apnea and PLMS did not significantly differ in elderly subjects and AD patients.[86]

Figure 20-3 shows mixed sleep apnea associated with significant oxygen desaturation in a 68-year-old man with advanced AD who was studied polysomnographically. In view of the recent documentation by Carskadon and associates (summarized by Miles and Dement[87]) of a high prevalence of apnea in asymptomatic ambulatory elderly volunteers, and the findings of Smallwood's group[81] it is difficult to estimate the true incidence of sleep apnea in AD patients.

Sleep-wake rhythm disturbances are common in AD.[88] The inability of patients to follow a normal schedule can present a significant management problem; "sundowning," an inversion of sleep schedule (wakefulness at night and somnolence in the daytime) is particularly troublesome. It may be that the suprachiasmatic nucleus of the hypothalamus, a well-established regulator of circadian activity rhythm in lower animals, likely plays a similar role in humans[89] and is involved in AD. Decreased REM sleep could also result from degeneration of brain

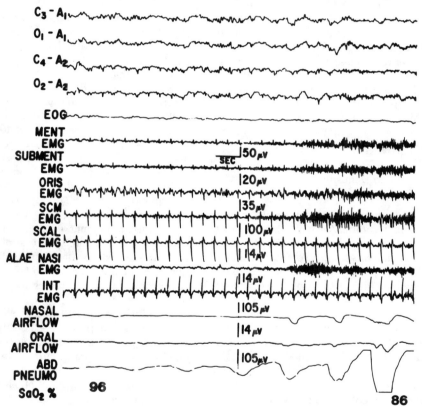

FIGURE 20-3. *PSG recording in a patient with advanced stage of Alzheimer's disease shows a portion of mixed apnea during stage 2 NREM sleep accompanied by oxygen desaturation. Top four channels represent EEG (Key: international electrode placement system). EOG, electrooculogram; EMG, electromyograms of mentalis (MENT), submental (SUBMENT), orbicularis (ORIS), sternocleidomastoid (SCM), scalenus anticus (SCAL), ALAE NASI and intercostal (INT) muscles are shown. Also shown are nasal and oral airflow, abdominal pneumogram (ABD PNEUMO) and oxygen saturation (SaO$_2$%). (Reproduced with permission from Chokroverty S. Sleep and breathing in neurological disorders. In: Edelman NH, Santiago TV, eds. Breathing Disorders of Sleep. New York: Churchill Livingstone, 1986;225–264.)*

stem neurons, such as noradrenergic neurons of the locus ceruleus, which are affected in AD,[90] and the cholinergic neurons of the brain stem. These neurons have been strongly implicated in the control of sleep-wake rhythm.[4,91]

Vitiello and coworkers[84,88] and others[74,75,78,92-95] reported sleep disturbances in AD associated with a decrease in slow-wave sleep and an increase in nighttime awakenings. In a study of 45 control subjects and 44 mild AD patients Vitiello's group[96] confirmed their previous findings of disturbed sleep-wake patterns in AD patients, but the phenomenon of sleep disturbances was not diagnostically useful for discriminating those with a mild stage of AD from control subjects.

In summary, it is now known that sleep dysfunction is common in AD. Given the current state of knowledge, however, it is unclear whether a specific set of sleep abnormalities will be found to be associated with AD that are different from those observed in other dementias. It has been shown that the abnormalities in dementia are significantly different from those of depressive pseudo-dementia.[75] Reynolds and coworkers[75] suggested that sleep dysfunction in AD may be related to progression of the disease and may cause ongoing deterioration of alertness, orientation, and cognitive function.

Sleep, Breathing, and Hemispheric-Diencephalic Stroke

Stroke is an acute neurologic deficit resulting from vascular injury to the brain. Vascular injury could be ischemic (thrombotic or embolic) or hemorrhagic. In this section sleep and breathing disorders in cerebral hemispheric and thalamic strokes are described. Those resulting from brain stem stroke are discussed in a later section.

There are a few scattered reports of sleep complaints after stroke and several reports of sleep-related breathing disorders after cerebral infarction, but there is a dearth of well-controlled studies of the relationship between sleep disorders and cerebral vascular disease. Such studies are important from prognostic and therapeutic points of view.

Hemispheric stroke

Kapen and coworkers[97] reported a high incidence of obstructive sleep apnea in hemispheric stroke patients, though, because of associated risk factors such as obesity and hypertension in most of these patients a definite causal relationship between obstructive apnea and stroke cannot be claimed. In a recent study[97a] of 53 stroke patients, these authors confirmed their previous reports of peak prevalence for the onset of stroke in the morning, during a

6-hour period after awakening from sleep. This is similar to the peak incidence in the morning hours for myocardial infarction and sudden cardiac death. Therefore, in all of these conditions there may be a combination of circadian increase of corticosteroids and catecholamines, increased blood pressure and heart rate in the morning, and increased platelet "aggregability." In several other studies, the incidence of stroke was highest during sleep at night[98] or during early morning hours, after awakening from nocturnal sleep.[99-102]

There is an association between hypertension and habitual snoring[103-106] and between habitual snoring and stroke.[102,106-110] Sleep apnea is noted more frequently in patients with multiple cerebral infarction than in patients with AD or normal healthy elderly persons.[111,112]

Normal subjects exhibit increased platelet aggregability in the early morning,[113] and this factor may contribute to the fact that myocardial infarction, sudden cardiac death, and stroke, all are more likely to occur at that time.

Stroke may predispose to a number of sleep disorders. Kleine-Levin syndrome can occur after multiple cerebral infarction.[114] Narcolepsy-cataplexy has also been reported to follow cerebral hypoxic-ischemia.[115] Insomnia is commonly noted after cerebral infarction, but this may be partly due to the depression that typically follows stroke.[116]

Korner and colleagues[117] made an important polysomnographic (PSG) study in a group of patients with infarction in the territory of the middle cerebral artery. They found marked attenuation of REM sleep after right cerebral hemispheric stroke and reduction of slow-wave sleep after left hemispheric stroke; however, the numbers are too few to be statistically significant and further studies are needed to confirm this conclusion.

Hachinski and colleagues[118] reported serial preischemic and poststroke PSG recordings for 1 year after stroke in a 70-year-old woman who suffered massive cerebral infarction in the left middle cerebral artery territory. Immediate post-infarction PSG showed deterioration of sleep architecture from both the affected and the unaffected hemisphere. Serial recordings showed gradual return of normal sleep EEG rhythms over both hemispheres and persistent delta activity over the affected hemisphere. The authors concluded that diaschisis was responsible for the rapid deterioration of the sleep EEG pattern on the undamaged side of the brain.

Diencephalic stroke

Thalamic stroke may cause ipsilateral loss of sleep spindles,[119] and bilateral paramedian thalamic infarcts may be associated with hypersomnia.[120]

Basal Ganglia and Basal Ganglia Plus Disorders

Sleep disturbances and sleep-related respiratory dysrhythmias are noted in many patients with basal ganglia disorders, but a systematic study to evaluate such dysfunction has not been undertaken in a large number of patients. A review of sleep and movement disorders is given in Chapter 19.

Disorders of Cerebellum and Brain Stem

Olivopontocerebellar atrophy

Olivopontocerebellar atrophy (OPCA) defines chronic progressive hereditary (mostly dominant, sometimes recessive, occasionally sporadic) cerebellar degeneration manifested by cerebellar-parkinsonian or parkinsonian-cerebellar syndrome and associated with atrophy of the pontine nuclei and cerebellar cortex, and degenerative lesions of the olivopontocerebellar regions.[121-123] There have been a few reports on sleep disturbances and sleep-related respiratory dysrhythmias in OPCA.

Cerebellar influence on the sleep-wakefulness mechanism has been clearly demonstrated in experimental animal studies.[124] The role of the cerebellum, however, on the respiratory control mechanism in sleep is not known. Brain stem neurons, which are known to be degenerated in OPCA,[122,123] lie close to the hypnogenic[39] and respiratory neurons.[50] Thus, dysfunction of the respiratory control, in parallel with the somatic structural dysfunction in OPCA, may be expected. The known morphologic changes of OPCA[122,123] are adequate to explain the sleep

disturbances and sleep apnea in this condition. Several authors[125-128] described EEG sleep alterations in degenerative cerebellar atrophy. Reduced or absent REM sleep, reduced slow-wave sleep, and increased awakenings are the essential PSG findings. In several cases of OPCA, REM sleep without muscle atonia accompanied by the typical features of REM behavior disorder have been described.[129-131] Jouvet and Delorme[132] produced REM sleep without atonia in cats by bilateral pontine tegmental lesions. A similar lesion in OPCA may be also responsible for REM behavior disorder in this condition. OPCA has also been associated with hyposomnia.[133]

Sleep apnea has been described in several cases of OPCA.[128,133-136] Chokroverty and colleagues[134] described five patients with OPCA and sleep apnea. PSG study showed repeated episodes of central, upper airway obstructive, and mixed apneas (Figure 20-4) during sleep; the apneic episodes lasted from 10 to 62 seconds and the apnea index was 30 to 55. Pure central apnea was noted in three patients, but all three types of apnea were seen in two, and most of the apneic episodes occurred during NREM sleep stage 2. Thus, these findings suggested central neuronal dysfunction in an area where respiratory and sleep-waking systems are closely interrelated, such as the nucleus tractus solitarius and the pontomedullary reticular formation. Salazar-Grueso and associates[128] described a 37-year-old man with a 19-year history of autosomal dominant OPCA and EDS whose PSG demonstrated episodes of mixed and central (predominantly central) sleep apnea and no sleep spindles or REM sleep. Trazodone treatment

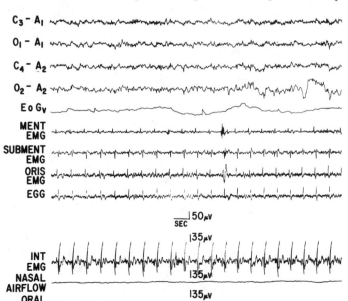

FIGURE 20-4. *PSG recording in a patient with OPCA showing a portion of an episode of mixed apnea (central followed by upper airway obstructive apnea) during stage 2 NREM sleep. EEGs are shown in the top four channels. Key: EOG$_V$: vertical electrooculogram; MENTAL, mentalis; EGG, electroglossogram. (Reproduced with permission from Chokroverty S, Sachdeo R, Masdeu J. Autonomic dysfunction and sleep apnea in olivopontocerebellar degeneration. Arch Neurol 1984;41:509–510.)*

normalized the sleep architecture and reduced the apneic episodes.

Occasionally, sleep disturbances are associated with other types of cerebeller lesions, though systematic studies are lacking. Bergamasco and colleagues[137] made a polygraphic study of a 13-year-old girl with a diagnosis of dyssynergia cerebellaris myoclonica (Ramsey-Hunt syndrome). All-night sleep study showed no REM sleep and increased slow-wave sleep. The EEG showed multiple spike-wave discharges accompanied by myoclonic generalized seizures, and on other occasions desynchronized EEG was noted during tonic seizure.

Brain Stem Lesions

Both the metabolic and autonomic respiratory neurons, and the lower brain stem hypnogenic neurons are located in the medulla. These neurons are influenced by the supramedullary respiration-controlling inputs and hypothalamic preoptic nuclei, as well as by the peripheral afferent inputs to the respiratory centers (see Chapter 5). Therefore, sleep and respiratory disturbances should be common manifestations of lesions in the brain stem, and many such cases have been described. Such affections have included brain stem vascular lesions, tumors, traumatic lesions, multiple sclerosis (MS), bulbar poliomyelitis, and postpolio syndrome, brain stem encephalitis, motor neuron disease affecting the bulbar nuclei, syringobulbia, and Arnold-Chiari malformation.[58] In addition, several cases in which brain stem lesions caused symptomatic or secondary narcolepsy have been described.[120,138–141] Generally, all the characteristic features of narcolepsy are not seen in the secondary syndrome. The causes have included infarction,[120] trauma, and tumors[138] (including third ventricle tumor[139]), and some cases have been associated with MS.[140,141]

Brain stem vascular lesions

Brain stem vascular lesions include infarction, hemorrhage, arterial compression, and localized brain stem ischemia. Sleep disturbances have been described in brain stem infarction by Markand and Dyken[142] and several other authors.[19,21,143,144] PSG findings generally consisted of increased wakefulness after sleep onset and decreased REM and slow-wave sleep. Several reports of EEG or PSG studies to document sleep disturbances have been described in patients with locked in syndrome (LIS), which is characterized by quadriplegia associated with deefferention and results from ventral pontine infarction. Patients are generally aware of the surroundings and are conscious. They cannot speak because of facial muscle paralysis but can respond by moving the eyes, whose control is spared. Sleep EEG recordings

of LIS patients have been reported by Feldman,[145] Freemon and coworkers,[146] Markand and Dyken,[142] Cummings and Greenberg,[147] and Oxenberg and colleagues.[148] Feldman[145] found in his patient reduced REM, stage 4 and total sleep time. Markand and Dyken[142] noted in five of seven LIS patients total absence of REM sleep and variable changes in NREM sleep. Cummings and Greenberg[147] described that one patient had reduced slow-wave sleep and the other reduced NREM sleep and no REM. Oxenberg's group[148] described a 35-year-old man with LIS who had three PSG recordings at intervals. Sleep patterns showed only minor alterations (e.g., a slight decrease of stage 2 and an increase of slow-wave and REM sleep) in their initial recording, in contrast to the more marked alterations noted in previous reports. The authors thought that the difference could be related to the extent of the lesion. Autret and coworkers[149] found a reduction of REM and NREM sleep in four patients after medial pontine tegmental stroke.

Kushida and associates[150] described, in a 24-year-old woman with a left pontine hematoma, marked asymmetry in the EEG of REM sleep, which suggested to the authors that a unilateral pontine lesion may cause disruption of the normal REM sleep EEG in the ipsilateral hemisphere. The lesion did not affect the other characteristics of REM sleep, such as REMs and muscle atonia.

The term *Ondine's curse*, or the *syndrome of primary failure of automatic respiration*, was coined by Severinghaus and Mitchell[151] to describe three patients who experienced long periods of apnea even when awake but could breathe on command. They became apneic following surgery involving the brain stem and high cervical spinal cord and required artificial ventilation while asleep. When their consciousness was altered by nitrous oxide or thiopental, they became apneic. Carbon dioxide response to breathing showed low sensitivity. One patient died in apnea and the two others improved in a week. The authors suggested that Ondine's curse resulted from damage to the medullary carbon dioxide chemoreceptors. It is notable that the term *Ondine's curse* was derived from the sea nymph in German mythology, whose curse rendered her unfaithful lover incapable of automatic respiratory function and caused his death. This eponymic syndrome generated considerable controversy and confusion.[152] The syndrome of the Ondine's curse is usually caused by bilateral lesions anywhere caudal to the fifth cranial nerve in the pons down to the upper cervical spinal cord in the ventrolateral region. However, Levin and Margolis[144] described a 52-year-old man with unilateral medullary infarction who lost automatic respiratory control. At autopsy the lesion was found to extend from the left lower pons through the left lateral medullary tegmentum to the upper cervical spinal cord and to involve the left paramedian pontine reticular formation. Thus, in some patients automatic respiratory control can reside unilaterally in the pontomedullary tegmentum.

Respiratory rate and pattern were studied by Lee and colleagues[19] by impedance pneumography in 14 patients with acute brain stem or cerebral infarction, and in a subsequent study[21] they reported on another 23 patients with acute brain stem infarction. They found frequent abnormalities of respiratory pattern and rate in such patients, and these abnormalities became worse during sleep. The abnormal pattern included Cheyne-Stokes and Cheyne-Stokes variant types of breathing, in addition to tachypnea and cluster breathing in some. In contrast to the observations of Plum and coworkers[11-13,69] that such breathing patterns are associated with bilateral cerebral hemispheric and diencephalic lesions but rarely with lesions in the upper pons, Lee's group[21] observed Cheyne-Stokes respiration in patients with extensive bilateral pontine lesions. They suggested that the size and the bilaterality of the lesions determined the types of respiratory pattern abnormalities.

Devereaux and coworkers[143] reported sleep apnea that required ventilatory support in two women who breathed normally while awake. Aged 36 and 59 years, they had bilateral infarctions limited to the lateral medullary tegmentum. One of these patients' carbon dioxide response was markedly depressed. Though the authors stated that acute automatic respiratory failure did not generally evolve into a chronic alveolar hypoventilation syndrome, their second patient continued to have sleep-induced apnea after many months.

Sleep apnea following bulbar stroke was also described by Askenasy and Goldhammer.[153] Their patient had a left-sided Wallenberg's syndrome (lateral medullary syndrome) and 2 nights' PSG recordings documented mostly obstructive or mixed apneas and hypopneas. This was a clinical diagnosis, and neuroimaging did not define the exact anatomy of the lesion. Their report, however, should direct attention to the possibility that unilateral brain stem lesions can cause sleep apnea syndrome. In such patients it is important to diagnose and promptly treat ventilatory dysfunction during sleep.

Miyazaki and associates[154] recently described a 5-year-old boy with central sleep apnea (documented by PSG recording) associated with compression of the ventral medulla by abnormal looping of the vertebral artery as documented by magnetic resonance imaging (MRI). The authors suggested that the aberrant vertebral artery might have compressed the respiratory center, though the hypercapnic ventilatory response, which reflects central chemoreceptor function, was normal during sleep in this case.

Periodic breathing, apnea, and cyanosis were described in a 57-year-old woman after carotid endarterectomy.[155] The authors suggested that respiratory depression resulted from midbrain hypoxia and edema.

Brain stem ischemic damage may also cause respiratory dysfunction. Beal and colleagues[156] described a 19-year-old man who had failure of automatic respiration and other signs of brain stem dysfunction after nearly drowning. He had sleep apneas, and PSG study confirmed the presence of central sleep apneas. During wakefulness his breathing was normal. Hypercapnic ventilatory response was markedly impaired, but hypoxic ventilatory response appeared to be normal. Autopsy findings 8 months later, following sudden death, documented marked bilateral neuron loss in the tractus solitarius, ambiguus, and retroambigualis nuclei. These most likely resulted from anoxia or ischemia.

Brain stem tumor

Brain stem glioma with automatic respiratory failure was mentioned by Plum.[13] A patient of mine with a medullary tumor that caused severe hypoventilation during sleep, required tracheostomy (unpublished observation). The central apneic episodes in the same patient became prolonged when the tracheostomy tube was occluded. Brain stem tumor may cause disorganization of the tonic and the phasic events of REM sleep, as described in a patient whose pontine tumor caused a marked decrease in the atonia of REM sleep.[157]

Brain stem trauma

North and Jennett[18] recorded irregular breathing patterns in patients with traumatic lesions of the medulla and pons. They did not, however, discuss the changes in the breathing patterns during sleep in these patients. In contrast to the findings of Plum and Posner,[69] they did not find that long- or short-cycle Cheyne-Stokes respirations helped localize the site of brain damage.

Demyelinating lesion in the brain stem

In persons with MS a demyelinating plaque may involve the hypnogenic and respiratory neurons in the brain stem, giving rise to sleep and to sleep-related breathing disorders. A few such cases have been described in MS patients. An interesting patient, a 38-year-old man, was described by Newsom Davis.[158] The patient had a clinical diagnosis of acute demyelinating lesion in the cervicomedullary junction. He had an autonomous breathing pattern, but he could neither take a voluntary breath nor stop breathing, thus illustrating the apparent independence of the mechanisms controlling metabolic and behavioral respiratory control systems. The patient of Rizvi and coworkers[159] whose brain stem dysfunction was consistent with MS became apneic when asleep but was able to breathe when awake. His hypercapnic and hypoxic ventilatory responses were normal. Boor and associates[160] described a 40-year-old patient with paralysis of automatic respiration. During relaxation, the patient had recurrent apnea, but the breathing was stable when the patient was alert. The discovery at postmortem examination of a large, demyelinating lesion in the central medulla involving the medullary respiratory neurons explained the respiratory failure.

Bulbar Poliomyelitis and Postpolio Syndrome

In the acute and convalescent stages of poliomyelitis respiratory disturbances commonly get worse during sleep. Some patients are left with the sequelae of respiratory dysrhythmia, particularly sleep-related apnea or hypoventilation requiring ventilatory support, especially at night. Another group of patients decades later develop symptoms that constitute *postpolio syndrome*. Sleep disturbances and sleep apnea or hypoventilation are also noted in postpolio syndrome. Medullary respiratory and hypnogenic neurons are involved directly by the poliovirus infection, and this explains the patients' symptoms.

Hypoventilation syndrome in bulbar poliomyelitis was first documented quantitatively by Sarnoff and colleagues.[161] They described four patients who could breathe voluntarily on command but hypoventilated during periods of sleep and quiescence. The authors described irregular rate and rhythm of respiration, incoordination of the muscles of respiration, and hypoventilation resulting from decreased sensitivity of the respiratory center to PCO_2 as a result of direct involvement of the respiratory center by the poliomyelitis virus. Two of their patients benefitted from electrophrenic respiration.

An extensive report on the clinical and physiologic findings in 20 of 250 poliomyelitis patients with central respiratory disturbances was given by Plum and Swanson.[16] These patients' respiratory disturbances could not be explained by involvement of the spinal motor neurons or airway obstruction. In acute bulbar poliomyelitis the disordered breathing progressed through three successive stages. Stage I was characterized by disorder of respiratory rhythm during sleep, when breathing became irregular in rate and depth with periods of apnea ranging from 4 to 12 seconds. During stage II, normal breathing required increasing effort and concentration, and strong auditory or painful stimuli were necessary to maintain respiratory rhythmicity. At this stage the

patients had impaired chemosensitivity of the central respiratory centers as evidenced by a reduction in ventilation and carbon dioxide retention after oxygen inhalation. Sleep exacerbated the breathing difficulty, and there were longer periods of apnea. The respiratory homeostasis was lost entirely in stage III, and there was no ventilatory responsiveness to reflex, chemical, or other neuronal stimuli. The respiratory pattern was chaotic, with varying periods of apnea. The patients required ventilatory support to maintain respiratory homeostasis. Severe inflammatory changes and small areas of necrosis in the ventrolateral reticular formation of the medulla were noted in two patients on neuropathologic examination. The breathing abnormalities in this series rarely lasted more than 2 weeks, but two patients had sleep-related irregular respiration that persisted many months after acute poliomyelitis. These two patients also demonstrated impaired hypercapnic ventilatory response and hypoventilation during administration of 100% oxygen. The physiologic abnormalities suggested severe and permanent dysfunction of the medullary respiratory neurons. In several convalescent spinal poliomyelitis patients, the authors also observed subnormal ventilatory response to carbon dioxide with reduction of maximum breathing capacity or vital capacity to less than 50% of predicted normal values. These findings implied that peripheral mechanisms that cause restriction of chest movements may also contribute to impaired ventilatory response to carbon dioxide.

Postpolio syndrome

Postpolio syndrome is manifested clinically by increasing weakness or wasting of the previously affected muscles and by involvement of previously unaffected regions of the body, fatigue, aches and pains, and sometimes symptoms secondary to sleep-related hypoventilation such as EDS and tiredness.[162,163] The exact mechanism of postpolio syndrome is not known.[164] Some of the symptoms (e.g., EDS and fatigue) could result from sleep-related hypoventilation or apnea and sleep disturbances.[165] Thus, it is important to be aware of sleep apnea in such patients. This syndrome has been described in patients who had poliomyelitis decades earlier. Guilleminault and Motta[166] reported on five such men who had a history of bulbar poliomyelitis 16 years earlier. All had EDS, and PSG study documented numerous episodes of apneas, which were predominantly central but also mixed and upper airway obstructive types associated with oxygen desaturation. Their longest apneas were seen during REM sleep. It is important to know that these patients resemble those with primary sleep apnea syndrome. Presumably, the lesions in these cases involved the medullary respiratory neurons and thus central lesions were responsible for all three types of apneas. The patients' symptoms improved and daytime somnolence decreased following ventilatory assistance at night. A 41-year-old woman with a history of bulbar poliomyelitis 20 years earlier was reported by Solliday and associates.[167] This patient had chronic hypoventilation with marked hypoxemia and hypercapnia during sleep. Hypercapnic ventilatory response was impaired, but the hypoxic ventilatory response was normal, suggesting that the patient had impaired central chemoreceptors but functioning peripheral chemoreceptors.

Steljes and coworkers[165] performed PSG examinations on 13 postpolio patients, five of whom used rocking beds for ventilatory assistance and eight no ventilatory assistance. Patients who required ventilatory assistance demonstrated severe sleep disturbances with decreased total sleep time, reduced sleep efficiency, decreased percentage of stage II, slow-wave sleep and REM sleep, but increased awakenings and percentage of stage 1 sleep. Respiratory abnormalities in these patients consisted of hypoventilation, apneas, and hypopneas associated with significant oxygen desaturation. These patients did not respond to continuous positive airway pressure (CPAP) treatment with the rocking bed, but they showed improvement in sleep structure and respiratory function following mechanical ventilation via nasal mask. Five of the eight patients who required no ventilatory assistance also showed impairment of sleep architecture similar to the other group's, but the findings were less severe. All but one patient from the second group had obstructive or mixed apneas, which were treated successfully with nasal CPAP. One patient with mixed apnea and marked hypoventilation improved following treatment with nasal ventilation by mask.

PSG and pulmonary function studies by Bye[168] and Ellis[169] and their respective coworkers documented respiratory failure and sleep hypoxemia, particularly during REM sleep, in patients with postpolio respiratory muscle weakness. Sleep studies by Ellis' group[169] under controlled conditions without respiratory support showed repeated arousals with disruption and fragmentation of REM-NREM cycle. Bye's group[168] and Howard's[170] found a direct relationship between forced vital capacity, sleep hypoxemia, and nocturnal hypoventilation in such patients.

Syringobulbia-myelia

Some patients with syringobulbia-myelia may have alveolar hypoventilation and sleep-related apneas or irregular breathing and stridor. Haponik and colleagues[171] described such a case. The patient was a 35-year-old woman whose polygraphic examination

showed 370 upper airway obstructive apneas lasting 10 to 170 seconds associated with hypoxemia during 7 hours of NREM stage 1 and 2 sleep. The patient died 9 months after the onset of the illness, and neuropathologic examination disclosed a syrinx that extended from the lower third of the medulla to the upper thoracic spinal cord.

Western equine encephalitis

Cohn and Kuida[172] and White and coworkers[173] described alveolar hypoventilation, central sleep apnea, EDS, and subnormal hypercapnic ventilatory response following western equine encephalitis. The respiratory center was thought to have been damaged by the virus.

Arnold-Chiari malformation

Central sleep apnea may result from Arnold-Chiari malformation.[174,175] On the basis of autopsy findings Papasozomenos and Roessman[174] suggested in their patient with Arnold-Chiari malformation that central sleep apnea resulted from brain stem compression and ischemia with vascular stretching. In their report of Chiari I malformation in children Dure and associates[175] did not have MRI or computed tomographic (CT) evidence of brain stem vascular compression. Upper airway obstructive sleep apnea has also been described in Arnold-Chiari malformation.[176] Earlier, Campbell[177] described two patients with Arnold-Chiari malformation who had profound hypoventilation. Bokinsky and colleagues[178] described an 18-year-old patient with Arnold-Chiari malformation and syringomyelia accompanied by dysfunction of the ninth, tenth, and twelfth cranial nerves. They noted absent hypoxic ventilatory response but normal hypercapnic ventilatory response in their patient. These findings are consistent with bilateral ninth cranial nerve dysfunction.

Diseases of the Spinal Cord

In spinal cord disorders, sleep disturbances occur as a result of sleep-related respiratory dysrhythmias causing sleep apneas, hypopneas, or hypoventilation associated with hypoxemia and repeated arousals. The voluntary or the behavioral respiratory control system descends via the corticospinal tracts, and the metabolic or automatic respiratory controlling system descends via the reticulospinal tracts, and the two systems are integrated in the spinal cord (see also Chapter 5). The behavioral system is located in the dorsolateral quadrant of the cervical spinal cord[13,14] and the automatic respiratory system in the ventrolateral quadrant. These two systems control the final common respiratory pathways of the spinal respiratory motor neurons, which send impulses along the phrenic and intercostal nerves to the main respiratory muscles. The anterior horn cells in the third, fourth, and fifth cervical spinal cord segments give rise to phrenic nerves and the intercostal nerves originate from the ventral rami from the anterior horn cells in the thoracic spinal cord. It is known that transection of either the dorsolateral or the ventrolateral quadrant of the spinal cord may independently affect the voluntary and the automatic respiratory controlling systems.[51] Most of the reports, however, refer to transection of the ventrolateral tracts giving rise to dysfunction of the metabolic respiratory control system. Direct involvement of the lower motor respiratory pathways, either in the anterior horn or in the phrenic and intercostal nerves, may also give rise to respiratory dysfunction. Several patterns of respiratory dysfunction have been summarized by Krieger and Rosomoff[179]: (1) efferent motor impairment (e.g., phrenic nerve paralysis causing diaphragmatic weakness) associated with reduced vital capacity; (2) impaired hypercapnic ventilatory response without significant chest wall or diaphragmatic weakness and with normal vital capacity; and (3) a mixture of these two abnormalities. The lesions that cause such dysfunction in the spinal cord may include spinal surgery, spinal trauma, amyotrophic lateral sclerosis, syringomyelia, cervical spinal cord tumor, and cervical myelitis (demyelinating or nonspecific myelitis).

Spinal surgery

Several cases of sleep apnea have been described following spinal surgery.[179-182] Belmusto and colleagues[180] noted ineffective breathing during sleep that required assisted ventilation in a patient treated with bilateral high cervical cordotomy for intractable pain. Damage to the reticulospinal tracts was thought to be responsible for the breathing difficulty. Tenicela's group[181] and Krieger and Rosomoff[179] also described sleep apnea after high cervical cordotomy. Krieger and Rosomoff[179] observed respiratory dysfunction within 24 to 48 hours of bilateral percutaneous cervical cordotomy in 10 patients. Sleep apnea was associated with impaired hypercapnic ventilatory response, and the respiratory dysrhythmia lasted from 3 to 32 days in those who survived (two of the patients died in their sleep). The patients' breathing was normal during wakefulness but they had intermittent apnea and irregular rate and depth of breathing during sleep. Though the authors concluded that the ascending reticular fibers in the ventrolateral segment of the spinal cord that relay afferent impulses to the medullary respiratory center had been damaged in their patients, it is most likely that selective damage to the descending automatic respiratory controlling fibers in the ventrolateral

quadrant of the spinal cord was the lesion responsible. In two other patients Krieger and Rosomoff[182] described sleep apnea which required assisted ventilation at night for several days following anterior spinal surgery at C3–4 interspace. Thus, these reports clearly document Ondine's curse as a sequela of high cervical spinal cord lesions.

Spinal trauma

Obstructive sleep apnea has also been described in patients with cervical spine fractures[183] or high spinal cord injury.[184,184a] Additionally, alterations of EEG sleep patterns after high cervical lesions have also been noted.[184b] Guilleminault[57] described eight victims of neck trauma who showed sleep apnea, hypoxemia, and EDS. The long-term prognosis of these patients is variable, and some may require tracheostomy. Guilleminault[57] suggested that mild compression of the lower medulla and upper cervical spinal cord might cause respiratory disturbances during sleep following severe whiplash injury or odontoid fractures.

Amyotrophic lateral sclerosis (ALS or motor neuron disease)

ALS is a degenerative central nervous system disease of middle aged and elderly persons. The illness is characterized by progressive degeneration of the ventral horn cells of the spinal cord, motor neurons of the bulbar nuclei, and upper motor neurons (primarily cortical), which produces a combination of lower and upper motor neuron signs. The natural history of the disease shows a relentless progression without impairment of mental function or sensation. Patients with ALS often have sleep complaints and sleep-related respiratory dysrhythmias. Weaknesses of the upper airway, diaphragm, and intercostal muscles secondary to involvement of the bulbar, phrenic, and intercostal nerve nuclei are the main contributing factors for sleep-disordered breathing in this condition. There may also be degeneration of the central respiratory neurons, accounting for both central and obstructive apneas in this condition. Literature on sleep disorders in ALS is sparse.

Respiratory failure in ALS generally occurs late, but occasionally it is a presenting feature and requires mechanical ventilation.[185] Thorpy and colleagues[186] described a 52-year-old man with spinal muscle atrophy and diaphragmatic paralysis who complained of nocturnal respiratory difficulty and progressive daytime somnolence for 10 years. Sleep-related nonobstructive hypoventilation associated with oxygen desaturation was noted on PSG examination. The patient's symptoms of hypersomnolence and daytime ventilation improved following assisted respiration at night. Newsom Davis' group[187] described eight patients with diaphragmatic paralysis resulting from a variety of motor disorders. One of their patients had Kugelberg-Welander syndrome, which is considered a variant of juvenile type motor neuron disease. The following features may be helpful in the diagnosis of diaphragmatic paralysis[58,187]: (1) breathlessness and EDS suggesting alveolar hypoventilation; (2) paradoxical inward movement of the abdomen with epigastric retraction instead of protrusion during inspiration; (3) an elevated diaphragm on chest radiography and paradoxical movement or decreased excursion of the diaphragm on fluoroscopy; (4) documentation of a very sensitive measurement showing a lack of change in the transdiaphragmatic pressure during a maximum inspiration; (5) diaphragmatic electromyographic (EMG) findings; (6) respiratory function tests with evidence of a restrictive pattern; (7) blood gases showing hypoxemia and hypercapnia, suggesting alveolar hypoventilation; and (8) documentation of sleep-related breathing abnormalities on PSG.

Serpick and colleagues[188] described a patient with ALS who had hypersomnolence, periodic breathing, hypercapnia, and hypoxia. The authors suggested that medullary dysfunction was responsible for ventilatory impairment. Sleep-related respiratory dysrhythmia in two patients with ALS was described by the present writer,[189] who since has seen several other cases of sleep apnea associated with motor

neuron disease. Polygraphic study of one of these patients (Figure 20-5) documents both central and upper airway obstructive apnea.

Gay and coworkers[190] performed PSG studies of 18 patients with ALS. This study emphasized sleep-disordered breathing and pulmonary functions rather than detailed descriptions of sleep architecture. In a brief report Ferguson and associates[191] described two consecutive overnight PSG findings in four men and three women with ALS whose manifestations were predominantly bulbar. Four patients had difficulty falling asleep and restless sleep; three had EDS. Their findings consisted of decreased sleep efficiency, frequent arousals with sleep fragmentation and sleep stage shifts but no significant obstructive apnea. In an early study, Minz and colleagues[192] described PSG findings in 12 ALS patients, six men and six women. Four patients had both central and obstructive apneas. Sleep structure was normal in eight, but others had frequent awakenings.

Bye's group[168] also studied, by PSG and pulmonary function tests, three patients with motor neuron disease. They noted hypoventilation, particularly during REM sleep.

Howard and colleagues[193] described 14 patients with motor neuron disease associated with respiratory dysfunction. Eleven received respiratory support, with considerable benefit. Seven of eight with typical features of ALS had mainly diaphragmatic

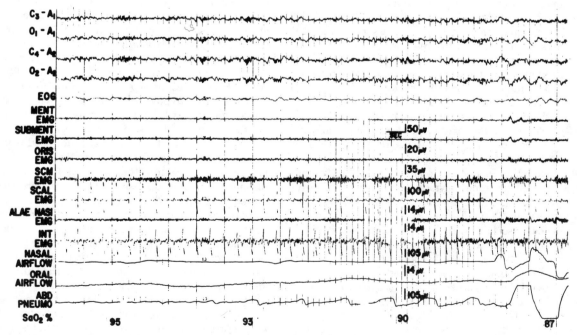

FIGURE 20-5. *PSG recording showing mixed apnea during stage 2 NREM sleep accompanied by oxygen desaturation in a patient with ALS. Channel key as for Figure 20-3. (Reproduced with permission from Chokroverty S. Sleep and breathing in neurological disorders. In: Edelman NH, Santiago TV, eds. Breathing Disorders of Sleep. New York: Churchill Livingstone, 1986; 225–264.)*

paralysis and one had generalized respiratory muscle weakness. Seven of these patients had negative pressure ventilation by Cuirass, which improved the respiratory problem and the quality of sleep. Three with mainly bulbar type had sleep apnea or hypoventilation; one of these patients with additional diphragmatic weakness was treated with a cuirass, CPAP, and later intermittent positive-pressure ventilation (IPPV) at night. Three patients with predominantly diaphragmatic paresis with sleep apnea were treated with nocturnal CPAP, cuirass, or IPPV with symptomatic relief. In the series by Howard and coworkers[193] were three patients with sleep apnea (all had obstructive apnea and one also had central apnea) and four who suffered nocturnal hypoventilation. The authors concluded that sleep-related respiratory dysrhythmia is a significant complication of motor neuron disease and may contribute to daytime hypersomnolence.

Sleep and Sleep-Disordered Breathing in Polyneuropathies

The cardinal manifestations of polyneuropathies are bilaterally symmetric, distal sensory symptoms and signs and muscle weakness and wasting (affecting the legs more often than the arms). Peripheral neuropathies may be caused by a variety of heredofamilial and acquired lesions. Affection of the phrenic, intercostal, and other nerves supplying the accessory muscles of respiration can cause weakness of the diaphragm, intercostal, and accessory respiratory muscles, giving rise to breathlessness on exertion, hypoxia, and hypercapnia. These respiratory dysrhythmias become worse during sleep. Sleep disturbances in polyneuropathies may result from painful neuropathies, partial immobility owing to paralysis of the muscles, or sleep-related breathing disorders.

Trauma, inflammatory polyneuropathy, and infiltrative lesions (e.g., neoplasms) may cause phrenic neuropathy. The commonest cause of respiratory dysfunction in polyneuropathy is acute inflammatory demyelinating polyradiculoneuropathy (Landry-Guillain-Barré-Strohl) syndrome. The characteristic clinical manifestations consist of predominantly motor deficits associated with rapidly progressive ascending paralysis beginning in the legs and being maximally manifest in 2 to 3 weeks. In about 20% to 25% of cases, severe respiratory involvement has been reported, and the critical period is usually the first 3 to 4 weeks of the illness. It is important to recognize and treat the ventilatory dysfunction. Even the mild respiratory dysrhythmia during wakefulness may worsen during sleep, causing sleep apnea and hypoventilation. Phrenic neuropathy may also be secondary to varicella-zoster virus infection or to the diphtheritic neuropathy.[194] Goldstein and colleagues[195] described

a patient with peripheral neuropathy and severe involvement of the phrenic nerves who presented with hypoventilation.

Diaphragmatic dysfunction has also been described in siblings with hereditary motor and sensory neuropathy (Charcot-Marie-Tooth disease).[196] Bilateral glossopharyngeal and vagal neuropathy can also cause respiratory dysfunction.[178]

Sleep and Breathing Disorders Associated with Primary Muscle Diseases

Myopathies are primary muscle disorders characterized by weakness and wasting of the muscles resulting from a defect in the muscle membrane or the contractile elements that is not secondary to a structural or functional derangement of the lower or upper motor neurons.[58] The characteristic clinical presentation consists of symmetric, proximal muscle weakness and wasting in the upper or lower limbs without sensory impairment or fasciculations. The causes include hereditary muscular dystrophies with or without myotonia, glycogen storage diseases, myoglobinuric myopathies, congenital nonprogressive myopathies with distinct morphologic characteristics, and various acquired metabolic, inflammatory, and noninflammatory myopathies. Some of these patients may report breathing disorders during sleep or worsening of the respiratory dysfunction during sleep. Generally, respiratory disorders show manifestations in the advanced stage, but a small number of them may present with respiratory failure at an early stage. In many such patients, the true incidence of the sleep disturbances and sleep-related respiratory dysrhythmias in these muscle disorders cannot be determined without a systematic PSG study. Factors responsible for breathing disorders associated with hypoventilation and sleep apnea in these patients may be summarized as follows[58]: impairment of chest bellows owing to weakness of the respiratory and chest wall muscles, increased work of breathing, and functional changes in the medullary respiratory neurons that could be due to hyporesponsive or unresponsive chemoreceptors acquired secondarily.[197] The other suggestion for carbon dioxide hyposensitivity is altered afferent input from the skeletal muscle receptors.[198] Sleep disturbances generally occur in muscle disorders secondary to sleep-related respiratory dysrhythmias. Alveolar hypoventilation, both during wakefulness and sleep, should be diagnosed early in these patients in order to prevent the fatal or dangerous hypoventilation during sleep or during administration of drugs, general anesthetic agents, and respiratory infections.[58] Complaints of daytime hypersomnolence and breathlessness should direct attention to the possibility of sleep-disordered breathing in these patients.

Muscular dystrophy

A few cases of muscular dystrophy with sleep complaints and sleep-related respiratory dysrhythmias have been described. Smith and associates[199] described 14 patients with Duchenne's muscular dystrophy who had sleep apneas or hypopneas associated with marked oxygen desaturation. These authors state that the severity of sleep-disordered breathing in Duchenne's dystrophy could not reliably be ascertained from daytime pulmonary function studies and assert that sleep studies are essential.

Bye's[168] and Ellis'[169] groups also included patients with muscular dystrophy in their reports of patients with neuromuscular disorders who also had sleep-related breathing disorders. The REM sleep showed significant oxygen desaturation. Sleep study[169] showed repeated arousals and sleep fragmentation.

Gross and coworkers[200] described a 22-year-old patient with Duchenne's dystrophy who was wheelchair bound and experienced breathlessness after meals. The blood gas studies showed hypercapnia and hypoxemia during wakefulness. A PSG study revealed nonapneic and hypopneic oxygen desaturation, which was more marked during REM than NREM sleep. Following progressive inspiratory muscle training and administration of oxygen at a rate of 2 liters per minute via nasal prongs, the patient's subjective daytime symptoms of fatigue and breathlessness subsided. Another patient with Duchenne's muscular dystrophy and alveolar hypoventilation that was worse during sleep was described by Buchsbaum and colleagues.[201]

Skatrud and coworkers[202] described a 45-year-old man with limb girdle muscular dystrophy and progressive daytime somnolence. Pulmonary function tests revealed evidence of restrictive pattern and diaphragmatic weakness (based on transdiaphragmatic pressure measurement). Sleep study showed REM-related hypoventilation associated with severe hypoxemias but no apneas. The authors concluded that these findings in this patient were secondary to the intercostal and accessory muscle inhibition.

Myotonic dystrophy

Dystrophica myotonica, or myotonic dystrophy, is an adult-onset, dominantly inherited muscular dystrophy associated with myotonia. Benaim and Worster-Drought[203] were most probably the first to describe alveolar hypoventilation in myotonic dystrophy. Alveolar hypoventilation associated with hypoxemia, hypercapnia, and impaired hypercapnic and hypoxic ventilatory responses may be present in both the early and late stages of the illness. A few authors[204-206] performed polygraphic studies that showed central, mixed, and upper airway

obstructive sleep apneas, and in some patients sleep-onset REM was noted. The latter finding may have been due to sleep deprivation secondary to sleep-related respiratory disturbances. Two fundamental mechanisms account for the sleep-related breathing disorders in this illness: (1) weakness and myotonia of the respiratory and upper airway muscles and (2) an inherited abnormality of the central control of ventilation, most likely related to a common generalized membrane abnormality of the muscles and other tissues, including brain stem neurons that regulate breathing and sleep.[205-208]

Sleep studies by Bye and colleagues[168] in four patients with myotonic dystrophy showed REM sleep–related oxygen desaturation and sleep disorganization. Several other authors have described alveolar hypoventilation, daytime somnolence, and periodic breathing in patients with myotonic dystrophy in single case reports and small series.[209-217]

The danger of administering anesthetic agents to these patients is demonstrated by Kaufman and colleagues[212]: five of 25 myotonic patients in this series had marked respiratory depression during operation, and another four died in the postoperative period.

Guilleminault's group[205] described six adult myotonic patients with EDS: two had obstructive, mixed, and central apneas associated with oxygen desaturation. Armagast and associates[217] described three women with myotonic dystrophy who complained of fatigue and daytime somnolence. All three had central apnea, but one also had obstructive and mixed apneas. The patients' symptoms and oxygen desaturation improved after treatment with dichlorphenamide, a carbonic anhydrase inhibitor and a respiratory stimulant.

Striano and coworkers[208] described predominantly obstructive sleep apnea associated with daytime hypersomnolence in a patient with dominantly inherited myotonia congenita. Because the patient was obese and also had obstructive pulmonary disease the relationship between sleep apnea and myotonia congenita remains inconclusive.

Acid maltase deficiency and other glycogen storage disorders

Alveolar hypoventilation has been described in several cases of mild to moderate myopathy associated with adult-onset acid maltase deficiency, a variant of glycogen storage disease.[187,197,218-220] In this condition, correct diagnosis can be established by performing respiratory function testing, EMG, and biochemical, histochemical, or morphologic examination of muscle biopsy samples. Hypoxemia, hypercapnia, and impaired hypercapnic ventilatory response may be seen in these patients. Diaphragmatic dysfunction may account for the alveolar hypoventilation. Rosenow and Engel[218] suggested that the hypoxemia in their patients was secondary to a combination of hypoventilation due to muscle weakness and an impairment of ventilation-perfusion ratio resulting from compression atelectasis due to elevated diaphragm. The patient of Martin's group[220] on polygraphic study showed prolonged periods of hypopnea accompanied by oxygen desaturation. The patient improved considerably following inspiratory muscle training.

Bye and coworkers[168] also described REM sleep–related hypoxemia and sleep disorganization in a patient with acid maltase deficiency and another with Pompe's disease.

Other varieties of congenital myopathies

Riley and coworkers[198] described alveolar hypoventilation in two patients with congenital myopathies (one with nemaline myopathy and the other with a myopathy of uncertain type). The patients' ventilatory response to carbon dioxide was absent, and the authors suggested that the alveolar hypoventilation may have been due to a primary defect in the central chemoreceptor control of breathing. Their other suggestion was that the sensory stimuli from skeletal muscle receptors (e.g., muscle spindles) may have played a role in the blunted hypercapnic ventilatory response by altering afferent input to the central nervous system.

Bye and colleagues[168] also studied a patient with central core myopathy who had sleep disruption and sleep hypoxemia. Kryger and colleagues[221] described two sisters with congenital muscular dystrophy who had central sleep apnea and blunted chemical drive to breathing in the index case. These abnormalities were thought to be out of proportion to the somatic and respiratory muscle weakness. The authors suggested that this patient's central control of breathing was defective. There are other reports of sleep hypoventilation in congenital myopathy.[222,223]

Miscellaneous myopathies

Sleep-related hypoxemia and sleep disturbances have also been described in patients with polymyositis[168] and mitochondrial encephalomyopathy.[224,225]

Neuromuscular Junction Disorders

Myasthenia gravis, myasthenic syndrome, botulism and tic paralysis are several neuromuscular junction disorders that are characterized by easy fatiguability of the muscles, including the bulbar and other respiratory muscles, owing to failure of neuromuscular junctional transmission of the nerve impulses. The most important of these conditions is myasthenia gravis, which is an autoimmune disease characterized by a reduction in the number of functional acetylcholine receptors in the postjunctional region. Acute respiratory failure is often a dreaded complication of myasthenia gravis, and patients need immediate assisted ventilation for life support.[58,226] The respiratory failure, moreover, may be mild during wakefulness but may deteriorate considerably during sleep.

An important study was recently reported by Quera-Salva and colleagues.[227] These authors reported the pulmonary function and PSG studies of 16 women and four men whose mean age was 40 years and who were diagnosed and treated for myasthenia gravis. PSG findings included moderately disturbed nocturnal sleep with an increase in stage 1 NREM and decreased slow-wave and REM sleep. Eleven patients had a respiratory disturbance index of 5 or higher. They had central, obstructive, and mixed apneas and hypopneas accompanied by decreased oxygen saturation. All patients with REM sleep–related apneas or hypopneas had disturbed nocturnal sleep with a sensation of breathlessness. Twelve patients lost sleep owing to awakening in the middle of the night. and early morning hours with a sensation of breathlessness. Four of the 12 patients also had daytime hypersomnolence. The authors suggested that those patients of advancing age, moderately increased body mass index, and abnormal pulmonary function results, and daytime blood gas concentrations are at particular risk for sleep-disordered breathing. Prior to this report, brief reports of sleep disruptions[228] and sleep apnea[229] appeared in the literature.

Myasthenic syndrome or Lambert-Eaton syndrome is a disorder of the neuromuscular junction in the presynaptic region and is often a paraneoplastic manifestation, mostly of oat cell carcinoma of the lungs. Patients complain of muscle weakness and fatigue involving the limbs accompanied by decreased or absent muscle stretch reflexes and characteristic electrodiagnostic findings that differentiate this from myasthenia gravis.

Botulism caused by *Clostridium botulinum* and tic paralysis caused by female wood tic *Dermacentor andersoni* may also cause neuromuscular junctional transmission defects, which are due to released toxin.

In all of these conditions, respiratory muscles may be affected and patients may require assisted ventilation. They can exhibit sleep hypoventilation and sleep apnea.

Sleep and Breathing in Autonomic Failure

Anatomically and functionally, sleep, breathing, and the autonomic nervous system are closely interrelated.[52,230–232] To understand sleep and breathing disorders in autonomic failure it is important to understand the functional anatomy of sleep, control of breathing, and the central autonomic network. A brief review of the functional anatomy of sleep is given in the beginning of this chapter, and the neurophysiology of sleep is also described extensively in Chapter 3. The control of breathing is described briefly in Chapter 5. In this section the central autonomic network and its integration with sleep and breathing will be reviewed briefly.

Sleep has a profound effect on the functions of the autonomic nervous system (ANS).[232,233] Sleep disorders and respiratory dysrhythmias during sleep in patients with autonomic failure are, therefore, logical expectations. Such sleep and breathing disorders have in fact been described in many patients with autonomic failure. It is also important to remember that the peripheral respiratory receptors, the central respiratory and lower brain stem hypnogenic neurons, are intimately linked by the ANS, making it easy to comprehend why sleep and breathing disorders should be associated with autonomic failure.

Central autonomic network

A central autonomic network was recently discovered in the brain stem that has ascending and descending reciprocally connected projections (see Figures 5-1 and 5-2).[230,231,234,235]

Nucleus tractus solitarius (NTS) may be considered a central station in the central autonomic network. NTS, located in the dorsal region of the medulla ventral to the dorsal vagal nucleus, is the single most important structure of the autonomic network and is influenced by higher brain stem, diencephalon, forebrain, and neocortical regions (see Figures 5-1 and 5-2). NTS receives important afferent fibers from the cardiovascular, respiratory, and gastrointestinal tracts for autonomic control of cardiac rhythm and rate, circulation, respiration, and gastrointestinal motility and secretion (see Figure 5-4). Efferent projections arise from NTS to the supramedullary structures, including hypothalamic and limbic regions, and to ventral medulla, which in turn sends efferent projections to the intermediolateral neurons of the spinal cord (see Figures 5-1 and 5-2). NTS thus orchestrates the central autonomic network for integrating various autonomic functions that maintain internal homeostasis. NTS also contains the lower brain stem hypnogenic and central respiratory neurons. Dysfunction of ANS thus may have a serious impact on human sleep and respiration.

The best-known condition of autonomic failure in which sleep and respiratory disturbances have been reported and well described is Shy-Drager syndrome, or multiple system atrophy with progressive autonomic failure. Familial dysautonomia (FD), a recessively inherited primary autonomic failure, is also known to be associated with sleep and breathing disturbances. A large number of neurologic and general medical disorders are associated with prominent secondary autonomic failure. Sleep and respiratory disturbance have been studied in some of these conditions, particularly polyneuropathies. In many neurologic conditions, sleep and respiratory disturbances result from an affection of the central hypnogenic or respiratory neurons.

Shy-Drager syndrome

In 1960, Shy and Drager[236] described a neurodegenerative disorder characterized by autonomic failure and multiple-system atrophy. Since their description, there have been many reports[52,55,121,232,237–243] of the condition, which has generally come to be known as Shy-Drager syndrome or multiple-system atrophy with progressive autonomic failure (MSA-PAF). Patients frequently manifest sleep and respiratory disturbances. Initially, they present with autonomic failure of both the sympathetic and parasympathetic systems. They may present with symptoms related to orthostatic hypotension (e.g., postural dizziness and faintness or even frank loss of consciousness in the erect posture), urinary sphincter dysfunction (e.g., frequency, urgency, hesitancy, dribbling, or overflow incontinence), hypohidrosis or anhidrosis, and impotence in men. After 2 to 6 years patients lapse into the second stage, showing some combination of pyramidal, extrapyramidal, upper motor neuron, and lower motor neuron dysfunction, including bulbar deficits. Most patients manifest a parkinsonian-cerebellar syndrome. In some, atypical parkinsonian features (e.g., bradykinesia, rigidity, postural instability) predominate; in others pancerebellar dysfunction predominates. In the later stages of the illness a variety of respiratory and sleep disturbances add to the progressive disability. Occasionally, respiratory dysfunction, particularly dysrhythmic breathing in wakefulness that becomes worse during sleep, manifests in the initial stage of the illness. In the final stage, progressive autonomic and somatic dysfunction are compounded by respiratory failure. Ventilatory disturbances now may be present in both wakefulness and sleep.

Sleep disturbances in this syndrome, as documented by PSG, may be summarized as follows[244]: reduction of total sleep time, REM, and slow-wave sleep, with increased sleep latency and increased number of awakenings during sleep. These sleep disturbances may result either from direct involvement of the brain stem and hypothalamic neurons or may be secondary to respiratory dysrhythmias that affect the sleep-facilitating neurons.

It is important to recognize alveolar hypoventilation during sleep in these patients, so that appropriate treatment can be instituted to prevent sudden death from fatal sleep apnea. The clinical manifestations secondary to sleep-disordered breathing were described in the beginning of this chapter.

Patients with Shy-Drager syndrome may have a variety of respiratory dysrhythmias similar to those observed in other neurologic conditions. The commonest types consist of the sleep apnea and hypopnea, dysrhythmic breathing, and nocturnal stridor. These have been confirmed in many reports.

Bannister and Oppenheimer[238] initially reported periodic inspiratory gasps resembling apneustic breathing in two patients with Shy-Drager syndrome.

The 54-year-old patient with the Shy-Drager syndrome described by Lockwood[245] had cluster breathing with periods of apnea as long as 20 seconds during wakefulness and 40 seconds during sleep. The patient died of sudden respiratory arrest at night. Neuropathologic findings included widespread diffuse lesions typical of Shy-Drager syndrome, in addition to gliosis in the pontomedullary reticular formation. This patient's hypercapnic ventilatory response was normal, and this finding suggested to the author that neurons responsible for respiratory rhythmogenesis functioned independently of the medullary chemoreceptors that controlled ventilation.

Castaigne and colleagues[246] described a 65-year-old man with Shy-Drager syndrome who had central alveolar hypoventilation, rhythmic respiration, numerous episodes of apnea, and probable apneustic breathing 4 years after onset of the illness. Postmortem findings were consistent with the diagnosis of Shy-Drager syndrome.

Laryngeal stridor and excessive snoring resulting from laryngeal abductor paralysis have been described in cases of Shy-Drager syndrome by groups led by Bannister,[237,239] Martin,[247] Israel,[248] Guilleminault,[249] Williams,[250] Kenyon,[251] and Munschauer.[252] The nocturnal stridor can be inspiratory, expiratory, or both. The stridor may cause a striking noise that may be likened to a donkey's braying.[241] Williams' group[250] noted this abnormality in 8 of 12 cases. The stridor was relieved by tracheostomy. Bannister and coworkers[239] described the clinical

and pathologic findings in 3 cases of Shy-Drager syndrome with laryngeal stridor requiring tracheostomy. Pathologically, there was marked atrophy of the abductors of the vocal chords but the cell count in the nucleus ambiguus was normal, implying that biochemical deficit may be the cause of atrophy of laryngeal muscles in at least some of these cases. The patient of Lehrman and colleagues[253] had about 450 predominantly upper airway obstructive apneas during sleep. Briskin and coworkers[254] described three patients with this syndrome. Polygraphic studies documented that more than 70% of the apneic episodes were obstructive in nature, and the mean apnea index was 75 to 79 in two of these patients. One patient needed resuscitation at night on two occasions because of respiratory arrest, and ultimately all three died at night of respiratory arrest. Hypercapnic ventilatory responses were normal in all three, but the hypoxic ventilatory responses were normal in two and severely impaired in the third. Sleep scoring showed very little stage 3 and 4 NREM sleep and almost total absence of REM sleep. Guilleminault and coworkers[255] described another four patients with Shy-Drager syndrome who had predominantly upper airway OSA. The respiratory disturbance index ranged from 12 to 62. The authors found no correlation between waking hypercapnic and hypoxic responses and the degree or the presence of sleep apnea. They also noted a clear dissociation between heart rate and respiratory response in these patients.

McNicholas and coworkers[61] described two patients with Shy-Drager syndrome whose impaired hypoxic and hypercapnic ventilatory responses suggested a defect in the metabolic respiratory control system. Their pattern of breathing during sleep was highly irregular. They had some 61 to 79 apneic episodes in all during NREM stages 1 and 2 but without oxygen desaturation. The apneic episodes were mostly central, but occasionally they had transient occlusion of the upper airway or transient uncoupling of intercostal and diaphragmatic muscle activity. The most striking abnormality was an irregular pattern of breathing during sleep, as documented by overnight PSG study. These findings suggested a defective autonomic respiratory rhythm generator in the brain stem.

In our early study of four patients with Shy-Drager syndrome[65] we observed periodic central apnea in the erect position and Cheyne-Stokes type breathing in one patient during the last stage of the illness. In one patient, hypercapnic ventilatory response in the supine position was impaired and the neuropathologic findings in the same patient—neuronal loss and astrocytosis in the pontine tegmentum—suggested involvement of the respiratory neurons in the brain stem. In our later studies[52] we described 10 other patients with Shy-Drager syndrome who showed central apnea, including Cheyne-Stokes or Cheyne-Stokes variant–type breathing and upper airway obstructive and mixed apneas accompanied by oxygen desaturation, predominantly during NREM sleep stages 1 and 2 and REM sleep (Figure 20-6). During sleep, seven patients had central apnea, two upper airway OSA, and three mixed apneas. The respiratory disturbance index varied from 20 to 80; the duration of apneas ranged from 10 to 65 seconds. The variation in the heart rate during apneic and eupneic cycles was not seen in these patients with evidence of cardiac autonomic denervation. This finding was in contrast to the bradyarrhythmias and tachyarrhythmias noted during apnea and immediately after resumption of normal breathing in patients with primary sleep apnea syndrome.[58] Four patients had several episodes of central apneas during relaxed wakefulness; it was as if the respiratory center "forgot" to breathe. Two patients had inspiratory gasps and two required tracheostomy for respiratory dysrhythmia. All night PSG studies in two patients revealed the following sleep abnormalities

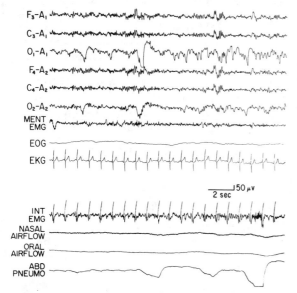

FIGURE 20-6. *A portion of an episode of mixed apnea during stage 2 NREM sleep associated with oxygen desaturation in a patient with the Shy-Drager syndrome. EEGs are shown in the top six channels. Also shown are EMG of the mentalis (MENT) and intercostal (INT) muscles, electrocardiogram (EKG), nasal and oral airflow, and abdominal pneumogram (ABD PNEUM). (Reproduced with permission from Chokroverty S. Sleep and breathing in neurological disorders. In: Edelman NH, Santiago TV, eds. Breathing Disorders of Sleep. New York: Churchill Livingstone, 1986; 225–264.)*

in addition to recurrent episodes of sleep apneas accompanied by oxygen desaturation: marked reduction of NREM sleep stages 3 and 4 and REM sleep; increased awakenings after sleep onset; snoring; excessive body movements and frequent arousal responses in the EEG. Impaired hypercapnic ventilatory response and mouth occlusion pressure response in one patient suggested impairment of the metabolic respiratory system, whereas normal hypercapnic and hypoxic ventilatory responses in another patient in presence of an abnormal respiratory pattern resembling that noted by Lockwood[245] suggest that the chemoreceptor control and respiratory pattern generator were probably subserved by different populations of neurons that were rendered selectively vulnerable in Shy-Drager syndrome. In eight of 10 patients dysrhythmic breathing occurred mostly during sleep though in four it was also present during wakefulness; this finding suggests that this type of respiratory dysrhythmia is very common in Shy-Drager syndrome. These observations are in agreement with the suggestion of McNicholas and colleagues[61] that such findings imply impaired respiratory pattern generator in these patients.

Chester and colleagues[256] described a patient with Shy-Drager syndrome and alveolar hypoventilation who on postmortem examination did not show lesions in the brain stem respiratory neurons. The authors suggested a peripheral mechanism for the abnormal breathing.

Munschauer and coworkers[252] studied respiration during sleep in seven patients with Shy-Drager syndrome whose respiratory symptoms ranged from inspiratory gasping during wakefulness to stridor during sleep. Their findings are similar to those of McNicholas' group[61] in showing significantly greater coefficients of variability in respiratory rate, tidal volume, and inspiratory flow rate in the patients than in controls. They found evidence of upper airway obstruction without significant oxygen desaturation in four of five nontracheostomized patients. Five patients died, three of them during sleep. Postmortem examination in four patients confirmed the diagnosis of Shy-Drager syndrome. Three patients showed marked loss of neurons in the region of the pontine tegmentum and medullary reticular formation, including neurons around the nucleus tractus solitarius.

What are the mechanisms of ventilatory dysrhythmia in Shy-Drager syndrome? There is ample evidence in the literature[121,236] of pathologic involvement of the pontine tegmentum, the reticular formation, NTS, nucleus ambiguus, hypoglossal nucleus, and in some patients anterior horn cells of the cervical and thoracic spinal cord. Lockwood[245] and Chokroverty and colleagues[65] correlated the physiologic and clinical findings of respiratory dysrhythmias with direct involvement of the regions of the brain stem that contain the respiratory neurons. In addition, physiologic studies of respiratory control[61] (also Chokroverty, unpublished data) showing impairment of hypercapnic and hypoxic ventilatory and mouth occlusion pressure responses indirectly suggested an impairment of the metabolic respiratory control system. Vagal and sympathetic denervation in these patients is firmly established.[121,236] These pathogenic mechanisms for the respiratory dysrhythmia of Shy-Drager syndrome include all that had been postulated in the beginning of this chapter for the respiratory dysrhythmias in neurologic disorders. Other mechanisms have been suggested in Shy-Drager syndrome[52]: interference with the forebrain, midbrain, and pontine inputs to the medullary respiratory neurons causing dysrhythmic and apneustic breathing; involvement of the direct projections from the hypothalamus and central nucleus of amygdala to the respiratory neurons in the NTS and nucleus ambiguus; involvement of the vagal afferents from the lower and upper airway receptors, which would reduce the input to the central respiratory neurons, causing respiratory dysrhythmia; sympathetic denervation of the nasal mucosa causing increased nasal resistance, thus promoting upper airway obstructive apnea; finally, discrete neurochemical alterations in Shy-Drager syndrome that may interfere with normal regulation of breathing. There is experimental evidence that noradrenaline, serotonin, and dopamine play distinct roles in the control of breathing.[257] Patients with Shy-Drager syndrome have been found to have low levels of dopamine and noradrenaline in the basal ganglia, the limbic-hypothalamic regions including the septal nuclei, and the locus ceruleus.[258] Furthermore, these patients may also have specific catecholamine enzyme deficits in the brain and sympathetic ganglia.[259]

Familial dysautonomia (Riley-Day syndrome)

Riley-Day syndrome is a recessively inherited disorder of autonomic failure. The condition usually presents in childhood and is peculiar to the Jewish population. The clinical features consist of a variety of autonomic and somatic manifestations[260]: autonomic, neuromuscular, cardiovascular, gastroesophageal, skeletal, renal, and respiratory abnormalities; absence of the fungiform papillae of the tongue; defective lacrimation and sweating; vasomotor instability and fluctuation of blood pressure (postural hypotension and paroxysmal hypertension); relative insensitivity to pain; and absent muscle stretch reflexes. Sleep dysfunction, associated with both central and obstructive apneas, has been described in most of these patients.[244,261] Sleep abnormalities consist of increased awakenings, delayed sleep onset, including prolonged REM sleep onset (but reduced REM sleep time), and sleep apneas. Patients with familial dysautonomia often have prolonged breath-holding spells, owing to defective responses of central respiratory neurons to changes in $PaCO_2$.

Gadoth and colleagues[261] performed PSG recordings of 13 patients (7 women and 6 men aged 5 to 31 years) with familial dysautonomia to investigate the role of ANS in sleep and breathing disorders in this condition. All had sleep apneas (average 73.5 per night): 11 central apnea and 2 OSA). REM latency was prolonged, with decreased amount of REM in some patients, and adults also had increased sleep latency. All had orthostatic hypotension, and cardiac responses during apnea were absent, indicating cardiac autonomic denervation.

Guilleminault and colleagues[255] described two adolescent girls with familial dysautonomia who had respiratory irregularities. One also had esophageal reflux during sleep that gave rise to sleep disturbances due to frequent awakenings. McNicholas and coworkers[61] described dysrhythmic breathing in a patient with familial dysautonomia similar to the irregular breathing noted in patients with Shy-Drager syndrome. Maayan and associates[262] described a 42-year-old woman with familial dysautonomia who had several episodes of apnea during both wakefulness and sleep. The patient had megaesophagus associated with constriction in the lower esophageal region, which caused recurrent aspiration and apnea. Following gastrostomy, no apneas were noted.

Secondary autonomic failure

A group of patients experience autonomic failure secondary to lesions in the central or peripheral nervous system, general medial disorders, drug effects, and other causes.[55,263]

An important example of an acquired nonprogressive dysautonomia syndrome was described by Frank and associates[264] in a 6-year-old girl who experienced subacute onset of hypoventilation and sleep apnea and gave evidence of dysautonomia. Frequent obstructive and central apneas were noted during all-night PSG study. The absence of variation in the heart rate suggested cardiac autonomic denervation. Postmortem findings 2 years after onset of the illness showed a ganglioneuroma of the lumbar sympathetic ganglia, neuron loss with gliosis in the locus ceruleus, the reticular formation of the brain stem, and the Edinger-Westphal nuclei.

Diabetic neuropathy and other peripheral autonomic neuropathies

Many medical and neurologic conditions have associated autonomic neuropathies with peripheral neuropathies, but in most of these conditions, sleep and respiratory dysfunctions have not been adequately studied. There are, however, many reports of such studies in diabetic polyneuropathies associated with autonomic neuropathy. This combination of somatic and autonomic neuropathies has been observed in some patients with acute inflammatory polyradiculoneuropathy (Guillain-Barré syndrome) and amyloidosis.

Rees and coworkers[265] observed 30 or more apneic episodes (in two patients mainly central and in one predominantly obstructive) during sleep at night in three of eight patients with diabetic autonomic neuropathy. In contrast, eight diabetes patients without autonomic neuropathy exhibited no sleep-related respiratory dysrhythmias. The authors speculate that sudden cardiorespiratory arrests that have been noted in some patients with diabetes may be related to autonomic failure and sleep apneas.

Guilleminault and coworkers[255] reported OSAs in two of four patients with juvenile diabetic autonomic neuropathy. One had central apnea and the other irregular breathing associated with sleep-related esophageal reflux. Of the patients with primary sleep apnea syndrome described by Chokroverty and Sharp,[56] four had diabetes mellitus.

Mondini and Guilleminault[266] obtained PSG recordings for 12 type I and seven type II diabetics. They found obstructive and central apneas and an irregular pattern of breathing in five of 12 type I patients. In only one of seven type II diabetics they noted OSA. Autonomic neuropathy was present in all three type I patients with diabetes.

The findings of Catterall and coworkers[267] do not support the findings reported here of patients with diabetic autonomic neuropathy. They studied 8 patients who had autonomic neuropathy and 8 who did not and found no significant difference in frequency of apnea between the two groups.

Miscellaneous Neurologic Disorders

Sleep apnea in narcolepsy syndrome

The narcolepsy syndrome is manifested by an irresistible desire to fall asleep at inappropriate times. Such attacks last a few seconds to as long as 20 to 30 minutes. They are often accompanied by cataplexy or other characteristic ancillary manifestations of narcolepsy (see Chapter 18). Sleep apnea is reported in some patients with narcolepsy syndrome.

Guilleminault's group[268] first reported central sleep apnea that lasted 20 to 90 seconds (during REM and NREM sleep) accompanied by oxygen desaturation in 2 patients with pure narcolepsy. In a later report, Guilleminault and colleagues[269] described 20 additional cases of narcolepsy with sleep apnea, which was predominantly central though five also had mixed and obstructive apneas. The authors speculated that a dysfunction of the CNS structures that control the sleep and respiratory centers was responsible for the combined syndrome of sleep apnea and narcolepsy. Laffont and colleagues[270] also described central, obstructive, and mixed apneas in five of 18 narcolepsy patients. Chokroverty[271] made a polygraphic observations in 16 patients with narcolepsy syndrome, 11 of whom showed central apneas and five upper airway obstructive apneas during both REM and NREM sleep stages associated with oxygen desaturation (Figures 20-7 and 20-8).

Kleine-Levin syndrome

An episodic disorder occurring mostly in adolescent boys (but also described in girls) and characterized by periodic hypersomnolence and bulimia was first described by Kleine[272] and later by Levin.[273] Critchley[274] gave a comprehensive description after analysis of 15 cases from the literature and 11 personal cases. The episodes usually occur three to four times a year, and each episode lasts days to weeks. During the sleep "attacks," patients sleep 16 to 18 hours a day or more, and on awakening they eat voraciously. Other behavior disturbances during the episode may include dull appearance, withdrawal, confusion, hallucinations, inattentiveness, memory impairment, and hypersexuality. In a recent report Billiard and Cadilhac[275] reviewed 123 cases collected from the literature. The condition is generally self-limited (though not always) and disappears by adulthood. PSG studies show normal sleep cycling and the Multiple Sleep Latency Test shows pathologic sleepiness without sleep-onset REM. The cause of the condition remains undertermined, although a limbic-hypothalamic dysfunction has long been suspected.

Idiopathic CNS hypersomnia

This condition of excessive somnolence has no known cause.[276] The disease occurs insidiously and generally is manifested between age 15 and 30 years. It closely resembles narcolepsy, and also sleep apnea. Though sometimes it is very difficulty to distinguish it from narcolepsy syndrome, the sleep pattern *is* different from that in narcolepsy or sleep apnea. The patient generally sleeps hours, and the sleep is not refreshing. The patient does not give a history of snoring or repeated awakenings throughout

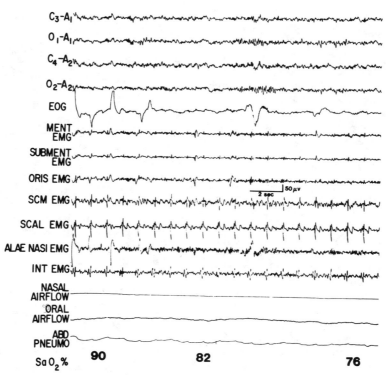

FIGURE 20-7. *PSG recording of a patient with narcolepsy showing four channels of EEG (C_3–A_1, O_1–A_1, C_4–A_2, O_2–A_2), vertical electrooculogram (EOG), electromyograms (EMG) of mentalis (MENT), submental (SUBMENT), orbicularis oris (ORIS), sternocleidomastoid (SCM), scalenus anticus (SCAL), alae nasi and intercostal (INT) muscles, nasal and oral airflow, abdominal pneumogram (ABD PNEUMO), and oxygen (Sao_2%) saturation (ear oximeter). The patient has central apnea (only 18 of 30 seconds is shown) during REM sleep. Note decrease of oxygen saturation from 90% to 76% during apnea.*

the night. Sleep drunkenness is often seen in these patients, and they manifest automatic behavior with amnesia for the event. Physical examination shows no abnormal neurologic or other findings. The condition is very disabling, and the patient is usually unable to function meaningfully in any employment. It is generally a lifelong condition. PSG examination shows normal sleep structure and sleep cycling with prolonged NREM sleep accompanied by decreased stage 1 and increased stages 3 and 4 NREM sleep. There is no sleep-onset REM. MSLT shows evidence of pathologic sleepiness without sleep-onset REM. Some patients may have a positive family history, and an occasional patient has a history of infectious mononucleosis, or rarely Guillain-Barré syndrome. The treatment is unsatisfactory and is somewhat similar to the stimulant treatment for narcolepsy syndrome.

Primary alveolar hypoventilation

Primary alveolar hypoventilation (PAH) is a syndrome of failure of automatic respiration without

any recognizable disorder of the central or peripheral nervous system. Central alveolar hypoventilation and central apnea syndrome associated with an organic neurologic disease should be differentiated from PAH.[277] The hallmark of PAH is a combination of arterial hypercapnia and hypoxemia during wakefulness that becomes worse during sleep.[278,279] Other manifestations include sleep apnea, congestive heart failure, pulmonary hypertension, and polycythemia. Central apnea is the usual type, but another feature of some cases is upper airway obstructive apnea. Impairment of hypercapnic ventilatory response is characteristic of this condition. The cause of the syndrome is unknown, and none of the reported cases of PAH showed evidence of CNS disease. Occasional postmortem reports showed no central nervous system structural lesions or nonspecific findings such as gliosis or mild loss of neurons in the medulla. A dysfunction of the medullary chemoreceptors is suspected, but no definite proof is available. Thus, the pathologic basis for PAH giving

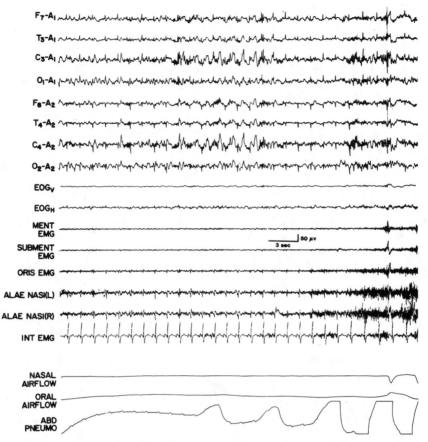

FIGURE 20-8. *PSG recording in a patient with narcolepsy and sleep apnea showing EEG (top eight channels), vertical (EOG$_V$ and horizontal electrooculograms (EOG$_H$), EMG of mentalis (MENT), submental (SUBMENT), orbicularis oris (ORIS), left (L) and right (R) alae nasi and intercostal (INT) muscles, nasal and oral airflow and abdominal pneumogram (ABD PNEUMO). Note mixed apnea (initial period of 13 seconds of central apnea followed by 19 seconds of OAS) during NREM sleep stage II.*

rise to the clinical manifestations of Ondine's curse syndrome remains undetermined. An important distinction from primary sleep apnea syndrome is that hypercapnic and hypoxic ventilatory responses during wakefulness are usually normal in primary sleep apnea syndrome.

Sleep and increased intracranial pressure[280]

Increased intracranial pressure (ICP) may result from a variety of neurologic disorders (e.g., tumor, large infarction, intracranial hemorrhage, head trauma, focal abscess, diffuse encephalitis). Cooper and Hulme[281,282] found that the ICP of patients with intracranial lesions rose during REM and stage 2 NREM sleep. This was probably due to a combination of factors[280] (e.g., variations in cerebral blood flow, neurogenic reflex, cerebral vasoconstriction,

enhanced brain metabolism). These observations have been confirmed by the findings of Munari and Calbucci[283] in 16 head trauma patients.

Headache syndromes

Dexter and Weitzman[284] made the first PSG recordings in patients with chronic migraine and cluster headaches and found a clear relationship between REM sleep and attacks of headache. Attacks occurred during REM or within 9 minutes after it terminated.

Kudrow and colleagues[285] found a high prevalence of central or obstructive sleep apnea syndromes in patients who suffer cluster headaches, especially episodic cluster headaches.

Dexter[286] reported PSG-documented sleep apnea in 11 patients with chronic recurring headache syndrome. Following surgical reconstruction in six patients with obstructive apneas, PSG demonstrated marked improvement in sleep apnea and considerable improvement in headache symptoms.

Sahota and Dexter[287] recently reviewed the relationship between headache syndromes and sleep. They also reported[288] long-term psychophysiologic insomnia in association with chronic cluster headache in a 35-year-old man. This disorder of difficulty initiating sleep gradually abated after the headaches resolved.

Another type of headache, chronic paroxysmal hemicrania (CPH), is probably a variant of cluster headache. The attacks of CPH occur unilaterally and are briefer and more frequent than cluster headaches. CPH is most commonly associated with REM sleep,[289] and it responds well to indomethacin.

Fatal familial insomnia

Lugaresi and associates[290] described a family (14 affected members in three generations) with an autosomal dominant progressive neurologic illness characterized by insomnia and dysautonomia that terminated in death—fatal familial insomnia (FFI). In two patients neuropathologic examination showed characteristic and selective destruction of the anterior and dorsomedial thalamic nuclei. PSG recordings documented an alternating pattern of wakefulness and REM-like states throughout the 24 hours, with no evidence of sleep spindles or slow-wave sleep. There was evidence of central autonomic failure on laboratory investigation.

In the most recent reports,[291,292] Lugaresi and coworkers reported the clinical, physiologic and other laboratory investigations of FFI patients who belonged to two unrelated Italian families. Neuropathologic examination was performed in nine patients. Age at onset was between 35 and 61 years, and the clinical course ran 7 to 36 months. Progressive insomnia, autonomic disturbances, and motor abnormalities (e.g., ataxia, myoclonus and pyramidal dysfunction) were present in every case. Severe neuron loss and reactive gliosis were seen in the anterior or anteroventral and dorsomedial thalamic nuclei. Other findings included gliosis of the cerebral cortex and olivocerebellar atrophy. The authors concluded that FFI is a multisystem disease and a prion disease marked by a mutation at codon 178 of the prion protein gene.[293,294]

LABORATORY INVESTIGATIONS

The laboratory tests should be directed toward a diagnosis of the primary neurologic disorder and an assessment of sleep disturbances resulting from the neurologic illness.

Laboratory Tests for the Primary Neurologic Disorders

It is beyond the scope of this chapter to delve into details of neurodiagnostic tests to assess the neurologic condition that gives rise to the sleep and sleep-related breathing disorders, so readers are referred to some excellent neurologic texts available.[295-297] Laboratory tests must subserve the findings of the history and physical examination, as discussed in Chapter 14. Laboratory tests are essential for diagnosis, prognosis, and treatment of the primary neurologic disorders. These investigations can be broadly divided into neurophysiologic tests, neuroimaging studies, examination of the cerebrospinal fluid, and general laboratory tests, including "blood work" and urinalysis. Special procedures such as tests to uncover autonomic deficits, neuroimmunologic, neurovirologic or neurourologic investigations, and brain biopsy are required to detect some neurologic disorders.

Neurophysiologic Tests

Neurophysiologic tests include EEG, evoked potential and nerve conduction velocity studies, and EMG. EEG, including 24-hour ambulatory and video-EEG examinations is necessary to detect seizure disorder, metabolic-toxic-nutritional encephalopathies, and dementing illnesses (e.g., AD, Jakob-Creutzfeldt disease). Evoked potential studies include sensory (somatosensory, brain stem auditory, and visual evoked responses) and motor evoked potentials, and may be indicated in certain neurologic disorders, particularly demyelinating diseases such as multiple sclerosis. Nerve conduction measurements and EMG studies are necessary for diagnosis of various neuromuscular disorders, including neuromuscular junction diseases.

Neuroimaging Studies

Cerebral angiography, including digital subtraction arteriography, may be necessary to investigate for strokes. CT and MRI are important studies for structural lesions of the CNS (e.g., tumors, infarctions, vascular malformations). CT and MRI are also helpful in patients with demyelinating and degenerative neurologic disorders that can be responsible for sleep and sleep-related breathing disturbances.

Positron emission tomography (PET) dynamically measures cerebral blood flow, oxygen uptake, and glucose utilization, and is helpful in diagnosis of dementing, degenerative (e.g., Parkinson's disease), and seizure disorders. It is, however, very expensive and is not available in most centers. Single-photon emission CT (SPECT), which dynamically measures regional cerebral blood flow, may be useful for patients with cerebral vascular disease, Alzheimer's disease, or seizure disorders. Doppler ultrasonography is an important test for investigation of stroke due to extracranial vascular disease. Myelography besides CT and MRI is important for diagnosis of diseases of the spinal cord.

Cerebrospinal Fluid Examination and Other Laboratory Tests

Cerebrospinal fluid examination is important for the diagnosis of meningoencephalitis, Lyme disease, and MS, all of which may give rise to sleep disturbances. Hematologic tests and biochemical studies of blood and urine, as well as tests to assess endocrine, pulmonary, and cardiac disorders, are essential to undercover general medical disorders that may result in metabolic or toxic encephalopathies.

Laboratory Tests to Investigate Sleep and Sleep-Related Breathing Disorders

Polysomnography

The importance of PSG in the diagnosis of sleep and sleep-related breathing disorders is discussed in Chapters 6 and 14. Sleep can adversely affect breathing, and, conversely, respiratory dysrhythmias can have deleterious effects on sleep (see Chapter 5). Both alterations can affect the severity and course of a neurologic illness, causing such sleep disturbances, and so the sleep architecture should be studied. The technique of PSG is described in detail in Chapter 6.

Multiple channels of EEG recordings are essential to document focal and diffuse neurologic lesions and to accurately localize epileptiform discharges in patients with seizure disorders (see Chapter 7). Multiple orofacial muscle EMGs, in addition to the standard chin EMG, may help assess upper airway muscle hypotonia (see Chapter 7). Multiple muscle EMGs, including tibialis anterior EMG, are essential for diagnosis of restless legs syndrome, periodic limb movements in sleep, and some parasomnias (e.g., REM behavior disorder and paroxysmal nocturnal dystonia).

Multiple sleep latency test

The MSLT is essential for objectively measuring daytime sleepiness. Sleep-onset latency of 5 minutes or less indicates pathologic sleepiness and may be seen in patients with narcolepsy, sleep apnea, idiopathic central nervous system hypersomnia, and other hypersomnic conditions. Additionally, sleep-onset REM during two of four or five recordings of MSLT is highly suggestive of narcolepsy. Further details about the recording technique and indications of MSLT are described in Chapter 10.

Video-polysomnography

This test is important for monitoring patients suspected of having epilepsy or parasomnias that may be associated with certain neurologic disorders (see Chapters 14 and 27).

EEG, including 24-hour ambulatory EEG:

These tests are essential if epilepsy is suspected, as it can cause sleep disturbances and which may sometimes be mistaken for parasomnias or sleep apneic episodes. For further details see Chapters 7 and 27.

Pulmonary function tests

(see Chapter 9): Pulmonary function tests exclude intrinsic bronchopulmonary disease which may affect sleep-related breathing disorders.[298]

Ventilatory functions: Forced expiratory volume in one second (FEV_1), forced vital capacity (FVC), FEV_1-FVC ratio, peak expiratory flow rate (PEFR), forced expiratory flow rate (FEF).

Measurement of lung volumes: Total lung capacity (TLC), residual volume (RV), functional residual capacity (FRC).

Gas distribution and gas transfer: Single-breath nitrogen test (SBN_2/L), diffusing capacity by the technique of single-breath apnea method using carbon monoxide and helium ($DL_{CO}SB$).

Arterial blood gases: PaO_2, $PaCO_2$.

Other tests that may be performed in special situations include exercise tests and measurements of lung volumes and ventilatory functions before and after a bronchodilator is used.

The respiratory muscle function of persons with neuromuscular disorders, should be specifically assessed. According to Black and Hyatt,[299] it is important to measure the maximal static inspiratory and expiratory pressures, which are more important than the dynamic values. Such measurements, which require cooperation, may be difficult in many patients with neurologic disorders.

Chemical control of breathing may be impaired if neurologic disease causes dysfunction of the metabolic respiratory controllers.[9] Such impairment may be detected by hypercapnic ventilatory response ($\dot{V}E/PaCO_2$), hypoxic ventilatory response ($\dot{V}E/PaO_2$), and mouth occlusion pressure ($P_{0.1}$) response, with or without load.[9] Central respiratory drive and the inspiratory muscle strength independent of pulmonary mechanical factors are reflected in the $P_{0.1}$ response.

Electrodiagnosis of the respiratory muscles

EMG of the upper airway, diaphragmatic, and intercostal muscles (see Chapters 5 and 7) may detect affection of these muscles in neurologic diseases. In patients with the Shy-Drager syndrome with laryngeal stridor it is important to perform laryngeal EMG, to detect laryngeal paresis.[300]

Phrenic nerve and intercostal nerve conduction study[301,302] may detect phrenic and intercostal neuropathy, which may cause diaphragmatic and intercostal muscle affections in some patients with neurologic disorders.

TREATMENT OF SLEEP AND RESPIRATORY DYSFUNCTION SECONDARY TO NEUROLOGIC DISORDERS

Treatment is discussed in two broad categories: (1) therapy for the primary neurologic illness and (2) therapy for the secondary sleep disturbance.

Treatment of Primary Neurologic Illness

First and foremost is accurate diagnosis of the primary neurologic disorder. This is followed by vigorous treatment and monitoring of the neurologic illness. Such treatment may improve the sleep disturbances. It is beyond the scope of this volume to discuss the treatment of the primary neurologic disorders, and readers are referred to some excellent texts.[295–297]

Treatment of Sleep Disturbances

Sleep disturbances in neurologic disorders include hypersomnia, insomnia, circadian rhythm sleep disturbances, and parasomnias. Treatment of these complaints is discussed in several chapters in this volume (see Chapters 16–19, 23–25, 27 and 28). In this section, treatment of hypersomnia mainly that results from sleep-related respiratory dysrhythmias in neurologic disorders is discussed. In the final paragraph, general principles of treatment for sleep disturbances not related to the respiratory dysrhythmias in dementias is briefly reviewed.

Treatment of Sleep-Related Breathing Disorders

The objective of treatment is twofold: (1) to improve the quality of life by improving the quality of sleep and (2) to prevent life-threatening cardiac arrhythmias, pulmonary hypertension, and congestive heart failure related to sleep-disordered breathing. The quality of sleep may be improved by eliminating repeated apneas during sleep and thus preventing repeated arousals, sleep fragmentation, nocturnal hypoxemia, and daytime hypersomnolence. The treatment modalities for sleep-related respiratory dysrhythmias resulting from neurologic illness may be divided into five categories: general measures, pharmacologic agents, mechanical devices, supplemental oxygen administration, and surgical treatment.

General Measures

These include reduction or elimination of risk factors that can aggravate sleep-related respiratory dysrhythmias. Avoidance of alcohol and sedative-hypnotic drugs[303] (e.g., benzodiazepines, barbiturates, narcotics) that can depress breathing during sleep is an important step in eliminating the risk factors. Alcohol is known to increase the frequency and duration of apneas, probably by two mechanisms[304–306]: (1) selective depression of the genioglossus and other upper airway muscles and (2) impairment of the arousal response by raising its threshold. For obese patients weight loss is another important step in eliminating risk factors for sleep-related respiratory dysrhythmia.

Drug Therapy

The three most important agents that had been tried for mild to moderate sleep apnea—with partial success—are protriptyline, medroxyprogesterone acetate and acetazolamide. Protriptyline may be used in a dose of 5 to 20 mg at bedtime. Suppression of REM sleep, a specific alerting property, and conversion of apnea to hypopnea are cited as mechanisms of action of this drug.[303] Anticholinergic effects and cardiac arrhythmias are the limiting side effects of this drug.

Medroxyprogesterone acetate has been tried in many patients with sleep apnea, but the results have been disappointing.[307–310] It is thought to act by increasing ventilatory drive. Impotence in men is a limiting side effect.

Acetazolamide has been used with some success in central apnea, but development of obstructive apnea or aggravation of orthostatic hypotension owing to its diuretic and natriuretic effects should be kept in mind during treatment.

Mechanical Devices

Nasal CPAP

An important therapeutic advance in the treatment of obstructive sleep apnea syndrome, CPAP is described in detail in Chapter 28. It should be given a trial in neurologic disease patients with upper airway obstructive apnea associated with intermittent central apnea or with mixed apneas. Such treatment often improves the quality of sleep and reduces daytime symptoms by eliminating or reducing sleep-related obstructive or mixed apneas and oxygen desaturation. The role of nasal CPAP for central apnea is highly controversial. Stanford group[311] found CPAP helpful for central apnea patients who had associated OSA or who showed sleep fragmentation and repeated sleep-wake changes.

Other ventilatory supports

Besides tracheostomy and diaphragmatic pacing, which is described under Surgical Treatment, two types of ventilatory supports are available for patients with sleep-related apnea or hypoventilation (see also chapter 28): negative-pressure and positive-pressure ventilators. Intermittent positive-pressure ventilation (IPPV) can be administered through a nasal mask. Tracheostomy and CPAP also deliver postive-pressure ventilation. Negative-pressure ventilation can be delivered from a tank respirator or a cuirass. The various mechanical ventilators have been used successfully in patients with neuromuscular disorders or chest wall deformity associated with respiratory failure, to relieve symptoms of daytime hypersomnolence, morning headache, and intellectual impairment, and to improve sleep architecture. Bye and colleagues[312] suggested a combination of a nasal mask and a positive-pressure ventilator for nocturnal ventilation of patients with respiratory failure associated with neuromuscular diseases.

Stanford group[311] has successfully used IPPV through a nasal mask during sleep in patients with central aveolar hypoventilation, muscle diseases that cause sleep hypoventilation and apnea, former poliomyelitis patients with kyphosis and associated sleep-related apneas and hypoventilation, and unilateral phrenic nerve lesions. Some of these patients may need negative-pressure ventilation (cuirass) with nasal CPAP, but IPPV is a better and more promising treatment. Using these methods, the Stanford group[311] and others were able to avoid tracheostomy associated with mechanical ventilation or diphragmatic pacing and were able to control sleep-related problems. It should be noted that correct diagnosis of central sleep apnea syndrome (by modern methods) and identification of the causes of such apnea by sleep-wake studies are essential to correct treatment.

Ellis and colleagues[169] also found that the treatment of respiratory failure—including alveolar hypoventilation—during sleep in patients with neuromuscular diseases (e.g., postpolio, ALS, muscle diseases) using positive-pressure ventilation through a nose mask, prevents severe hypoxemia and hypercapnia. Such treatment also improves patients' subjective sleep quality, though at the same time REM sleep rebound is seen. Negative-pressure ventilation improves these patients' ventilation during NREM sleep but produces upper airway obstruction during REM sleep, causing severe hypoxemia and hypercapnia.

Nocturnal positive-pressure ventilation via nasal mask has also been used successfully by Kerby and coworkers[313] in patients with chronic respiratory failure from neuromuscular diseases and nocturnal hypoventilation.

According to Howard and colleagues[170] patients with neuromuscular disease may benefit from negative-pressure ventilation. This type of treatment improves ventilation and allows intermittent rest of the residual respiratory muscles. Nine patients in their series used a cuirass and enjoyed considerable improvement of sleep and of daytime symptoms. It should be noted that acute respiratory failure needs positive-pressure ventilation, but later these patients may be weaned from positive-pressure ventilation and transferred to negative-pressure ventilation using an iron lung or cuirass.

For sleep apnea and hypoventilation in patients with ALS, ventilatory support at night is needed. Some of these patients may need the negative-pressure ventilation by cuirass, which improves respiratory problems and sleep quality. Some with general respiratory muscle weakness, including diaphragmatic paresis, may require a combination of cuirass, CPAP, and later IPPV at night.

Howard's group[193] treated patients with motor neuron disease with mechanical ventilation, with considerable benefit. Seven patients with mainly diaphragmatic muscle weakness were treated with negative-pressure ventilation by cuirass, which improved the respiratory problems and the quality of sleep. Patients with sleep apnea or hypoventilation due to bulbar muscle weakness as well as diaphragmatic weakness were treated with cuirass, CPAP, and later with IPPV at night and got symptomatic relief.

In severe cases of poliomyelitis or postpolio syndrome ventilatory support is required to maintain respiratory homeostasis. Some postpolio patients—those who have predominantly central apnea—require a rocking bed[165] for ventilatory assistance.

They do not respond to CPAP, but they do show improved sleep architecture and respiratory function following mechanical ventilation via nasal mask. Some patients may have obstructive or mixed apneas, and they improve with CPAP. Patients with hypoventilation improve following treatment with nasal ventilation via a mask.

Oxygen

Supplemental oxygen therapy may decrease the severity of obstructive sleep apnea in certain patients.[314] The recommended treatment of nocturnal hypoxemia is administration of oxygen at a low flow rate (1 to 2 l per minute) via a nasal cannula (see Chapter 22). Oxygen administration may not be safe for all patients with sleep apnea syndrome. Motta and Guilleminault[315] and Chokroverty and coworkers[316] observed prolongation of apneas after oxygen administration during sleep in patients with OSA syndrome.

Surgical Treatment

Diaphragmatic pacing or electrophrenic respiration

Sarnoff and coworkers[317] first used electrophrenic stimulation in patients with poliomyelitis in 1951, but the technical difficulties at that time prevented its being used regularly for such treatment. Glenn and associates[318] improved the technique and studied extensively the electrophrenic respiration by diaphragmatic pacing. This form of treatment is used successfully in patients with respiratory center involvement with central sleep apnea syndrome. Superimposed obstructive sleep apnea may complicate the procedure, which may then require both electrophrenic respiration and tracheostomy for treating such patients. Glenn's group[318] have used such treatment successfully in three groups of neurologic disease patients: those with respiratory center involvement, either direct or through interruption of the afferent or efferent neurons to the respiratory center; those with high cervical spinal cord lesions; and those with primary alveolar hypoventilation. This form of treatment has not been very popular because of precipitation of upper airway obstructive apneas in these patients.

Tracheostomy

Tracheostomy remains the only effective measure for emergency treatment of patients with marked respiratory dysfunction with severe hypoxemia, patients with sudden respiratory arrest after resuscitation by intubation, and patients with severe laryngeal stridor due to laryngeal abductor paralysis. This used to be the most definitive treatment for patients with severe obstructive sleep apnea syndrome, but this has been largely replaced by CPAP, since it became available. Following improvement after emergency tracheostomy patients may later be weaned from tracheostomy.

Treatment of Sleep Disturbances in Alzheimer's Disease and Related Dementias

Treatment of acute confusional states associated with dementia has been described in Chapter 25. In this section, general principles of treatment of sleep disturbance in patients with dementia are outlined. Medications that could have an adverse effect on sleep and breathing should be reduced in dose or changed. Associated conditions that could interfere with sleep (e.g., pain due to arthritis and other causes) should be treated with analgesics. Depression is often an important feature in patients with Alzheimer's disease, and a sedative antidepressant may be helpful. Frequency of urination in such patients may result from infection or enlarged prostate and may disturb sleep at night. Appropriate treatment should be directed toward such conditions. Patients should be encouraged to develop good sleep habits. They should be discouraged from taking daytime naps and should be encouraged to exercise (e.g., walking during the day). They should not drink caffeine before bedtime or in the evening. For sleeplessness, a trial with intermediate-acting benzodiazepines should be tried for a short period (see Chapter 17). For extreme agitation, patients should be treated with haloperidol, as for confusional episodes (see Chapter 25).

CONCLUSION

The science of sleep is beginning to advance and probe even deeper into the significance and pathogenesis of sleep and its disorders. Dement[319] stated so aptly that sleep medicine focuses on the sleeping brain and on all phenomena and pathologic effects that derive therefrom. This chapter has summarized how sleep, sleep disorders, and breathing interact in the brain and other neural structures, and how dysfunctions result in sleep and sleep-related breathing disturbances. Further research holds great promise to unravel the mysteries of sleep even further and to direct our attention to finding more promising therapies for the unfortunate millions suffering from chronic disorders of sleep and wakefulness.

REFERENCES

1. Steriade M, McCarley RW. Brainstem Control of Wakefulness and Sleep. New York: Plenum, 1990.
2. Vertes RP. Brainstem control of the events of REM sleep. Progr Neurobiol 1984;22:241–288.
3. Moruzzi G. The sleep waking cycle. Ergeb Physiol 1972;64:1–165.
4. Hobson JA, Lydic R, Baghdoyan HA. Evolving concepts of sleep cycle generation: From brain centers to neuronal populations. Behav Brain Sci 1986;9:371–448.
5. Jouvet M. The role of monoamines and acetylcholine containing neurons in the regulation of the sleep-waking cycle. Ergeb Physiol 1972;64:166–307.
6. Bulow K. Respiration and wakefulness in man. Acta Physiol Scand Suppl 1963;59:1–110.
7. Phillipson EA. Control of breathing during sleep. Am Rev Respir Dis 1978;118:909–939.
8. Phillipson EA. Respiratory adaptations in sleep. Ann Rev Physiol 1978;40:133–156.
9. Phillipson EA, Bowes G. Control of breathing during sleep. In: Fishman AF, Cherniack NS, Widdicombe JG, eds. Handbook of Physiology, vol II, Part 2, Sect 3: The respiratory system. Bethesda, Md.: American Physiological Society, 1986; 649–689.
10. McGinty DJ, Beahm EK. Neurobiology of sleep. In: Saunders NA, Sullivan C, eds. Sleep and Breathing. New York: Marcel Dekker, 1984;1–89.
11. Plum F, Brown HW. The effect on respiration of central nervous system disease. Ann NY Acad Sci 1963;109:915–931.
12. Plum F. Breathlessness in neurological disease: The effects of neurological disease on the act of breathing. In: Howell JBL, Campbell EJM, eds. Breathlessness. Oxford: Blackwell Scientific Publications, 1966;203–222.
13. Plum F. Neurological integration of behavioral and metabolic control of breathing. In: Porter R, ed. Ciba Foundation Symposium on Breathing. Herine-Breuer Centenary Symposium. London: J & A Churchill, 1970;159–181.
14. Nathan PW. The descending respiratory pathway in man. J Neurol Neurosurg Psychiatry 1963;26:487–499.
15. Heyman A, Birchfield RI, Sieker HO. Effects of bilateral cerebral infarction on respiratory center sensitivity. Neurology 1958;8:694.
16. Plum F, Swanson AG. Abnormalities in central regulation of respiration in acute and convalescent poliomyelitis. Arch Neurol Psychiatry 1958;80:267–285.
17. Plum F, Brown HW, Snoep E. Neurologic significance of post-hyperventilation apnea. JAMA 1962;181:1050.
18. North JB, Jennett S. Impedance pneumography for the detection of abnormal breathing patterns associated with brain damage. Lancet 1972;2:212.
19. Lee MC, Klassen AC, Resch JA. Respiratory pattern disturbances in ischemic cerebral vascular disease. Stroke 1974;5:612.
20. North JB, Jennett S. Abnormal breathing patterns associated with acute brain damage. Arch Neurol 1974;31:338.
21. Lee MC, Klassen AC, Heaney LM, et al. Respiratory rate and pattern disturbances in acute brain stem infarction. Stroke 1976;7:382.
22. Von Economo C. Die Pathologie des Schlafes. In: Bethe A, Bergmann G, Embden G, eds. Handbuch der normalen und pathologischen Physiologie. Berlin: Springer-Verlag, 1926;591–610.
23. Von Economo C. Encephalitis Lethargica. Its Sequelae and Treatment. London: Oxford University Press, 1931.
24. Hess WR. Le sommeil. CR Soc Biol (Paris) 1931;107:1333.
25. Nauta WJH. Hypothalamic regulation of sleep in rats. An experimental study. J Neurophysiol 1946;9:285.
26. Bremer F. Cerveau "isolé" et physiologie du sommeil. CR Soc Biol (Paris) 1935;118:1235–1241.
27. Moruzzi G, Magoun HW. Brain stem reticular formation and activation of the EEG. Electroencephalogr Clin Neurophysiol 1949;1:455–473.
28. Moruzzi G. Active processes in the brain stem during sleep. Harvey Lect 1963;58:233–297.
29. Batini C, Magni F, Palestini M, et al. Neural mechanisms underlying the enduring EEG and behavioral activation in the mid-pontine pretrigeminal preparation. Arch Ital Biol 1959;97:1–12.
30. Batini C, Moruzzi G, Palestini M, et al. Effect of complete pontine transections on the sleep-wakefulness rhythm: The mid-pontine pretrigeminal preparation. Arch Ital Biol 1959;97:1–12.
31. Jouvet M. Neurophysiology of the states of sleep. Physiol Rev 1967;47:117–177.
32. Magnes J, Moruzzi G, Pompeiano O. Synchronization of the EEG produced by low-frequency electrical stimulation of the region of the solitary tract. Arch Ital Biol 1961;99:33.
33. Sterman MB, Clemente CD. Forebrain inhibitory mechanisms: Cortical synchronization induced by basal forebrain stimulation. Exp Neurol 1962;6:103.
34. Sterman MB, Clemente CD. Forebrain inhibitory mechanisms. Sleep patterns induced by basal forebrain stimulation. Exp Neurol 1962;6:91.
35. Lucas EA, Sterman MB. Effect of a forebrain lesion on the polycyclic sleep-wake cycle and sleep-wake patterns in the cat. Exp Neurol 1975;46:368.
36. McGinty DJ, Sterman MB. Sleep suppression after basal forebrain lesions in the cat. Science 1968;160:1253.
37. Ricardo JA, Koh ET. Anatomical evidence of direct projections from the nucleus of the solitary tract to the hypothalamus, amygdala, and other forebrain structures in the rat. Brain Res 1978;153:1.
38. Jones BE. Basic mechanisms of sleep-wake states. In: Kryger MH, Roth T, Dement WC, eds. Principles and Practice of Sleep Medicine. Philadelphia: WB Saunders, 1989;121–138.
39. Bremer F. Cerebral hypnogenic centers. Ann Neurol 1977;2:1–6.
40. Steriade M, Glenn LL. Neocortical and caudate projections of intralaminar thalamic neurons and their synaptic excitation from the midbrain reticular cord. J Neurophysiol 1982;48:352–371.

41. Steriade M, Oakson G, Ropert N. Firing rates and patterns of midbrain reticular neurons during stead and transitional states of sleep-waking cycle. Exp Brain Res 1982;46:37–51.

42. Jouvet M. Recherches sur les structures nerveuses et les mecanismes responsables des differentes phases du sommeil physiologique. Arch Ital Biol 1962;100:125–206.

43. Sallanon M, Denoyer M, Kitahama K, et al. Long-lasting insomnia induced by preoptic neuron lesions and its transient reversal by muscimol injection into the posterior hypothalamus in the cat. Neuroscience 1989;32:669–683.

44. Szymusiak R, McGinty D. Sleep-related neuronal discharge in the basal forebrain of cats. Brain Res 1986;370:82–92.

45. Detari L, Juhasz G, Kukorelli T. Neuronal firing in the pallidal region: Firing patterns during sleep-wakefulness cycle in cats. Electroencephalogr Clin Neurophysiol 1987;67:159–166.

46. Buzsaki G, Bickford RG, Ponomareff G, et al. Nucleus basalis and thalamic control of neocortical activity in the freely moving rat. J Neurosci 1988;8:4007–4026.

47. Mesulam MM, Mufson EJ, Levey AI, et al. Atlas of cholinergic neurons in the forebrain and upper brainstem of the macaque based on monoclonal choline acetyltransferase immunohistochemistry and acetylcholinesterase histochemistry. Neuroscience 1984;12:669–686.

48. Swanson LW, Mogenson GJ, Simerly RB, et al. Anatomical and electrophysiological evidence for a projection from the medial preoptic area to the "mesencephalic and subthalamic locomotor regions" in the rat. Brain Res 1987;405:108–122.

49. Mitchell RA, Berger AJ. Neural regulation of respiration. Am Rev Respir Dis 1975;111:206–244.

50. Berger AJ, Mitchell RA, Severinghaus JW. Regulation of respiration. N Engl J Med 1977;297:92–97,138–143,194–201.

51. Mitchell RA. Neural regulation of respiration. Clin Chest Med 1980;1:3–12.

52. Chokroverty S. The spectrum of ventilatory disturbances in movement disorders. In: Chokroverty S, ed. Movement Disorders. Costa Mesa, Calif.: PMA, 1990;365–392.

53. Hugelin A, Cohen MI. The reticular activating system and respiratory regulation in the cat. Ann NY Acad Sci 1963;109:586–603.

54. Chokroverty S. Sleep apnea and respiratory disturbances in multiple system atrophy with progressive autonomic failure (Shy-Drager syndrome). In: Bannister R, ed. Autonomic Failure, ed. 2. London: Oxford University Press, 1988;432–450.

55. Chokroverty S. The Shy-Drager syndrome. Neurol Neurosurg Update 1986;7:1–8.

56. Chokroverty S, Sharp JT. Primary sleep apnea syndrome. J Neurol Neurosurg Psychiatry 1981;44:970–982.

57. Guilleminault C. Sleep and breathing. In: Guilleminault C ed. Sleeping and Waking Disorders: Indications and Techniques, Menlo Park, Calif.: Addison-Wesley, 1982;155–182.

58. Chokroverty S. Sleep and breathing in neurological disorders. In: Edelman NH, Santiago TV, ed. Breathing Disorders of Sleep. New York: Churchill Livingston, 1986;225–264.

59. Cherniack NS, Longobardo GA. Abnormalities in respiratory rhythm. In: Fishman AF, Cherniack NS, Widdicombe JG, eds. Handbook of Physiology, vol II, part 2, Section 3: The Respiratory System.Bethesda, Md.: American Physiological Society, 1986; 729–749.

60. Browne HW, Plum F. The neurologic basis of Cheyne-Stokes respiration. Am J Med 1961;30:849–860.

61. McNicholas WT, Rutherford R, Grossman R, et al. Abnormal respiratory pattern generation during sleep in patients with autonomic dysfunction. Am Rev Respir Dis 1983;128:429–433.

62. Lumsden T. Observations on the respiratory centers in the cat. J Physiol (London) 1923;57:153–160.

63. Wang SC, Ngai SH, Frumin MJ. Organization of central respiratory mechanisms in the brainstem of the cat: Genesis of normal respiratory rhythmicity. Am J Physiol 1957;190:333–342.

64. Cohen MI. Neurogenesis of respiratory rhythm in the mammal. Physiol Rev 1979;59:1105–1173.

65. Chokroverty S, Sharp JT, Barron KD. Periodic respiration in erect posture in Shy-Drager syndrome. J Neurol Neurosurg Psychiatry 1978;41:980–986.

66. Guilleminault C, Tilkian A, Dement WC. The sleep apnea syndromes. Annu Rev Med 1976;27:465.

67. Aldrich MS. Sleep and degenerative neurological disorders involving the motor system. In: Thorpy MJ, ed. Handbook of Sleep Disorders. New York: Marcel Dekker, 1990;673–692.

68. Nomura Y, Segawa M. Anatomy of RETT syndrome. Am J Med Genet 1986;24:289–303.

69. Plum F, Posner JB. The Diagnosis of Stupor and Coma, ed. 3. Philadelphia: FA Davis, 1980.

70. Katzman R, Terry R. The Neurology of Aging. Philadelphia: FA Davis, 1983.

71. McKhann G, Drachman D, Folstein M, et al. Clinical diagnosis of Alzheimer's disease: Report of the NINCDS-ADRDA work under the auspices of Department of Health and Human Services Task Force on Alzheimer's Disease. Neurology 1984;34:939–944.

72. Hoch CC, Reynolds CF III, Kupfer DJ, et al. Sleep-disordered breathing in normal and pathologic aging. J Clin Psychiatry 1986;47:499–503.

73. Erkinjuntti T, Partinen M, Sulkava R, et al. Sleep apnea in multi-infarct dementia and Alzheimer's disease. Sleep 1987;10:419–425.

74. Loewenstein RJ, Weingartner H, Gillin JC, et al. Disturbances of sleep and cognitive functioning in patients with dementia. Neurobiol Aging 1982;3:371–377.

75. Reynolds CF III, Kupfer DJ, Houck PR, et al. Reliable discrimination of elderly depressed and demented patients by electroencephalographic sleep data. Arch Gen Psychiatry 1988;45:358–264.

76. Allen SR, Seiler WO, Stahelin HB, et al. 72-hour polygraphic and behavioral recordings of wakefulness and sleep in a hospital geriatric unit: Comparison between demented and nondemented patients. Sleep 1987;10:143–159.

77. Feinberg I, Koresko RL, Heller N. EEG sleep patterns as a function of normal and pathological aging in man. J Psychiatr Res 1967;5:107–144.

78. Prinz PN, Peskind ER, Vitaliano PP, et al. Changes in sleep and waking EEGs of non-demented and demented elderly subjects. J Am Geriatri Soc 1982;30:86–93.

79. Billiard M, Abboundi G, Dermenghem M, et al. Sleep apneas and mental deterioration in the elderly subjects. Rev Electroencephalogr Clin Neurophysiol 1981;10:290–296.

80. Moldofsky H, Goldstein R, McNicholas WT, et al. Disordered breathing during sleep and overnight intellectual deterioration in patients with pathological aging. In: Guilleminault C, Lugaresi E, eds. Sleep/Wake Disorders: Natural History, Epidemiology and Long-Term Evolution. New York: Raven Press, 1983;143–150.

81. Smallwood RG, Vitiello MV, Giblin EC, et al. Sleep apnea: Relationship to age, sex and Alzheimer's dementia. Sleep 1983;6:16–22.

82. Smirne S, Francschi M, Bareggi SR, et al. Sleep apnea in Alzheimer's disease. In: Sleep 1980, 5th European Congress on Sleep Research, Amsterdam. Basel: Karger, 1981;442–444.

83. Reynolds CF, et al. Sleep apnea in Alzheimer's dementia: Correlation with mental deterioration. J Clin Psychiatry 1985;46:7.

84. Vitiello M, Prinz P, Williams D, et al. Sleep related respiratory dysfunction in normal healthy aged individuals, Alzheimer's disease and major depressive disorder patients. Sleep Res 1987;16:453.

85. Mant A, Saunders NA, Eyland AE, et al. Sleep-related respiratory disturbance and dementia in elderly females. J Gerontol 1988;43:M140–144.

86. Ancoli-Israel S, Kripke DF, Mason W, et al. Sleep apnea and periodic movements in an aging sample. J Gerontol 1985;40:419–425.

87. Miles LE, Dement WC. Sleep and aging. Sleep 1980;3:119–220.

88. Vitiello MV, Prinz PN. Sleep/wake patterns and sleep disorders in Alzheimer's disease. In: Thorpy MJ, ed. Handbook of Sleep Disorders. New York: Marcel Dekker, 1990;703–718.

89. Moore-Ede MC. The circadian timing system in mammals: Two pacemakers preside over many secondary oscillators. Fed Proc 1983;42:2802–2808.

90. Tomlinson BE, Irving D, Blessed G. Cell loss in the locus coeruleus in senile dementia of the Alzheimer type. J Neurol Sci 1981;49:419–428.

91. Baghdoyan HA, McCarley RW, Hobson JA. Cholinergic manipulation of brainstem reticular systems: Effects on desynchronized sleep generation. In: Waquier A, Monti J, Gaillard JP, et al., eds. Sleep: Neurotransmitters and Neuromodulators. New York: Raven Press, 1985;15–27.

92. Prinz P, Vitalianoi P, Vitiello M, et al. Sleep, EEG and mental functions changes in mild, moderate and severe senile dementia of the Alzheimer's type. Neurobiol Aging 1982;3:361–370.

93. Bliwise D. Sleep in normal aging and dementia. Review. Sleep 1993;16:40–81.

94. Reynolds C, Kupfer D, Taska L, et al. Slow wave sleep in elderly depressed, demented and healthy subjects. Sleep 1985;8:151–159.

95. Martin P, Loewenstein R, Kay W, et al. Sleep EEG in Korsakoff's psychosis and Alzheimer's disease. Neurology 1986;36:411–414.

96. Vitiello MV, Prinz PN, Williams DE, et al. Sleep disturbances in patients with mild stage Alzheimer's disease. J Gerontol 1990;45:M131–M138.

97. Kapen S, Park A, Goldberg J, et al. The incidence and severity of obstructive sleep apnea in ischemic cerebrovascular disease. Neurology 1991;41(suppl 1):125.

97a. Kapen S, Goldberg J, Diskin C, et al. The circadian rhythm of ischemic stroke and its relationship to obstructive sleep apnea. Sleep Res 1992;21:216.

98. Marshall J. Diurnal variation in occurrence of strokes. Stroke 1977;8:230–231.

99. Agnoli A, Manfredi M, Mossuto L, et al. Rapport entre les rythmes héméronyctaux de la tension artérielle et sa pathogenie de l'insuffisance vasculaire cérébrale. Rev Neurol (Paris) 1975;131:597–606.

100. Tsementzis SA, Gilla JS, Hitchcock ER, et al. Diurnal variation of the activity during the onset of stroke. Neurosurgery 1985;17:901–904.

101. Mitler MM, Hajdukovic RM, Shafor R, et al. When people die? Cause of death versus time of death. Am J Med 1987;82:266–274.

102. Palomaki H, Partinen M, Juvela S, et al. Snoring as a risk factor for sleep-related brain infarction. Stroke 1989;20:1311–1315.

103. Lugaresi E, Cirignotta F, Coggagna G, et al. Some epidemiological data on snoring and cardiocirculatory disturbances. Sleep 1980;3:221–224.

104. Norton PG, Dunn EV. Snoring as a risk factor for disease: An epidemiological survey. Br Med J 1985;291:630–632.

105. Koskenvuo M, Kaprio J, Partinen M, et al. Snoring as a risk factor for hypertension and angina pectoris. Lancet 1985;1:893–896.

106. Koskenvuo M, Kaprio J, Telakivi T, et al. Snoring as a risk factor for ischaemic heart disease and stroke in men. Br Med J 1987;294:16–19.

107. Partinen M, Palomaki H. Snoring and cerebral infarction. Lancet 1985;2:1325–1326.

108. Palomaki H, Partinen M, Erkinjuntti T, et al. Snoring, sleep apnea syndrome and stroke. Neurology 1992;42 (suppl 6):75–82.

109. Spriggs D, French JM, Murdy JM, et al. Historical risk factors for stroke: A case-control study. Age Ageing 1990;19:280–287.

110. Palomaki H. Snoring and risk of ischemic brain infarction. Stroke 1991;22:1021–1025.

111. Erkinjuntti T, Partinen M, Sulkava R, et al. Are sleep apneas more common in vascular dementia than in Alzheimer's disease? Acta Neurol Scand 1984;69 (suppl):228–229.

112. Manni R, Marchioni E, Romani A, et al. Sleep-apnea in vascular and primary degenerative dementia. In: Koella WP, Obal F, Schulz H, et al., eds. Sleep '86. Stuttgart: Gustav Fischer Verlag, 1988;427–429.

113. Tofler GH, Brezinski D, Schafer AI, et al. Concurrent morning increase in platelet aggregability and the risk

of myocardial infarction and sudden cardiac death. N Engl J Med 1987;316:1514–1518.

114. Drake ME Jr. Kleine-Levin syndrome after multiple cerebral infarctions. Psychosomatics 1987;28:329–330.

115. Rivera VM, Meyer JS, Hata T, et al. Narcolepsy following cerebral hypoxic ischemia. Ann Neurol 1986; 19:505–508.

116. Partinen M. Cerebrovascular disorders and sleep. In: Thorpy MJ, ed. Handbook of Sleep Disorders. New York: Marcel Dekker, 1990;693–702.

117. Korner E, Flooh E, Reinhart B, et al. Sleep alterations in ischemic stroke. Eur Neurol 1986;25(suppl 2):104–110.

118. Hachinski VC, Mamelak M, Norris JW. Clinical recovery and sleep architecture degradation. Can J Neurol Sci 1990;17:332–335.

119. Chatrian GE, White LE Jr, Daly D. Electroencephalographic patterns resembling those of sleep in certain comatose states after injury to the head. Electroencephalogr Clin Neurophysiol 1963;15–272–280.

120. Castaigne P, Lhermitte F, Buge A, et al. Paramedian thalamic and midbrain infarcts: Clinical and neuropathological study. Ann Neurol 1981;10:127–148.

121. Chokroverty S. Autonomic dysfunction in olivopontocerebellar atrophy. In: Duvoisin RC, Plaitakis A, eds. The Olivopontocerebellar Atrophies. New York: Raven Press, 1984;105–151.

122. Eadie MJ. Olivopontocerebellar atrophy. In: Vinken PJ, Bruyn GW, eds. Handbook of Clinical Neurology. Amsterdam: Elsevier North-Holland, 1975;21:415–457.

123. Oppenheimer DR. Diseases of the basal ganglia, cerebellum and motor neurons. In: Blackwood W, Corsellis JAN, eds. Greenfield's Neuropathology, ed 3. London: Edward Arnold, 1976;608–651.

124. Cunchillos JD, DeAndres I. Participation of the cerebellum in the regulation of the sleep-wakefulness cycle: Results in cerebellectomized cats. Electroencephalogr Clin Neurophysiol 1982;53:549–558.

125. Neil JF, Holzer BC, Spiker DG, et al. EEG sleep alterations in olivopontocerebellar degeneration. Neurology 1980;30:660–662.

126. Osorio I, Daroff RB. Absence of REM and altered NREM sleep in patients with spinocerebellar degeneration and slow saccades. Ann Neurol 1980;7:277–280.

127. Cicirata F, Scrofani A, Biondi R. Spindle and EEG sleep alterations in subjects affected by cortical cerebellar atrophy. Eur Neurol 1987;26:120–125.

128. Salazar-Grueso EF, Rosenberg RS, Roos RP. Sleep apnea in olivopontocerebellar degeneration: Treatment with trazodone. Ann Neurol 1988;23:399–401.

129. Quera-Salva MA, Guilleminault C. Olivopontocerebellar degeneration, abnormal sleep, and REM sleep without atonia. Neurology 1986;36:576–577.

130. Shimizu T, Sugita Y, Teshima Y, et al. Sleep study in patients with spinocerebellar degeneration and related diseases. In: Koella WP, ed. Sleep 1980. Basel: S Karger, 1981;435–437.

131. Mahowald MW, Schenck CH. REM sleep behavior disorder. In: Kryger MH, Roth T, Dement WC, eds. Principles and Practice of Sleep Medicine. Philadelphia: WB Saunders, 1989;389–401.

132. Jouvet M, Delorme F. Locus coeruleus et sommeil paradoxal. CR Soc Biol 1965;159:895–899.

133. Bergonzi P, Gigli GL, Laudisio A, et al. Sleep and human cerebellar pathology. Int J Neurosci 1981;15:159–163.

134. Chokroverty S, Sachdeo R, Masdeu J. Autonomic dysfunction and sleep apnea in olivopontocerebellar degeneration. Arch Neurol 1984;41:926–931.

135. Adelman S, Dinner DS, Goren H, et al. Obstructive sleep apnea in association with posteria fossa neurologic diseases. Arch Neurol 1984;41:509–510.

136. Katayama S, Yokoyama S, Hirano Y, et al. TRH and sleep abnormalities in spinocerebellar degeneration (SCD). In: Sobue I, ed. TRH and Spinocerebellar Degeneration. Amsterdam; Elsevier, 1986;227–236.

137. Bergamasco B, Bergamini L, Mutani R. Spontaneous sleep abnormalities in a case of dyssynergia cerebellaris myoclonica. Epilepsia 1967;8:271–281.

138. Stahl SM, Layzer RB, Aminoff MJ, et al. Continuous cataplexy in a patient with a midbrain tumor: The limp man syndrome. Neurology 1980;30:1115–1118.

139. Anderson M, Salmon MV. Symptomatic cataplexy. J Neurol Neurosurg Psychiatry 1977;40:186–191.

140. Berg O, Hanley J. Narcolepsy in two cases of multiple sclerosis. Acta Neurol Scand 1963;39:252–257.

141. Ekbom K. Familial multiple sclerosis associated with narcolepsy. Arch Neurol 1966;15:337–344.

142. Markand ON, Dyken ML. Sleep abnormalities in patients with brainstem lesions. Neurology 1976;26: 769–776.

143. Devereaux MW, Kleane JR, Davis RL. Automatic respiratory failure associated with infarction of the medulla. Arch Neurol 1973;29:46–52.

144. Levin B, Margolis G. Acute failure of autonomic respirations secondary to unilateral brain stem infarct. Ann Neurol 1977;1:583–586.

145. Feldman MH. Physiological observations in a chronic case of "locked-in" syndrome. Neurology 1971;21: 459–478.

146. Freemon FR, Salinas-Garcia RF, Ward JW. Sleep patterns in a patient with a brain stem infarction involving the raphe nucleus. Electroencephalogr Clin Neurophysiol 1974;36:657–660.

147. Cummings JL, Greenberg R. Sleep patterns in the "locked-in" syndrome. Electroencephalogr Clin Neurophysiol 1977;43:270–271.

148. Oxenberg A, Soroker N, Solzi P, Reider-Groswasser I. Polysomnography in locked-in syndrome. Electroencephalogr Clin Neurophysiol 1991;78:314–317.

149. Autret A, Laffont F, De Toffol B, et al. A syndrome of REM and non-REM sleep reduction and lateral gaze paresis after medial tegmental pontine stroke. Arch Neurol 1988;45:1236–1242.

150. Kushida CA, Rye DB, Nummy D, et al. Cortical asymmetry of REM sleep EEG following unilateral pontine hemorrhage. Neurology 1991;41:5981.

151. Severinghaus JW, Mitchell RA. Ondine's curse—Failure of respiratory center automaticity while awake. Clin Res 1962;10:122.

152. Comroe JH Jr. Frankenstein, Pickwick and Ondine. Am Rev Respir Dis 1975;111:689–692.

153. Askenasy JJM, Goldhammer I. Sleep apnea as a feature of bulbar stroke. Stroke 1988;19:637–639.

154. Miyazaki M, Hashimoto T, Sakurama N, et al. Central sleep apnea and arterial compression of the medulla. Ann Neurol 1991;29:564–565.

155. Beamish D, Wildsmith JAW. Ondine's curse after carotid endarterectomy. Br Med J 1978;2:1607.

156. Beal MF, Richardson EP Jr, Brandstetter R, et al. Localized brain stem ischemic damage and Ondine's curse after near-drowning. Neurology 1983;33:717.

157. de Barros-Ferreira M, Chodkiewicz JP, Lairy GC, et al. Disorganized relations of tonic and phasic events of REM sleep in a case of brain-stem tumour. Electroencephalogr Clin Neurophysiol 1975;38:203–207.

158. Newsom Davis J. Autonomous breathing. Report of a case. Arch Neurol 1974;30:480.

159. Rizvi SS, Ishikawa S, Faling LJ, et al. Defect in automatic respiration in a case of multiple sclerosis. Am J Med 1974;56:443.

160. Boor JW, Johnson RJ, Canales L, et al. Reversible paralysis of automatic respiration in multiple sclerosis. Arch Neurol 1977;34:686.

161. Sarnoff SJ, Whittenberger JL. Affeldt JE: Hypoventilation syndrome in bulbar poliomyelitis. JAMA 1951;147:30.

162. Speier JL, Owen RR, Knapp M, et al. Occurrence of post-polio sequelae in an epidemic population. In: Halstead LS, Wiechers DO, eds. Research and Clinical Aspects of the Late Effects of Poliomyelitis. White Plains, NY: March of Dimes Birth Defects Foundation, 1987.

163. Codd MB, Mulder DW, Kurland LT, et al. Poliomyelitis in Rochester, Minnesota, 1935–1955: Epidemiology and long-term sequelae: a preliminary report. Research and Clinical Aspects of the Late Effects of Poliomyelitis. White Plains, NY: March of Dimes Birth Defects Foundation, 1987.

164. Halsted LS, Rossi CD. New problems in old polio patients: Results of a survey of 539 polio survivors. Orthopedics 1985;845–850.

165. Steljes DG, Kryger MH, Kirk BW, et al. Sleep in post-polio syndrome. Chest 1990,81:133–140.

166. Guilleminault C, Motta J. Sleep apnea syndrome as a long-term sequela of poliomyelitis. New York: Alan R Liss, 1978;309–315.

167. Solliday NH, Gaensler EA, Schwaber R, et al. Impaired central chemoreceptor function and chronic hypoventilation many years following poliomyelitis. Respiration 1974;31:177.

168. Bye PTP, Ellis ER, Issaq FG, et al. Respiratory failure and sleep in neuromuscular disease. Thorax 1990;45:241–247.

169. Ellis ER, Bye PTP, Bruderer JW, et al. Treatment of respiratory failure during sleep in patients with neuromuscular disease: Positive pressure ventilation through a nose mask. Am Rev Respir Dis 1987;135:148–152.

170. Howard RS, Wiles CM, Spencer GT. The late sequelae of poliomyelitis. Q J Med 1988;66:219–232.

171. Haponik EF, Givens D, Angelo J. Syringobulbia-myelia with obstructive sleep apnea. Neurology 1983;33:1046.

172. Cohn JE, Kuida H. Primary alveolar hypoventilation associated with western equine encephalitis. Ann Intern Med 1962;56:633.

173. White D, Miller F, Erickson R. Sleep apnea and nocturnal hypoventilation following western equine encephalitis. Am Rev Respir Dis 1983;127:132–133.

174. Papasozomenos S, Roessman U. Respiratory distress and Arnold-Chiari malformation. Neurology 1981;91:97–100.

175. Dure LS, Percy AK, Cheek WR, et al. Chiari type I malformation in children. J Pediatr 1989;115:573–576.

176. Balk RA, Hiller FC, Lucas EA, et al. Sleep apnea and the Arnold-Chiari malformation. Am Rev Respir Dis 1985;132:929–930.

177. Campbell EJM. Respiratory failure. Br Med J 1965;1:1451.

178. Bokinsky GE, Hudson LD, Weil JV. Impaired peripheral chemosensitivity and acute respiratory failure in Arnold-Chiari malformation and syringomyelia. N Engl J Med 1973;288:947.

179. Krieger AJ, Rosomoff HL. Sleep-induced apnea. Part 1: A respiratory and autonomic dysfunction syndrome following bilateral percutaneous cervical cordotomy. J Neurosurg 1974;40:168.

180. Belmusto L, Woldring S, Owens G. Localization and patterns of potentials of the respiratory pathway in the cervical spinal cord in the dog. J Neurosurg 1965;22:277.

181. Tenicela R, Rosomoff HL, Feist J, et al. Pulmonary function following percutaneous cervical cordotomy. Anesthesiology 1968;29:7.

182. Krieger AJ, Rosomoff HL. Sleep-induced apnea. Part 2: Respiratory failure after anterior spinal surgery. J Neurosurg 1974;39:181.

183. Star AM, Osterman AL. Sleep apnea syndrome after spinal cord injury. Spine 1988;13:116–117.

184. Bonekat HW, Anderson G, Squires J. Obstructive disordered breathing during sleep in patients with spinal cord injury. Paraplegia 1990;28:292–298.

184a. Short DJ, Stradling JR, Williams SJ. Prevalence of sleep apnea in patients over 40 years of age with spinal cord lesions. J Neurol Neurosurg Psychiatr 1992;55:1032–1036.

184b. Adey WR, Bors E, Porter RW. EEG sleep patterns after high cervical lesions in man. Arch Neurol 1968;19:377–383.

185. Parhad IM, Clark AW, Barron KD, Staunton SB. Diaphragmatic paralysis in motor neuron disease. Report of two cases and a review of the literature. Neurology 1978;28:18.

186. Thorpy MJ, Schmidt-Nowara WW, Pollak C, Weitzman ED. Sleep-induced non-obstructive hypoventilation association with diaphragmatic paralysis. Ann Neurol 1982;12:308.

187. Newsom Davis J, Goldman M, Loh L, et al. Diaphragm function and alveolar hypoventilation. Q J Med 1976;45:87.

188. Serpick AA, Baker EL, Woodward TE. Motor system disease. Arch Intern Med 1965;115:192.

189. Chokroverty S. Sleep apnea in neurodegenerative diseases. Electroencephalogr Clin Neurophysiol 1982;53:22P.

190. Gay PC, Westbrook PR, Daube JR, et al. Effect of alterations in pulmonary function and sleep variables

on survival in patients with amyotrophic lateral sclerosis. Mayo Clin Proc 1991;66:686–694.

191. Ferguson KA, Strong MJ, Ahmad D, et al. Sleep dysfunction in amyotrophic lateral sclerosis. Sleep Res 1992;21:291.

192. Minz M, Autret A, Laffont F, et al. A study of sleep in amyotrophic lateral sclerosis. Biomedicine 1979;30:40–46.

193. Howard RS, Wiles CM, Loh L. Respiratory complications and their management in motor neuron disease. Brain 1989;112:1155–1170.

194. Tanner CM. Respiratory dysfunction and peripheral neuropathy. In: Weiner WJ, ed. Respiratory Dysfunction in Neurologic Disease. Mount Kisco, NY: Futura, 1980;83.

195. Goldstein RFL, Hyde RW, Lapham LW, et al. Peripheral neuropathy presenting with respiratory insufficiency as the primary complaint. Am J Med 1974;56:443.

196. Chan CK, Mohsenin V, Loke J, et al. Diaphragmatic dysfunction in siblings with hereditary motor and sensory neuropathy (Charcot-Marie-Tooth Disease). Chest 1987;91:567–570.

197. Bellamy D, Newsom Davis J, Hickey BP, et al. A case of primary alveolar hypoventilation associated with mild proximal myopathy. Am Rev Respir Dis 1975;112:867.

198. Riley DJ, Santiago TV, Danielle RP, et al. Blunted respiratory drive in congenital myopathy. Am J Med 1977;63:459.

199. Smith PEM, Calverley PMA, Edwards RHT. Hypoxemia during sleep in Duchenne Muscular dystrophy. Am Rev Respir Dis 1988;137:884–888.

200. Gross D, Ladd HW, Riley EJ, et al. The effect of training on strength and endurance of the diaphragm in quadriplegia. Am J Med 1980;68:27–35.

201. Buschsbaum HW, Martin WA, Turino GM, et al. Chronic alveolar hypoventilation due to muscular dystrophy. Neurology 1968;18:319–327.

202. Skatrud J, Iber C, McHugh W. Determinants of hypoventilation during wakefulness and sleep in diaphragmatic paralysis. Am Rev Respir Dis 1980; 121:587–593.

203. Benaim S, Worster-Drought C. Dystrophia myotonica with myotonia of diaphragm causing pulmonary hypoventilation with anoxaemia and secondary polycythaemia. Med Illus 1954;8:221–226.

204. Coccagna G, Mantovani M, Parchi C, et al. Alveolar hypoventilation and hypersomnia in myotonic dystrophy. J Neurol Neurosurg Psychiatry 1975;38:977–984.

205. Guilleminault C, Cummiskey J, Motta J, et al. Respiratory and hemodynamic study during wakefulness and sleep in myotonic dystrophy. Sleep 1978;1:19–31.

206. Hansotia P, Frens D. Hypersomnia associated with alveolar hypoventilation in myotonic dystrophy. Neurology 1981;31:1336–1337.

207. Harper PS. Myotonic Dystrophy. Philadelphia: WB Saunders, 1979.

208. Striano S, Meo R, Bilo L, et al. Sleep apnea syndrome in Thomsen's disease. A case report. Electroencephalogr Clin Neurophysiol 1983;56:332.

209. Bashour F, Winchell P, Reddington J. Myotonia atrophica and cyanosis. N Engl J Med 1955;252:768–770.

210. Kilburn KH, Eagan JT, Heyman A. Cardiopulmonary insufficiency associated with myotonic dystrophy. Am J Med 1959;26:929–935.

211. Kohn NN, Faires JS, Rodman T. Unusual manifestations due to involvement of involuntary muscle in dystrophia myotonica. N Engl J Med 1964;271:1179–1183.

212. Kaufman L. Anaesthesia in dystrophia myotonica. A review of the hazards of anesthesia. Proc R Soc Med 1966;53:183–188.

213. Gillam PMS, Heaf PJD, Kaufman L, et al. Respiration in dystrophia myotonica. Thorax 1964;19:112–120.

214. Coccagna G, Martinelli P, Lugaresi E. Sleep and alveolar hypoventilation in myotonic dystrophy. Acta Neurol Belg 1982;82:185–194.

215. Carroll JE, Zwillich CW, Weil JV. Ventilatory response in myotonic dystrophy. Neurology 1977;27:1125–1128.

216. Begin R, Bureau MA, Lupien L, et al. Pathogenesis of respiratory insufficiency in myotonic dystrophy: The mechanical factors. Am Rev Respir Dis 1982;125:312–318.

217. Armagast SJ, Ringel SP, Martin RJ. The effects of dichlorphenamide on sleep apnea in patients with myotonic dystrophy. Clin Res 1983;31:70A.

218. Rosenow EC, Engel AG. Acid maltase deficiency in adults presenting as respiratory failure. Am J Med 1978;64:485.

219. Sivak ED, Salanga VD, Wilbourn AJ, et al. Adult-onset acid maltase deficiency presenting as diaphragmatic paralysis. Ann Neurol 1981;9:613.

220. Martin RJ, Sufit RL, Ringel SP, et al. Respiratory improvement by muscle training in adult-onset acid maltase deficiency. Muscle Nerve 1983;6:201–203.

221. Kryger MH, Steljes DG, Yee W-C, et al. Central sleep apnoea in congenital muscular dystrophy. J Neurol Neurosurg Psychiatry 1991;54:710–712.

222. Maayan C, Springer C, Armon Y, et al. Nemaline myopathy as a cause of sleep hypoventilation. Pediatrics 1986;77:390–395.

223. Wilson DO, Sanders MH, Dauber JH. Abnormal ventilatory chemosensitivity and congenital myopathy. Arch Intern Med 1987;147:1773–1777.

224. Tatsumi C, Takahashi M, Yorifugi S, et al. Mitochondrial encephalomyopathy with sleep apnea. Eur Neurol 1988;28:64–69.

225. Carroll JE, Zwillich C, Weil JV, et al. Depressed ventilatory response in oculocraniosomatic neuromuscular disease. Neurology 1976;26:146.

226. Mier-Jedrzejowicz A, Brophy C, Green M. Respiratory muscle function in myasthenia gravis. Am Rev Respir Dis 1988;138:867–873.

227. Quera-Salva MA, Guilleminault C, Chevret S, et al. Breathing disorders during sleep in myasthenia gravis. Ann Neurol 1992;31:86–92.

228. Mennumi G, Morante MT, Scoppeta, et al. Night sleep organization in myasthenic patients not undergoing therapy. Sleep Res 1983;12:84.

229. Shiozawa Z, Shintani S, Tsunoda S, et al. Sleep apnea in well-controlled myasthenia gravis. Sleep Res 1987;16:301.

230. Chokroverty S. Functional anatomy of the autonomic nervous system: Autonomic dysfunction and disorders of the CNS. In: American Academy of Neurology Course No. 144, Boston, Mass., 1991; 77–103.

231. Loewy AD, Spyer KM. Central Regulation of Autonomic Functions. New York: Oxford University Press, 1990.

232. Chokroverty S. Sleep apnea and autonomic failure. In: Low PA, ed. Clinical Autonomic Disorders. Boston: Little, Brown, 1993;589–603.

233. Parmeggiani PL, Morrison AR. Alterations of autonomic functions during sleep. In: Loewy AD, Spyer KM, eds. Central Regulation of Autonomic Functions. New York: Oxford University Press, 1990;367–386.

234. Loewy AD. Central autonomic pathways. In: Low PA, ed. Clinical Autonomic Disorders. Boston: Little, Brown, 1993;88–103.

235. Barron KD, Chokroverty S. Anatomy of the autonomic nervous system: Brain and brainstem. In: Low PA, ed. Clinical Autonomic Disorders. Boston: Little, Brown, 1993;3–15.

236. Shy GM, Drager GA. A neurological syndrome associated with orthostatic hypotension. Arch Neurol 1960;2:511–527.

237. Bannister R, Ardill L, Fentem P. Defective autonomic control of blood vessels in idiopathic orthostatic hypotension. Brain 1967;90:725–746.

238. Bannister R, Oppenheimer DR. Degenerative disease of the nervous system associated with autonomic failure. Brain 1972;95:457–474.

239. Bannister R, Gibson W, Michaels L, Oppenheimer DR. Laryngeal abductor paralysis in multiple system atrophy. Brain 1981;104:351–368.

240. Chokroverty S, Barron KD, Katz FH, et al. The syndrome of primary orthostatic hypotension. Brain 1969;92:743–768.

241. Chokroverty S. The assessment of sleep disturbances in autonomic failure. In. Bannister R, Mathias C, eds. Autonomic Failure, ed 3. Oxford: Oxford University Press, 1992;443–461.

242. Cohen J, Low P, Fealey R, et al. Somatic and autonomic function in progressive autonomic failure and multiple system atrophy. Ann Neurol 1987;22:692–699.

243. Quinn N. Multiple system atrophy—the nature of the beast. J Neurol Neurosurg Psychiatry 1989;52:S78–S89.

244. Wooten V. Medical causes of insomnia. In: Kryger MN, Roth T, Dement WC, eds. Principles and Practice of Sleep Medicine. Philadelphia: WB Saunders, 1989;456–475.

245. Lockwood AH. Shy-Drager syndrome with abnormal respirations and antidiuretic hormone release. Arch Neurol 1976; 33:292–295.

246. Castaigne P, Laplane D, Autrel A, et al. Syndrome de Shy et Drager avec troubles du rhythme respiratoire et de la vigilance. Rev Neurol (Paris) 1977;133:455–456.

247. Martin JB, Travis RH, Van Den Noort S. Centrally mediated orthostatic hypotension. Arch Neurol (Chicago) 1968;19:163–173.

248. Israel RH, Marino JM. Upper airway obstruction in the Shy-Drager syndrome. Ann Neurol 1977;2:83.

249. Guilleminault C, Tilkian A, Lehrman K, et al. Sleep apnoea syndrome: States of sleep and autonomic dysfunction. J Neurol Neurosurg Psychiatry 1977;40:718–725.

250. Williams A, Hanson D, Calne DB. Vocal cord paralysis in the Shy-Drager syndrome. J Neurol Neurosurg Psychiatry 1979;42:151–153.

251. Kenyon GS, Apps MCP, Traub M. Stridor and obstructive sleep apnea in Shy-Drager Syndrome treated by laryngofissure and cord lateralization. Laryngoscope 1984;94:1106–1108.

252. Munschauer FE, Loh L, Bannister R, et al. Abnormal respiration and sudden death during sleep in multiple system atrophy with autonomic failure. Neurology 1990;40:677–679.

253. Lehrman KL, Guilleminault C, Schroeder JS, et al. Sleep apnea syndrome in a patient with Shy-Drager syndrome. Arch Intern Med 1978;138:206–209.

254. Briskin JG, Lehrman KL, Guilleminault C. Shy-Drager syndrome and sleep apnea. In: Guilleminault C, Dement WC, eds. Sleep Apnea Syndromes. New York: Alan R Liss, 1978;316–322.

255. Guilleminault C, Briskin JG, Greenfield MS, et al. The impact of autonomic nervous system dysfunction on breathing during sleep. Sleep 1981;4:263–278.

256. Chester CS, Gottfried SB, Camerson DI, et al. Pathophysiological findings in a patient with Shy-Drager and alveolar hypoventilation syndromes. Chest 1988;94:212–214.

257. Dempsey JA, Olson EB Jr, Skatrud JB. Hormones and neurochemicals in the regulation of breathing. In: Fishman AF, Cherniack NS, Widdicombe JG, eds. Handbook of Physiology, vol II, part I, Section 3: The Respiratory System. Bethesda, Md.: American Physiological Society, 1986;181–221.

258. Spokes EG, Bannister R, Oppenheimer DR. Multiple system atrophy with autonomic failure: Clinical, histological and neurochemical observations on 4 cases. J Neurol Sci 1979;43:59–82.

259. Black IB, Petito CK. Catecholamine enzymes in the degenerative neurological disease idiopathic orthostatic hypotension. Science 1976;192:910–912.

260. Brunt PW, McKusick V. Familial dysautonomia. Medicine 1970;49:343–374.

261. Gadoth N, Sokol J, Lavie P. Sleep structure and nocturnal disordered breathing in familial dysautonomia. J Neurol Sci 1983;60:117–125.

262. Maayan C, Oren A, Goldin E, et al. Megaesophagus and recurrent apnea in an adult patient with familial dysautonomia. Am J Gastroenterology 1990;85:729–732.

263. Chokroverty S. Functional anatomy of the autonomic nervous system correlated with symptomatology of neurologic disease. In: American Academy of Neurology Course No. 246, San Diego, Calif.: 1992;49–76.

264. Frank Y, Kravath RE, Inoue K, et al. Sleep apnea and hypoventilation syndrome associated with acquired

nonprogressive dysautonomia: Clinical and pathological studies in a child. Ann Neurol 1980;10:18–22.

265. Rees PJ, Prior JG, Cochrane GM, et al. Sleep apnoea in diabetic patients with autonomic neuropathy. JR Soc Med 1981;74:192–195.

266. Mondini S, Guilleminault C. Abnormal breathing patterns during sleep in diabetes. Ann Neurol 1985; 17:391–395.

267. Catterall JR, Calverley PMA, Ewing DJ, et al. Breathing, sleep and diabetic autonomic neuropathy. Diabetes 1984;33:1025–1027.

268. Guilleminault C, Eldridge F, Dement WC. Insomnia, narcolepsy and sleep apneas. Bull Physiopathol Respir 1972;8:1127–1138.

269. Guilleminault C, Hoed JVD, Mitler MM. Clinical overview of the sleep apnea syndromes. In: Guilleminault C, Dement WC, eds. Sleep Apnea Syndromes. New York: Alan R Liss, 1978;1–12.

270. Laffont F, Minz AM, Beillevaire T, et al. Sleep respiratory arrhythmias in control subjects, narcoleptics and non-cataplectic hypersomniacs. Electroencephalogr Clin Neurophysiol 1978;44:697.

271. Chokroverty S. Sleep apnea in narcolepsy. Sleep 1986;9:250–253.

272. Kleine W. Periodische Schlafsucht. Mschr Psychiatr Neurol 1925;57:285–320.

273. Levin M. Periodic somnolence and morbid hunger: A new syndrome. Brain 1936;59:494—504.

274. Critchley M. Periodic hypersomnia and megaphagia in adolescent males. Brain 1962;85:627–657.

275. Billiard M, Cadilhac J. Les hypersomnies recurrentes. Rev Neurol (Paris) 1988;144:249–258.

276. Guilleminault C. Idiopathic central nervous system hypersomnia. In. Kryger MN, Roth T, Dement WC, eds. Principles and Practice of Sleep Medicine. Philadelphia: WB Saunders, 1989;347–350.

277. Reichel J. Primary alveolar hypoventilation. Clin Chest Med 1980;1:119.

278. Fishman AP, Goldring RM, Turino GM. General alveolar hypoventilation: A syndrome of respiratory and cardiac failure in patients with normal lungs. QJ Med 1966;35:261.

279. Fishman AP. The syndrome of chronic alveolar hypoventilation. Bull Physiopath Resp 1972;8:971.

280. Martin RJ. Neuromuscular and skeletal abnormalities with nocturnal respiratory disorders. In: Martin RJ, ed. Cardiorespiratory Disorders during Sleep. Mount Kisco, NY: Futura, 1990;251–281.

281. Cooper R, Hulme A. Intracranial pressure and related phenomena during sleep. J Neurol Neurosurg Psychiatry 1966;29:564–570.

282. Cooper R, Hulme A. Changes of the EEG, intracranial pressure and other variables during sleep in patients with intracranial lesions. Electroencephalogr Clin Neurophysiol 1969;27:12–22.

283. Munari C, Calbucci F. Correlations between intracranial pressure and EEG during coma and sleep. Electroencephalogr Clin Neurophysiol 1981;51:170–176.

284. Dexter JD, Weitzman E. The relationship of nocturnal headaches to sleep stage patterns. Neurology 1970;20: 513–518.

285. Kudrow L, McGinty DJ, Phillips ER, et al. Sleep apnea in cluster headache. Cephalalgia 1984;4:33–38.

286. Dexter JD. Headache as a presenting complaint of sleep apnea syndrome. Headache 1984;24:171.

287. Sahota PK, Dexter JD. Sleep and headaches syndromes: A clinical review. Headache 1990;1:80–84.

288. Sahota PK, Dexter JD. Reversible physiological insomnia associated with cluster headache. Sleep Res 1992;21:307.

289. Kayed K, Godtlibsen OB, Sjaastad O. Chronic paroxysmal hemicrania. IV. "REM Sleep locked" nocturnal headache attacks. Sleep 1978;1:91–95.

290. Lugaresi E, Medori R, Montagna P, et al. Fatal familial insomnia and dysautonomia with selective degeneration of thalamic nuclei. N Engl J Med 1986;315:997–1003.

291. Manetto V, Medori R, Cortelli P, et al. Fatal familial insomnia and pathological study of five new cases. Neurology 1992;42:312–219.

292. Lugaresi E. The thalamus and insomnia. Neurology 1992;42(suppl 6):28–33.

293. Medori R, Montagna P, Tritschler HJ, et al. Fatal familial insomnia. A second kindred with mutation of prion protein gene at codon 178. Neurology 1992;42:669–670.

294. Medori R, Tritschler J, LeBlanc A, et al. Fatal familial prion protein gene. N Engl J Med 1992;326:444–449.

295. Bradley WG, Daroff RB, Fenichel GM, et al. eds. Neurology in Clinical Practice, vols I and II. Boston: Butterworth/Heinemann, 1991.

296. Adams RD, Victor M. Principles of Neurology, ed 4. New York: McGraw-Hill, 1989.

297. Rowland LP, ed. Merritt's Textbook of Neurology, ed 8. Philadelphia: Lea & Febiger, 1989.

298. Bates DV. Respiratory Function in Disease, ed 3. Philadelphia: WB Saunders, 1989;106–151.

299. Black LF, Hyatt RE. Maximal static respiratory pressures in generalized neuromuscular disease. Am Rev Respir Dis 1971;103:641–650.

300. Guindi GM, Bannister R, Gibson W, et al. Laryngeal electromyography in multiple system atrophy with autonomic failure. J Neurol Neurosurg Psychiatry 1981;44:49–53.

301. Markand ON, Kincaid JC, Pourmand RA, et al. Electrophysiologic evaluation of diaphragm by transcutaneous phrenic nerve stimulation. Neurology 1984;34:604–614.

302. Chokroverty S, Olney RK. Magnetic stimulation of human peripheral nervous system and roots: An AAEM workshop. Rochester, Minn.: AAEM, 1992.

303. Sanders MH. The management of sleep disordered breathing. In: Martin RJ, ed. Cardiorespiratory Disorders During Sleep. Mt. Kisco, NY: Futura, 1990;141–187.

304. Issa FG, Sullivan CE. Upper airway closing pressures in snorers. J Appl Physiol 1984;57:528–535.

305. Krol RC, Knuth SL, Bartlett D Jr. Selective reduction of genioglossal muscle activity by alcohol in normal human subjects. Am Rev Respir Dis 1984;129:247–250.

306. Taasan VC, Block AJ, Boysen PG, et al. Alcohol increases sleep apnea and oxygen desaturation in asymptomatic men. Am J Med 1981;71:240–245.

307. Hensley MJ, Saunders NA, Strohl KP. Medroxyprogesterone treatment of obstructive sleep apnea. Sleep 1980;3:441–446.

308. Rajagopal KR, Abbrecht P, Jabbari P. Effects of medroxyprogesterone acetate in obstructive sleep apnea. Chest 1986;90:815–821.

309. Skatrud JB, Dempsey JA, Kaiser DG. Ventilatory response to medroxyprogesterone acetate in normal subjects: Time, course and mechanisms. J Appl Physiol 1978;44:939–944.

310. Strohl KP, Hensley M, Saunders NA, et al. Progesterone administration and progressive sleep apneas. JAMA 1981;245:1230–1232.

311. Guilleminault C, Kowall J. Central sleep apnea in adults. In: Thorpy MJ, ed. Handbook of Sleep Disorders. New York: Marcel Dekker, 1990;337–351.

312. Bye PTB, Ellis ER, Donnelly PD, et al. Role of sleep in the development of respiratory failure in neuromuscular disease. Am Rev Respir Dis 1985;131:108.

313. Kerby DY, Meyer LS, Tingleton SK. Nocturnal positive pressure ventilation via nasal mask. Am Rev Respir Dis 1987;135:738–740.

314. Martin RJ, Sanders MA, Gray BA, et al. Acute and long term ventilatory affects of hyperoxia in the adult sleep apnea syndrome. Am Rev Respir Dis 1982;125:175–180.

315. Motta A, Guilleminault C. Effects of oxygen administration in sleep-induced apneas. In: Guilleminault C, Dement WC, eds. Sleep Apnea Syndrome. New York: Alan R Liss, 1978;137–144.

316. Chokroverty S, Barrocas M, Barron KD, et al. Hypoventilation syndrome and obesity: A polygraphic study. Trans Am Neurol Assoc 1969;94:240–242.

317. Sarnoff SJ, Whittenberger JL, Affeldt JA. Hypoventilation syndrome in bulbar poliomyelitis. JAMA 1951;147:30.

318. Glenn WWL, Phelps M, Gersten LM. Diaphragm pacing in the management of central alveolar hypoventilation. In: Guilleminault C, Dement WC, eds. Sleep Apnea Syndromes. New York: Alan R Liss, 1978;333–344.

319. Dement WC. A personal history of sleep disorders medicine. J Clin Neurophysiol 1990;7:17–47.

21

Sleep Disorders in Psychiatric Illness

Virgil Wooten

Links between psychopathology and poor sleep have been made many times in the literature. Often, physicians who have exhausted all routine laboratory assessments and medical interventions in the effort to diagnose and treat a person with an undiscovered sleep problem refer the patient to a psychiatrist. Patients who present to sleep disorders centers frequently exhibit symptoms of psychopathology, which may or may not be due to true psychiatric illness. In a study by Mosko and colleagues, 66.5% of 206 patients presenting to one sleep disorders center reported one episode of major depression in the previous 5 years and 25.7% described themselves as depressed on presentation.[1] Studies such as this one suggest that symptoms of apnea and other sleep disorders overlap with symptoms of psychiatric disturbance and that the treatment of the organic sleep disturbance may eliminate psychiatric symptoms.

According to the Epidemiological Catchment Area (ECA) study of the National Institute of Mental Health (NIMH) consisting of 18,571 people aged 18 years and older, 15.4% of the population had a mental disorder within 1 month of initial interview—5.1% an affective disorder, 7.3% an anxiety disorder, and 3.8% a substance abuse disorder.[2] The respective lifetime prevalence in these groups was estimated at 8.3%, 14.6% and 16.4%. A survey of 7954 people in scattered major U.S. cities between 1981 to 1985 as part of the NIMH/ECA study also revealed that 40% of those with insomnia and 46.5% of those with hypersomnia met the American Psychiatric Association's Diagnostic and Statistical Manual (3rd edition) (DSM-III-R) criteria for mental illness.[3] Ten percent of the sample complained of insomnia and 3.2% of hypersomnia. Fourteen percent of the patients with insomnia met criteria for major depression, compared to 9.9% of those with hypersomnolence. The rate of new psychiatric disorders at 1-year follow-up was greater among respondents with sleep complaints. The numbers in this study were thought to be low owing to strict criteria for defining insomnia and the omission of generalized anxiety disorder and personality disorders from the survey.

Other studies have also identified substantial risks for patients with sleep disorders of developing major depression and generalized anxiety. Mellinger and coworkers reported that 21% of insomniacs had symptoms of major depression and another 13% symptoms of generalized anxiety.[4] Kales and colleagues suggested that older insomniacs had more psychopathology.[5] Data from the ECA/NIMH study and other studies do not support the assertion that psychopathology is more prevalent among elderly persons.[6] However, the study agreed with Kales and colleagues that insomnia is likely to be associated with psychopathology.

REM SLEEP STUDIES OF PSYCHOPATHOLOGY

Studies of rapid eye movement (REM) sleep architecture in various psychopathologic states have been conducted since Dement first evaluated REM sleep in schizophrenic patients. In more recent times, REM sleep changes have most often been correlated with affective disorders. Subsequently, numerous studies have attempted to use measures of REM sleep latency, REM density, and REM sleep distribution to link affective disorders to various other psychopathologic states such as schizophrenia, eating disorders, personality disorders, and substance abuse disorders. Others have attempted to use these same measures to distinguish various psychopathologic states from major depression. Unfortunately, a great deal of confusion has resulted from various methodologic issues and diagnostic uncertainties in psychiatric patients. Examples of methodologic differences in studies include the number of consecutive nights patients are studied, determination of the time between sleep onset and REM sleep onset, the definition of increased REM density, psychotropic drugs, period of withdrawal from psychotropic medications, and the severity of the illness. Just as important is the lack of specificity found in the DSM III-R and Research Diagnostic Criteria (RDC) classifications for various mental disorders. Psychiatric diagnoses are not always as clear as proponents of these classification systems sometimes maintain, mostly because of a great overlap in the symptoms among

TABLE 21-1.   Prevalence of Insomnia and Hypersomnia in Association with Psychiatric Disorders

Disorder	Insomnia (%)	Hypersomnolence (%)
Dysthymia	8.6	8.5
Anxiety disorder	23.9	27.6
Alcohol abuse	7.0	6.2
Drug abuse	4.2	4.7
Other psychiatric disorders	5.1	5.2

various psychiatric diagnoses. Additionally, it is not uncommon for patients with psychiatric illness to have more than one diagnosis. For example, a patient with panic disorder may also develop major depression.

MAJOR DEPRESSION

Major depression is the psychiatric disorder most studied by sleep researchers, and several theories of the mechanisms involved have been published.[7] Great efforts have been made to distinguish major depression from other psychopathologic states by use of sleep electroencephalography (EEG) and other biologic markers. The primary well-documented changes in sleep architecture include shortened REM sleep onset latency, increased REM density, reduced total sleep time, reduced sleep efficiency, increased awakenings, decreased slow-wave sleep, and a shift of slow-wave sleep from the first non-REM (NREM) cycle to the second. The causes of these alterations are the subject of much speculation.

Changes in sleep architecture, particularly in REM sleep and deep NREM sleep are more pronounced with age. Prepubertal depressed children are less likely to show changes in sleep architecture than postpubertal depressives.[8,9] There has been some conflict in the literature about whether REM sleep latency in depressed children is normal or shortened.[10] The difference in findings has been suggested to be due to the presence of affective illness in families of depressed children (i.e., reduced REM sleep latency may be more likely to occur in children with a family history of affective disorder).[11] Changes in sleep architecture in adolescents also appear to depend on the severity of the illness. In one study, adolescents who were inpatients or suicidal were found to exhibit the typical changes of major depression, whereas the sleep of adolescents who were not as severely depressed was no different from that of normal controls.[12] Naylor and associates supported the reflection of severity in REM sleep changes

in adolescents.[13] In this study group, psychotic, depressed adolescents had a shorter REM sleep latency than nonpsychotic adolescents.

Aging has a marked shortening influence on REM sleep latency; elderly depressed patients not uncommonly having REM sleep onset of less than 10 minutes. Older patients with a history of suicide attempts have longer sleep-onset latency, reduced sleep efficiency, and increased REM density than "nonattempters."[14]

A study of gender differences in subjects aged 20 to 70 years showed that depressed men have less slow-wave sleep than depressed women; however, this is the only difference that has been demonstrated.[15] Approximately 90% of the time major depression results in insomnia. Only a small percentage of patients with major depression complain of excessive sleepiness; most are adolescents and young adults.[16] While depressed adolescents and young adults may be more prone to be "long sleepers," studies of older depressed patients with the complaint of hypersomnolence have failed to show evidence of pathologic sleepiness.[17]

Studies of the acute effects of antidepressant medication on REM sleep measures in patients with major depression have suggested that when an immediate antidepressant-induced prolongation of the REM sleep latency, reduction of total REM sleep time, and REM density is observed, the clinical response is better.[18] The occurrence of sleep-onset REM sleep episodes and shorter REM sleep episode duration during maintenance treatment with antidepressants has been associated with increased risk of relapse during treatment.[19] Studies of the effects of electroconvulsive therapy (ECT) on REM sleep architecture suggest that they are not as pronounced as those observed with most antidepressants.[20]

PANIC DISORDER

Panic disorder is a condition that has been given many other names. In addition to *mitral valve prolapse syndrome* and *cardiovascular dysautonomia* it has also been recently called *sleep choking syndrome*. Which name is assigned often depends on whether the patient is seen by a psychiatrist, cardiologist, sleep specialist, or another practitioner. The diagnosis also often depends on the degree of psychiatric symptoms, as opposed to cardiovascular symptoms. As many as 70% of patients with panic disorder have difficulty with sleep onset and maintenance insomnia.[21] Patients with panic disorder often have prolonged sleep onset latency, lower sleep efficiency, and more movement time than control subjects.[22] Panic attacks can occur in any stage of sleep, but most occur during NREM sleep. It has been suggested that a number of substances and situations provoke panic attacks, such as caffeine, nicotine, over-the-counter cold remedies, cannabis, cocaine, sleep deprivation, excessive sugar intake, exercise, relaxation, hyperventilation, stress, and even fluorescent lighting.[23] Nocturnal panic attacks may occur in as many as 69% of patients with panic disorder.[24] Nocturnal panic symptoms are usually more intense than those of daytime attacks. Patients with nocturnal panic attacks experience worse daytime panic attacks and more somatic symptoms than daytime-only panic disorder patients.[25] Symptoms similar to nocturnal panic attacks may be observed in patients with sleep apnea[26] and paroxysmal dystonia.[27] In a study of 70 patients with panic disorder, 63.5% reported frequent nocturnal panic attacks; a surprising 46% reported sleep paralysis, and another 42.6% reported hypnagogic hallucinations.[28]

Early studies suggested that increased central medullary carbon dioxide receptor sensitivity was at fault, particularly in nocturnal panic attacks.[29] However, a study by Craske and Barlow showed no difference between sleep panic and daytime-only panic patients in response to carbon dioxide challenge.[30] It has been suggested that patients with only sleep panic have more frequent depression than panic disorder patients who do not experience sleep-related panic attacks.[31] Other associations have been drawn between panic disorders and major depression. Uhde and colleagues found that panic disorder patients had decreased REM sleep latency but reduced REM density.[32] Contrasting this, another study reported that patients with mixed major depression and panic disorder have longer REM sleep onset and higher REM density than depressed patients without panic disorder.[33] Patients with major depression with panic disorder may have earlier age onset of illness, longer episode duration, worse symptoms, and more impairment. The sleep-onset latency is longer in patients with major depression and major depression with panic disorder than in normals.[34] Primary major depressives have shorter REM sleep latency and a higher percentage of REM sleep than controls or panic disorder patients, though, as previously mentioned, panic disorder patients are also often noted to have shorter REM sleep onset than controls.

GENERALIZED ANXIETY DISORDER

Patients with generalized anxiety disorder typically have prolonged sleep-onset latency, increased stage 1 and 2 sleep, less slow-wave sleep, a smaller REM sleep percentage, and increased or normal REM sleep latency.[35,36] One report suggested that REMs are decreased in patients with generalized anxiety disorder.[35] Compared to patients with major depression, patients with generalized anxiety disorder have fewer awakenings.[37] No difference has been found between patients with generalized anxiety disorder alone and those with generalized anxiety disorder and depression.

OBSESSIVE COMPULSIVE DISORDER

Patients with obsessive compulsive disorder show decreased total sleep time, increased number of awakenings, reduced stage 4 sleep, and reduced sleep efficiency. It has also been suggested that there is comparable reduced REM sleep latency in patients with bipolar depression, but lower REM density and higher stage 1 and 3 sleep.[38]

EATING DISORDERS

Most studies of bulimics show very little change in REM sleep measures as compared to controls. In one study by Hudson and coworkers, bulimics had the same sleep architecture as controls except for a trend toward increased REM density in the first REM sleep episode.[39] Another study by Weiberg and colleagues showed that normal-weight bulimics had long REM sleep latency.[40] REM sleep architecture studies of patients with anorexia nervosa have been more contradictory: some report no change in REM sleep parameters[41] while others suggest that there are changes similar to those seen in major depression.[42] Patients with severe untreated anorexia nervosa often show reduced total sleep time, decreased sleep efficiency, increased wakefulness after sleep onset, and increased stage 1 and decreased slow-wave sleep. Sleep normalizes after weight is gained.[43,44] One study suggested that perhaps there is initial shortening of the REM sleep latency with severe weight loss but that with recovery of weight the REM sleep latency returns to normal.[45]

SCHIZOPHRENIA

Patients with acute manifestations of schizophrenia often sleep worse. In a study of young adult schizophrenics it was found that total sleep time and total REM sleep were decreased immediately on withdrawal of neuroleptics.[46] Patients with tardive dyskinesia had earlier onset of REM suppression after withdrawal of medication. Mean REM sleep latency was shorter, and total REM sleep time was greater in patients with tardive dyskinesia than in those without tardive dyskinesia. NREM sleep parameters improved more upon withdrawal of medication than REM sleep parameters. All had prolonged sleep onset latency. Slow-wave sleep was more abundant in patients without tardive dyskinesia.

In patients with chronic schizophrenia, normal sleep latency has been observed. Studies show no differences in sleep quality and quantity of older schizophrenics and other older adults.[47] Two studies have suggested an inverse relationship between stage 4 sleep and brain ventricle size.[48,49]

The first attempt to establish a connection between REM sleep abnormalities and schizophrenia was reported by Dement in 1955.[50] This study, done before the advent of neuroleptics, found shortened REM sleep latency but no difference in eye movement activity in schizophrenics. Despite subsequent conflicts in the literature about whether there is shorter REM sleep latency in schizophrenia,[51-56] the relationship between the hallucinatory activity that normally occurs in REM sleep and the hallucinations of schizophrenics have continued to intrigue investigators. Dement[50] was the first to propose that there may be a link.

Acute schizophrenics have no REM sleep rebound after REM sleep deprivation, whereas chronic schizophrenics without active symptoms have more rebound than normal.[51,57] A subsequent hydraulic "leakage" theory of schizophrenia was developed, which posited that the hallucinatory activity of REM sleep "leaked" into wakefulness in schizophrenics.[58] This theory was developed because studies showed that there were reductions in intricate themes, clarity, and vividness in the dreams of these patients.[50,59]

Another theory later developed by Dement and coworkers holds that schizophrenics have hallucinations resulting from ponto-geniculo-occipital (PGO) discharges in the waking state due to serotonin depletion in the brain.[60] Recordings of waking periorbital potentials and middle ear muscle activity during sleep showed no increased activity compared to normals; however no sleeping comparisons were performed.[61]

Models from artificial intelligence theory suggested that the central nervous system (CNS) malfunction in schizophrenia occurs because of ineffective REM sleep. REM sleep was theorized to be necessary to eliminate "parasitic states" in which too many neural connections interfere with information processing and memory.[62] One of the most recent studies that attempted to link REM sleep to schizophrenia was done by Weiler and colleagues.[63] Brain glucose metabolism was evaluated in 49 schizophrenics, 30 awake controls, and 12 controls during

REM sleep by positron emission tomography. No relationship was found between glucose utilization in REM sleep for awake schizophrenics and controls in REM sleep, including patients with active hallucinations. The glucose utilization in awake schizophrenics most closely resembled that of awake controls.[63]

A better-accepted theory of schizophrenia is that it is due to an imbalance of dopamine and acetylcholine in key CNS structures. Dopaminergic activity has been shown to increase in the psychotic phase, and a compensatory increased of muscarinic acetylcholine activity in turn results in increased negative symptoms. In a study of the effects on REM sleep latency in schizophrenics and controls of biperiden, an antimuscarinic M-1 agent, it was found that the psychotic patients had a smaller increase in REM latency. Biperiden also increased positive symptoms and decreased negative ones.[64] It has also been reported that prolactin secretion is increased during sleep in schizophrenics. This may reflect abnormalities in the dopaminergic system.[65] One study also linked decreased REM sleep latency and increased REM density with the negative symptoms of schizophrenia and attributed these changes to increased CNS muscarinic activity.[66]

Assuming that the dopaminergic/acetylcholinergic imbalance theory is correct, variations in REM sleep parameters that have been reported by numerous investigators could be explained by the phase of the illness, the degree of neurotransmitter imbalance, and the influence of short- and long-term use of medication. Sleep apnea has been reported to aggravate schizophrenia symptoms,[67] and incidence of paranoid psychosis is increased in narcoleptics, especially following stimulant use.[68] As both narcolepsy and schizophrenia have been linked to abnormalities in the dopaminergic-acetylcholinergic system, investigation of the shared mechanisms of psychosis may yield important information.

BORDERLINE PERSONALITY DISORDER

Borderline personality disorder as defined by the *DSM III-R* encompasses a number of symptoms of other psychiatric disorders, including major depression. In numerous studies of borderline personality disorder, it has been shown repeatedly that the sleep architecture changes are very similar to those observed in patients with major depression.[69-72] Borderline personality disorder patients have less total sleep time, less sleep efficiency, reduced slow-wave sleep, increased stage 2 sleep, reduced REM sleep latency, and increased REM density. Subjects with borderline personality disorder have also been shown to have abnormalities of other biologic markers associated with depression.[73]

BIPOLAR DISORDER, MANIC PHASE

Patients in the manic phase of bipolar disorder have been shown to have much reduced total sleep time, which gradually extends as the manic phase passes.[74] There is also a reduction in stage 3 and 4 sleep. No consistent change in REM sleep has been found,[74,75] probably owing to excitability and subsequent reduction of total sleep in these patients. It has been suggested that the switch from euthymia or depression into the manic phase occurs during sleep.[76] Lithium, which is the primary drug used to treat the manic phase of bipolar disorder, has been found to increase slow-wave sleep and reduce REM sleep.

POSTTRAUMATIC STRESS DISORDER

Posttraumatic stress disorder is caused by involvement in events not normally experienced by the average person, usually by exposure to combat, torture, or other situations involving physical and psychological abuse. It has been associated with increased sleep-onset latency, decreased sleep efficiency, increased wakefulness after sleep onset, decreased total sleep time, reduction in stage 2 sleep, and increased stage 1 sleep.[77] Frequent nightmares are a hallmark of posttraumatic stress disorder, involving both reliving of true experiences and nightmares of gruesome or life-threatening content. Controversy over effects on REM sleep exists: some authors report normal REM sleep parameters[77] while others report reduced REM sleep latency and increased REM density.[78,79] Nightmare experiences have been found to occur during both NREM and REM sleep.[80,81] REM sleep behavior disorder has also been associated with posttraumatic stress disorder.[82,83] Ross and coworkers speculated that post-traumatic stress disorder may be a disorder of REM sleep mechanisms and suggested that potent REM-suppressing medications, such as monoamine oxidase inhibitors, are responsible for the improvement seen in nightmares and flashbacks.[84]

MEDICATION EFFECTS AND SUBSTANCE ABUSE

The reader is referred to Table 21-2 for a review of the acute, chronic, and withdrawal effects on sleep parameters of various medications and substances of abuse.

APPROACH TO SLEEP DISORDERS PATIENTS WITH SYMPTOMS OF PSYCHIATRIC ILLNESS

Patients with sleep disorders frequently have symptoms of psychiatric illness. It is the task of the sleep disorders specialist to determine whether there is an underlying organic disorder such as sleep apnea, restless legs syndrome, or periodic limb movements that may be entirely responsible for the symptoms. Conversely, though many sleep disorders practitioners have inadequate training in psychiatry to appropriately diagnose and treat psychiatric disorders, it behooves nonpsychiatrist sleep disorders medicine specialists to gain enough experience in recognizing and treating psychiatric illness to help mental health workers appropriately care for patients with psychiatric illness and sleep disturbance. Psychiatrists may not be aware that tricyclic antidepressants may aggravate restless legs syndrome or that certain newer-generation antidepressants such as fluoxetine, which has an alerting effect, may lead to insomnia. Psychiatrists may also need the guidance of a sleep specialist in selecting the proper sedative hypnotic for their patient. Specifically, they may need help understanding the pharmacologic properties—onset of action, duration of action, relative toxicity, drug interactions, and withdrawal effects.

As most sleep practitioners do not have extensive psychiatric training, it is often necessary to engage the assistance of a psychiatrist or psychologist to evaluate a patient with suspected or known psychiatric illness. Psychological tests such as the Minnesota Multiphasic Personality Inventory are useful for screening patients with sleep disorders for psychopathology. However, these tests alone are somewhat limited. Many patients with untreated organic sleep disorders such as narcolepsy show changes in psychological tests that are suggestive of psychopathology, but the changes may resolve following effective treatment. Though there is currently little objective data that shows that behavioral techniques are useful in improving insomnia in patients with psychiatric illness, it is this author's experience that patients with a variety of psychiatric disorders can benefit from behavioral methods. Data have recently become available showing that patients with chronic sleep onset insomnia have sustained benefit with[85] and without[86] adjunctive sedative administration.

As evidenced in the preceding sections on various psychopathologic states, the severity of the insomnia of a psychiatric patient often parallels the severity of the illness. The aggressiveness of medication and behavioral management of insomnia in psychiatric patients should parallel the severity of psychiatric symptoms present. Patients with severe sleep disturbances and aggressiveness due to schizophrenia or affective psychosis often require very

TABLE 21-2.   Drugs That Affect Sleep

Drug		Effects on sleep	Comments
Barbiturates	Acute:	↑ TST	Rapid development of tolerance
		↓ Wake after sleep onset (WASO)	Withdrawal insomnia
		↓ REM	Daytime sedation
		↑ Stage 2, ↑ spindles	
		↑ or ↓ delta	
	Withdrawal:	↓ TST	
Benzodiazepines	Acute:	↓ SL (most agents)	Agents vary in onset and duration of action
		↑ TST	Daytime sedation (with long acting agents)
		↓ WASO	Tolerance develops (with short-acting agents)
		↓ REM	Withdrawal insomnia (with short-acting
		↑ Stage 2, ↑ spindles	agents)
		↓ Delta (most agents;	
		some ↑ delta)	
	Withdrawal:	↓ TST	
Chloral hydrate		↑ TST	Little information on tolerance or withdrawal
		→REM	
		→Stage 2	
		→Delta	
L-Tryptophan		→or ↑ TST	Effects are mild and inconsistent, and may be
		→or ↓ REM	delayed
		↑ Delta	
Alcohol	Acute:	↑ TST (1st half of night;	Acute effects variable
		↓ 2nd half)	
		↓ WASO (1st half of night;	
		↑ 2nd half)	
		↓ REM (1st half of night)	
		↑ Delta	
	Chronic:	→TST	
		→REM	
		↓ Delta	
	Withdrawal:	↓ TST	Degree of REM rebound may correlate with
		↑ WASO	likelihood of withdrawal delirium
		↑ REM	
		↓ Delta	
Narcotics	Acute:	↑ WASO	Effects vary with specific agents
		↓ REM	
		↓ Delta (total), with	
		↑ delta "bursts"	
	Chronic:	→WASO	Hypersomnolence may occur during with-
		→Delta	drawal
	Withdrawal:	↓ WASO	
Aspirin	Acute:	↓ Delta	May act via prostaglandin inhibition and
			temperature effects
Amphetamine	Acute	↓ TST	Sleep-wake cycle may be severely disrupted
		↑ WASO, ↑ movements	during acute use and withdrawal
		↓ REM	
		↓ Delta	
	Withdrawal:	↑ TST	
		↑ REM	
Caffeine		↑ SL	May have effects on sleep EEG even when no
		↓ TST	subjective disturbance occurs
		↑ WASO	
		↓ REM	
		↓ Delta (1st half of night)	
Miscellaneous stimulants		↑ SL	
(nicotine, cocaine,		↓ TST	
pemoline, methylphenidate)		↓ REM	

TABLE 21-2.   *(Continued)*

Drug		Effects on sleep	Comments
Antidepressants (tricyclic and monoamine oxidase inhibitors)	Acute:	↓ WASO ↓ REM ↑ Stage 2 ↑ Delta	Sleep effects vary with sedative potential of specific agent; MAOIs may cause ↑ WASO
	Withdrawal:	↑ WASO ↑ REM	
Lithium		↓ REM ↑ Delta	
Phenothiazines		↑ TST ↑ Delta	Effects mild and variable, according to specific agent; REM effects inconsistent
Reserpine		↑ WASO ↑ REM ↑ Delta	Can cause insomnia, nightmares
Yohimbine		↑ REM ↓ Delta	
Clonidine		→TST ↑ WASO ↑ Stage shifts ↓ REM	Can cause insomnia, daytime sedation
α-Methyldopa		↑ REM (1st half of night) ↓ Delta	Can cause nightmares
Diuretics		↑ WASO	Probably acts via nocturia, hemodynamic effects
Cimetidine		↑ Delta	Can cause daytime sedation
Baclofen		↑ TST	
L-Dopa		→TST →or ↑ REM →Delta	In toxic doses, causes insomnia, delirium
Methysergide		→TST →or ↑ REM ↑ Delta	
γ-Hydroxybutyrate		↑ TST	
Steroids		↑ WASO	

Key: SL, sleep latency; WASO, wakefulness after sleep onset; REM, rapid eye movement sleep; TST, total sleep time.
↑ = increased; ↓ = decreased; → = unchanged.
From Buysse DJ, Reynolds CF. Insomnia. In: Thorpy MJ, ed. Handbook of Sleep Disorders. New York, Marcel Dekker, 1990;18:373–434.

sedating neuroleptics as well as adjunctive sedative-hypnotics. Patients with schizophrenia and affective disorders with nocturnal hallucinations may need additional neuroleptic medication to reduce nighttime hallucinations. Chronic psychiatric illnesses with associated insomnia are much more difficult to manage and may require long-term administration of benzodiazepines, including sedative hypnotics of that class. Others whose psychiatric illnesses are intermittent, like major depression, may require sedative hypnotics only during the active phase of the illness.

In milder cases, in which the individual is often considered essentially normal, there may be obsessional characteristics or traits that result in chronic insomnia. DuPont has even suggested that there is a subset of persons with chronic insomnia who develop performance anxiety specifically about sleep that can benefit from benzodiazepines.[87] In addi-

tion, DuPont and Saylor believe that the anxiolytic effects of the benzodiazepines are sustained for months or years and that individuals may be able to function well on small doses of benzodiazepines without tending to abuse the drug or increase the dose.[88]

In some instances, medications used in psychiatric patients aggravate an existing organic sleep problem or aggravate insomnia. Antidepressants, antipsychotics, and antihistamines may tend to aggravate restless legs syndrome. Sometimes, nocturnal akathisia is caused by neuroleptic compounds and has symptoms almost identical to restless legs syndrome. Medications such as the monoamine oxidase inhibitors fluoxetine, sertraline, bupropion, protriptyline, and buspirone, which have stimulant properties, may aggravate insomnia.

It is not unusual for patients with psychiatric illness, particularly schizophrenia, to have "pseudo insomnia." The underlying cause for the inability to perceive sleep when it occurs is unknown in these patients but is often vexing to the patient, the family, and the physician. The problem is often easily identified because the patient complains of little or no sleep but paradoxically has no daytime fatigue or other impairment. Although the patient is rarely reassured by an overnight study that confirms adequate sleep, the family and health care providers are often relieved to have the information. In addition, it is not uncommon to see patients with undetected psychiatric symptoms who exhibit alpha intrusion throughout the sleep EEG. Alpha intrusion has been identified in patients with obsessive characteristics and illnesses associated with somatic complaints. Patients with chronic insomnia and the finding of alpha intrusion often warrant more thorough psychological assessment. When obsessive characteristics are identified, medications with specific antiobsessive effects such as clomipramine and the serotonin reuptake inhibitors are sometimes quite helpful.

The appropriate selection of a sedative-hypnotic for patients with psychiatric illness is often more difficult than for the general population. There is greater potential for adverse drug interactions between multiple psychotropic medications than between most sedative-hypnotics alone and medications used for other medical conditions. Particular attention has to be paid to the duration of action of sedatives in patients who have anxiety. There may be a tendency for rebound anxiety in patients taking short- and intermediate-acting sedative hypnotics. This problem can be circumvented by using longer-acting sedative hypnotics such as flurazepam or quazepam at bedtime, relying on the long-life (80 and 20 hours, respectively) to reduce anxiety during the day. Alternative approaches include using multiple doses of intermediate-acting benzodiazepines (e.g., alprazolam, oxazepam) and using that same medication at bedtime as a sedative. Another approach is to use a long-acting antianxiety agent such as diazepam, clonazepam or chlordiazepoxide less frequently during the day and also as a sedative. As most of the intermediate and long-acting benzodiazepines antianxiety agents have delayed onset, it is often best that they be given about an hour before bedtime for the sedative properties to have enough time to take effect. Patients with nocturnal panic attacks may benefit from benzodiazepines such as alprazolam, estazolam, or clonazepam. In addition, various antidepressants, β-blockers, calcium channel blockers, and α-agonists may be useful.

In patients with chronic psychiatric illness with associated chronic insomnia it is very important for the patient to be followed carefully, to ensure that no long-term adverse effects result from psychotropic drugs and, in cases where abusable medications are necessary, that the patient does not develop tolerance leading to excessive usage. When a patient presents to the sleep disorders center taking excessive amounts of sedative-hypnotics with abuse potential, it is very important to determine whether there is a psychiatric illness or any underlying tendency to abuse drugs. Unfortunately, some patients who begin with sleep disorders such as persistent psychophysiologic insomnia and periodic limb movements never have the underlying causes of their insomnia identified, and resort to long-term use of sleeping medications. These persons may increase the dose of the sedative to quite large amounts to achieve sleep yet do not experience the craving or euphoria often associated with substance abuse. For them, it is quite important to identify the underlying causes of the sleep problem. With long-term use of large doses of sedative-hypnotics, it is very important that the patient be gradually tapered by as little as one-fourth the therapeutic dose per week until the medication is eliminated. After treatment of underlying organic sleep disorders and training in sleep hygiene and relaxation skills, these patients are often able to sleep without the help of excessive amounts of medication.

REFERENCES

1. Mosko S, Zetin M, Glen S, et al. Self-reported depressive symptomatology, mood ratings, and treatment outcome in sleep disorders patients. J Clin Psychology 1989;45:51–60.
2. Regier DA, Burke JD, Christie KA. Comorbidity of affective and anxiety disorders in population based studies: The NIMH Epidemiological Catchment Area (ECA) program. In: Maser JD, Cloninger CR, eds. Comorbidity of Anxiety and Depressive Disorders. Washington, D.C.: American Psychiatric Press, 1990.
3. Ford DE, Kamerow DB. Epidemiological study of sleep disturbances and psychiatric disorders. JAMA 1989;262:1479–1484.
4. Mellinger GD, Balter MB, Uhlenmuth EH. Insomnia and its treatment: Prevalence and correlates. Arch Gen Psychiatry 1985;42:225–232.
5. Kales A, Caldwell AB, Soldatos CR, et al. Biopsychobehavioral correlates of insomnia.II. Pattern specificity and consistency with the Minnesota Multiphasic Personality Inventory. Psychosomat Med 1983;45:341–356.
6. Bliwise NG, Bliwise DL, Dement WC. Age and psychopathology in insomnia. Clin Gereontologist 1985; 4:3–9.
7. Gillin JC: Sleep studies in affective illness. Diagnostic, therapeutic and pathophysiological implication. Psychiatr Ann 1983;13:367–384.
8. Puig-Antich J, Goetz R, Hanlon C, et al. Sleep architecture and REM sleep measures in prepubertal major depressives during an episode. Arch Gen Psychiatry 1982;39:932–939.

9. Young W, Knowles JB, MacLean AW. The sleep of childhood depressives: Comparison with age-matched controls. Biol Psychiatry 1982;17:1163–1169.

10. Emslie GJ, Roffwarg HP, Rush AJ, et al. Children with major depression show reduced rapid eye movement latencies. Arch Gen Psychiatry 1990;47:119–123.

11. Giles DE, Roffwarg HP, Kupfer DJ. Secular trend in unipolar depression: A hypothesis. J Affect Dis 1989; 14:51–59.

12. Dahlre, Puig-Antich J, Ryan N, et al. EEG sleep in adolescents with major depression: The role of suicidality and inpatient status. J Affect Disord 1990;19:63–75.

13. Naylor MW, Shain BN, Shipley JE. REM latency in psychotically depressed adolescents. Biol Psychiatry 1990;28:161–164.

14. Sabo E, Reynolds CF, Kupfer DJ, et al. Sleep, depression and suicide. Psychiatry Res 1991;36:265–277.

15. Reynolds CF, Kupfer DJ, Thase ME, et al. Sleep, gender and depression: An analysis of gender effects on the electroencephalographic sleep of 302 depressed outpatients. Biol Psychiatry 1990;28:673–684.

16. Hawkins DR, Taub JM, Van de Castle RL. Extended sleep (hypersomnia) in young, depressed patients. Am J Psychiatry 1985;142:905–910.

17. Nofzinger EA, Thase ME, Reynolds CF, et al. Hypersomnia in bipolar depression: A comparison with narcolepsy using the multiple sleep latency test. Am J Psychiatry 1991;148:1177–1181.

18. Reynolds CF. Sleep and affective disorders. A minireview. Psychiatr Clin North Am 1987;10:583–591.

19. Hoch CC, Buysse DJ, Reynolds CF. Sleep and depression in late life. Clin Geriatr Med 1989;5:259–274.

20. Dealy RS, Reynolds CF, Spiker DG, et al. Effect of ECT on EEG sleep measures in depression. Sleep Res 1982;11:119.

21. Sheehan DV, Ballenger J, Jacobsen G. Treatment of endogenous anxiety with phobic, hysterical, and hypochondriacal symptoms. Arch Gen Psychiatry 1980;37:51–59.

22. Mellman TA, Uhde TW. Electroencephalographic sleep in panic disorder. Arch Gen Psychiatry 1989;46:178–184.

23. Roy-Byrne PP, Uhde TW. Exogenous factors in panic disorder. Clinical and research implications. J Clin Psychiatry 1988;49:56–61.

24. Mellman TA, Uhde TW. Sleep in panic and generalized anxiety disorders, In: Ballenger JC ed. Neurobiological Aspects of Panic Disorder. New York: Alan R Liss, 1987;5:94–100.

25. Craske MG, Barlow DH. Nocturnal panic. J Nerv Ment Dis 1989;177:160–167.

26. Edlund MJ, McNamara EM, Millman RP. Sleep apnea and panic attacks. Compr Psychiatry 1991;32:130–132.

27. Stoudemire A, Ninan PT, Wooten V. Hypnogenic paroxysmal dystonia with panic attacks responsive to drug therapy. Psychosomatics 1987;28:280–281.

28. Patterson WM, Koplan AL, Shehi GM, et al. Clinical correlates in patients with panic disorder: Depression, sleep disturbances, memory recall and rage reactions. Presented to the 34th annual meeting of the Academy of Psychosomatic Medicine, Nov 12–15, 1988. Kalamazoo, Mich: Upjohn, 1989.

29. Gorman JM, Askanazi J, Liebowitz MR, et al. Response to hyperventilation in a group of patients with panic disorder. Am J Psychiatry 1984;141:857–861.

30. Craske MG, Barlow DH. Nocturnal panic: Response to hyperventilation and carbon dioxide challenge. J Abnorm Psychol 1990;99:302–307.

31. Mellman TA, Uhde TW. Sleep panic attacks: New clinical findings and theoretical implications. Am J Psychiatry 1989;146:1204–1207.

32. Uhde TW, Roy-Byrne P, Gillin JC, et al. The sleep of patients with panic disorder: A preliminary report. Psychiatry Res 1985;12:251–259.

33. Grunhaus L, Rabin D, Harel Y, et al. Simultaneous panic and depressive disorders: Clinical and sleep EEG correlates. Psychiatry Res 1986;17:251–259.

34. Dube S, Jones DA, Bell J, et al. Interface of panic and depression: Clinical-EEG correlates. Psychiatry Res 1986;19:119–133.

35. Reynolds CF, Shaw DH, Newton TF, et al. EEG sleep in outpatients with generalized anxiety: A preliminary comparison with depressed outpatients. Psychiatry Res 1983;8:81–89.

36. Papadimitriou GN, Kerkhofs M, Kempenaers C, et al. EEG sleep studies in patients with generalized anxiety disorder. Psychiatry Res 1988;26:183–190.

37. Papadimitriou GN, Linkowski P, Kerkhofs M, et al. Sleep EEG recordings in generalized anxiety disorder with significant depression. J Affect Disord 1988; 15:113–118.

38. Insel TR, Gillin JC, Moore A, et al. The sleep of patients with obsessive compulsive disorders. Arch Gen Psychiatry 1982;39:1372–1377.

39. Hudson JI, Pope HG, Jonas JM, et al. Sleep EEG in bulimia. Biol Psychiatry 1987;22:820–828.

40. Weiberg JB, Stakes JW, Brotman A, et al. Sleep architecture in bulimia: A pilot study. Biol Psychiatry 1985;20:225–228.

41. Lauer C, Zulley J, Krieg JC, et al. EEG sleep and the cholinergic induction test in anorexic and bulimic patients. Psychiatry Res 1988,26:171–181.

42. Katz JL, Kuperberg A, Pollack CP, et al. Is there a relationship between eating and affective disorders? New evidence from sleep recordings. Am J Psychiatry 1984;141:753–759.

43. Neil JF, Merikangas JR, Foster FG, et al. Waking and all-night sleep EEGs in anorexia nervosa. Clin Electroencephalographer 1980;11:9–15.

44. Lacey JH, Crips AH, Kalucey RS, et al, Weight gain and the sleeping electroencephalogram: Study of ten patients with anorexia nervosa. Br Med J 1975;4:556–558.

45. Bergiannaki JD, Soldatos CR, Sakkas PN, et al. Longitudinal studies of biologic markers for depression in male anorectics. Psychoneuroendocrinology 1987;12:237–239.

46. Thaker GK, Wagman AMI, Tamminga CA. Sleep polygraphy in schizophrenia: Methodological issues. Biol Psychiatry 1990;28:240–246.

47. Paul PK, Ancoli-Israel S, Jeste DV, et al. Sleep in older schizophrenic patients. Presented at the 6th Annual

Meeting of the Association of Professional Sleep Societies. Rochester, Minn., June 2, 1992. APSS Meeting Abstracts 1992;128.

48. van Kammen DP, van Kammen WB, Peters J, et al. Decreased slow wave sleep and enlarged lateral ventricles in schizophrenia. Neuropsychopharmacology 1988;1:265–271.

49. Benson KL, Zarcone VP. Slow wave sleep and brain structural imaging in schizophrenia. Presented at the 6th Annual Meeting of the Association of Professional Sleep Societies. Rochester, Minn., June 2, 1992. APSS Meeting Abstracts 1992;128.

50. Dement WC. Dream recall and eye movements in schizophrenics and normals. J Nerv Ment Dis 1955;122:263–269.

51. Gulevich GD, Dement WC, Zarcone VP. All night sleep recordings of chronic schizophrenics in remission. Compr Psychiatry 1967;8:141–149.

52. Jus K, Bouchard M, Jus AK, et al. Sleep EEG variables in untreated long-term schizophrenic patients. Arch Gen Psychiatry 1973;29:386–390.

53. Hiatt JF, Floyd TC, Katz PH, et al. Further evidence of abnormal non-rapid-eye-movement sleep in schizophrenia. Arch Gen Psychiatry 1985;42:797–802.

54. Caldwell DF, Domino DF. Electroencephalographic and eye movement patterns during sleep in chronic schizophrenia. Electroencephalogr Clin Neurophysiol 1967;22:414–420.

55. Reich L, Weiss BL, Coble P, et al. Sleep disturbance in schizophrenia: A revisit. Arch Gen Psychiatry 1975; 32:51–55.

56. Ganguli R, Reynolds CF, Kupfer DJ. Electroencephalographic sleep in young never-medicated schizophrenics. Arch Gen Psychiatry 1987;44:36–44.

57. Azumi K: A polygraphic study of sleep in schizophrenics. Seishin Shinkeigaku Zasshi 1966. 68:1222–1241.

58. Wyatt R, Termini BA, Davis J. A review of the literature 1960–1970. Part II. Sleep studies. Schizophr Bull 1969;1:45–66.

59. Cartwright RD. Sleep fantasy in normal and schizophrenic persons. J Abnorm Psychol 1972;80:275–279.

60. Dement WC, Zarcone VP, Feruson J, et al. Some parallel findings in schizophrenic patients and serotonin depleted cats. In: Sankar S, ed. Schizophrenia: Current Concepts and Research. Hicksville, NY: PJD, 1969;1: 775–811.

61. Benson, KL, Zarcone VP. Testing the REM sleep phasic event intrusion hypothesis of schizophrenia. Psychiatry Res 1985;15:163–172.

62. Crick F, Michelson G. The function of dream sleep. Nature 1983;304;111–114.

63. Weiler MA, Buchsbaum MS, Gillin JC, et al. Explorations in the relationship of dream sleep to schizophrenia using position emission tomography. Neuropsychobiology 1990;23:109–118.

64. Tandon R, Shipley JE, Greden JF, et al, Muscarinic cholinergic hyperactivity in schizophrenia. Relationship to positive and negative symptoms, Schizophrenia Res 1991;4:23–30.

65. Cauter EV, Linkowski P, Kerkhofs M, et al. Circadian and sleep-related endocrine rhythms in schizophrenia. Arch Gen Psychiatry 1991;48:348–356.

66. Tandon R, Shipley JE, Eiser AS, et al. Association between abnormal REM sleep and negative symptoms, in schizophrenia. Psychiatry Res 1988;27:359–361.

67. Berrettini WH. Paranoid psychosis and sleep apnea syndrome. Am J Psychiatry 1980;137:493–494.

68. Leong GB, Shaner AL, Silva JA. Narcolepsy, paranoid psychosis and analeptic abuse. 1989;14:481–483.

69. Akiskal HS: Subaffective disorders. Dysthymic, cyclothymic and bipolar II disorders in the borderline realm. Psychiatr Clin North Am 1981;4:25–46.

70. Akiskal HS, Yerevanian BI, Davis GC, et al. The nosologic status of borderline personality: Clinical and polysomnographic study. Am J Psychiatry 1985;142: 192–198.

71. Reynolds, CF, Soloff PH, Taska LS, et al. EEG sleep evaluation of depression in borderline patients: A prospective replication. Sleep Res 1984;13:124.

72. Bell J, Lycaki H. Jones D. et al. Effect of preexisting borderline personality disorder on clinical and EEG sleep correlates of depression. Psychiatry Res 1983; 9:115–123.

73. Lahmeyer HW, Val E, Gaviria FM, et al. EEG sleep, lithium transport, dexamethasone suppression, and monoamine oxidase activity in borderline personality disorder. Psychiatry Res 1988;25:19–30.

74. Hartman E. Longitudinal studies of sleep and dream patterns in manic-depressive patients. Arch Gen Psychiatry 1968;19:312–329.

75. Hudson JI, Lipinski JF, Frankenburg FR, et al. Electroencephalographic sleep in mania. Arch Gen Psychiatry 1988;45:267–273.

76. Bunny WE, Wehr TR, Gillin JC, et al. The switch process in manic-depressive psychosis. Ann Inter Med 1977;87:319–335.

77. van Kammen W, Christiansen C, Van Kammen D, et al. Sleep and the POW experience. Sleep Res 1987;16:291.

78. Greenberg R. Pearlman CA, Gampel D. War neuroses and the adaptive function of REM sleep. Br J Med Psychol 1972;1972:27–33.

79. Kauffman CD, Reist C, Djenderedjian A, et al. Biological markers of affective disorders and post traumatic stress disorder: A pilot study with desipramine. J Clin Psychiatry 1987;48:366–367.

80. Schlosberg A, Benjamin M. Sleep patterns in three acute combat fatigue cases. J Clin Psychiatry 1978;39:546–549.

81. van der Kolk B, Blitz R, Burr W, et al. Nightmares and trauma: A comparison of nightmares after combat with lifelong nightmares in veterans. Am J Psychiatry 1984;41: 187–190.

82. Hefez A, Metz L, Lavie P. Long term effects of extreme situational stress on sleep and dreaming. Am J Psychiatry 1987;144:344–347.

83. Schenck CH, Hurwitz TD, Mahowal MW. REM sleep behavior disorder. Am J Psychiatry 1988;145:652.

84. Ross RJ, Ball WA, Sullivan KA, et al. Sleep disturbances as the hallmark of post traumatic stress disorder. Am J Psychiatry 1989;146:697–707.

85. Milby JB, Williams V, Wooten V, et al. Effectiveness of combined triazolam-behavioral therapy for treatment of persistent disorders of initiating and maintaining sleep. Accepted for publication. Am J Psychiatry 1993.

86. McClusky HY, Milby JB, Switzer PK, et al. Efficacy of behavioral versus triazolam treatment in persistent sleep-onset insomnia. Am J Psychiatry 1991;149:121–125.

87. DuPont RL. Overcoming Sleep Disorders. A Guide for Insomniacs. Rockville, Md.: Institute for Behavior and Health, 1990;1:1–29.

88. DuPont RL, Saylor KE. Sedatives/hypnotics and benzodiazepines. In: Clinical Textbook of Addictive Disorders. Frances RV, Miller SI, eds. New York: Guilford Press, 1991;1:69–102.

22

Sleep and Other Medical Disorders

Sudhansu Chokroverty

Sleep disturbances associated with seven medical disorders are listed under the category of medical-psychiatric sleep disorders in the International Classification of Sleep Disorders (ICSD)[1]: sleeping sickness, nocturnal cardiac ischemia, chronic obstructive pulmonary disease, sleep-related asthma, sleep-related gastroesophageal reflux, peptic ulcer disease, and fibrositis syndrome. A number of other medical disorders may cause severe disturbances of sleep and breathing that have important practical implications, in terms of diagnosis, prognosis, and treatment. These other medical disorders not listed in the ICSD are also briefly reviewed in this chapter, to give an overview of sleep disturbances in the general medical disorders. The reason for their inclusion is that sleep disturbance itself may adversely affect the course of the medical illness, and, of course, the medical disorders and drugs prescribed to treat these may also have deleterious effects on sleep and breathing.

When a patient presents to a sleep specialist, with sleep disturbance, either with the complaint of insomnia or hypersomnia, the first important step is to obtain a detailed medical history and other histories, followed by physical examination to uncover a cause for the sleep disturbance. Often, the patient presents to an internist, who may then refer for a consultation to a sleep specialist if there are sleep complaints. Therefore, a comprehensive knowledge of major medical disorders that may present with sleep disturbance is essential, and in this section a brief outline of the salient clinical diagnostic points is offered, followed by some key laboratory investigations of some important medical disorders presenting with sleep disturbance.

Gislason and Almqvist[2] made an epidemiologic study in a random sample of 4064 Swedish men aged 30 to 69 years. Difficulty initiating or maintaining sleep and too little sleep were the major complaints, followed by excessive daytime somnolence (EDS) or too much sleep. Sleep maintenance problems became more frequent with increasing age. The following conditions were associated with the sleep complaints: systemic hypertension, bronchitis and bronchial asthma, musculoskeletal disorders, obesity, and diabetes mellitus. The authors suggested that the reported increased in mortality among patients with sleep complaints might be related to the intercurrent somatic diseases.

In a questionnaire survey of 100 adult male medical and surgical patients in a teaching hospital in Melbourne, Australia, Johns and coworkers[3] found sleep duration to be the same as that in the general population. The sleep duration decreased from age 20 to 50 years, then increased again after age 60. Daytime sleep duration increased with age. In their survey they found that increasing age and ischemic heart disease were mostly associated with long-term sleep disturbances.

EXAMPLES OF THE MEDICAL DISORDERS THAT CAUSE SLEEP DISTURBANCES:

A brief description of the clinical features of some of the medical disorders associated with sleep disturbances is given in this section, but for further details readers should consult general textbooks of internal medicine.

Cardiovascular diseases: cardiac arrhythmia; congestive cardiac failure; ischemic heart disease; nocturnal angina

Intrinsic respiratory disorders: chronic obstructive pulmonary disease (COPD), asthma including nocturnal asthma, restrictive lung disease

Gastrointestinal diseases: peptic ulcer disease and reflux esophagitis

Endocrine diseases: hyperthyroidism, hypothyroidism, diabetes mellitus, growth hormone deficiency and excess

Renal disorders: chronic renal failure, sleep disturbances associated with renal dialysis

Hematologic disorders

Rheumatic disorders, including fibromyalgia syndrome

Miscellaneous disorders: acquired immunodeficiency syndrome, Lyme disease, medical and surgical disorders of patients in medical and surgical intensive care units (ICU), chronic fatigue syndrome, sleeping sickness.

MECHANISM OF SLEEP DISTURBANCES IN MEDICAL DISORDERS

Sleep disturbance itself may have an added adverse effect on the course of the medical illness. Thus, a vicious cycle may result from the effect of sleep disturbance on the medical disease and the effect of the medical illness on sleep architecture, and these effects are relevant for treating patients.

Sleep may be disturbed in medical disorders by a variety of mechanisms, listed here:

Indirect effects on the hypnogenic and respiratory neurons in the brain stem by metabolic disturbances (e.g., renal, hepatic, or respiratory failure, electrolyte disturbances, hypoglycemia, hyperglycemia, ketosis, toxic states)

Adverse effects on sleep organization and sleep structure by drugs used to treat medical illness

Disturbances of circadian rhythm (i.e., sleep-wake schedule)

Effects on the peripheral respiratory mechanism (including respiratory muscles) causing respiratory sleep disorder

Sleep disturbances by esophageal reflux, which may be due to the following factors: prolongation of acid clearance of the lower esophagus; aspiration; and reflex mechanism (see also Chapter 5).

GENERAL FEATURES OF SLEEP DISTURBANCES IN MEDICAL ILLNESS

Sleep architecture and sleep organization may be affected in a variety of medical illnesses. Patients may present with either insomnia or hypersomnolence, but most medical disorders present with insomnia. Some patients may have a mixture of insomnia and hypersomnolence (e.g., those with COPD or nocturnal asthma).

Patients with insomnia may complain of lack of initiation of sleep, inability to maintain sleep, repeated arousals at night, early morning awakening. Daytime symptoms of fatigue, inability to concentrate, irritability, anxiety, and sometimes depression[4] may be related to the sleep deprivation. Polysomnographic (PSG) findings are these[5]: prolonged sleep latency, reduction of the rapid eye movement (REM) sleep and slow-wave sleep, more than 10 awakenings per night, frequent stage shifts (15 to 20 per

night, i.e., three to four times the normal number); early morning awakening; increased waking after sleep onset (WASO); and increased percentage of wakefulness and stage 1 non-REM (NREM) sleep.

Patients with hypersomnolence may present with repeated daytime somnolence, fatigue, depression, headache, and intellectual deterioration related to repeated sleep-related disordered breathing and hypoxemia.[6–9] PSG findings consist of these[6–9]: sleep-disordered breathing, repeated arousals with oxygen desaturation at night, sleep fragmentation, sleep stage shifts, reduced slow-wave sleep, shortened sleep onset latency on Multiple Sleep Latency Tests (MSLT), and sometimes REM sleep abnormalities.

Systemic medical disorders may cause neurologic disturbances, which in turn may cause sleep disturbances either directly by affecting sleep-wake systems in the central nervous system (CNS) or indirectly by affecting breathing. Sleep-related breathing dysfunction and neurologic illness are described in Chapter 20.

SPECIFIC MEDICAL DISORDERS AND SLEEP DISTURBANCES

Cardiovascular Diseases

It is generally well-known that sleep disturbances may occur in cardiovascular diseases, particularly in patients with ischemic heart disease, myocardial infarction, or congestive cardiac failure. Cardiac arrhythmias and sudden cardiac death at night are also known to occur, though adequate objective tests, including PSG study to document such disturbances, are lacking.

Ischemic heart disease

A careful inquiry into history is most important in making the diagnosis. The patient complains of a sense of tightness in the middle of the chest and a bandlike feeling around the chest. The pain is often induced by exertion and relieved by rest. Generally it lasts only a few minutes. When the patient complains of pain on lying supine, it is known as angina decubitus, whereas pain that awakens the patient at night is known as "nocturnal angina." Infrequently, the pain results from coronary artery spasm accompanied by transient ST elevation in the electrocardiogram (ECG), and the entity is then known as Prinzmetal's or variant angina. The condition is most common in middle-aged men but may affect postmenopausal women. Complications include cardiac arrhythmias, left ventricular failure, acute myocardial infarction, and sudden cardiac, often nocturnal, death.

Sleep disturbances are very common in patients with ischemic heart disease. Pain may awaken the patient, causing frequent awakenings and reduced sleep efficiency. Sometimes, obstructive sleep apnea syndrome is associated with arterial hypoxemia causing cardiac ischemia. Simultaneous recording of ECG may show ST depression at least 1 mm below the horizontal, whereas in Prinzmetal's or variant angina there is ST elevation. Often, the patient complains of discomfort in the arms during the retrosternal pain. Pain may sometimes radiate to the epigastrium or to the neck and the jaw. It may be accompanied by shortness of breath. For the diagnosis of ischemic heart disease or myocardial infarction ECG is essential. Coronary angiography provides information about the site of coronary artery occlusion.

The treatment consists of avoiding exertion for patients susceptible to angina attacks and administration of drugs such as nitrates, β-blockers, and calcium antagonists. Patients with severe symptoms that persist despite medical treatment may need surgical treatment in the form of coronary artery bypass grafting.

Nocturnal angina and sleep disturbance.   Nocturnal angina is known to occur during both REM and NREM sleep stages. Karacan and coworkers[10] found increased sleep onset latency, reduced stage 3 and 4 NREM sleep, decreased sleep efficiency, and very little change in REM sleep on PSG study in 10 patients with a history of nocturnal angina.

Nowlin and colleagues[11] noted increased number of nocturnal anginal attacks (32 of 39 attacks associated with REM sleep) associated with ECG changes of ST segment depression in four patients with a history of angina. King and workers[12] described Prinzmetal's or variant angina during REM sleep. On the other hand, Stern and Tzivoni[13] recorded ECG continuously for 24 hours in 140 patients with ischemic heart disease and they could not ascribe ST segment changes to dreaming, though they did not record electroencephalography (EEG) or electrooculography (EOG) to document sleep stages objectively. Murao and colleagues,[14] following all-night polygraphic studies in 12 patients with nocturnal angina, found more episodes of ischemic ECG changes during REM sleep.

Epidemiologically, there is a clear relationship between increased cardiovascular morbidity and mortality and sleep disturbances associated with sleep-disordered breathing. Kripke and associates,[15] in an important study, noted increased mortality rates among patients with ischemic heart disease, stroke, and cancer who slept no more than 4 hours or more than 10 hours. Wingard and Berkman[16] in their study of about 7000 adults over a period of 9 years also found excessive mortality from ischemic heart disease in short sleepers (less than 7 hours) and long sleepers (more than 9 hours). Poor sleep is, therefore, associated with increased risk of future cardiovascular morbidity or mortality.[15-17]

Sleep in Myocardial Infarction Patients.   In 12 patients who had suffered acute myocardial infarction studied in the ICU, Broughton and Baron[18] found decreased sleep efficiency, increased sleep stage shifts, increased awakenings, and decreased REM sleep. Sleep pattern became normal by the ninth day of the illness. Circadian susceptibility to myocardial infarction—between midnight and 6:00 A.M.—has been noted.[19,20]

Karacan and coworkers[21] also studied four patients with myocardial infarction in the ICU continuously from the second to the sixth day and found increased wakefulness, reduced REM sleep, absent stage 3 and 4 NREM sleep, and a partial breakdown in the circadian cycling.

Sleep in congestive cardiac failure.   Sleep disturbances, periodic breathing, and hypoxemia at night have been described in patients with congestive cardiac failure (CCF)[22,23] but there is a dearth of PSG studies that might document sleep architecture changes in such patients.

Sleep and Cardiac Arrhythmias

An understanding of the interaction between the autonomic nervous system, cardiac innervation, and sleep is important to appreciating the effects of sleep on cardiac rhythms. Readers are referred to Chapters 5 and 20 for such review. A relationship between sleep and atrioventricular arrhythmias has been noted, but reports in the literature are somewhat contradictory. Atrial arrhythmias, such as atrial flutter, atrial fibrillation, and paroxysmal atrial tachycardia,[24] and first- and second-degree atrioventricular block[25] have been described in normal subjects during REM sleep, but no clear relationship between different sleep stages and atrial arrhythmias has emerged. A prominent sinus arrhythmia has been noted in several studies in normal subjects using Holter monitoring.[26] Brodsky and colleagues[27] monitored 24-hour continuous ECG in 50 male medical students with no apparent heart disease and observed sinus pauses of 1.8 to 2 seconds' duration in 30% of them, and another 6% had episodes of second-degree heart block (Mobitz type I). Guilleminault and associates[28] noted 42 episodes of sinus arrest in four young, healthy adults that lasted 2 to 9 seconds during REM sleep. No associated apneas or significant oxygen desaturation were observed. The incidence of nocturnal bradyarrhythmias decreases with advancing age.[29]

Contradictory results have been noted in human studies of the effects of sleep on ventricular arrhythmia, but the majority showed an antiarrhythmic effect of sleep on ventricular premature beats.[30] Ventricular arrhythmias are also noted to occur during arousal from sleep.[30] A classic example was provided by Wellens and colleagues,[31] who described a 14-year-old girl awakened from sleep by a loud auditory stimulus who had ventricular tachyarrhythmia. The authors postulated that increased sympathetic activity triggered these episodes, because they could be prevented by the β-blocker propranolol.

Holter monitoring may reveal several different ECG changes during sleep in patients with ischemic heart diseases: ST segment depression and T-wave inversion.[13] In some middle-aged men and postmenopausal women during sleep, cardiac ischemia at night associated with ST segment depression or elevation has been noted. In contrast, subjects with normal ECG findings showed no ST segment changes.[32]

Lown's group[33] noted reduction of ventricular premature beats (VPB) by at least 50% in 22 subjects and 25% to 35% in 13 others during sleep. De Silva and coworkers[34] noted reduction in VPB in all stages except REM sleep, and stage 3 and 4 NREM sleep were most affected. Pickering and colleagues[35] described 12 untreated patients with frequent ventricular extrasystoles who showed a significant decrease in both the heart rate and extrasystoles during sleep. Intravenous propranolol (a β-blocker), and to a lesser extent intravenous phenylephrine, during wakefulness produced similar decrease in the heart rate and ventricular arrhythmias. These changes appear to be mediated by the autonomic nervous system, the sympathetic system dominating over the parasympathetic system. They found that the frequency of ventricular arrhythmias was similar in both REM and NREM sleep. Their findings are similar to those of Lown and colleagues.[33] In contrast, Rosenblatt's group[36] observed arrhythmias during stage 3 and 4 NREM sleep. They noted VPBs with similar frequency during wakefulness and REM sleep.

It is known that there is an imbalance between sympathetic and parasympathetic tone during REM and NREM sleep. Gillis and colleagues[37] observed no group difference in the frequency of ventricular premature depolarization (VPD) during REM and NREM sleep. After studying 14 patients with ventricular arrhythmias, they concluded that heart rate determined the diurnal variation of VPD. The reduction of VPD frequently correlated with the reduction in the heart rate and was independent of sleep state or wakefulness.

The observations of Pickering's group[35] also contrast with those of Smith and coworkers,[38] who studied 18 patients in a coronary care unit to document frequency of cardiac arrhythmias in wakefulness and sleep. They found no significant difference in the occurrence of ventricular or atrial premature contractions during sleep and wakefulness. Disturbed sleep in coronary care patients[18] may explain the discrepancies in these data.

Sleep and sudden cardiac death

An analysis of the time of sudden cardiac death in 2203 persons by Muller and associates[19] revealed a low incidence during the night and a high incidence from 7:00 to 11:00 A.M. Similarly, nonfatal myocardial infarction and myocardial ischemic episodes are also more likely to occur in the morning. It is known that sympathetic activity increases in the morning, causing increased myocardial electrical instability; thus, sudden cardiac death may result from a primary fatal arrhythmia.

LaRovere and associates[39] correlated increased cardiovascular mortality among patients with a first myocardial infarction with reduced baroreflex sensitivity (BRS). Reduced BRS is defined as less slowing in heart rate for a given rise in arterial blood pressure, which indicates reduced vagal tone.

McWilliam[40] first suggested that ventricular fibrillation is the cause of sudden death and that sympathetic discharges play an important role in causing this fatal arrhythmia. During sleep, cardiovascular hemodynamic activity is decreased, as are heart rate and blood pressure, owing to withdrawal of sympathetic tone and increased vagal tone (see Chapter 5).

Reduced vagal tone, as measured by decreased heart rate variability in 24-hour Holter monitoring, was found by Kleiger and colleagues[41] to be a powerful predictor of increased mortality and sudden cardiac death after myocardial infarction. Autonomic imbalance (either sympathetic overactivity or parasympathetic underactivity) may trigger ventricular arrhthymias.[42]

Sleep and hypertension

There is a high prevalence (22% to 48%) of sleep apnea and related symptoms (e.g., EDS) in patients with systemic hypertension.[43–46] In contrast, studies by Escourrou and colleagues[47] found no significant difference between 21 hypertensive and 29 normotensive patients, in terms of sleep stage distribution and disorganization, apnea-hypopnea index and duration, and oxygen saturation. These 50 patients did not have airway obstruction as evidenced by FEV_1 value or daytime hypoxemia and were selected from 65 patients referred to the sleep clinic complaining of daytime hypersomnolence and snoring. The prevalence of hypertension in sleep apnea patients is about 50% to 90%.[6,48-51]

Intrinsic Respiratory Disorders

Chronic obstructive pulmonary disease

In order to understand sleep disturbances it is important to have some knowledge of gas exchange during sleep.[52] In COPD patients during sleep SaO_2 and PaO_2 fall and $PaCO_2$ rises; these values become worse during REM sleep.[53-56] Some patients' sleep-disordered breathing (e.g., apnea, hypopnea, or periodic breathing) is associated with reduced SaO_2 saturation, which is generally short-lived (less than 1 minute) and mild to moderate in intensity.[57-59] Episodes of SaO_2 desaturation during REM sleep last more than 5 minutes and are more severe than in NREM sleep.[57,60,61] Physiologic changes in respiration, respiratory muscles, and control of breathing (see Chapter 5) during sleep adversely affect breathing in these patients.

Other groups at risk for hypoxemia include those of advancing age (particularly middle-aged and elderly men), postmenopausal women, and obese persons.[52] In addition, diminished ventilatory response to hypoxia and hypercapnia in some COPD patients contribute to increasing nocturnal oxygen desaturation.[52] Nocturnal hypoxemia causes repeated disruption and fragmentation of sleep architecture.[52]

COPD includes chronic bronchitis and emphysema. The salient clinical features include chronic cough, exertional dyspnea, tightness in the chest, and sometimes wheeze. Physical examination reveals inspiratory and expiratory rhonchi and crepitations. Patients with resting hypoxemia and hypercapnia may exhibit cyanosis. Investigations should include radiographic examination of the chest and pulmonary function tests. Complications include polycythemia, pulmonary hypertension, car pulmonale, and cardiac arrhythmias.

COPD patients are traditionally divided into two groups, "pink puffers" and "blue bloaters."[62,63] The pink puffers generally have normal blood gases and have no hypoxemia or hypercapnia, they have hyperinflated lungs and do not have cardiomegaly or cor pulmonale.[52] On the other hand, blue bloaters are generally hypoxemic, hypercapnic, and have cor pulmonale, polycythemia, enlarged heart, and reduced ventilatory response to hypoxemia and hypercapnia.[52] In general, blue bloaters have more severe hypoxemia of longer duration than pink puffers.[64,65] It should be noted that oxygen saturation for both groups is somewhat similar during wakefulness and in the upright position but is markedly different during sleep. The worse value is noted in blue bloat-

ers. There are no absolute criteria for determining which groups of COPD patients have more severe nocturnal hypoxemia except to monitor patients at night, which is impractical considering the large number of patients who should be monitored.

Changes in sleep architecture

Disturbances in sleep architecture in COPD patients have been reported by several authors.[54,66-69] These disturbances may be summarized as follows: reduction of sleep efficiency, delayed sleep onset, increased WASO, frequent stage shifts, and frequent arousals. In the report of Arand and coworkers[66] they correlated these findings with EDS.

What are the causes of disturbed EEG sleep patterns? A number of factors cause sleep disturbances in these patients[70]: the use of the drugs, such as methylxanthines, which have a sleep-reducing effect, increased nocturnal cough resulting from accumulated bronchial secretions, and associated hypoxemia and hypercapnia. In a study by Calverly,[71] administration of two l per minute supplemental oxygen by nasal cannula during sleep improved both oxygen saturation at night and sleep architecture, in terms of decreasing sleep latency and increasing all stages of sleep including REM and slow-wave sleep. Other reports did not note improved sleep quality but the nocturnal hypoxemia did improve after oxygen administration.[66,67]

Cardiac arrhythmias

There are several reports of increasing prevalence of cardiac arrhythmias, particularly during sleep, in COPD patients. According to Flick and Block[72] the peak incidence of premature ventricular contractions is between 3:00 and 5:00 A.M. and 6:00 and 7:00 A.M. In a recent study by Shepard and colleagues[73] a relationship between nocturnal oxygen desaturation and cardiac arrhythmias has been established in 42 COPD patients. They found premature ventricular contractions in 64% of patients, and in six patients with oxygen desaturation below 80% during REM sleep there was a 150% increase in premature ventricular contractions. The authors concluded that factors such as hypoxemia, hypercapnia, elevation of systemic blood pressure with increased myocardial oxygen demands, and increased catecholamines contributed to increasing irritability.

Treatment of nocturnal oxygen desaturation

Recently investigators became aware of severe nocturnal hypoxemia in many patients with COPD.[53-56] This nocturnal hypoxemia may or may not be accompanied by sleep-related apnea, hypopnea, or periodic breathing and impairment of gas exchange.[57-59] It is clear that repeated or prolonged oxygen desaturation at night may cause cardiac arrhythmias and may lead to pulmonary hypertension and cor pulmonale.[73] In addition, patients with COPD show changes in sleep[54,66-69] architecture that may be related to the poor quality of sleep or may be secondary to nocturnal hypoxemia causing disruption of nocturnal EEG sleep stages. Oxygen desaturation during sleep in COPD patients can be identified only if PSG, using sleep staging or continuous monitoring of oxygenation, is performed. Several studies show episodes of oxygen desaturation during sleep in COPD patients. An important study by Wynne's group[57] showed that oxygen desaturation could be associated with two types of patients: those with oxygen desaturation and sleep-disordered breathing (apnea and hypopnea) and those not associated with such breathing. In patients with SDB the desaturation usually lasts less than 1 minute and is mild. In the other group, the desaturation lasts longer than 1 minute (up to 30 minutes) and is associated with a profound decrease in oxygen saturation. The maximum episodes, lasting longer than 5 minutes, occur during REM sleep. Similar episodes of nocturnal oxygen desaturation have been described in patients with kyphoscoliosis,[74,75] in young patients with cystic fibrosis,[61,76,77] and in patients with interstitial lung disease.[78,79]

Modern treatment of nocturnal hypoxemia is administration of oxygen by nasal cannula at a slow flow rate, usually less than 2 l per minute. The multiple-center study by the Nocturnal Oxygen Therapy Trial Group[80] and the Medical Research Council Working Party study[81] showed increased longevity for patients who used continuous home supplemental oxygen.

Particular indications for supplemental oxygen can be summarized as follows: Patients whose daytime PaO_2 fell below 55 mm Hg and those with a daytime PaO_2 between 55 and 60 mm Hg showing signs of right-sided heart failure, unexplained polycythemia or other laboratory evidence of pulmonary hypertension, and cor pulmonale.[70,82] Oxygen administration may also improve sleep architecture.[71]

The question of safety of oxygen administration has to be determined.[52] Some patients become more hypercapnic after oxygen administration.[54] Furthermore, Motta and Guilleminault[83] showed the worsening effects of administration of oxygen at night in patients with obstructive sleep apnea syndrome. Many patients with COPD may have obstructive sleep apnea (the two entities are then grouped under the term *overlap syndrome*),[54] so physicians must be careful during administration of oxygen. Kearly and colleagues[84] had shown that administration of oxygen

at 2 l per minute reduced the episodic desaturation. Fleetham and associates[85] confirmed this finding, but Guilleminault and coworkers[59] contradicted these findings in five patients with excessive sleepiness associated with chronic obstructive airflow disease. However the multiple-institution studies by the Nocturnal Oxygen Therapy Trial Group[80] showed the relative safety of oxygen therapy, including home oxygen.

Some patients with COPD and nocturnal hypoxemia benefit from treatment with medroxyprogesterone actate, a respiratory stimulant,[86,87] but the results have not been consistent. Similarly, acetazolamide, which improves sleep hypoxemia and periodic breathing in patients with acute mountain sickness,[88] has not been found effective in the majority of patients with COPD.

Recently, almitrine[70,89-91] was found to improve ventilation in COPD patients. Almitrine acts by stimulating peripheral chemoreceptors, thus improving hypoxic ventilatory drive. A dangerous side effect of almitrine noted both in animals and humans with COPD is acute rise of pulmonary artery pressure, as reported recently by MacNee and coworkers.[91] The long-term effect, in terms of morbidity and mortality, of the drug treatment, as well as the natural history of COPD, must be clearly assessed before recommending judicious use of these drugs.

Bronchial asthma (including nocturnal asthma)

The characteristic clinical triad of asthma is the paroxysm of dyspnea, wheezing, and cough. The paroxysmal attacks of wheezing and breathlessness may occur at any hour of the day or night, and the nocturnal attacks are distributed at random without any relationship to a particular sleep stage. Breathing is characterized by prolonged expiration accompanied by wheezing and unproductive cough. There may be tightness of the chest and palpitation. The attacks last for 1 to 2 hours, or sometimes last hours, in which case the term *acute severe asthma* or *status asthmaticus* is applied. That is a life-threatening condition because of extreme respiratory distress and arterial hypoxemia.

Pulmonary function tests and radiographic examination of the chest are important for confirming the diagnosis. Abnormalities of certain pulmonary function tests (FEV_1, VC, PEF) suggest airflow obstruction. Chest radiography may reveal hyperinflated lungs and emphysema.

Sleep disturbances in bronchial asthma.   A variety of sleep disturbances have been noted in patients with asthma. Janson and associates,[92] using questionnaires and sleep diaries, studied the prevalence of sleep complaints and sleep disturbances prospectively in 98 consecutive adult asthma patients attending an outpatient clinic in Uppsala, Sweden.

Compared with 226 age- and sex-matched controls, they found a high incidence of sleep disturbances in asthma patients—early morning awakening, difficulty in maintaining sleep, and EDS. Sleep disturbances in general consist of a combination of insomnia and hypersomnia. PSG studies may reveal disruption of sleep architecture as well as sleep apnea in some patients.

Nocturnal exacerbation of symptoms during sleep is a frequent finding in asthma patients. In an important study by Turner-Warwick[93] 94% of 7729 asthmatics surveyed woke up at least once a night with symptoms of asthma; 74% at least one night a week, 64% at least 3 nights a week, and 39% every night. Nocturnal asthma is a potentially serious problem, as there is a high incidence of respiratory arrests and sudden death in adult asthmatics between midnight and 8:00 A.M.[94,95]

In order to understand the relationship between the attacks of asthma and sleep stage and time of the night Kales and colleagues[96] studied six men and six women aged 20 to 45 years by PSG, each for 2 or 3 consecutive nights. They observed a total of 93 asthma attacks in these patients, 73 during NREM sleep and 18 during REM. They did not find a relation between asthma attacks and sleep stage or time of night. Sleep pattern showed less total sleep time, frequent awakenings after sleep onset, and early final awakenings and reduced stage 4 sleep. Kales' group[97] observed similar findings in a PSG study of 10 asthmatic children.

Montplaisir and colleagues[98] studied 12 asthmatics, eight of whom showed nocturnal attacks on sleep studies (six women and two men aged 20 to 51 years). Twenty-six attacks were documented. No attacks occurred in stage 3 or 4 sleep, nor were attacks more frequent during REM than NREM sleep. Thus, stage 3 and 4 sleep was "protective." Sleep efficiency was decreased. The number and duration of apneas were not significantly greater in asthmatics than in controls. Episodes of oxygen desaturation occurred only in the asthmatics. Sleep efficiency and waking time after sleep onset were altered in asthmatics. When there were no attacks, no difference in sleep architecture was noted between the controls and the patients, which suggested that sleep disturbances are characteristic of unstable asthma with nocturnal attacks.

Several pathogenic mechanisms for sleep disturbances and nocturnal excerabations of asthma have been suggested[92,99,100]:

Sleep deprivation[101]
Impaired ventilatory function in the supine posture[102]
A decrease in circulating epinephrine at night, with an increase in histamine[103]

Gastroesophageal reflux[104] (a recent study by Tan and associates[105] casts doubt on this),
Marked fluctuation in airway tone during REM sleep[106]
Theophylline, a commonly used asthma drug which may cause insomnia[107,108] and increase episodes of gastroesophageal reflux[109,110] (a study by Hubert's group[111] found no such increase in asthmatics taking theophylline)
Prolonged administration of corticosteroids in some asthmatics, which may have adverse effects on sleep and daytime functioning because of increased incidence of obstructive sleep apnea[112]
Increased cellular inflammatory response in the bronchopulmonary region at night[99,113]
Miscellaneous factors[99]—allergens (e.g., houe dust); increased bronchial secretions combined with suppression of cough, especially during REM sleep; airway cooling at night; increased pulmonary resistance; altered bronchial reactivity; normal propensity for worsening of lung function during sleep; normally increased vagal tone during sleep; suppressed arousal response to bronchoconstriction in severe nocturnal asthma.
Certain circadian factors.[99,100]

Evidence for the contribution of circadian factors is this:

1. Peak expiratory flow rate (PEFR) normally is highest at 4:00 P.M. and lowest at 4:00 A.M.[99] The variation is typically about 5% to 8%, but if it reaches 50%, as it can in some asthmatics, there is the danger of respiratory arrest.[99] This circadian variation in PEFR is related to sleep and not to recumbency or the hour.[99,100]
2. Airway resistance as measured breath by breath is not increased in normal persons at night, but asthmatics show a circadian rhythm of increased airway resistance at night that is related to the duration of the sleep and not to sleep stages.[99,114]
3. Similar to patients with sleep apnea syndrome and COPD, nocturnal asthma is also associated with sleep-disturbed breathing[115] (hypopneas more than apneas of mixed, obstructive, or central type) accompanied by awakening, which is worse during REM sleep.

Treatment of bronchial asthma[99]

Treatment of bronchial asthma, including nocturnal asthma, consists of judicious use of bronchodilators and corticosteroids, preferably inhaled in a compressor; oral theophylline, maximizing the serum concentration at around 4 A.M. when most nocturnal attacks occur; and, for a small subset of patients who show the lowest plasma cortisol levels accompanied by the lowest peak expiratory flow rate at night or early morning, nocturnal steroids.[116] Other measures include treating the reversible factors, such as allergens, nasal congestion, or bronchopulmonary infections and use of humidified air.[99]

Sleep in Restrictive Lung Disease

Restrictive lung disease is characterized functionally by a reduction of total lung capacity, functional residual capacity, vital capacity, expiratory reserve volume, and diffusion capacity but preservation of the normal ratio of FEV_1 to FVC.[79] This may be due to intrapulmonary restriction (e.g., interstitial lung disease) or extrapulmonary restriction resulting from diseases of the chest wall (e.g., kyphoscoliosis) or pleura, neuromuscular diseases, obesity, or pregnancy, which may abnormally elevate the diaphragm.

Interstitial lung disease

Etiopathogenesis. Interstitial lung disease may result from a variety of causes, for example, idiopathic pulmonary fibrosis, fibrosing alveolitis associated with connective tissue disorders, pulmonary sarcoidosis, occupational dust exposure, pulmonary damage resulting from drugs, or radiotherapy to the thorax.[117] The common features of all these conditions include alveolar thickening due to fibrosis, cellular exudates or edema, increased stiffening of the lungs causing reduced compliance and ventilation-perfusion mismatch giving rise to hyoxemia, hyperventilation and hypocapnia.

Clinical features. Features of interstitial lung disease include progressive exertional dyspnea, often a dry cough, clubbing of the fingers, and pulmonary crepitations on auscultation of the lungs. The diagnosis is based on a combination of characteristic clinical features, radiographic findings, (e.g., diffuse pulmonary fibrosis), and pulmonary function test results.

Sleep abnormalities. Bye[78] and Perez-Padilla and their coworkers[118] reported on sleep studies on this condition. Sleep abnormalities consist of repeated arousals with sleep fragmentation and multiple sleep stage shifts, increased stage 1 and reduced REM sleep accompanied by oxygen desaturation during REM and NREM sleep owing to episodic hypoventilation and ventilation-perfusion mismatch, and occasionally obstructive sleep apnea.

Treatment. For about 30% of cases of interstitial lung disease corticosteroids are effective. George and Kryger[79] advocate symptomatic treatment with sup-

plemental nocturnal oxygen therapy, according to the guidelines developed by the Nocturnal Oxygen Therapeutic Trial Group.[80]

Kyphoscoliosis. Kyphoscoliosis is a thoracic cage deformity that causes extrapulmonary restriction of the lungs and gives rise to impairment of pulmonary functions, as described above for restrictive lung diseases. The condition may be primary, idiopathic, or secondary to neuromuscular diseases, spondylitis, or Marfan's syndrome.[79]

In severe cases of kyphoscoliosis, breathing disorders during sleep (e.g., central, obstructive, and mixed apneas associated with oxygen desaturation) and sleep disturbances (e.g., disrupted night sleep, reduced NREM stages 2 through 4 and REM sleep, and EDS) have been described.[74,75,79]

Continuous positive airway pressure or tracheostomy may benefit those with moderate to severe obstructive apnea. Some patients may also require nighttime mechanical ventilation.[119] Patients with mild respiratory failure may benefit from medical treatment with acetazolamide, medroxyprogesterone, or almitrine, as discussed above for COPD patients.

Gastrointestinal Diseases

Peptic ulcer disease

A peptic ulcer is one in the lower esophagus, stomach, or duodenum. The prevalence of peptic ulcer in the general population is fairly high—approximately 10% of the adult population—and men are most often affected. The commonest presentation of peptic ulcer is episodic pain localized to the epigastrium that is relieved by food or antacids or other acid-suppressant agents. The pain has a characteristic periodicity and extends over many years. The patient generally can localize the pain to the epigastrium. Occasionally, however, it is referred to the interscapular region at the lower chest and is usually described as burning or gnawing. Duodenal pain is often described as "hunger pain" and is relieved by taking food. An important feature is that the pain awakens patients 2 to 3 hours after they retire to bed, disturbing sleep. An important physical sign is the so-called pointing sign and localized epigastric tenderness.

The natural history of the disease is its episodic occurrence over a course of days or weeks, after which the pain disappears, to recur weeks or months later. Between attacks the patient feels well. Sometimes the presentation may be secondary to complications of ulcer, such as an acute episode of bleeding or perforation, or even an episode of gastric obstruction. The differential diagnosis of ulcer pain should include cholecystitis, angina, gastroesophageal reflux, and esophagitis or pancreatitis. Definitive diagnosis is established by barium examination of the gastroduodenal tract, and if necessary by endoscopic examination and biopsy.

Sleep, nocturnal acid secretion, and duodenal ulcer

To understand the role of nocturnal gastric acid secretion in duodenal ulcer, Dragstedt[120] studied hourly collections of nocturnal gastric acid from patients with duodenal ulcer and from normal subjects. They found three to 20 times greater volumes of nocturnal acid secretion in patients than in normal controls. Vagotomy abolished this increased secretion and improved healing of ulcers. Studies by Orr and colleagues[121] have shown that patients with duodenal ulcer exhibit failure of inhibition of gastric acid secretion during the first 2 hours after onset of sleep.

Sleep disturbances in duodenal ulcer patients characteristically result from episodes of nocturnal epigastric pain. These symptoms cause arousals and repeated awakenings, thus fragmenting and disturbing the sleep considerably in these patients. Gastroenterologists are beginning to be aware of the importance of sleep-related hypersecretion of acid in peptic ulcer patients, and appropriate therapeutic measures in the form of nocturnal acid suppression by use of histamine H_2 receptor antagonist (cimetidine or ranitidine) are being applied in such patients with benefit.[122]

Treatment.   Treatment of peptic ulcer disease consists of a combination of avoidance of tobacco and alcohol and administration of antacids and histamine H_2 receptor antagonists such as cimetidine or ranitidine.[122-125] These two drugs heal duodenal ulcer in 80% of cases and gastric ulcer 70% of the time if taken for 4 weeks. The drugs are generally given twice a day with a third dose at night. Those patients with intractable ulcer may require elective surgery.

The importance of nocturnal acid suppression in the healing of duodenal ulcer and in preventing the reoccurrence of such ulcers in patients is well-established.[122] It has been found that some patients treated with cimetidine remain symptomatic, and in these patients acid secretion remains high. When these patients are treated with ranitidine, a more potent acid-suppressant agent, both the symptoms and the amount of acid secretion decreased considerably. Furthermore, patients who show little improvement in response to medical treatment have subsequently undergone vagotomy, which suppressed the acid secretion and relieved symptoms and healed the ulcers.[126] Also, maintenance of nocturnal acid suppression by ranitidine

prevents the recurrence of duodenal ulcers.[127-129] These therapeutic measures clearly document the importance of the nocturnal acid secretion and its suppression in the pathogenesis of duodenal ulcer.[122] Other factors, such as mucosal resistance, may also play a role.[122]

Gastroesophageal reflux and reflux esophagitis

Clinical features.   Gastroesophageal reflux frequently occurs in middle-aged and elderly women, and sometimes in younger women during pregnancy. Hiatus hernia is often associated with reflux esophagitis. The characteristic symptom is heartburn, described as retrosternal burning pain exacerbated by lifting or straining or when the patient lies down at night.[130,131] The burning pain causes difficulty in initiating sleep, frequent awakenings, and fragmentation of sleep. The nocturnal pain is characteristically relieved by sitting up or ingesting food or by acid-suppressant agents. An important differential diagnosis would be angina, particularly when the pain radiates to the neck, jaws, and arms, but an important point to remember is that the esophageal pain is usually not related to the exertion. Other symptoms include transient or persistent dysphagia if the patient has developed stricture and regurgitation of gastric contents associated with coughing, wheezing, and shortness of breath due to the aspiration of the gastric contents into the bronchopulmonary region.[130] A serious complication of repeated episodes of gastroesophageal reflux and esophagitis is Barrett's esophagus, which may be a precursor to esophageal adenocarcinoma.[131-134] The other complication includes exacerbation of nocturnal asthma.

Differential diagnosis.   Peptic ulcer disease, ischemic heart disease, sleep apnea, abnormal swallowing, and sleep choking syndromes, may be mistaken for gastroesophageal reflux or reflux esophagitis.

Pathogenesis.   Several factors are important in the pathogenesis of gastroesophageal reflux.[122,131] The most important factor is the acid clearance time, in addition to the frequency of swallowing and the secretion of saliva. The diagnosis of gastroesophageal reflux and prolonged acid secretion can be made by continuous monitoring of lower esophageal pH.[122,135] When the pH falls below 4, gastroesophageal reflux occurs.[136] Repeated prolonged episodes of gastroesophageal reflux during sleep at night can cause esophagitis.[137] Suppression of saliva, decreased swallowing frequency, and prolonged mucosal contact with the gastric acid all contribute to the development of esophagitis.[122] Following repeated prolonged episodes of gastroesophageal reflux at night after many years such patients may develop Barrett's esopha-gus, which results from replacement of the squamous epithelium of the lower esophagus by the columnar epithelium of the stomach.[131-134] Docu-mentation of spontaneous gastroesophageal reflux and prolonged acid clearance is important for diag-nosis and treatment of esophagitis resulting from repeated episodes of gastroesophageal reflux. Ad-ministration of acid suppressant agents (cimetidine or ranitidine) two to three times a day plus a night-time dose, combined with elevation of the head end of the bed, decreases the acid clearance time in the ma-jority of patients and improves the symptoms of gas-troesophageal reflux and esophagitis.[122,131]

Role of gastroesophageal reflux in bronchopulmonary disease. In some patients with asthma and chronic bronchitis or COPD spontaneous gastroesophageal reflux at night plays a role in the pathogenesis of symptoms such as nocturnal wheeze, cough, or shortness of breath.[122,138-141] In such patients in-traesophaogeal pH monitoring has shown prolonged acid clearance.[139] This is important from a therapeu-tic point of view, because administration of acid suppressant agents to such patients improves the pulmonary symptoms.[122] On the other hand, a study by Tan and coworkers[142] casts doubt on the rele-vance of gastroesophageal reflux to asthma.

The mechanisms of pulmonary symptoms in gas-troesophageal reflux associated with asthma and bronchitis may include these[122,143,144]: 1. Aspira-tion of the gastric contents in the lungs causes pneu-monitis and 2. Acid contact to the lower esophagus initiates reflex stimulation of the vagus nerve which causes bronchoconstriction. Actual aspiration of gastric contents into the lungs can be documented by the method used by Chernow and associates.[141] These authors used a scintigraphic technique. They instilled a radionuclide into the stomach before sleep. A lung scan made the next morning showed the radioactive material in the lung, suggesting noc-turnal pulmonary aspiration. It should be noted that children with asthma and bronchopulmonary dis-ease, in addition to the other complications of gas-troesophageal reflux may have sleep apena.[145] In some cases of sudden infant death syndrome gas-troesophegeal reflux has been implicated, causing apnea and sudden death, but this occurs in only a small percentage of patients.[145,146]

Diagnostic tests. No single test is diagnostic, but a combination of tests to assess the potential for reflux damage to the esophagus and actual presence of reflux is necessary to make the diagnosis. The diag-nosis is confirmed by barium examination, and if necessary by endoscopic examination and biopsy.

Measurement of lower esophageal sphincter pres-sure and a diagnosis of hiatus hernia may detect potential risk factors for reflux.[131] A damage to the esophagus may be assessed by Bernstein's test (acid perfusion test), esophagography, esophagoscopy, and mucosal biopsy.[131] The actual presence of re-flux may be diagnosed by the following tests: esoph-agography, acid reflux test, prolonged esophageal pH monitoring, and gastroesophageal scintigraphy.[131] The importance of 24-hour ambulatory esophageal pH monitoring has been emphasized recently by Triadafilopoulos and Castillo.[147]

Treatment.[122,131] Treatment includes general mea-sures such as avoidance of fatty foods and stooping, weight reduction, and elevation of the head end of the bed to reduce reflux at night. Smoking should also be avoided. Antacids and acid-suppressing agents such as cimetidine or ranitidine may relieve the symptoms. Recently, omeprazole, an agent that inhibits gastric acid secretion by inhibiting $H+/K+$-ATPase activity, is found to be superior to histamine H_2 receptor antagonists (e.g., cimetidine or raniti-dine) in many patients with reflux esophagitis.[147a] For patients who fail to respond to medical treat-ment, antireflux surgery (e.g., fundoplication) is indicated.

In conclusion, an awareness of the role of sleep in the pathogenesis and treatment of peptic disease, particularly duodenal ulcer and esophageal reflux, is important for diagnosis and treatment. Facilities for all-night PSG study and 24-hour esophageal pH monitoring have contributed to an understanding of this association in these diseases. These are also some examples of diseases that benefit from a mul-tidisciplinary approach to patient management by a gastroenterologist, a pulmonologist, and a sleep spe-cialist. This review also shows that sleep adversely affects patients with reflux esophagitis by increasing the episodes of reflux and prolonging the acid clear-ance time. Furthermore, repeated spontaneous reflux episodes adversely affect sleep by causing arousals and frequent awakenings and sleep fragmentation.

Endocrine Diseases

Thyroid disorders

It is important to be aware of the association between thyroid disorders, disordered breathing, and sleep disturbances. History and physical examination may direct attention to a thyroid disorder, in which case thyroid function tests should be performed to con-firm the clinical diagnosis.

Hypothyroidism

The salient diagnostic features suggestive of myxedema consist of presentation in a middle-aged or elderly person of fatigue, weight gain, decrease of physical and mental faculties, dryness and coarsening of the skin, pretibial edema, hoarse voice, cold sensitivity (sometimes presenting with hypothermia), constipation, and bradycardia or evidence of ischemic heart disease in the ECG.

Both upper airway obstructive[148] and central sleep apneas[149] have been described in patients with myxedema. They disappeared following thyroxine treatment. Mechanisms include deposition of mucopolysaccharides in the upper airways as well as central respiratory dysfunction as evidenced by impaired hypercapnic ventilatory response in such patients.

Rajagopal and coworkers[150] made an important observation of obstructive sleep apnea in nine of 11 consecutive hypothyroid patients (apnea index 17 to 176). They noted improvement after thyroid replacement treatment.

In the sleep EEG study of myxedema patients, Kales and colleagues[151] noted a reduction of slow-wave sleep, which normalized following treatment.

Hyperthyroidism

Clinical features suggestive of thyrotoxicosis are presentation in a woman (8:1 woman-man ratio) of apparent increased energy, weight loss despite increased appetite, staring or bulging of the eyes, exophthalmos, tachycardia or atrial fibrillation, heat intolerance with excessive sweating, feelings of warmth, and a fine tremor of the outstretched fingers.

Few sleep studies have been made in patients with thyrotoxicosis. Dunleavy and colleagues[152] observed an increased amount of slow-wave sleep, which returned to normal after treatment. In contrast, Passouant and colleagues[153] did not find any change in slow-wave sleep but described an increase in sleep onset latency in hyperthyroid patients. Johns and Rinsler[154] found no relationship between stages of sleep and alteration of thyroid function.

Diabetes mellitus

For sleep disturbance and sleep apnea in diabetes see the section on autonomic neuropathy in Chapter 20.

Growth hormone deficiency and sleep

In 8 adults with isolated growth hormone (GH) deficiency (aged 18 to 28 years) Astrom and Lindholm[155] found a reduction of stage 4 sleep but increases in stage 1 and 2 NREM sleep, with a net

result of an increase of total sleep time. In a later paper, Astrom and others[156] studied these patients after daily treatment with GH for 6 months and found a decrease in total sleep time that was due mainly to a reduction in stage 2 sleep but unchanged slow waves and an increase in REM sleep time. In contrast to these findings in adults, Wu and Thorpy[157] found normal stage 4 sleep but increased stage 3 NREM sleep in seven children with GH deficiency.

Excessive growth hormone release and sleep. Sullivan and colleagues[158] reported sleep apnea in association with GH release from the pituitary in patients with acromegaly. The commonest explanation for sleep apnea in these patients is enlargement of the tongue and pharyngeal wall which causes narrowing of the upper airway. Sullivan's group[158] studied 40 patients with acromegaly and observed central sleep apnea in 30%. There is increased respiratory drive with increased hypercapnic ventilatory response. Sandostatin, a somatostatin analog, cured central apnea and normalized the ventilatory response.

Grunstein and coworkers[159] studied 53 patients with acromegaly who were consecutively referred for consultation. Sleep apnea was a reason for referral of 33 patients, and 20 patients were referred without any suspicion of apnea. Thirty-one patients of the group of 33 referred for apnea had sleep apnea; in contrast 12 of 20 patients referred without suspected apnea were found to have apnea. Central apnea was predominant in 33% of patients. The authors concluded that sleep apnea is common in persons with acromegaly and central sleep apnea is associated with increased disease activity as reflected by biochemical measurement. They speculated that alteration of the respiratory control may be a mechanism for sleep apnea in these patients.

Renal Disorders

Although sleep complaints and sleep disturbances have been reported in patients with chronic renal failure (CRF), with or without hemodialysis, only a limited number of studies have been performed to document these objectively.

Sleep disturbances and chronic renal failure

Sleep disturbances, in the form of reduced total and slow-wave sleep, have been described in patients with CRF as well as in those receiving long-term hemodialysis or peritoneal dialysis. In the studies by Williams[160] and Karacan's group[161] sleep disturbances remained unchanged in patients on dialysis, even those who underwent renal transplantation, suggesting that an irreversible CNS deficit causes

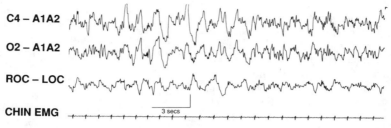

FIGURE 22-1.   *Portion of a PSG recording. Note alpha intrusion into NREM sleep (alpha-delta sleep) in the EEG channels.*

sleep dysfunction. An interesting finding in the EEG studies[160,161] of Karacan's group is the presence of alpha-delta sleep. Daly and Hassall[162] reported that subjective sleep complaints became worse on dialysis nights.

Disturbed sleep, as manifested by reduced sleep efficiency, increased sleep fragmentation, decreased slow-wave sleep, and increased daytime somnolence, has been reported in patients with uremia.[160,161,163–165] Strub and colleagues[164] found worsening of symptoms after dialysis, but they did not have PSG studies. Passouant's group[163] studied the night sleep of 18 patients with CRF polygraphically and found difficulty in maintenance of sleep, frequent awakenings, decreased slow-wave sleep, disorganization of the sleep cycle, and myoclonic jerks. Dialysis improved nighttime sleep and the sleep abnormalities.

Sleep apnea in patients receiving dialysis

Many CRF patients on and off dialysis suffer from sleep apnea syndrome and may have periodic limb movements in sleep.[166–168] Kimmel and associates found by PSG sleep apnea in 73% of 22 patients with CRF whose history also suggested sleep apnea.

Mendelson and colleagues[169] observed significant sleep apnea in six of 11 patients. Unfortunately six of their 11 patients had diabetes mellitus, which is known to be associated with sleep apnea. They did not find any alteration after hemodialysis in the sleep architecture and the number of sleep-related disordered breathing events (both obstructive and central sleep apneas), though they did find an increase in the percentage of obstructive apnea time on the night following hemodialysis, which may have been due to modulation of chemical control of ventilation.

Millman and colleagues[168] studied 29 men on long-term dialysis. In 12 (41%) their symptoms suggested sleep apena—EDS, repeated arousals at night, and morning headache. By PSG six of these patients had obstructive sleep apnea. The authors

did not find any significant effect of testosterone on sleep apnea. It should be noted that testosterone is often given to CRF patients to stimulate erythropoiesis.

Kimmel and colleagues[166] performed a PSG study of 26 patients with CRF treated with hemodialysis. Twenty-two had a history suggestive of sleep apnea, and 16 of these symptomatic (73%) patients had sleep apnea syndrome. In nine of 16 patients the sleep apnea was of obstructive type. The authors concluded that EDS in some patients with CRF may be related to the disturbed nocturnal sleep and sleep apnea.

The following mechanisms have been suggested for the pathogenesis of sleep apnea in CRF:

Upper airway edema causing partial airway obstruction coupled with decreased muscle tone during sleep[170]

CNS depression during sleep resulting from so-called uremic toxins causing excessive reduction of upper airway muscle tone.[170] (persistence of sleep apnea after dialysis speaks against this suggestion)

Disturbance of the ventilatory control of breathing in renal failure and hemodialysis[171,172] may make the respiratory control unstable, causing an imbalance between diaphragmatic and upper airway muscle

Congestive cardiac failure, which may occur in association with CRF, may itself cause sleep-disordered breathing[173]

Chronic metabolic acidosis, as noted in patients with CRF, may be responsible[174] (however, in the study by Kimmel's group[166] they did not find any relationship between disordered breathing events and hydrogen ion concentrations or carbon dioxide tension in the symptomatic patients)

An alteration of the hydrogen ion set point for stimulation of respiration.[171])

Anatomic narrowing of the upper airway (but this has not been documented by computed tomography in CRF patients.[166])

Hypertension associated with CRF

Rheumatic Diseases

Fibrositis or fibromyalgia syndrome

According to Goldenberg[175] an estimated 3 to 6 million Americans are afflicted with fibromyalgia syndrome (FMS), a syndrome characterized by diffuse muscle aches and pains not related to diseases of the joints, bones, or the connective tissues. Common sites of these aches and pains include the neck and shoulder joints and the sacrospinal and gluteal regions. Yunus and colleagues[176] listed specific diagnostic criteria for FMS. An important item in the differential diagnosis is polymyalgia rheumatica, which is also characterized by diffuse muscle aches and pains but is often associated with accelerated erythrocyte sedimentation rate and evidence of temporal arteritis.

Sleep disturbance is very common in FMS, and the characteristic PSG finding is intermittent alpha activity during NREM sleep giving rise to the characteristic alpha-delta or alpha-NREM sleep in the PSG recording (Figure 22-1). Another important association is the presence of periodic limb movements in sleep on PSG examination. It should be noted that though alpha-delta sleep is seen in this condition, this variant is not specific for the syndrome. Alpha-NREM sleep has also been reported in other rheumatic disorders,[177] in febrile illness and postviral fatigue syndrome,[178] in psychiatric patients,[179] and even in normal persons.[180,181]

Hematologic Disorders

The only hematologic disorder that may be adversely affected by sleep is paroxysmal nocturnal hemoglobinuria (PNH). Hansen[182] noted increased levels of plasma hemoglobin in five of seven patients with PNH and the maximum values were found at midnight or at 4:00 A.M. The author did not, however, record EEG or EOG to document any relationship with different sleep stages. Occasionally, patients with sickle cell anemia show reduced arterial oxygen saturation during sleep.[183]

Miscellaneous Disorders

Sleep of intensive care unit (ICU) patients (medical and surgical)[160,184]

Generally, patients are admitted to the medical ICU because of acute respiratory failure resulting from COPD, bronchial asthma, sleep apnea syndrome, restrictive lung disease, acute cardiovascular disorders (e.g., ischemic heart disease with or without myocardial infarction, cardiac arrhythmias, congestive cardiac failure), acute neurologic disorders causing respiratory disturbances (e.g., brain stem lesion, status epilepticus, high cervical cord lesions, neuromuscular disorders), renal failure, or gastroesophageal reflux causing acute respiratory tract symptoms. All of these conditions can be associated with sleep disturbances (insomnia and hypersomnia and sleep-related respiratory dysrhythmia), which become intense in severely ill patients admitted to the ICU who require life-saving cardiorespiratory support.

Other factors may aggravate sleep and sleep-related respiratory disturbances in the ICU; for example, a variety of drugs used in the ICU. The ICU environment itself is deleterious to normal sleep and conducive to sleep deprivation (with its attendant complications such as ICU psychosis). In addition to sleep deprivation, physiologic and physical factors contribute to ICU psychosis. Noise, bright light, constant activity on the part of the ICU personnel for monitoring and drug administration also play a significant role in disturbing the sleep of ICU patients.

In the surgical ICU, patients are usually admitted in the postoperative period, when they are recovering from anethesia, beginning to suffer from pain and to have metabolic disturbances, or sometime if they have an infection related to surgical care. All these factors may cause severe disturbance of sleep and breathing.

The physicians and the paramedical personnel who take care of the patients in the ICU must be aware of these problems, so that correct diagnosis and management of secondary complications can be effected promptly (in addition to treatment of the primary disorders).

Several authors have studied ICU patients by PSG to document disruption of sleep structure.[185–188] Briefly, these disturbances consist of marked diminution of stage 3 and 4 NREM and REM sleep, frequent awakenings, sleep fragmentation, and reduced total sleep time.

Treatment

The most important point for treatment is awareness of the sleep problems of such patients, so that factors that contribute to sleep disturbances can be prevented or minimized. In addition to treating the primary disorder, it is important to treat secondary sleep-related respiratory problems. If a sleep disturbance persists after the patient leaves the ICU, a primary sleep disorder may be suspected and appropriate investigations, such as PSG study and MSLT, should be performed to document such problems.

Acquired immunodeficiency syndrome

AIDS is a multisystem disorder caused by infection with human immunodeficiency virus (HIV). Its manifestations are protean. Neurologic manifestations include both CNS and peripheral neuromuscular dysfunction. Encephalitis, due to either opportunistic infection or direct invasion by the virus may cause a variety of disorders, such as memory impairment, seizures, and pyramidal or extrapyramidal manifestations. Some patients have sleep disturbances.

Norman and colleagues[189] studied a group of asymptomatic HIV-positive homosexual men and found an increase in slow-wave sleep and a disruption of the NREM-REM cycle. A follow-up study[190] of 17 of these patients 19 to 63 months later showed a decrease in the slow-wave sleep, an increase of sleep fragmentation, and disruption of the NREM-REM cycle as the disease became symptomatic.

Moller and associates[191] obtained nocturnal PSG recordings for 14 patients with HIV infection. They found increased sleep-onset latency, short total sleep time, reduced sleep efficiency, increased time in wakefulness and stage 1, and reduced stage 2 sleep. They found that asymptomatic patients had similar sleep abnormalities. The authors suggested that sleep study may be a sensitive method for detecting and monitoring CNS infection in HIV-positive patients.

Whether PSG can document significant and specific abnormalities in asymptomatic persons or warn of the development of encephalopathy remains to be determined. A systematic study needs to be done of a large number of cases to answer these questions.

Lyme disease[192–195]

Lyme disease is a multisystem disease caused by the spirochete *Borrelia burgdorferi* and transmitted to humans by tick bite. The clinical manifestations may be divided into acute, subacute, and chronic stages. Initially, there is a characteristic skin lesion, erythema migrans. This is followed in the course of time by a febrile illness. Later, patients may have arthritis or arthralgias, and even cardiac involvement (conduction disturbance or cardiomyopathy) and hepatic failure. In the subacute and chronic stages neurologic manifestations may present as axonal polyneuropathy, radiculoneuropathy, cranial neuropathy (particularly affecting the facial nerve), lymphocytic meningitis, encephalitis, or encephalopathy. Encephalitis is rare. Patients with CNS manifestations may have sleep disturbances. No large-scale study utilizing PSG is available to characterize the sleep disturbances in this condition. Because Lyme disease is treatable, every attempt should be made to diagnose it accurately. Diagnosis depends on the serologic detection of antibodies against *B. burgdorferi* in the serum (or, in case of CNS infection, in cerebrospinal fluid samples). The usual method of testing is the enzyme-linked immunosorbent assay,

but antibodies usually are not detectable until 4 to 6 weeks after the initial infection. Diagnosis may be complicated by false positive results and by lack of a standardized technique to assay for antibodies. Recently, polymerase chain reaction has been shown to be useful in demonstrating *B. burgdorferi* DNA in clinical material. The disease shows an excellent response to antibiotic therapy.

Chronic fatigue syndrome

A recently described but ill-defined heterogeneous condition is chronic fatigue syndrome (CFS).[196] Certain diagnostic criteria, both major and minor, have been established for it.[197] Two major manifestations are (1) insidious onset of fatigue for at least 6 months and (2) no evident cause for the fatigue despite extensive laboratory investigation. The minor manifestations include arthralgias, myalgias, headache, and sleep disturbances. The cause is undetermined. Various psychological and psychiatric illnesses (e.g., major affective disorder) may present as CFS. On the other hand, in many cases of CFS depression is one of the minor manifestations. A variety of viruses, particularly herpes simplex, enterovirus, retroviruses, and Epstein-Barr virus, have been incriminated without any firm evidence. Sleep disturbances (e.g., disturbed nighttime sleep, sleep disorganization, EDS) are important problems in some patients, but in many cases these have not been adequately characterized by PSG studies.

African sleeping sickness (trypanosomiasis)

African sleeping sickness is caused by *Trypanosoma gambiense* or *Trypanosoma rhodesiense* and is transmitted to humans by the bite of tsetse flies. The clinical features are characterized by lymphadenopathy, fever, and later, after several months or years, excessive sleepiness due to encephalopathy or encephalitis. On PSG study,[198–200] the NREM sleep stages cannot be easily recognized because of the presence throughout the recording of diffuse delta waves in the EEG. Sleep-onset REM is frequently documented in this condition. Buguet and colleagues[201] performed a 24-hour PSG study of a patient with sleeping sickness due to *T. gambiense*. The patient had eight sleep episodes during the daytime, and the patient showed characteristic daytime sleepiness and nighttime restlessness. REM latency was found to be reduced, and two sleep-onset REM episodes were observed. Their findings agree with the previous reports on sleep disorganization with loss of monophasic sleep at night and slow-wave activity invading the NREM sleep stage.

REFERENCES

1. Diagnostic Classification Steering Committee. The International Classification of Sleep Disorders: Diagnostic and Coding Manual. Rochester, Minn.: American Sleep Disorders Association, 1990;259–280.

2. Gislason T, Almqvist M. Somatic diseases and sleep complaints. An epidemiological study of 3201 Swedish men. Acta Med Scand 1987;221:475–481.

3. Johns MWW, Egan P, Gay TJ, et al. Sleep habits and symptoms in male medical and surgical patients. Br Med J 1970;2:509–512.

4. Aldrich MS. Cardinal manifestations of sleep disorders. In: Kryger MH, Roth T, Dement WC, eds. Principles and Practice of Sleep Medicine. Philadelphia WB Saunders, 1989;313–319.

5. Wooten V. Medical causes of insomnia. In: Kryger MH, Roth T, Dement WC, eds. Principles and Practice of Sleep Medicine. Philadelphia: WB Saunders, 1989;456–475.

6. Guilleminault C, Hoed JVD, Mitler MM. Clinical overview of the sleep apnea syndromes. In: Guilleminault C, Dement WC, eds. Sleep Apnea Syndromes. New York: Alan R Liss, 1978;1–12.

7. Remmers JE, Anch AM, deGroot WJ. Respiratory disturbances during sleep. Clin Chest Med 1980;1:57–71.

8. Guilleminault C, Tilkian A, Dement WC. The sleep apnea syndromes. Ann Rev Med 1976;27:465–484.

9. Chokroverty S. Sleep and breathing in neurological disorders. In: Edelman NH, Santiago TV, eds. Breathing Disorders of Sleep. New York: Churchill Livingstone, 1986;225–264.

10. Karacan I, Williams RL, Taylor WJ. Sleep characteristics of patients with angina pectoris. Psychosomatics 1969;10:280–284.

11. Nowlin JB, Troyer WG, Collins WS, et al. The association of nocturnal angina pectoris with dreaming. Ann Intern Med 1965;63:1040–1046.

12. King MJ, Zir LM, Kaltman AJ, et al. Variant angina associated with angiographically demonstrated coronary artery spasm and REM sleep. Am J Med Sci 1973;265:419–422.

13. Stern S, Tzivoni D. Dynamic changes in the ST-T segment during sleep in ischemic heart disease. Am J Cardiol 1973;32:16–20.

14. Murao S, Harumi K, Katayama S, et al. All-night polygraphic studies of nocturnal angina pectoris. Jpn Heart J 1972;13:295–306.

15. Kripke D, Simons R, Garfinkel L, et al. Short and long sleep and sleeping pills. Arch Gen Psychiatry 1979;36:103–116.

16. Wingard DL, Berkman LF. Mortality risk associated with sleep pattern among adults. Sleep 1983;6:102–107.

17. Partinen M, Putkonen PTS, Kaprio J, et al. Sleep disorders in relation to coronary heart disease. Acta Med Scand (Suppl) 1982;660:69–83.

18. Broughton R, Baron R. Sleep of acute coronary patients in an open ward type intensive care unit. Sleep Res 1973;2:144.

19. Muller JE, Stone PH, Turi ZG, et al. Circadian variation in the frequency of onset of acute myocardial infarction. N Engl J Med 1985;313:1315–1322.

20. Mitler MM, Kripke DF. Circadian variation in myocardial infarction. N Engl J Med 1986;314:1187–1188.

21. Karacan I, Green JR, Taylor WJ, et al. Sleep characteristics of acute myocardial infarct patients in an ICU. Sleep Res 1973;2:159.

22. Dark DS, Pingleton SK, Kerby GR, et al. Breathing pattern abnormalities and arterial oxygen desaturation during sleep in the congestive heart failure syndrome. Chest 1987;91:833–836.

23. Baylor P, Tayloe D, Owen D, et al. Cardiac failure presenting as sleep apnea: Elimination of apnea following medical management of cardiac failure. Chest 1988;94:1298–1300.

24. Otsuka K, Ichimaru Y, Yanaga T. Studies of arrhythmias by 24-hour polygraphic recordings: Relationship between artrioventricular block and sleep states. Am Heart J 1983;105:934–940.

25. Nevins DB. First- and second-degree A-V heart block with rapid eye movement sleep. Ann Intern Med 1972,76:981–983.

26. Parish JM, Shepherd JW, Jr. Cardiovascular effects of sleep disorders. Chest 1990;97:1220–1226.

27. Brodksy M, Wu D, Denes P, et al. Arrhythmias documented by 24-hour continuous electrocardiographic monitoring in 50 male medical students without apparent heart disease. Am J Cardiol 1977;39:390–395.

28. Guilleminault C, Pool P, Motta J. Sinus arrest during REM sleep in young adults. N Engl J Med 1984;311:1006–1010.

29. Fleg JC, Kennedy HL. Cardiac arrhythmias in a healthy elderly population. Chest 1982;81:302–307.

30. Verrier RL, Kirby DA. Sleep and cardiac arrhythmias. Ann NY Acad Sci 1988;533:238–251.

31. Wellens HJJ, Vermeulen A, Durrer D. Ventricular fibrillation occurring on arousal from sleep by auditory stimuli. Circulation 1971;46:661–665.

32. Tzivoni D, Stern S. Electrocardiographic changes during sleep in normal individuals. Clin Res 1972;20:401.

33. Lown V, Tykocinski M, Gartein A, et al. Sleep and ventricular premature beats. Circulation 1973;48:691–701.

34. De Silva RA. Central nervous system risk factors for sudden coronary death. Ann NY Acad Sci 1982;382:143–161.

35. Pickering TG, Johnston JM, Honour AJ. Comparison of the effects of sleep, exercise and autonomic drugs on ventricular extrasystoles, using ambulatory monitoring of electrocardiogram and electroencephalogram. Am J Med 1978;65:575–583.

36. Rosenblatt G, Zwillig G, Hartman E. Electrocardiographic changes during sleep in patients with cardiac abnormality [Abstr]. Psychophysiology 1969;6:233.

37. Gillis AM, MacLean KE, Guilleminault C. The QT interval during wake and sleep in patients with ventricular arrhythmias. Sleep 1988;11:333–339.

38. Smith R, Johnson L, Rothfield D, et al. Sleep and cardiac arrhythmias. Arch Intern Med 1972;130:751–753.

39. LaRovere MT, Specchia G, Mortara A, et al. Baroreflex sensitivity, clinical correlates and cardiovascular mortality among patients with a first myocardial infarction: A prospective study. Circulation 1988;78:816–824.

40. McWilliams JA. Ventricular fibrillation and sudden death. Br Med J 1923;2:215.

41. Kleiger RE, Miller JP, Bigger JWT, et al. Decreased heart rate variability and its association with increased mortality after acute myocardial infarction. AM J Cardiol 1987;59:256–262.

42. Verrier RL. Mechanisms of behaviorally induced arrhythmias. Circulation 1987;76:I48–I56.

43. Kales A, Bixler EO, Cadieux RJ, et al. Sleep apnoea in a hypertensive population. Lancet 1984;ii:1005–1008.

44. Lavie P, Ben-Yosef R, Rubin AE. Prevalence of sleep apnea syndrome among patients with essential hypertension. Am Heart J 1984;108:373–376.

45. Fletcher EC, DeBehnke RD, Lovoi MS, et al. Undiagnosed sleep apnea in patients with essential hypertension. Ann Intern Med 1985;103:190–195.

46. Williams AJ, Houston D, Finberg S, et al. Sleep apnea syndrome and essential hypertension. Am J Cardiol 1985;55:1019–1022.

47. Escourrour P, Jirani A, Nedelcoux H, et al. Systemic hypertension in sleep apnea syndrome. Chest 1990;98:1362–1365.

48. Tilkian AG, Guilleminault C, Schroeder JS, et al. Hemodynamics in sleep-induced apnea studies during wakefulness and sleep. Ann Intern Med 1976;85:714–719.

49. Burach B, Pollack C, Borowiecki B, et al. The hypersomnia–sleep apnea syndrome: A reversible major cardiovascular hazard. Circulation 1977;56:177.

50. Guilleminault C, Simmons FB, Motta J, et al. Obstructive sleep apnea syndrome and tracheostomy: Longterm follow-up experience. Arch Intern Med 1981;141:985–988.

51. Lugaresi E, Coccagna G, Cirignotta F. Breathing during sleep in man in normal and pathological conditions. Adv Exp Med Biol 1978;99:33–45.

52. Wynne JW. Gas exchange during sleep in patients with chronic airway obstruction. In: Saunders NA, Sullivan CE, eds. Sleep and Breathing. New York: Marcel Dekker, 1984;485–515.

53. Pierce AK, Jarret CE, Werkle G Jr, et al. Respiratory function during sleep in patients with chronic obstructive lung disease. J Clin Invest 1966;45:631–636.

54. Leitch AJ, Clancy LJ, Leggett RJ, et al. Arterial blood gas tensions, hydrogen ion, and electroencephalogram during sleep in patients with chronic ventilatory failure. Thorax 1976;31:730–735.

55. Coccagna G, Lugaresi E. Arterial blood gases and pulmonary and systemic arterial pressure during sleep in chronic obstructive pulmonary disease. Sleep 1978;1:117–124.

56. Koo KW, Sax DS, Snider GL. Arterial blood gases and pH during sleep in chronic obstructive pulmonary disease. Am J Med 1975;58:663–670.

57. Wynne JW, Block AJ, Hemenway J, et al. Disordered breathing and oxygen desaturation during sleep in patients with chronic obstructive lung disease (COLD). Am J Med 1979;66:573–579.

58. Littner MR, McGinty DJ, Arand DL. Determinants of oxygen desaturation in the course of ventilation during sleep in chronic obstructive pulmonary disease. Am Rev Respir Dis 1980;122:849–857.

59. Guilleminault C, Cummiskey J, Motta J. Chronic obstructive airflow disease and sleep studies. Am Rev Respir Dis 1980;122:397–406.

60. Douglas NJ, Calverley PM, Leggett RJ, et al. Transient hypoxemia during sleep in chronic bronchitis and emphysema. Lancet 1979;i:1–4.

61. Francis PW, Muller NL, Gurwitz D, et al. Hemoglobin desaturation: Its occurrence during sleep in patients with cystic fibrosis. Am J Dis Child 1980;134:734–740.

62. Fletcher CM, Hugh-Jones P, McNicol MW, et al. The diagnosis of pulmonary emphysema in the presence of chronic bronchitis. QJ Med 1963;123:33–49.

63. Filley GF, Beckwitt HJ, Reeves JT, et al. Chronic obstructive bronchopulmonary disease. II. Oxygen transport in two clinical types. Am J Med 1968;44:26–38.

64. Flenley DC, Claverly PM, Douglas NJ, et al. Nocturnal hypoxemia and long-term domiciliary oxygen therapy in "blue and bloated" bronchitics. Physiopathological correlations. Chest 1980;77:305–307.

65. DeMarco FJ, Wynne JW, Block AJ, et al. Oxygen desaturation during sleep as a determinant of the "blue and bloated" syndrome. Chest 1981;79:621–625.

66. Arand DL, McGinty DJ, Littner MR. Respiratory patterns associated with hemoglobin desaturation during sleep in chronic obstructive pulmonary disease. Chest 1981;80:183–190.

67. Fleetham JA, Bradley CA, Kryger MH, et al. The effect of low flow oxygen therapy in chemical control of ventilation in patients with hypoxemic COPD. Am Rev Respir Dis 1980;122:833–840.

68. Brezinova A, Catterall JR, Douglas NJ, et al. Night sleep of patients with chronic ventilatory failure and sage matched controls: Number and duration of the EEG episodes of intervening wakefulness and drowsiness. Sleep 1982;5:123–130.

69. Fletcher EC, Martin RJ, Monlux RD. Disturbed EEG sleep patterns in chronic obstructive pulmonary disease. Sleep Res 1982;11:186.

70. Fletcher EC. Respiration during sleep and cardiopulmonary hemodynamics in patients with chronic lung disease. In: Martin RJ, ed. Cardiorespiratory Disorders During Sleep. Mount Kisco, NY: Futura, 1990;215–249.

71. Calverley PMA, Brezinova V, Douglas NJ, et al. The effect of oxygenation on sleep quality in chronic bronchitis and emphysema. Am Rev Respir Dis 1982;126:206–210.

72. Flick MR, Block AJ. Nocturnal vs. diurnal cardiac arrhythmias in patients with chronic obstructive pulmonary disease. Chest 1979;75:8–11.

73. Shepard JW Jr, Garrison MW, Grither DA, et al. Relationship of ventricular ectopy to nocturnal oxygen desaturation in patients with chronic obstructive pulmonary disease. Am J Med 1985;78:28–34.

74. Mezon BL, West P, Israel J, et al. Sleep breathing abnormalities in kyphoscoliosis. Am Rev Respir Dis 1980;122:617–621.

75. Guilleminault C, Kurland G, Winkle R, et al. Severe kyphoscoliosis, breathing and sleep. Chest 1981;79:626–630.

76. Muller NL, Francis PW, Gurwitz D, et al. Mechanism of hemoglobin in desaturation during rapid-eye-movement sleep in normal subjects and in patients with cystic fibrosis. Am Rev Respir Dis 1980;121:463–469.

77. Stokes DC, McBride JT, Wall MA, et al. Sleep hypoxemia in young adults with cystic fibrosis. Dis Child 1980;134:741–743.

78. Bye PT, Issa F, Berthan-Jones M, et al. Studies of oxygenation during sleep in patients with interstitial lung disease. Am Rev Respir Dis 1984;129:27–32.

79. George CF, Kryger MH. Sleep in restrictive lung disease. Sleep 1987;10:409–418.

80. Nocturnal Oxygen Therapy Trial Group. Continuous or nocturnal oxygen therapy in hypoxemic chronic obstructive lung disease. Ann Intern Med 1980;93:391–398.

81. Medical Research Council Working Party. Long-term domiciliary oxygen therapy in chronic hypoxic cor pulmonale complicating chronic bronchitis and emphysema. Lancet 1981;i:681–686.

82. Fulmer JD, Snider GL. ACCP-NHLBI national conference on oxygen therapy. Chest 1984;86:234–247.

83. Motta J, Guilleminault C. Effects of oxygen administration in sleep-induced apneas. In: Guilleminault C, Dement WC, eds. Sleep Apnea Syndrome. New York: Alan R. Liss, 1978;137–144.

84. Kearley RW, Wynne JW, Bock AJ, et al. Effects of low flow oxygen on sleep disordered breathing in patients with COPD. Chest 1980;78:682–685.

85. Fleetham JA, Conway W, West P, et al. The effect of oxygen therapy on sleep profile and arousal frequency in hypoxemic COPD patients. Am Rev Respir Dis 1981;123(suppl):72.

86. Tyler JM. The effect of progesterone on the respiration of patients with emphysema and hypercapnia. J Clin Invest 1960;39:34–41.

87. Dolly R, Block AJ. Medroxyprogesterone and COPD: Effect on breathing and oxygenation in sleep and awake patients. Chest 1983;84:394–398.

88. Sutton JR, Gray GW, Houston CS, et al. Effects of duration at altitude and acetazolamide in ventilation and oxygenation during sleep. Sleep 1980;3:445–464.

89. Prefaut C, Bourgouin-Karaouni D, Ramonatxo M, et al. Blood gases and pulmonary haemodynamic follow-up during a one-year double blind bismesylate almitrine therapy in COPD patients. Am Rev Respir Dis 1985;131:A71.

90. Connaughton JJ, Douglas NJ, Morgan AD, et al. Almitrine improves oxygenation when both awake and asleep, in patients with hypoxia and CO_2 retention due to chronic bronchitis and emphysema. Am Rev Respir Dis 1985;132:206–210.

91. MacNee W, Connaugton JJ, Hayhurst MD, et al. The effects of almitrine on pulmonary artery pressure and right ventricular performance in chronic bronchitis and emphysema. Respiration 1984;46:157–158.

92. Janson C, Gislason T, Boman G, et al. Sleep disturbances in patients with asthma. Respir Med 1990;84:37–42.

93. Turner-Warwick M. Epidemiology of nocturnal asthma. Am J Med 1988;85:6–8.

94. Cochrane GM, Clark TJH. A survey of asthma mortality in patients between ages 35 and 65 in the greater London hospitals in 1971. Thorax 1975;30:300–315.

95. Hetzel MR, Clark TJH, Branthwaite MA. Asthma: Analysis of sudden deaths and ventilatory arrests in hospital. Br Med J 1977;1:808–811.

96. Kales A, Beall GN, Bajor GF, et al. Sleep studies in asthmatic adults: Relationship of attacks to sleep stage and time of night. J Allergy 1968;41:164–173.

97. Kales J, Kales JD, Sly R, et al. Sleep patterns of asthmatic children: All night electroencephalographic studies. J Allergy 1970;46:300–308.

98. Montplaisir J, Walsh J, Malo JL. Nocturnal asthma: Features of attacks, sleep and breathing patterns. Am Rev Respir Dis 1982;125:18–22.

99. Martin RJ. Nocturnal asthma. In: Martin RJ, ed. Cardiorespiratory Disorders During Sleep. Mount Kisco, N.Y.: Futura, 1990;189–214.

100. Clark TJH, Hetzel MR. Diurnal variation of asthma. Br J Dis Chest 1977;71:87–92.

101. Catterall JR, Rhind GB, Stewart IC, et al. Effect of sleep deprivation on overnight bronchoconstriction in nocturnal asthma. Thorax 1986;41:676–680.

102. Jonsson E, Mossberg B. Impairment of ventilatory function by supine posture in asthma. Eur J Respir Dis 1984;65:496–503.

103. Barnes PJ, Fitzgerald G, Brown M, et al. Nocturnal asthma and changes in circulating epinephrine, histamine and cortisol. N Engl J Med 1980;303:263–267.

104. Goodall RJR, Earis JE, Cooper DN, et al. Relationship between asthma and gastrooesophageal reflux. Thorax 1981;36:116–121.

105. Tan WC, Ballard RD, Martin RJ, et al. The role of gastroesophageal reflux in nocturnal asthma. Am Rev Respir Dis 1988;137:55.

106. Sullivan CE, Zamel N, Kozar LF, et al. Regulation of airway smooth muscle tone in sleeping dogs. Am Rev Respir Dis 1979;119:87–99.

107. Rhind GB, Connaughton JJ, McFie J, et al. Sustained release choline theophyllinate in nocturnal asthma. Br Med J 1985;291:1605–1607.

108. Janson C, Gislason T, Almqvist M, et al. Theophylline disturbs sleep mainly in caffeine-sensitive persons. Pulm Pharmacol 1989;2:125–129.

109. Berquist WE, Rachelefsky GS, Kadden M, et al. Effect of theophylline on gastroesophageal reflux in normal adults. J Allergy Clin Immunol 1981;67:407–411.

110. Stein MR, Towner TG, Weber RW, et al. The effect of theophylline on the lower esophageal sphincter pressure. Ann Allergy 1980;45:238–241.

111. Hubert D, Gaudric M, Guerre J, et al. Effect of theophylline on gastroesophageal reflux in patients with asthma. J Allergy Clin Immunol 1988;81:1168–1174.

112. Guilleminault C, Silvestri R. Aging, drugs and sleep. Neurobiol Aging 1982;3:379–386.

113. Martin RJ, Cicutto LC, Smith HR, et al. Airway inflammation in nocturnal asthma. Am Rev Respir Dis 1991;143:351–357.
114. Ballard RD, Saathoff MC, Patel DK, et al. The effect of sleep on nocturnal bronchoconstriction and ventilatory patterns in asthmatics. J Appl Physiol 1989;67:243–249.
115. Catterall JR, Douglas NJ, Calverley PMA. Irregular breathing and hypoxemia during sleep in chronic stable asthma. Lancet 1982;1:301–314.
116. Šoutar CA, Costello J, Ijuduola O, et al. Nocturnal and morning asthma. Thorax 1975;30:436–440.
117. Warren CPW. Lung restriction. In: Kryger M, ed. Pathophysiology of Respiration. New York: John Wiley & Sons, 1981;43–69.
118. Perez-Padilla RR, West P, Lertzman M, et al. Breathing during sleep in patients with interstitial lung disease. Am Rev Respir Dis 1985;132:224–229.
119. Hoeppner VH, Cockcroft DW, Dosman JA, et al. Nighttime ventilation improves respiratory failure in secondary kyphoscoliosis. Am Rev Respir Dis 1984;129:240–243.
120. Dragstedt LR. A concept of the etiology of gastric and duodenal ulcers. Gastroenterology 1956;30:208–220.
121. Orr WC, Hall WH, Stahl ML, et al. Sleep patterns and gastric acid secretion in duodenal ulcer disease. Arch Intern Med 1976;136:655–660.
122. Orr WC. Gastrointestinal disorders. In: Kryger MH, Roth T, Dement WC, eds. Principles and Practice of Sleep Medicine. Philadelphia: WB Saunders, 1989; 622–629.
123. Kildebo S, Aronsen O, Bernersen B, et al. Cimetidine 800 mg at night, in the treatment of duodenal ulcers. Scand J Gastroenterol 1985;20:1147–1150.
124. McGuigan JE. Peptic ulcer and gastritis. In: Wilson JD, Braunwald E, Isselbacher KJ, et al., eds. Harrison's Principles of Internal Medicine, ed 2 New York: McGraw-Hill, 1991;1229–1248.
125. Howden CW, Jones DB, Hunt RH. Nocturnal doses of H₂ receptor antagonists for duodenal ulcer. Lancet 1985;i:647–648.
126. Gledhill T, Buck M, Paul A, et al. Comparison of the effects of proximal gastric vagotomy, cimetidine, and placebo on nocturnal intragastric acidity and acid secretion in patients with cimetidine resistance duodenal ulcer. Br J Surg 1983;70:704–706.
127. Gough KR, Bardhan KD, Crowe JP, et al. Ranitidine and cimetidine in prevention of duodenal ulcer relapse. Lancet 1984;2:659–662.
128. Silvis SE. Final report on the United States multicenter trial comparing ranitidine to cimetidine as maintenance therapy following healing of duodenal ulcer. J Clin Gastroenterol 1985;7:482–487, 1985.
129. Santana IA, Sharma BK, Pounder RE, et al. 24-Hour intragastric acidity during maintenance treatment with ranitidine. Br Med J 1984;289:1420.
130. Klauser AG, Schindlbeck NE, Muller-Lissner SA. Symptoms in gastroesophageal reflux disease. Gut 1988;29:886–889.
131. Richter JE, Castell DO. Gastroesophageal reflux. Ann Intern Med 1982;97:93–103.
132. Barrett NR. Chronic peptic ulcer of the oesophagus and "oesophagitis." Br J Surg 1950;38:175–182.
133. Allison PR, Johnstone AS. The osophagus lined with gastric mucous membrane. Thorax 1953;8:87–101.
134. Bozymski EM, Herlihy KJ, Orlando RC. Barrett's esophagus. Ann Intern Med 1982;97:103–107.
135. Johnsson F, Joelsson B. Reproducibility of ambulatory oesophageal pH monitoring. Gut 1988;29:886–889.
136. Johnson LF, DeMeester TR. Twenty-four hour pH monitoring of the distal esophagus. Am J Gastroenterol 1974;62:325–332.
137. DeMeester R, Johnson LF, Guy JJ, et al. Patterns of gastroesophageal reflux in health and disease. Ann Surg 1976;184:459–470.
138. Allen CJ, Newhouse MT. Gastroesophageal reflux and chronic respiratory disease. Am Rev Respir Dis 1984;129:645–647.
139. David P, Denis P, Nouvet G, et al. Lung function and gastroesophageal reflux during chronic bronchitis. Bull Eur Physiopathol Respir 1982;18:81–86.
140. Orringer MB. Respiratory symptoms and esophageal reflux. Chest 1979;76:618–619.
141. Chernow B, Johnson LF, Janowitz WR, et al. Pulmonary aspiration as a consequence of gastroesophageal reflux: A diagnostic approach. Dig Dis Sci 1979;24:839–844.
142. Tan WC, Martin RJ, Pandey R, et al. Effects of spontaneous and simulated gastroesophageal reflux on sleeping asthmatics. Am Rev Respir Dis 1990;141:1394–1399.
143. Mansfield LE. Gastroesophageal reflux and respiratory disorders: A review. Ann Allergy 1989;62:158–163.
144. Pack AI. Acid: A nocturnal brochoconstrictor? Am Rev Respir Dis 1990;141:1391–1392.
145. Herbst JJ, Minton SD, Book LS. Gastroesophageal reflux causing respiratory distress and apnea in newborn infants. J Pediatr 1979;95:763.
146. Herbst JJ, Book LS, Bray PF. Gastroesophageal reflux in the "near miss" sudden infant death syndrome. J Pediatr 1978;92:73.
147. Triadafilopoulos G, Castillo T. Nonpropulsive esophageal contractions and gastroesophageal reflux. Am J Gastroenterol 1991;86:153–159.
147a. Maton PN. Drug therapy: Omeprazole. N Engl J Med 1991;324:965–975.
148. Skatrud J, Iber C, Ewart R, et al. Disordered breathing during sleep in hypothyroidism. Am Rev Respir Dis 1981; 124:325–329.
149. Millman RP, Bevilacqua J, Peterson DD, et al. Central sleep apnea in hypothyroidism. Am Rev Respir Dis 1983;127:504–507.
150. Rajagopal KR, Abbrecht PH, Derderian SS, et al. Obstructive sleep apnea in hypothyroidism. Ann Intern Med 1984;101:491–494.
151. Kales A, Heuser G, Jacobson A, et al. All-night sleep studies in hypothyroid patients before and after treatment. J Clin Endocrinol 1967;27:1593–1599.
152. Dunleavy DLF, Oswald I, Brown P, et al. Hyperthyroidism, sleep and growth hormone. Electroencephalogr Clin Neurophysiol 1974;36:259–263.

153. Passouant P, Passouant-Fountaine T, Cadilhac J. L'influence de l'hyperthyroidie sur le sommeil. Etude clinique et experimentale. Rev Neurol 1966;115:353–366.

154. Johns MW, Rinsler MG. Sleep and thyroid function. Further studies in healthy young men. J Psychosomat Res 1977;21:161–166.

155. Astrom C, Lindholm J. Growth hormone–deficient young adults have decreased deep sleep. Neuroendocrinology 1990;51:82–84.

156. Astrom C, Pedersen SA, Lindholm J. The influence of growth hormone on sleep in adults with growth hormone deficiency. Clin Endocrinol 1990;33:495–500.

157. Wu RHK, Thorpy MJ. Effect of growth hormone treatment on sleep EEGs in growth hormone deficiency children. Sleep 1988;11:425–429.

158. Sullivan CE, Parker S, Grunstein RR, et al. Ventilatory control in sleep apnea: A search for brain's neurochemical defects. In: Issa FG, Suratt PM, Remmers JE, eds. Sleep and Respiration. New York: Wiley-Liss, 1990;325–334.

159. Grunstein RR, Ho KY, Sullivan CE. Sleep apnea in acromegaly. Ann Intern Med 1991;115:527–532.

160. Williams RL. Sleep disturbances in various medical and surgical conditions. In: Williams RL, Karacan I, Moore CA, eds. Sleep Disorders. New York: John Wiley & Sons, 1988;265–291.

161. Karacan I, Williams RL, Bose J, et al. Insomnia in Hemodialytic and Kidney Transplant Patients. Abstracts of Papers Presented to the Eleventh Annual Meeting of the Association for the Psychophysiological Study of Sleep. Psychophysiology 1972;9:137.

162. Daly RJ, Hassall C. Reported sleep on maintenance haemodialysis. Br Med J 1970;2:508–509.

163. Passouant P, Cadihac J, Baldy-Moulinier M, et al. Etude du sommeil nocturne chez des uremiques chroniques soumis a une epuration extrarenale. Electroencephalogr Clin Neurophysiol 1970;29:441–449.

164. Strub B, Schneider-Helment D, Gnirss F, et al. Sleep disorders in patients with chronic renal insufficiency in long-term hemodialysis treatment. Schweiz Med Wochenschr 1982;112:824–828.

165. Fraser C, Arieff AI. Nervous system complications in uremia. Ann Intern Med 1988;109:143–153.

166. Kimmel PL, Miller G, Mendelson WB. Sleep apnea syndrome in chronic renal disease. Am J Med 1989;86:308–314.

167. Kimmel PL. Sleep apnea in end-stage renal disease. Semin Dialys 1991;4:52–58.

168. Millman RP, Kimmel PL, Shore ET, et al. Sleep apnea in hemodialysis patients: The lack of testosterone effect on its pathogenesis. Nephron 1985;40:407–410.

169. Mendelson WB, Wadhwa NK, Greenberg HE, et al. Effects of hemodialysis on sleep apnea syndrome in end-stage renal disease. Clin Nephrol 1990;33:247–251.

170. Fein AM, Niederman MS, Imbriano L, et al. Reversal of sleep apnea in uremia by dialysis. Arch Intern Med 1987;147:1355–1356.

171. Anderton J, Harris E, Robson J. The ventilatory response to carbon dioxide and hydrogen ion in renal failure. Clin Sci 1965;28:251–258.

172. Hamilton R, Epstein P, Henderson L, et al. Control of breathing in uremia: Ventilatory response to CO_2 after hemodialysis. J Appl Physiol 1976;41:216–222.

173. Crabb JE, Pingleton SK, Gollub S, et al. Sleep-disordered breathing in decompensated congestive heart failure [Abstr]. Am Rev Respir Dis 1985;105:68.

174. Ingbar DH, Gee BL. Pathophysiology and treatment of sleep apnea. Annu Rev Med 1985;36:365–395.

175. Goldenberg DL. Fibromyalgia syndrome: An emerging but controversial condition. JAMA 1987;257:2782–2787.

176. Yunus M, Masi AT, Calabro JJ, et al. Primary fibromyalgia (fibrositis): Clinical study of 50 patients with matched normal controls. Semin Arthritis Rheum 1981;11:151–172.

177. Moldofsky H, Lue FA, Smythe H. Alpha EEG sleep and morning symptoms of rheumatoid arthritis. J Rheumatol 1983;10:373–379.

178. Moldofsky H, Saskin P, Lue FA. Sleep and symptoms in fibrositis syndrome after a febrile illness. J Rheumatol 1988;15:1701–1704.

179. Hauri P, Hawkins H. Alpha-delta sleep. Electroencephalogr Clin Neurophysiol 1973;34:233–237.

180. Scheuler W, Kubicki ST, Marquardt J, et al. The alpha sleep pattern—quantitative analysis and functional aspects. In: Koella WP, et al. eds. Sleep 86. Stuttgart: Gustav Fischer, 1988;284–286.

181. Horne JA, Shackett BS. Alpha-like EEG activity in non-REM sleep and the fibromyalgia (fibrositis) syndrome. Electroencephalogr Clin Neurophysiol 1991;79:271–276.

182. Hansen NE. Sleep related plasma haemoglobin levels in paroxysmal nocturnal haemoglobinuria. Acta Medica Scand 1968;184:547–549.

183. Scharf MB, Lobel JS, Cadwell E, et al. Nocturnal oxygen desaturation in patients with sickle cell anemia. JAMA 1983;249:1753–1755.

184. Hara KS, Shepard JW Jr. Sleep and critical care medicine. In: Martin RJ, ed. Cardiorespiratory Disorders During Sleep. Mount Kisco, N.Y.: Futura Publishing Company, 1990;323–363.

185. Richards KC, Bairnsfather L. A description of night sleep patterns in the critical care unit. Heart Lung 1988;17:35–42.

186. Orr WC, Stahl ML. Sleep disturbances after open heart surgery. Am J Cardiol 1977;39:196–201.

187. Karacan I, Green JR Jr, Taylor WJ, et al. Sleep in postmyocardial infarction patients. In: Eliot RS, ed. Stress and the Heart: Contemporary Problems in Cardiology. Mt Kisco, N.Y.: Futura, 1974;163–195.

188. Aurell J, Emlqvist D. Sleep in the surgical intensive care unit: Continuous polygraphic recording of sleep in nine patients receiving postoperative care. Br Med J 1985;290:1029–1032.

189. Norman SE, Chediak AD, et al. Sleep disturbances in HIV-infected homosexual men. AIDS 1990;4:775–781.

190. Norman SE, Chediak AD. Longitudinal analysis of sleep disturbances in HIV-infected men. Sleep Res 1992;21:304.

191. Moller WM, Schreiber W, Krieg J-C, et al. Alterations of nocturnal sleep in patients with HIV infection. Acta Neurol Scand 1991;83:141–142.

192. Logigian EL, Kaplan RF, Steere AC. Chronic neurologic manifestations of Lyme disease. N Engl J Med 1990;323:1438–1444.

193. Halperin JJ. Neurological applications of Lyme disease. Neurol Chron 1992;1:1–4.

194. Dinerman H, Steere AC. Lyme disease associated with fibromyalgia. Ann Intern Med 1992;117:281–285.

195. Steere AC, Beraidi VP, Weeks KE, et al. Evaluation of the intrathecal antibody response to *Borrelia burgdorferi* as a diagnostic test for Lyme neuroborreliosis. J Infect Dis 1990;161:1203–1209.

196. Krupp LB, Mendelson WB, Friedman R. An overview of chronic fatigue syndrome. J Clin Psychiatry 1991;52:403–410.

197. Holmes GP, Kaplan JE, Gantz NM, et al. Chronic fatigue syndrome: A working case definition. Ann Intern Med 1988;108:385–389.

198. Bert J, Collomb H, Fressy J, et al. Etude électro-encéphalographique du sommeil nocturne au cours de la trypanosomiase humaine africaine. In: Fischgold H, ed. Le Sommeil de Nuit Normal et Pathologique. Etudes Electroencéphalographiques. Paris: Masson, 1965;334–352.

199. Schwartz BA, Escande C. Sleeping sickness: Sleep study of a case. Electroencephalogr Clin Neurophysiol 1970;29:83–87.

200. Billiard M. Other hypersomnias. In: Throphy MJ, ed. Handbook of Sleep Disorders. New York: Marcel Dekker, 1990;353–371.

201. Buguet A, Gati R, Sevre JP, et al. 24-Hour polysomnographic evaluation in a patient with sleeping sickness. Electroencephalogr Clin Neurophysiol 1989;72:471–478.

23

Circadian Rhythm Disorders

Kevin A. O'Connor
Mark W. Mahowald
Milton G. Ettinger

Chronobiology, the study of biologic rhythms, both normal and abnormal, is a field whose time has come. Giant strides have been made; much remains to be learned. The staggering medical, social, and economic consequences of chronobiologic dysfunction are imperatives for further advancement of this exciting field.

Disorders of these rhythms are of more than academic interest; they affect alertness, concentration, and performance that can be crucial for safety in occupations such as transportation and manufacturing. The recently released *Report of the National Commission on Sleep Disorders Research* has underscored the startling socioeconomic consequences of sleepiness in our society, at the personal, national, and international level.[1] The wake-sleep scheduling conditions figure large in these disastrous consequences. Job-related and social demands on wake-sleep schedules may result in circadian rhythm disorders that can be life threatening. Studies have shown a circadian pattern of motor vehicle accidents: the incidence is several times higher in early morning hours and peak again (though not as high) in the afternoon.[2] Human death and birth show circadian patterns: both tend to occur in the late night or early morning.[3,4] Other circadian rhythm disorders may not have any obvious cause, but they can nevertheless result in significant impairment if affected persons are required to perform when sleepy or fatigued as they attempt to adjust to the geophysical world.

Most living creatures follow a relentless and pervasive daily rhythm of activity and rest that is, ultimately, linked to the periodic energy flow from the sun to a spot on Earth as it rotates. Plants, animals, even unicellular organisms, show daily variations in metabolic activity, locomotion, feeding, and many other functions.[5-7] When isolated from time cues such as sunlight, many creatures show intrinsic rhythms of nearly, but rarely exactly, 24 hours. Certain mice, for example, run on an exercise wheel for several hours about once every 24 hours when kept in an environment with constant lighting.[7] Such a near–24-hour rhythm is called a *circadian* rhythm, a term coined by Franz Halberg, from the Latin *circa* (about) and *dies* (day).[8]

In humans and other mammals the suprachiasmatic nucleus (SCN) of the hypothalamus controls most circadian rhythms, such as rest-activity rhythm[9] and drinking rhythm. The SCN does not appear to mediate food-anticipatory activity, however.[10,11] The recent discovery of a retinohypothalamic tract in animals indicated that the biologic clock may be directly influenced by environmental light.[12-15] This led to the application of bright light to rest rhythms of activity in animal studies and the wake-sleep cycle in humans.[16,17] The timing of exposure to bright light, with respect to the animal's intrinsic rhythm, controls the nature of the resetting. For example, in a diurnal (day-active) animal, bright light administered just as activity is beginning, say at 6:00 A.M., typically advances the onset of the next active period, which might occur at 5:00 A.M. the next day. Bright light administered in the middle of the day, say at 1:00 P.M., usually has no effect on the timing of the next day's activity. The interval of little effect is called the *dead zone*. Bright light administered at the end of the day, a few hours before sleep onset, say at 8:00 P.M. often delays the activity rhythms. The animal experiences a delay in activity onset, which in this example might not occur until 7:30 A.M. instead of the usual 6:00 A.M.

This has lead to the concept of the phase response curve (PRC), which indicates the various responses of advance, dead zone, and delay of the cycle.[18-20] The PRC is determined by exposing an individual or a population to the bright light or another stimulus at a variety of clock times in the free-running condition and noting the effects on subsequent activity onsets. The same stimulus has dramatically different effects on the underlying rhythm, depending on when in the rhythm it is administered. The effect is much greater during the subjective night and may be negligible during the day. Light at the beginning of the "night" delays the rhythm; administered toward the end of the night it advances it.[16,21,22] The PRC may differ substantially between individuals, and differs systematically with the intensity of the light stimulus.

The importance of the light-dark cycle on the human biologic clock is underscored by the fact that only a third of totally blind humans become entrained to the environment. One-third have a cycle of 24 hours but out of phase with the environment, and the remaining third experiencing a free-running pattern longer than 24 hours.[23] In fact, treating totally blind people with a variety of agents may be useful in demonstrating their effects on biologic rhythms.[24] In addition to light, a variety of other stimuli can affect rest-activity rhythms and others, resulting in a variety of PRCs.[25–28]

In human beings, too, many biologic variables show circadian rhythms in isolation studies: temperature, sleep, serum potassium, sodium, and calcium, urine output, white blood cell count, attention, short-term memory, ability to perform calculations, and performance. Such isolation studies have been carried out for decades. Typically they require a subject to live in a set of rooms sequestered from external time cues for weeks or longer without windows, clocks, radios, televisions, current newspapers, or magazines. Instruments record activity, core temperature, and sleep electroencephalography (EEG). The laboratory may obtain a variety of other tests, such as serum electrolytes, cortisol, and melatonin.[5]

Figure 23-1 displays a schematic example of the sleep-wake pattern typical of a free-running study. This is not from an actual recording but is contrived to illustrate some conventions and terms that are used in the following discussion of circadian rhythm disorders. Black bars represent sleep, double plotted to highlight patterns. Two 24-hour intervals extend to the right of each number, which represents a day of the study. The left end of the first bar represents the first sleep onset, which occurs at about 11:00 P.M. on day 1. Just below that, on day 2, sleep begins also at 11:00 P.M. The second sleep onset is represented to the right of the first and also below it. During the first six days of the study, the subject is entrained, or synchronized, with external time cues (*Zeitgebers*). The sleep onsets virtually all line up at 11:00 P.M.

On day 7 isolation begins, after which sleep onset is delayed to about 00:30 on day 8. From day 7 through day 17 there is a fairly constant delay of about 1 hour per day. Sleep onsets occur throughout the hours of the day. The average time between sleep onsets, which is one measured of the "period" of the cycle, is about 25 hours, typical for humans in free-running conditions. Such a free-running pattern is observed briefly during the transition from the cha-

otic wake-sleep pattern of newborn infants to the well-developed wake-sleep and day-night pattern in normal adults.[29]

In addition to overall circadian wake-sleep schedule abnormalities, there may be ultradian (less than 24-hour) dysrhythmias of state (wakefulness, rapid eye movement [REM] sleep, non-REM [NREM] sleep). These are beyond the scope of this review.[30]

CLINICAL EVALUATION

The wake-sleep schedule disorders fall into two categories: primary (malfunction of the biologic clock per se) and secondary (due to environmental effects on the underlying clock). The secondary disorders (such as jet lag and that induced by shift work) are usually immediately apparent on questioning the patient. The primary disorders may be much more difficult to diagnose, as they typically masquerade as other disorders, such as hypersomnia, insomnia, substance (sedative-hypnotic or stimulant) abuse, or psychiatric conditions.

Clinical evaluation must include a thorough medical and psychiatric history, physical examination, and a detailed analysis of the wake-sleep pattern. Careful attention must be given to medications (prescription and other). A most important piece of historical information is that, once sleep has begun, it is uninterrupted and normal. It is not the sleep per se, but rather the timing of sleep, that is abnormal. The patient's report of what the pattern would be (or has been) under free-running conditions may be invaluable. Even if there has been no opportunity to run free, the patient may be amazingly accurate when asked to speculate about what the pattern would likely be if he or she were to spend 2 weeks on a South Seas Island with absolutely no environmental time constraints (work, school, meals, family obligations). When the patient is running free, it is usually clear that the issue is the timing, not the duration or quality, of sleep.

A subjective log reflecting at least 2 weeks of the patient's wake-sleep pattern should be available for the initial interview. Often, analysis of such a sleep diary is sufficient to suspect or establish a tentative diagnosis. If not, objective data may be invaluable. Such data may be obtained by actigraphy, a recently developed technique that provides an objective record of activity that supplements the log. For actigraphy a small wrist-mounted device is worn for a week or two, during which the device records the activity per time epoch, which is often 1 minute for a 1-week study. In one model of actigraphy, the recorded unit is the number of zero-crossings of a voltage that is affected by movements of a tiny beam

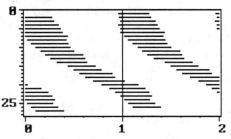

FIGURE 23-1. *Schematic example of a free-run study. See text for details.*

within the actigraph. Like a seismometer, the beam moves with respect to the actigraph, when the actigraph moves with the subject's wrist. There are different models of the actigraph, whose principles are reviewed elsewhere.[31] When data collection is completed, the results are transferred into a personal computer, where software permits display of activity versus time. Figure 23-2 shows an actigraphic report and demonstrates how the pattern is apparent at a glance. There is high correlation between the rest and activity recorded by the actigraph and the wake-sleep pattern.[32,33]

TREATMENT MODALITIES

Until recently, the circadian rhythm disorders were of only academic interest, as no proven effective treatments existed. Fortunately, this has changed,

and the majority of patients with these often incapacitating disorders benefit from accurate diagnosis and appropriate treatment. The mainstays of treatment are phototherapy and chronotherapy. In addition, promising new pharmacologic treatments are on the horizon.

Chronotherapy

In chronotherapy, the desirable total sleep time is determined by sleep logs during a free-running period. The patient then delays or advances sleep onset by a few hours every day and sleeps only the predetermined number of hours until sleep onset occurs at the desired time, at which point the patient attempts to maintain that time.[34-36] This method requires several days of free time and can be derailed if sleeping quarters cannot be kept dark and quiet during the several daytime sleeps required.[37]

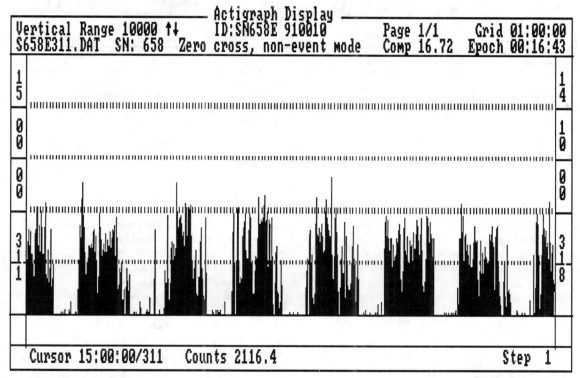

A

FIGURE 23-2. *Typical actigraphic reports. The vertical bars represent activity levels plotted over seven consecutive 24-hour periods, permitting rapid assessment of the objective rest/activity pattern, which correlates with the sleep/wake pattern. The difference between that of a normal adult female (A) and an adult male with a chaotic wake/sleep pattern (B) is immediately apparent.*

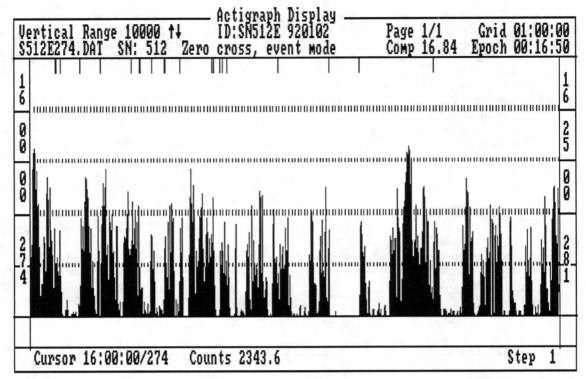

B

FIGURE 23-2.   *(continued)*

Phototherapy

It was recently discovered that exposure to bright light at strategic times of the wake-sleep cycle results in a change in the underlying rhythm. This has afforded an opportunity to treat circadian dysrhythmias very effectively.[16,21,37] The timing of the phototherapy and the duration depend on the diagnosis and individual response. The patient sits at a prescribed distance from a bright light, furnishing an illuminance of more than 2500 lux at that distance. Fluorescent lights are commonly used. Commercially available light boxes for treatment of seasonal affective disorders typically provide 5000 to 10,000 lux, depending on the model. Distance from the light is critical in determining the illuminance, according to the inverse square law. Doubling the distance cuts the illuminance to one-fourth. The effect of light on human rhythms varies with intensity, wavelength, timing, and duration of exposure. Much remains to be learned about these variables and the effectiveness of phototherapy in the clinical setting.[38,39]

The light should be angled with respect to the patient's eyes, to diminish eyestrain. Patients with a history of eye disorders should consult their ophthalmologist before beginning treatment. Light units should be safety tested electrically and should include measures to screen ultraviolet.[40]

Adverse effects include headache, eyestrain, and excessive advance of sleep onset. Possible remedies for these problems include analgesics, change in light position, and decrease in exposure time, respectively. Bright light exposure has been reported to precipitate mania in persons with bipolar disorder.[41,42] In such cases, light therapy should be discontinued immediately and appropriate measures instituted to control the mania, such as neuroleptics, other mood-stabilizing medication, and hospitalization. Candidates for light therapy should be questioned about both personal and family history of psychiatric disorders and should be warned about the possible precipitation of mania.

Little information exists on the interaction of light and a variety of commonly used medications.

Caution is urged in the use of light with medications that are said to cause photosensitization.[43,44]

PHARMACOLOGIC MANIPULATIONS

A number of exciting therapeutic possibilities are in development. Although promising, pharmacologic manipulation of biologic rhythms is still in its developmental phase. None of these potential treatments has efficacy for any given clinical application, and thorough review is beyond the scope of this chapter. There are compelling data that suggest that benzodiazepines are capable of affecting biologic rhythms.[45-48] There have been scattered reports of the effect of vitamin B_{12} on some circadian rhythms.[49-52] Tricyclic antidepressants, monoamine oxidase inhibitors, and lithium may also influence biologic rhythms.[53]

One of the most promising pharmacologic treatment hopefuls is melatonin. Melatonin is secreted by the pineal gland, and secretion is suppressed by exposure to light and is entrained by the light-dark cycle. It is coupled to the wake-sleep cycle and to circadian cortisol rhythm and is a valuable marker of the underlying wake-sleep period. Melatonin likely plays an important role in biorhythms, and there is evidence that administration of exogenous melatonin may alter them—an effect that could have most important therapeutic clinical applications.[24,54,55] The recent discovery of melatonin receptors in the suprachiasmatic nucleus of humans suggests its importance in biologic rhythms.[56] The timing of melatonin administration results in variable changes in the underlying rhythm (resulting in a PRC similar to that produced by exposure to light) though in the opposite direction (melatonin at the beginning of the "night" advances the sleep phase and vice versa).[55,57]

CHRONOPHARMACOLOGY

Not only may pharmacologic agents influence biologic rhythms, but, conversely, the timing of administration of a large variety of (perhaps all) medications and other therapies (such as irradiation) may have profound effects on their efficacy and toxicity. Many drugs exhibit circadian rhythms in therapeutic effectiveness or toxicity.[58,59] There is substantial work that demonstrates that the therapeutic benefits may be maximized and the toxic side effects minimized by administering the drug at the appropriate time of day. Circadian rhythms in rates of metabolism and inactivation have been demonstrated,[60] along with variation in rates of excretion of drug

products.[61] Circadian variations in blood volume and extracellular fluid volume, resulting in varying degrees of dilution of the drug and variations in the susceptibility of the target organ or organs to the circulating drug, all contribute to the net effect of circadian variation in response to a specific medication.

There has been very little work, to date, on the circadian considerations of drugs utilized in the treatment of sleep disorders, but there is compelling evidence from other areas—cancer chemotherapy, anesthetics and antiepilepsy drugs, steroid administration[62]—of the importance of considering time of day in drug administration.

Narcolepsy is a good example of a sleep disorder requiring lifelong stimulant therapy. No data are currently available to help plan timing of medication to maximize therapeutic effects and minimize toxic effects. This concept presents a challenging new opportunity for investigation of drug therapy in sleep disorders.

RELATIONSHIP WITH MAJOR PSYCHIATRIC DISORDERS

Although it is beyond the scope of this chapter, the striking relationship between circadian rhythms and psychiatric disorders, particularly seasonal affective disorder, primary depression, and bipolar affective disorder, must be mentioned.[63] These disorders are often associated with abnormalities of the wake-sleep cycle and of the cycling of REM and NREM sleep within that cycle.[64,65] Interestingly, many of the treatment modalities for these conditions affect the wake-sleep cycle and the REM-NREM cycle (sleep deprivation, phototherapy, and many medications such as the tricyclic antidepressants, monoamine oxidase inhibitors, and lithium).[53,66-68]

PRIMARY CIRCADIAN DYSRHYTHMIAS

Delayed Sleep Phase Syndrome

In delayed sleep phase syndrome (DSPS) the patient falls asleep late and rises late. There is a striking inability to fall asleep at an earlier, more desirable time. For example, a college student is habitually unable to fall asleep until 2:00 A.M. and has great difficulty getting up in time for her 8:00 A.M. class Monday through Friday. She finds herself dozing off during morning classes. On Saturday and Sunday she sleeps in until about 10:00 A.M. and feels rested on arising, with no episodes of dozing during the day.

This disorder may represent 5% to 10% of cases with presenting complaints of insomnia at some sleep disorders centers.[69] It often begins during adolescence, but some patients report onset in childhood. A history of DSPS in family members has been noted clinically. DSPS may follow head trauma.[70]

Some persons suffer disruption of school and work. The complications depend partly on the tolerance of the patient's environment. A lenient employer and a flexible schedule may allow a worker to perform unimpaired if he is permitted to begin and end work a few hours later than others. More demanding or rigid work or school regimens may not allow this and will require the patient to drop out if treatment is not possible. Disruption of family life may also result if other family members do not have a similar schedule. The pervasive misperception that sleeping in is an undesirable personality characteristic such as laziness, slothfulness, or avoidance behavior often leads to interpersonal stress and hostility. Driving or operating machinery when sleepy can result in accidents. Victims of DSPS may use alcohol and sedative-hypnotics in an attempt to induce sleep earlier, sometimes developing alcohol or drug dependency.[71]

The differential diagnosis includes irregular sleep-wake pattern and psychiatric disorders that are associated with disturbed sleep such as major depression, mania, dysthymia, obsessive-compulsive disorder, and schizophrenia, as well as obstructive sleep apnea syndrome, narcolepsy (particularly during its development in adolescents),[72] and the periodic limb movement disorder, with or without the restless legs syndrome. It may be very difficult to differentiate true physiologic DSPS from "sleep phase delay," which is a volitional wake-sleep schedule adopted by an individual to avoid family contact, school, or work.[73]

Exposure to bright light upon awakening (toward the end of the PRC) has been shown to be effective in advancing both sleep onset and temperature rhythm in a placebo-controlled study. The patient is asked to sit near a bright light, furnishing 5000 to 10,000 lux, for about an hour upon awakening every day. The response may not be evident for two weeks, and the treatment may have to be continuous.[37]

Other treatments for DSPS includes chronotherapy and schedule change. For example, the patient goes to sleep at 2:00 A.M. the first night, then at 5:00 A.M., then at 8:00 A.M., and so on, until bedtime is reaching 10:00 P.M. Patients are not always able to stop at the desired time, but keep delaying, sometimes ending up where they started.[74] There are case reports of persons who developed non-24-hour cycle disorder while attempting chronotherapy for DSPS. Their sleep onset never stopped changing once they were progressively delayed.[75]

Some persons with DSPS report temporary resolution in environments with strong time cues, for example when staying with friends or relatives who set limits on staying up late and who help the patient arise at the desired time. There are isolated reports of response to vitamin B_{12},[49] benzodiazepines,[76] and melatonin.[77] The (often unconscious) secondary gain in the intentional sleep phase delay syndrome can make this condition very difficult to treat.

Advanced Sleep Phase Syndrome

Persons suffering from advanced sleep phase syndrome (ASPS) fall asleep early and awaken early. They are unable to remain awake until the desired time, falling asleep in the early evening and awakening in the very early hours of the morning.

There are no studies of the prevalence or incidence of this disorder, but clinical experience suggests that it may be less common than DSPS. The onset of the disorder occurs in later years. Most patients are older than 50 years. ASPS may be responsible for some of the deterioration in the wake-sleep pattern experienced by elderly persons.

Patients complain of interruption of evening activities by sleepiness. They may avoid evening social activities, fearing the intrusive sleepiness. They are also distressed by the very early awakenings. Driving and operating machinery while sleepy (particularly in the evening) can result in accidents.

The differential diagnosis includes psychiatric disorders with sleep disturbance. The early morning awakenings are often erroneously assumed to be a manifestation of depression. The early evening hypersomnia may be misinterpreted as a symptom of a primary sleep disorder such as obstructive sleep apnea syndrome or narcolepsy.

Bright light administered in the late afternoon or early evening (in the early portion of the PRC) has been reported to be effective in delaying both sleep onset and temperature rhythm.[78] The technique is the same as that for DSPS, except for the timing of exposure. Adverse effects are similar, though there is no advance of sleep onset. Instead sleep onset may be long delayed, for example until the early hours of the morning. Briefer light exposure may prevent this. Some flexibility may be needed to establish the timing of the exposure, as the patient may have social activities in the early evening. Occasionally exposure just before supper is convenient and effective. Chronotherapy with a 3-hour advance every other day until the desired sleep-onset time has been reached, may be effective.[79]

Non–24-Hour Sleep-Wake Disorder

Persons who suffer from this disorder, which is also known as hypernycthemeral syndrome, cannot maintain a regular bedtime but find their sleep onset wandering around the clock. Most patients experience a gradually increasing delay in sleep onset, often about 1 hour per sleep-wake cycle. A typical pattern of sleep onsets might be 9:00 P.M. in the first cycle, then 10:00 P.M. then 11:30 P.M., then midnight, then 1:30 A.M., then 3:00 A.M., and so on, eventually progressing through daytime hours into the evening again. This likely reflects the fact that most humans have an intrinsic circadian rhythm of about 25 hours, slightly longer than the 24-hour geophysical day. Rarely, patients experience a gradually increasing advance in sleep-onset time. These persons lack the ability to be entrained, or synchronized, by the usual time cues, such as sunlight and social activity.

This disorder is apparently extremely uncommon. Our three patients have had a major psychiatric diagnosis including recurrent major depression, panic disorder with agoraphobia, and posttraumatic stress disorder. Two had a history consistent with DSPS before the onset of the non–24-hour sleep-wake disorder. In one, the onset of the non–24-hour sleep-wake disorder followed a period of shift work. The course is chronic, and many patients report years of this disturbance.

Structural lesions of the central nervous system such as hypothalamic tumors have been associated with the disorder. Magnetic resonance imaging studies of the head, with special attention to the hypothalamic and pituitary regions, are recommended for them.[80] Totally blind persons who have lost or suffered impairment of their retinohypothalamic pathway frequently experience this disorder. About a third of blind subjects in one series showed the disorder.[23]

Complications include severe disruptions of work or studies, and accidents due to attempting to drive or operate machinery while sleepy. As with DSPS, the tolerance of the patient's environment plays an important role in determining the degree of disruption. Some with a flexible work schedule (such as freelance writers) may experience no disruption of work, which they perform when it is convenient. Others are disabled by this disorder and have been fired from work or expelled from school as a result of poor performance when sleepy or as a result of tardiness or absences associated with inopportune episodes of sleep.

The differential diagnosis includes the irregular sleep-wake pattern, DSPS, psychiatric disorders associated with changes in the wake-sleep patterns, and primary sleep disorders such as narcolepsy and obstructive sleep apnea.

Treatment attempts have included strengthening time cues, and one person reported temporary resolution of symptoms while she lived with a relative who enforced strict schedule for her. Phototherapy,[81] benzodiazepine,[82] and vitamin B$_{12}$[49,83,84]

have all been successful in isolated cases, but controlled studies are not available.

Irregular Sleep-Wake Pattern

Some persons show a disorganized sleep-wake pattern with variable sleep and wake lengths. They complain of insomnia or excessive daytime sleepiness, or both. Sleep onset may occur at a variety of clock times. To meet the official criteria for this diagnosis, there must be at least three sleep episodes per 24-hour period.[85] The disturbance must be present at least 3 months. The average total sleep time per 24 hours is normal for age. There must be objective evidence of disturbed rhythms by 24-hour polysomnographic monitoring or by 24-hour temperature monitoring. The patient currently suffers no medical or psychiatric disorder that could explain the symptoms and does not suffer from another sleep disorder that would account for insomnia or excessive daytime sleepiness. Patients may complain of insomnia or excessive sleepiness, cognitive disturbance, and fatigue.

The incidence and prevalence of this disorder are unknown. It may occur in association with central nervous system disorders such as senile dementia of the Alzheimer's type, head injury,[86] hypothalamic lesions,[87] or developmental disabilities.[88] It may also occur independent of such disorders. Nursing home residents and elderly persons not in nursing homes receive very little exposure to natural light, spending nearly all day inside.[89] This relative lack of exposure to time cues may contribute to the development of the disorder. Some associated diagnoses in patients at our center include alcohol abuse in remission and major depression.

This uncontrollably irregular pattern of sleep may interfere with work and family activity. These disorders may have a high cost to society by forcing institutionalization of a demented or developmentally impaired person who previously lived at home. One major reason for institutionalizing demented elderly persons is the inability of caregivers at home to monitor the irregular, round-the-clock activity of their impaired relative.[88] The title of a popular manual for caregivers alludes to these demands.[90]

Other sleep disorders, such as obstructive sleep apena syndrome, narcolepsy, periodic limb movement disorder, and restless legs syndrome, could result in irregular patterns of sleeping and wakefulness and should be ruled out. Medical disorders that cause multiple awakenings, such as those of bladder or bowel dysfunction, could produce a similar pattern.

Stronger social time cues help some patients resume a regular 24-hour pattern. In uncontrolled reports, bright light exposure[91] or vitamin B$_{12}$ administration[92] has reportedly been effective.

SECONDARY CIRCADIAN DYSRHYTHMIAS

In contrast to the primary circadian dysrhythmias that represent malfunctioning of the biologic clock within the conventional geophysical environment, the secondary circadian dysrhythmias occur *because* the biologic clock is working properly but is functioning out of phase owing to an imposed shift in the geophysical environment. Technologic advances such as electric lights and jet planes have allowed us to override or intentionally ignore our physiologic biorhythms. The numbers of people involved in transmeridian flight and shift work are startling (nearly a fourth of all workers in industrialized countries work unconventional shifts). This, coupled with the well-documented impairment of performance and judgment attendant on trying to buck the biologic clock, has staggering implications at personal, national, and international levels.[1] The changes associated with time zone crossing are transient and self-limited; those with shift work persist as long as the shift work does. The symptoms of these disorders have been experienced by most of us and are thoroughly reviewed elsewhere.[93,94] Schedule-induced decrements in alertness and performance have enormous implications for shuttle diplomats, traveling athletic teams, and shift workers. Effective treatment to reduce or minimize the devastating consequences of the secondary circadian dysrhythmias is in the developmental stage and includes chronotherapy,[95] benzodiazepines,[96-98] phototherapy,[99] and melatonin administration.[100] Such chronobiologic, phototherapeutic, and pharmacologic manipulations (particularly melatonin administration) are most promising.

CONCLUSION AND FUTURE DIRECTIONS

The study of chronobiology has taught us much about circadian rhythms, both normal and abnormal. The dire consequences of all types of circadian dysrhythmias are just now being appreciated. The biologic clock is a powerful physiologic force, and when it is out of synchrony with the environment can cause disabling and even dangerous symptoms. In the primary disorders, the clock is defective; in the secondary ones, there is difficulty or delay in the clock's adjustment to a sudden shift in environmental time cues.

With the advent of effective treatments, the identification of these disorders is of utmost importance. The primary circadian dysrhythmias are undoubtedly much more prevalent than was previously thought and are masquerading as psychiatric, substance abuse, or primary sleep disorders. Careful history taking, and the use of sleep diaries and actigraphy, usually lead to a proper diagnosis that has practical therapeutic implications. Like any field in its infancy, chronobiology is exploding with excitement as new treatments emerge. Few fields have such important implications for so many people.

REFERENCES

1. National Commission on Sleep Disorders Research. Report of the National Commission on Sleep Disorders Research. DHHS Publ. Washington, D.C.: U.S. Government Printing Office, 1992.
2. Mitler MM, Carskadon MA, et al. Catastrophes, sleep, and public policy: Consensus report. Sleep 1988; 11:100–109.
3. Smolensky M, Halberg F, Sargent F. Chronobiology of the life sequence. In: Ito S, Ogata K, Yoshimura H, eds. Advances in Climatic Physiology. Tokyo: Igaku Shoin, 1972;281–318.
4. Kaiser IH, Halberg F. Circadian periodic aspects of birth. Ann NY Acad Sci 1962;98:1056–68.
5. Wever RA. The Circadian System of Man: Results of Experiments Under Temporal Isolation. New York: Springer-Verlag, 1979.
6. Minors DS, Waterhouse JM. Circadian Rhythms and the Human. Bristol: Wright-PSG, 1981;332.
7. Moore-Ede MC, Sulzman FM, Fuller CA. The Clocks That Time Us: Physiology of the Circadian Timing System. Cambridge, Mass.: Harvard University Press, 1982;448.
8. Halberg F. Physiologic 24-hour periodicity in human beings and mice, the lighting regimen and daily routine. In: Withrow RB, ed. Photoperiodism and related phenomena in plants and animals. Washington, D.C.: American Association for the Advancement of Science, 1959;803–878.
9. Ibuka N, Kawamura H. Loss of circadian rhythm in sleep-wakefulness cycle in the rat by suprachiasmatic nucleus lesions. Brain Res 1975;96:76–81.
10. Boulos Z, Rosenwasser AM, Terman M. Feeding schedules and the circadian organization of behavior in the rat. Behav Brain Res 1980;1:39–65.
11. Stephan FK. Limits of entrainment to periodic feeding of rats with suprachiasmatic lesions. J Comp Physiol A 1981;143:401–410.
12. Moore RY. Retinohypothalamic projections in mammals: A comparative study. Brain Res 1973;49:403–409.
13. Rawson KS. Homing behavior and endogenous activity rhythms. Ph.D. thesis, Harvard University 1956 [cited in reference 3].
14. Burchard JE. Re-setting a biological clock. Ph.D. thesis, Princeton University 1958 [cited in reference 3].
15. Pittendrigh CS, Bruce VG. An oscillator model for biological clocks. In: Rudnick D, ed. Rhythmic and Synthetic Processes in Growth. Princeton: Princeton University Press, 1957;75–109.
16. Czeisler CA, Kronauer RE, Allan JS, et al. Bright light induction of strong (type 0) resetting of the human circadian pacemaker. Science 1989,244:1328–1333.

17. Lewy AJ, Wehr TA, Goodwin FK, et al. Light suppresses melatonin secretion in humans. Science 1980:210:1267–1269.

18. DeCoursey PJ. Daily activity rhythms in the flying squirrel. Ph.D. thesis, University of Wisconsin 1959 [cited in reference 3].

19. DeCoursey PJ. Daily light sensitivity rhythm in a rodent. Science 1960;131:33–35.

20. Pittendrigh CS. Circadian rhythms and the circadian organization of living systems. Cold Spring Harb Symp Quant Biol 1960;25:159–182.

21. Eastman CI. Squashing versus nudging circadian rhythms with artificial bright light: Solutions for shift work? Perspect Biol Med 1991;34:181–195.

22. Moore-Ede MC, Czeisler CA, Richardson GS. Circadian timekeeping in health and disease. Part 1. Basic properties of circadian pacemakers. N Engl J Med 1983; 309:469–476.

23. Sack RL, Lewy AJ, Blood ML, et al. Circadian rhythm abnormalities in totally blind people; incidence and clinical significance. J Clin Endocrinol Metab 1992;75: 127–34.

24. Sack RL, Lewy AJ, Blood ML, et al. Melatonin administration to blind people: Phase advances and entrainment. J Biol Rhythms 1991;6:249–261.

25. Ehret CF, Potter VR, Dobra KW. Chronotypic action of theophylline and of pentobarbital as circadian *Zeitgebers* in the rat. Science 1975;188:1212–1215.

26. Enright JT. The internal clock of drunken isopods. Z Vergl Physiol 1971;75:332–346.

27. Edgar DM, Martin CE, Dement WC. Activity feedback to the mammalian circadian pacemaker: Influence on observed measures of rhythm period length. J Biol Rhythms 1991;6:185–199.

28. Welsh DK, Richardson GS, Dement WC. Effect of running wheel availability on the circadian pattern of sleep and wakefulness in the mouse. Sleep Res 1985;14:316.

29. Kleitman N. Sleep and Wakefulness. Chicago: University of Chicago Press, 1963:137.

30. Mahowald MW, Schenck CH, O'Connor KA. Dynamics of sleep/wake determination—normal and abnormal. Chaos 1991;1:287–298.

31. Tryon WK. Activity Measurement in Psychology and Medicine. New York: Plenum, 1991.

32. Brown A, Smolensky M, D'Alonzo G, et al. Circadian rhythm in human activity objectively quantified by actigraphy. In: Hayes DK, Pauly JE, Reiter RJ, eds. Chronobiology: Its Role in Clinical Medicine, General Biology, and Agriculture. New York: Wiley-Liss, 1990; Part A:77–83.

33. Brown AC, Smolensly MH, D'Alonzo GE, et al. Actigraphy: A means of assessing circadian patterns in human activity. Chronobiol Int 1990;7:125–133.

34. Moore-Ede MC, Czeisler CA, Richardson GS. Circadian timekeeping in health, and disease. Part 2. Clinical implications of circadian rhythmicity. N Engl J Med 1983;309:530–536.

35. Czeisler CA, Richardson GS, Coleman RM, et al. Chronotherapy: Resetting the circadian clocks of patients with delayed sleep phase insomnia. Sleep 1981;4: 1–21.

36. Weitzman ED, Czeisler CA, Coleman RM, et al. Delayed sleep phase syndrome. A chronobiological disorder with sleep-onset insomnia. Arch Gen Psych 1981;38: 737–746.

37. Rosenthal NE, Joseph-Vanderpool JR, Levendosky AA, et al. Phase-shifting effects of bright morning light as treatment for delayed sleep phase syndrome. Sleep 1990;13:354–361.

38. Lewy AJ, Sack RL. Intensity, wavelength, and timing: Three critical parameters for chronobiologically active light. In: Kupfer DJ, Monk TH, Barchas JD, eds. Biological Rhythms and Mental Disorders. New York: Guilford Press, 1988:197–217.

39. Terman M. Light therapy. In: Kryger MH, Roth T, Dement WC, eds. Principles and Practice of Sleep Medicine. Philadelphia: WB Saunders, 1988:717–722.

40. Terman M, Williams JB, Terman JS. Light therapy for winter depression: A clinician's guide. In: Keller PA, ed. Innovations in Clinical Practice: A Source Book, vol 10. Sarasota, Fla.: Professional Resource Exchange, 1991.

41. Kripke DF. Timing of phototherapy and occurrence of mania. Biol Psychiatry 1991;29:1156–1157.

42. Schwitzer J, Neudorfer C, Blecha HG, et al. Mania as a side effect of phototherapy. Biol Psychiatry 1990;28:523–524.

43. Roberts JE, Reme CE, Dillon J, et al. Exposure to bright light and the concurrent use of photosensitizing drugs. N Engl J Med 1992;326:1500.

44. Terman M, Reme CE, Rafferty B, et al. Bright light therapy for winter depression: Potential ocular effects and theoretical implications. Photochem Photobiol 1990;51:781–793.

45. Turek FW, Losee-Olson S. Entrainment of the circadian activity rhythm to the light-dark cycle can be altered by a short-acting benzodiazepine, triazolam. J Biol Rhythms 1987;2:249–260.

46. Turek FW. Manipulation of a central circadian clock regulating behavioral and endocrine rhythms with a short-acting benzodiazepine used in the treatment of insomnia. Psychoneuroendocrinology 1988;13:217–232.

47. Alvarez B, Dahlitz MJ, Vignau J, et al. The delayed sleep phase syndrome: Clinical and investigative findings in fourteen subjects. J Neurol Neurosurg Psychiatry 1992;55:665–670.

48. Ozaki N, Iwata T. Itoh A, et al. A treatment trial of delayed sleep phase syndrome with triazolam. Jpn J Psychiatry Neurol 1989;43:51–55.

49. Okawa M, Mishima K, Nanami T, et al. Vitamin B_{12} treatment for sleep-wake rhythm disorders. Sleep 1990;13:15–23.

50. Tshjimaru S, Kideaki E, Honma G, et al. Effects of vitamin B_{12} on the period of free-running rhythm in rats. Jpn J Psychiatry Neurology 1992;46:225–226.

51. Ohta T, Iwata T, Kayukawa Y, et al. Daily activity and persistent sleep-wake schedule disorders. Prog Neuropsychopharmacol Biol Psychiatry 1991;16:529–537.

52. Ohta T, Ando K, Iwata T, et al. Treatment of persistent sleep-wake schedule disorders in adolescents with methylcobalamin (vitamine B_{12}). Sleep 1991;12:414–418.

53. Hallonquist JD, Goldberg MA, Brandes JS. Affective disorders and circadian rhythms. Can J Psychiatry 1986;31:259–272.

54. Erlich SS, Apuzzo MLJ. The pineal gland: Anatomy, physiology, and clinical significance. J Neurosurg 1985;63:321–341.

55. Lewy AJ, Sack RL, Singer CM. Melatonin, light and chronobiological disorders. In: Photoperiodisim, Melatonin, and the Pineal. London: Pitman, 1985:231–252.

56. Reppert SM, Weaver DR, Rivkees SA, et al. Putative melatonin receptors in a human biological clock. Science 1988;242:78–81.

57. Lewy AJ, Ahmed S, Latham Jackson JM, et al. Melatonin shifts human circadian rhythms according to a phase-response curve. Chronobiol Int 1992;9:380–392.

58. Halberg F. Chronobiology. Ann Rev Physiol 1969; 31:675–725.

59. Moore-Ede MC. Circadian rhythms of drug effectiveness and toxicity. Clin Pharmacol Ther 1973;14:925–935.

60. Radzialowski FM, Bousquet WF. Daily rhythmic variation in hepatic drug metabolism in the rat and mouse. J Pharmacol Exp Ther 1968;163:229–238.

61. Reinberg A. The hours of changing responsiveness or susceptibility. Perspect Biol Med 1967;11:111–126.

62. Koren G, Ferrazzini G, Sohl H, et al. Chronopharmacology of methotrexate: Pharmacokinetics in childhood leukemia. Chronobiol Int 1992;9:434–438.

63. Rosenthal NE, Blehar MC, eds. Seasonal Affective Disorders and Phototherapy. New York: Guilford Press, 1989.

64. Wehr TA. Effects of wakefulness and sleep on depression and mania. In: Montplaisir J, Godbout R, eds. Sleep and Biological Rhythms. Basic Mechanisms and Applications to Psychiatry. New York: Oxford University Press, 1990:42–86.

65. Kupfer DJ, Monk TH, Barchas JD, eds. Biological Rhythms and Mental Disorders. New York: Guilford Press, 1988.

66. Schigen B, Tolle R. Partial sleep deprivation as therapy for depression. Arch Gen Psychiatry 1980;37:267–271.

67. Rosenthal NE, Sack DA, Gillin JC, et al. Seasonal affective disorder. A description of the syndrome and preliminary findings with light therapy. Arch Gen Psychiatry 1984;41:72–80.

68. Wehr TA, Jacobsen FM, Sack DA, et al. Phototherapy of seasonal affective disorder. Arch Gen Psychiatry 1986; 43:870–875.

69. Diagnostic Classification Steering Committee. International Classification of Sleep Disorders: Diagnostic and Coding Manual. Rochester, Minn. American Sleep Disorders Association, 1990:128–133.

70. Patten SB, Lauderdale WM. Delayed sleep phase disorder after traumatic brain injury. J Am Acad Child Adolesc Psychiatry 1992;31:100–102.

71. Institute of Medicine, National Academy of Sciences. Sleeping Pills, Insomnia and Medical Practice. Washington, D.C.: NAS Office of Publications, 1971.

72. Guilleminault C. Narcolepsy and its differential diagnosis. In: Guilleminault C, ed. Sleep and its Disorders in Children. New York: Raven Press, 1987;181–194.

73. Ferber R, Boyle MP. Delayed sleep phase syndrome versus motivated sleep phase delay in adolescents. Sleep Res 1983;12:239.

74. O'Connor KA. Personal communication.

75. Orem DA, Wehr TA. Hypernycthemeral syndrome after chronotherapy for delayed sleep phase syndrome. N Engl J Med 1992;327:1762.

76. Uruha S, Mikami A, Teshima Y, et al. Effect of triazolam for delayed sleep phase syndrome. Sleep Res 1987;16:650.

77. Dahlitz M, Alvarez B. Vignau J, et al. Delayed sleep phase syndrome response to melatonin. Lancet 1991; 337:1121–1124.

78. Campbell SS, Dawson D. Bright light treatment of sleep disturbance in older subjects. Sleep Res 1991;20:448.

79. Moldofsky H, Musisi S, Phillipson EA. Treatment of a case of advanced sleep phase syndrome by phase advance chronotherapy. Sleep 1986;9:61–65.

80. Diagnostic Classification Steering Committee. International Classification of Sleep Disorders: Diagnostic and Coding Manual. Rochester, Minn. American Sleep Disorders Association, 1990;137–140.

81. Hoban TM, Sack RL, Lewy AJ, et al. Entrainment of a free-running human with bright light. Chronobiol Int 1989;6:347–353.

82. Wollman M, Lavie P, Peled R. A hypernycthemeral sleep-wake syndrome: A treatment attempt. Chronobiol Int 1985;2:277–280.

83. Kamgar-Parsi B, Wehr TA, Gillin JC. Successful treatment of human non–24-hour sleep-wake syndrome. Sleep 1983;6:257–264.

84. Sugita Y, Ishikawa H, Mikami A, et al. Successful treatment for a patient with hypernycthemeral syndrome. Sleep Res 1987;16:642.

85. Diagnostic Classification Steering Committee. International Classification of Sleep Disorders: Diagnostic and Coding Manual. Rochester, Minn. American Sleep Disorders Association, 1990;125–128.

86. Okawa M, Takahashi K, Sasaki H. Disturbance of circadian rhythms in severely brain-damaged patients correlated with CT findings. J Neurol 1986;233:274–282.

87. Cohen RA, Albers HE. Disruption of human circadian and cognitive regulation following a discrete hypothalamic lesion: A case study. Neurology 1991;41:726–279.

88. Bliwise DL. Sleep in normal aging and dementia. Sleep 1993;16:40–81.

89. Ancoli-Israel S, Kripke DF, Williams-Jones D, et al. Light exposure and sleep in nursing home patients. Society for Light Treatment and Biological Rhythms Abstracts 1991;3:18.

90. Mace NL, Rabins PV. The 36-Hour Day. Baltimore: Johns Hopkins University Press, 1981.

91. Satlin A, Vilicer L, Ross V, et al. Bright light treatment of behavioral and sleep disturbances in patients with Alzheimer's disease. Am J Psychiatry 1992;149:1028–1032.

92. Mishima K, Okawa M, Hishikawa Y. Effect of methylcobalamin (VB$_{12}$) injection on sleep-wake rhythm in demented patients. Jpn J Psychiatry Neurol 1992; 46:227–228.

93. Biological Rhythms: Implications for the Worker. Washington DC: Office of Technology Assessment, US Congress, 1991.

94. Loat CER, Rhodes EC. Jet-lag and human performance. Sports Med 1989;8:226–238.

95. Czeisler CA, Moore-Ede MC, Coleman RM. Rotating shift work schedules that disrupt sleep are improved by applying circadian principles. Science 1982;217:460–463.

96. Cohen AS, Seidel WF, Yost D, et al. Triazolam used in the treatment of jet lag: Effects on sleep and subsequent wakefulness. Sleep Res 1991;20:61.

97. Walsh JK, Sugerman JL, Muehlbach MJ, et al. Physiological sleep tendency on a simulated night shift: Adaptation and effects of triazolam. Sleep 1988;11:251–264.

98. Bonnet MH, Dexter JR, Gillin JC, et al. The use of triazolam in phase-advanced sleep. Neuropsychopharmacology 1988;1:225–234.

99. Czeisler CA, Johnson MP, Duffy JF, et al. Exposure to bright light and darkness to treat physiologic maladaptation to night work. N Engl J Med 1990;322:1253–1259.

100. Samel A, Wegmann H-M, Vejvoda M, et al. Influence of melatonin treatment on human circadian rhythmicity before and after a simulated 9-hr. time shift. J Biol Rhythms 1991;6:235–248.

24

Parasomnias
Roger J. Broughton

The parasomnias may be defined as events that occur intermittently or episodically during the night, in contrast to other sleep disorders, which are characterized by an overall increase or decrease in the normal sleep amount or which relate to abnormalities of circadian sleep-wake regulation. Though the most recent classification of sleep disorders[1] lists and describes 24 distinct parasomnias, a number of these are either exceedingly rare (e.g., sleep-related abnormal swallowing syndrome, congenital central hypoventilation syndrome) or are not behavioral disorders (e.g., rapid eye movement [REM]–related sinus arrest). This chapter restricts itself to the major classical behavioral parasomnias.

Parasomnias may be classified according to the sleep-wake state in which they mainly, or exclusively, occur: sleep onset; deep slow-wave sleep; REM sleep (fully formed or dissociated); light sleep stages; or all sleep stages indiscriminately. The 13 main parasomnias that are discussed here are organized according to this approach in Table 24-1.

THE BEHAVIORAL PARASOMNIAS

Wake-Sleep Transition Disorders

Sleep starts

Sleep starts—often referred to as *hypnagogic jerks, hypnic jerks,* or *predormital myoclonus*—consist of bilateral, and sometimes asymmetric, brief body jerks, usually in isolation, but occasionally several in succession, that coincide with sleep onset. They principally involve the legs but may also affect the arms and head. Sleep starts may be spontaneous or be evoked by stimuli. At times they are accompanied by sensory symptoms such as a flash of light, a feeling of falling, or more organized hypnagogic hallucinations. The violence of the contraction may cause an abrupt cry. Rarely, mild injury such as bruises may occur.

One of the earliest careful descriptions of hypnagogic jerks was that of S. Weir Mitchell[2] in 1890, who described as well the possibility of particularly intense and frequent jerks leading to a form of sleep-onset insomnia with consequent sleep deprivation.

The early French neurologist Roger[3] also fully recognized the phenomenon.

The cause of the intensification of this otherwise normal physiologic event is often unknown. It has at times been related to intake of stimulants (including excessive caffeine), excessive exercise, or stress. There are no known familial cases; and the sexes appear to be equally affected.

Electroencephalographic (EEG) correlates were first described by Oswald,[4] who noted the presence of stage 1 drowsiness with at times a vertex sharp wave occurring at the time of the jerk. Superficial electromyographic (EMG) changes were subsequently described by Gastaut and Broughton[5]: brief 75- to 250-msec high-amplitude potentials occurring bilaterally and synchronously over homologous muscles in the affected regions (Figure 24-1). Broughton[6] has polygraphically confirmed the possible consequence of sleep-onset insomnia.

From a pathophysiologic point of view, clinically significant sleep starts appear to represent simple intensification of an otherwise normal event. It is pertinent to recall that during the sleep-onset process hypnagogic brain structures actively inhibit those responsible for wakefulness, thereby creating an unstable state before sleep maintenance mechanisms become fully functional. During this transitional state, synchronous volleys occur in the pyramidal tracts, which may form the basis of the phenomenon.

The differential diagnosis includes a number of other motor phenomena that may occur at sleep onset. The fragmentary partial myoclonus described by De Lisi[7] and documented polygraphically by Loeb and coworkers[8] and Gastaut and Broughton[5] involves very local areas of musculature independently and asynchronously in various body regions. Excessive startling in the hyperekplexia syndrome[9] is characterized by pathologic responsiveness to sensory stimuli during wakefulness and during sleep, including deep non-REM (NREM) sleep.[10] Brief epileptic myoclonus is associated with a coexisting EEG discharge,[11] and the patient typically also has waking seizures. In so-called periodic movements in sleep[12] the contractions last much longer, occur throughout various sleep stages, and show pseudo-periodic repetition every 20 to 60 seconds. Restless

TABLE 24-1. A Classification of the Parasomnias

Wake-sleep transition disorders
    Sleep starts (hypnic jerks)
    Rhythmic movement disorder (jactatio capitis
      nocturna)
NREM sleep disorders
    Confusional arousals (nocturnal sleep drunkenness)
    Sleepwalking (somnambulism)
    Sleep terrors (pavor nocturnus, incubus)
    Nocturnal paroxysmal dystonia
REM sleep disorders
    Nightmares, (terrifying dreams, anxiety dreams)
    REM sleep behavior disorder
    Sleep paralysis, isolated form
    Painful erections
Light sleep disorders (stage 1, 2, REM)
    Sleep talking
    Bruxism (tooth grinding)
Diffuse sleep disorders (no stage preference)
    Enuresis nocturna (bedwetting)

legs syndrome[13] consists of crampy dysethesias in the lower legs during the presleep and sleep-onset periods that produce an almost irresistible urge to move the legs and that are improved by getting out of bed and walking about.

Treatment of intense hypnagogic jerks involves mainly avoidance of precipitating factors such as stimulants or very irregular sleep-wake patterns. The condition is often self-limiting and disappears spontaneously. Rarely, patients require intermittent treatment with a benzodiazepine hypnotic, the most effective ones being clonazepam and diazepam in the usual hypnotic doses.

Rhythmic movement disorder
(jactatio capitis nocturna)

Rhythmic movement disorder consists of repetitive stereotyped movements involving large body areas, usually of the head and neck (head banging) or the entire body (body rocking), that typically occur just prior to sleep onset and persist into light sleep. Early descriptions include those of Zappert[14] in 1905, who introduced the term *jactatio capitis nocturna*, and of Cruchet.[15] Several recent comprehensive reviews exist.[16–18] The phenomenon is much more common in children, though adult cases are well-documented.

In the head-banging form, the patient often lies prone and repeatedly lifts the head or entire body, then bangs the head down onto the pillow or mattress. The head may also be struck rhythmically against the headboard. At times, a sitting posture is associated with backward banging of the occiput. In typical body rocking, the entire body is most usually rolled forward and backward from a sitting position, or side-to-side from a supine position. Such move-

ments are repeated rhythmically with a frequency of ½ to 2 seconds in long clusters. Rhythmic chanting or other vocalizations may occur during head banging or body rocking.

The condition is relatively common in infants and young children, the majority of affected children being otherwise normal.[19] The rare persistence into, or appearance during, later childhood or adulthood is more often associated with significant psychopathology including autism and mental retardation. At all ages, the condition has been found to predominate in males by a ratio of about 3:1.[19] Genetic factors are occasionally involved, and the condition has been described in twins. Older patients, in particular, may have organic brain disease.

When particularly persistent or intense, significant complications may ensue. These include scalp and other body wounds, subdural hematoma, retinal petechiae, skull callus formation, and significant family and psychosocial problems.

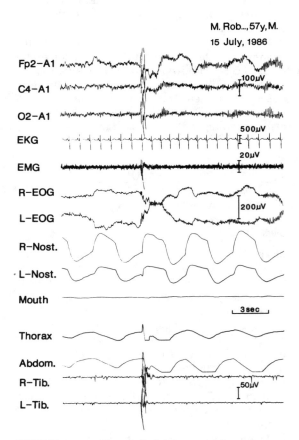

FIGURE 24-1. *Hypnic jerk in stage 1 drowsiness. The jerk involved both legs synchronously and created an artifact on the respiratory channel as well as in the EEG. The EEG was that of stage 1 drowsiness succeeded by a microarousal with return of alpha rhythm.*

Polysomnography (PSG) has shown the presence of rhythmic movement artifacts, mainly in the immediate presleep period, during light stages 1 and 2 sleep, as reported by Gastaut and Broughton[5] and confirmed by others.[20-22] Head rolling has also been described as sometimes occurring mainly[23] or exclusively[24,25] during REM sleep. In very serious cases, persistence in deep slow-wave sleep has also been noted.[5] A remarkable aspect is the typical absence of any EEG signs of arousal during, or immediately after, intense rocking movements (Figure 24-2).

Diagnosis seldom poses a problem, owing to the very stereotypical nature of the movements. In infants and in very young children it may have to be distinguished from bruxism (tooth grinding), thumb sucking, and other such disorders. Periodic movements in sleep are easily differentiated, as they appear only after sleep begins, involve mainly the legs, and, though "pseudorhythmic," show several seconds or dozens of seconds between individual contractions. Epileptic behaviors, including infantile spasms, are distinguished by an associated EEG discharge.

For the majority of infants and children no treatment is required and the parents can be reassured. Padding the bed area or a protective helmet is sometimes indicated. Restraining is, in general, ineffec-

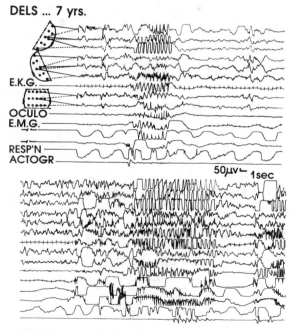

DELS ... 7 yrs.

E.K.G.

OCULO
E.M.G.

RESP'N
ACTOGR

50μv ⌐ 1sec

FIGURE 24-2. *Body rolling in sleep (jactatio capitis nocturna) all-night form. This 7-year-old mentally handicapped girl rolled with a 1- to 3-second frequency in all stages of sleep. Rhythmic artifacts from total body movement are shown in both stage 2 sleep (above) and SWS (below), without significant arousal.*

tive. Behavior modification procedures[26,27] have been used, with varying degrees of success. After early childhood, psychiatric and neurologic evaluation may be needed. Benzodiazepine and tricyclic medication have occasionally been helpful.[18]

NREM Sleep Disorders (Including SWS Arousal Disorders)

Confusional arousals (nocturnal sleep drunkenness)

Episodes of marked confusion during and following arousal from sleep, but without sleepwalking or sleep terror qualities, have been referred to as *nocturnal sleep drunkenness* or as *excessive sleep inertia*. Such episodes arise most typically from a deep sleep state in the first part of the night.

Early descriptions include those of Marc,[28] physician to the King of France, who called it *l'ivresse du sommeil*, and of von Gudden,[29] who employed the parallel term *Schlaftrunkenheit*. During episodes the subject awakens only partially and exhibits marked confusion with slow mentation, disorientation in time and place, and perceptual impairment. Behavior is often quite inappropriate. Rarely, aggressive behavior is observed, and there are several well-documented cases of homicide being committed immediately on sudden arousal from deep sleep.[30] The confusion lasts several minutes to hours. Memory for the episode is typically totally absent. Confusional arousals are more common in children[5] and perhaps are universal before about age 5 years.[5,31] They are then usually relatively benign and disappear with age. In adults, however, the condition can be more serious and is usually stable, varying only with the precipitating causes.

Any factor that deepens sleep or impairs ease of awakening can predispose the amnesic confusional arousals. The major factors are young age, recovery from prior sleep deprivation, fever, and central nervous system (CNS) depressant medications, including hypnotics and tranquilizers. Confusional arousals can be associated with medical diseases characterized by deep or disturbed sleep, including metabolic, toxic, and other encephalopathies; idiopathic hypersomnia; symptomatic hypersomnias; and sleep apnea syndrome. In cases of idiopathic confusional arousal, a family history of the episodes, and of deep sleepers, is common.

PSG recordings have shown that the episodes typically have their onset during slow-wave sleep.[5,31,32] They most commonly occur in the first third of nocturnal sleep but have also been described during afternoon naps. They rarely, if ever, accompany arousal from REM sleep, after which rapid return to clear mentation is usual. During confusional episodes, the EEG may show some residual slow-wave activity, stage 1 theta patterns, repeated microsleeps, or a diffuse and poorly reactive alpha rhythm,[5] all indicating incomplete awakening. Cerebral evoked potentials have also been described as being altered during such confusion accompanying experimental forced arousals from slow-wave sleep.[32,33]

Confusional awakenings must be distinguished from four other parasomnias that occur during sleep and have amnesic qualities: (1) sleepwalking, which consists of complex motor automatisms with walking about; (2) sleep terrors, in which there are signs of acute fear and usually a blood-curdling cry; (3) REM sleep behavior disorder, with its explosive movements such as fighting or diving out of bed; and, (4) very rarely, nocturnal epileptic seizures of complex partial type associated with ictal EEG discharges and usually with similar attacks in daytime wakefulness.

Treatment is rarely necessary for the confusional arousals of children, who typically outgrow them. Parents may be reassured and should be told to let the events run themselves out, rather than trying to abort them. Avoidance of precipitating causes (sleep deprivation, CNS depressants, stress) is indicated. Treatment of the rarely associated metabolic or other disease is indicated for symptomatic forms. Exceptionally, efforts to lighten sleep of very deep sleepers by a mild stimulant medication has proven useful.[34]

Sleepwalking

Sleepwalking or somnambulism consists of recurrent episodes in which the subject arises from a deep sleep, typically in the first third of the night, and, without awakening, exhibits complex automatic behaviors, which include walking for some distance.[15] Communication with sleepwalkers is difficult or impossible: the behavior seems to have to play itself out. A pattern of repetitive behavior may occur that has obvious symbolic meaning, such as a child repeatedly crawling into the parents' bed or a housewife trying to prepare meals. Rarely, eating may occur and the patient may present as a sleep-related eating syndrome. Mumbling or even comprehensible speech may occur as, rarely, may aggression, especially as a response to attempts to restrict the sleepwalker's mobility. Injury may arise from walking into dangerous situations or from cuts or burns. Rarely, a sleep terror immediately precedes and evolves into a sleepwalking episode. The episodes may terminate either spontaneously or by forced awakening. The patient is usually very hard to awaken and, once aroused, shows mental confusion with amnesia for the event.

Sleepwalking can occur at any age after a person learns to walk. It is most common in children aged 4

to 6 years[35] and frequently disappears during adolescence. Adult cases, however, are not infrequent. A strong family history is common[36,37]; and there is often a family or personal history of other arousal disorders from slow-wave sleep, specifically sleep terrors and confusional arousals.[38]

A number of so-called precipitating factors have been identified that increase the probability of an episode on a particular night. These are mainly factors that deepen sleep, particularly sleep deprivation and CNS depressant medication. The presence of factors that disrupt slow-wave sleep, including extreme stress, pain, sleep apnea, or distended bladder, can also trigger an attack. In chronic sleepwalkers, episodes can at times be precipitated by simple forced arousal during deep sleep in the early part of the night.[5]

PSG recordings, first reported by Gastaut and coworkers[39] and Gastaut and Broughton[5] and soon confirmed by the Los Angeles group,[40,41] found that episodes arise in deep stage 3 or 4 sleep (Figure 24-3), most often at the end of the first or second episode of slow-wave sleep. EEG during sleepwalking has been recorded by both long cables[40] and telemetry.[5] It has typically shown lightening to stage 1 patterns or an abnormal diffuse and slow alpha rhythm that is unresponsive to bright light stimulation. The marked autonomic activation characteristic of sleep terrors is absent. On nights without episodes, PSG often shows three or more direct slow-wave–wakefulness transitions,[42] a finding that only infrequently occurs in normals. There is also evidence of more frequent and higher-amplitude delta bursts during incomplete arousals from NREM sleep[40,43] and of a higher frequency of brief microarousals.[44]

Diagnosis is seldom a problem, though "escape" behaviors during certain sleep terrors or REM sleep behavior disorder must be distinguished. Sleep-related partial complex seizures with ambulatory automatisms are exceedingly rare[45]; they are associated with an ictal EEG discharge, and similar episodes usually occur in the daytime.

Treating[46] young children for sleepwalking is often unnecessary. The parents may be reassured that the child will most likely outgrow the episodes. When the behavior seriously distresses the patient and the family or risks injury, treatment should be instituted. Precipitating factors should be carefully avoided. Efforts should be made to minimize possible injury by locking doors and windows, removing sharp objects, and so forth. Hypnosis and psychotherapy have both been reported to have a favorable effect on some patients. Drug treatment, especially benzodiazepines, (diazepam, clonazepam, oxazepam) or tricyclic medication (clomipramine, imipramine), may be helpful for relatively short drug trials during periods of frequent attacks. The tricyclic antidepressant

FEV ... 20 yrs.

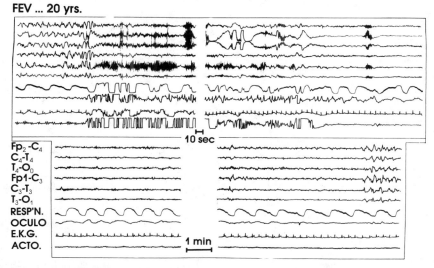

FIGURE 24-3.   *Sleepwalking in a 26-year-old adult male was recorded by cable electrodes. The upper left fragment shows onset in slow-wave sleep, followed by arousal and movement artifact, as the sleeper got out of bed. Some 10 seconds of recording is removed, followed by a quiescent stage 1 pattern (continued below) after the patient went back to bed. One minute later he was in stage 2 sleep (lower right).*

amineptine has been described as being particularly effective.[47] Adult cases are typically more difficult to treat than childhood ones, and psychopathology is much more frequent.

Sleep terrors

Sleep terrors typically consist of sudden sitting up during sleep and emitting a piercing scream. The sufferer appears to be in a state of acute terror, shows tachypnea, tachycardia, mydriasis, and increased muscle tone, and is impossible to console.[1,5] The attacks seem to run themselves out. Sleep terrors characteristically begin during the deep sleep in the first third of the night[5]; however, when episodes are very frequent they may be diffusely distributed across the sleep period. As attacks may also occur during daytime naps, the term *sleep terror* is preferable to *night terror*. Once awake, the subject often remembers having difficulty breathing or marked palpitations, but recall of mental activity is rare. If present, it consists almost always of a static scene like a single photograph[5,48] rather than a progressive succession of images as in a typical dream.

Attacks in children are sometimes referred to as *pavor nocturnus* (Latin for sleep terror) and in adults as *incubus* attacks. They have also been referred to as nightmares, but this creates a confusion with the true terrifying dream or REM nightmare. The latter has been known at least since Ernest Jones[48] to be a

distinctly different parasomnia. Both the words *incubus* (Latin *in*, upon; *cubare* to press) and nightmare (*mar*, Teutonic for devil) reflect the medieval belief that sleep terrors are caused by a devil sitting or pressing on the chest of the sleeper, which leads to the breathing difficulties and acute terror.[31]

The attacks can occur from young childhood on. The prevalence is low: the condition afflicts approximately 3% of children and 1% of adults. Sleep terrors are sometimes familial[49] and are associated with increased personal and family incidence of sleepwalking and confusional arousals. Males are more frequently affected than females. In children, psychopathology is very rare, and the attacks tend to disappear in adolescence. In adulthood, psychopathology is common; and adult attacks are most frequent in the 20- to 30-year range and less frequent in old age.

Sleep terrors were first shown to occur mainly during arousals from slow-wave sleep (Figure 24-4 A + B) by Gastaut and Broughton[5] and Broughton[32] and confirmed by Fisher and colleagues.[50,51] When many occur during a single night they may occasionally present in stage 2 sleep also. Marked tachycardia, polypnea, and reduced skin resistance are all present[5] and testify to an acute autonomic discharge. There is a correlation between the amount of prior slow-wave sleep and that of autonomic intensity as measured by degree of tachycardia,[50] which often doubles. In predisposed subjects, attacks may

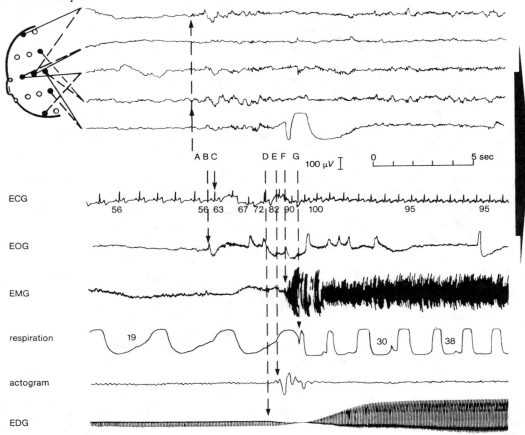

FIGURE 24-4.   *(A) Sleep terror beginning in stage 2 sleep was one of many experienced in a single night (spindles recorded shortly before). Sequential onset of PSG changes is indicated by letters: a series of delta waves or K complexes (A), eye movements (B), tachycardia (C), reducing skin resistance in electrodermography (D), bed movement by actigraphy (E), increase in submental EMG activity (F), and tachypnea (G).*

be elicited experimentally by forced arousals during monitored slow-wave sleep.[5,32,50,51]

A distinction must be made between terrifying dreams and sleep terrors. The former typically occur in the last (rather than first) third of the night, do not have the same intensity of terror, autonomic arousal, or motor activity, and are not followed by such intense mental confusion. Moreover, the person typically recalls an organized dream that evolved in theme and became personally threatening. Nocturnal anxiety related to obstructive sleep apnea, nocturnal cardiac ischemia, sleep-related epileptic seizures, or other such events rarely is a problem of differential diagnosis.

When attacks are rare, treatment is often unnecessary. Parents of young patients may be reassured that, even if the terror episodes are dramatic, they seldom cause injury and are often outgrown. Diazepam at bedtime in the usual hypnotic doses is effective in suppressing the attacks.[52] Though it was introduced because it reduces slow-wave sleep,

there is no correlation between the sleep architecture effect and the timing or degree of the clinical effect.[52] The latter appears more likely to be related to diazepam's suppressant effect on the autonomic, or motor, responsiveness to arousing stimuli.[53] Other benzodiazepines may be effective, as, in adults, may also be tricyclic antidepressants.[54,55] Psychotherapy[56] and general stress reduction are at times effective, particularly in adults.

Sleep drunkenness, sleepwalking, and sleep terrors all occur during abnormal arousals from slow-wave sleep, and all can be experimentally induced in a proportion of sufferers by simple attempts at force awakenings during slow-wave sleep in the first third of the night. This has led to the proposal that they represent disorders of arousal.[5] Moreover, attacks with intermediate or combined features of the classical forms occur, and there is a degree of genetic overlap. These, together, indicate that they are part of a continuum.

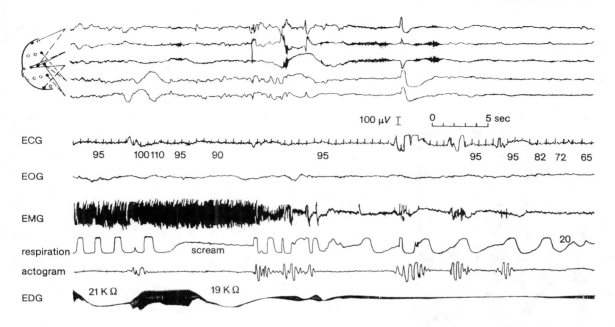

100 µV   0   5 sec

ECG   95   100 110   95   90   95   95   95   82   72   65

EOG

EMG

respiration   scream   20

actogram

EDG   21 K Ω   19 K Ω

FIGURE 24-4. *(B) Continuation of the recording. The EEG is desynchronized, heart rate doubles to 110 beats per minute, an intense, piercing scream was uttered, as indicated, during sustained expiration, and skin resistance continues to decrease (sweating). The attack is terminated by several body movements that are visible in the actigraphic and EMG channels.*

Nocturnal paroxysmal dystonia

This distinct parasomnia consists of repeated dystonic or dyskinetic (ballistic, choreoathetoid) movement episodes that are repeated in stereotypical fashion during sleep.[57,58] Two varieties exist: a short-lived form lasting 15 to 60 seconds and often repeated several times per night and a prolonged form that lasts up to 1 hour.[59] The nature of the movements is similar in both varieties. The attacks arise from tranquil sleep and consist of such dystonic movements as rotation of the head or trunk, often with abductor limb posturing, in either extension or flexion. The eyes are open but unresponsive. The sleeper may sit up and subsequently fall back, or may exhibit opisthotonus. Vocalization may occur; and the dystonic posturing is at times associated with wild ballistic or slower choreoathetoid movements. Subjects can remain asleep during episodes, or they may awaken, in which case they are usually coherent and have no difficulty going back to sleep.

The movements are intense and can cause severe sleep disruption with secondary daytime sleepiness. The sleeper or sleeping partner may be injured. Episodes typically occur most nights, and in the brief form several times per night. They can begin in childhood to late middle age and may persist in old age. Birth history, neurologic status, and psychological examination findings are typically all normal. Especially patients with the brief form may have a

history of daytime generalized tonic-clonic or other epileptic seizures, though ictal EEG discharges have not been recorded to date at the time of the dystonic episodes. The attacks typically persist years without showing any tendency to spontaneous remission.

PSG recordings[57–60] show that the attacks occur exclusively in NREM sleep, typically in stage 2 (Figure 24-5) but at times in stage 3 or 4. There is desynchronization of the EEG, indicating arousal without evident discharge. Increased muscle tone rapidly obscures the brainwave patterns. Just before an episode, a central respiratory pause, slowing of heart rate, or change in electrodermal activity may occur.

Differentiation from other parasomnias is seldom difficult, given the unusual dystonic nature of the movements and the characteristic PSG. Epileptic seizures of frontal lobe origin most closely resemble nocturnal paroxysmal dystonia, but then an ictal EEG discharge is usually recorded and patients usually have similar episodes in the daytime.[59]

Treatment is usually required. Attacks do not respond to normal tranquilizers, sedatives, barbiturates, or diphenylhydantoin, but most patients with the short form of attacks are controlled by carbamazapine, in the usual clinical dose of about 15 mg/kg daily.[56,58] Serum drug levels should be monitored, as should hematologic status for possible side effects. There appears some possibility that the short form of attacks are indeed occult epileptic seizures[59,60]

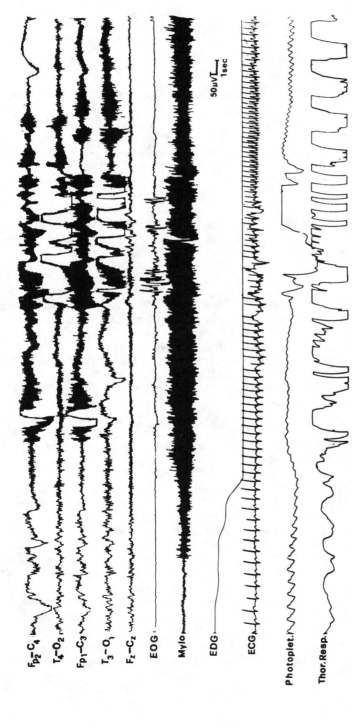

50μV └
1sec

FdP2 – C4
T4 – O2
Fp1 – C3
T3 – O1
Fz – Cz
EOG
Mylo
EDG
ECG
Photoplet.
Thor.Resp.

FIGURE 24-5.   *Paroxysmal nocturnal dystonia begins in stage 2 sleep. The EEG shows desynchronization with some alpha and then is obscured by sustained EMG artifact. A marked increase in muscle tone is visible in the submental EMG (mylohyoid muscle), associated with decreasing skin resistance, tachycardia, decreased pulsation (photoplethysmography), and hyperpnea with tachypnea. (Courtesy of Prof. Elio Lugaresi.)*

though this has not been proven, whereas the longer forms may represent dyskenesia of neurochemical origin.

REM Sleep Disorders

Nightmares (terrifying dreams)

The term *nightmare* is best reserved for dreamlike mental activity during sleep that exhibits a progressive content that becomes frightening to the sleeper and leads to awakening.[50,51,61] The term has also at times been used to designate sleep terror, though they are distinctly different parasomnias. Terrifying dreams occur mainly in the second half of the night in REM sleep. Movements, mumbling, or vocalizations may occur during sleep prior to awakening. The awakening itself is seldom accompanied by the piercing cry typical of a sleep terror, and palpitations or laboured breathing, if present, are much less marked. The sensorium is relatively intact with little of the confusion and disorientation that are characteristic of sleep terrors. Above all, typically there is detailed recall of a long succession of dream images whose content became threatening to the dreamer. Subjective perception of imminent injury or death is not infrequent. Nightmares never evolve into sleepwalking as sleep terrors can.

Nightmares are not uncommon in children and have been said to occur in 10% to 50% of 3- to 6-year-olds.[61] They may persist into, or initially appear in, adolescence or adulthood. Some 40% to 50% of adults admit to at least occasional nightmares. Certain personality characteristics appear associated with lifelong nightmares. Hartmann[62] and Kales and coworkers[63] have noticed an increased frequency of borderline personality disorder, schizoid personality disorder, and schizophrenia. Patients may feel that their childhood was unusually difficult, though often no specific major trauma occurred. Sufferers are often vulnerable persons with soft ego boundaries and marked artistic tendencies. In military personnel with combat shock, nightmares may be particularly intense and recurrent, and the relationship to life stresses is evident.[64,65] A number of drugs also predispose to nightmares including β-adrenergic blockers, L-dopa, and related medications, as does withdrawal from REM-suppressant medications such as tricyclic antidepressants, monoamine oxidase inhibitors, alcohol, and certain stimulants and sedative-hypnotics. In 50% of sufferers no psychiatric or other medical diagnosis can be made, and the nightmares appear to be related simply to daytime stress.

PSG recordings[50,51,61] show changes in REM sleep followed by the awakening, which occurs prior to recall of the dream sequence. Within REM sleep the amount of actual eye movement activity and of EMG brief "twitch potentials" may be increased. There may be a mild increase in frequency or variability in heart rate or of respiratory rate; but, on awakening, the explosive tachycardia and tachypnea characteristic of the sleep terror are absent (Figure 24-6). Especially after severe trauma, a typical nightmare report may follow awakenings from NREM sleep, especially stage 1 or 2.

The principal item of differential diagnosis is the sleep terror, the distinguishing features of which have already been detailed but which include, above all, typical occurrence in the first third of the night, intense piercing cry, marked tachycardia and tachypnea, and lack of recall of a detailed dream sequence. Occasionally, differentiation from REM sleep behavior disorder poses a problem. That condition is more common in elderly persons, some of whom have known CNS lesions. Their explosive, violent movements, markedly increased muscle tone, frequent intense myoclonus, and typical PSG features help make the distinction.

Treatment[66] of recurrent disturbing nightmares is often necessary. Stresses that appear recurrently and are related to precipitation of nightmares should be avoided. Drugs known to promote nightmares should, wherever possible, be substituted. Psychotherapy, including strengthening ego boundaries by assertiveness training, insight into dream content analysis, and techniques to acquire some degree of dream content control have all been helpful in individual cases. In patients with irregular sleep-wake patterns, a simple sleep hygiene regimen may reduce the frequency of nightmares. Rarely, patients with severe recurrent nightmares require a REM suppressant medication (tricyclics, MAO inhibitors), though later such drugs should be withdrawn very slowly, to avoid recurrence during the REM-rebound period.

REM sleep behavior disorder

A condition recently documented by Schenck, Mahowald, and colleagues[67–69] is characterized by intermittent absence of the normal atonia of REM sleep associated with the appearance of very intense motor activity associated with dream mentation. The movements are often explosive, with sudden jerking, leaping, or diving from the bed, rapid ambulatory collisions with walls or furniture, and other wild behaviors that often appear to represent dream enactment. Injury to self or to the bed partner is common. Similar but less violent movements, such as hand and arm waving, reaching gestures, and punching or kicking may occur while the patient remains in bed. Episodes may repeat only a few times a week; though if several occur each night they

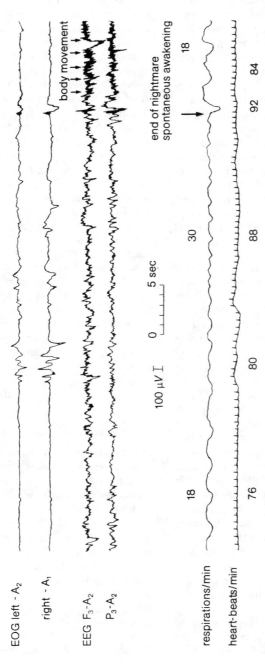

FIGURE 24-6.   *A REM nightmare in a chronic adult sufferer. Some mild to moderate increase in heart rate and respiratory rate in REM sleep are followed by body movement and an awakening. The patient subsequently described a detailed dream sequence in which he came to be attacked by man-sized cats. (Reprinted with permission from the late Dr. Charles Fisher.)*

may reappear in cyclic fashion about every 90 minutes after sleep onset. On awakening, recall of an intense dream is usual. It often contains elements of fighting back in self-defense or of attempting to flee. The violent nocturnal behavior is typically discordant with the dreamer's daytime personality.

In at least a third of patients, a prodromal period of sleep talking, yelling, or vigorous movements in sleep precedes the full-blown episodes by a number of years.[69] In a similar proportion, there is a history of significant neuropathology, such as dementia, subarachnoid hemorrhage, stroke, olivopontocerebellar degeneration, multiple sclerosis, or Guillain-Barré syndrome. The condition is common during, and was first identified in, chronic alcoholics.[70] Despite this variety of possible associations with pathology, at least 60% of cases are idiopathic. No associated psychopathology has been documented.

Whether or not CNS lesions are provable, it is believed that the condition is generally organic and due to dysfunction of the brain stem mechanisms that are responsible for the normal suppression of muscle tone in REM sleep. A similar behavior has long been described after dorsal pontine lesions in cats.[71] The precise prevalence is unknown, but the condition is far more common in males, and, though it can occur at any age, it is most frequent after age 60 years.

PSG recordings show a number of characteristic features.[67-69] During REM sleep there are recurrent periods of persistent muscle tone. Marked increases of phasic motor activity are present during REM sleep, and particularly during the episodes. These include eye movements, brief twitch potentials, and longer $\frac{1}{2}$- to 2-second phasic EMG potentials. During the actual episodes, such phasic increases are superimposed on marked sustained tonic increases in background EMG tone (Figure 24-7).

The differential diagnosis is quite extensive and includes posttraumatic stress syndrome, classic REM nightmares, sleep terrors, nocturnal paroxysmal dystonia, sleep-related epileptic seizures, and nocturnal delirium. Though the history is often suggestive, definitive diagnosis is based on the characteristic PSG features.

This parasomnia is treated with drugs.[68,69] Most cases respond to the benzodiazepine clonazepam, 1

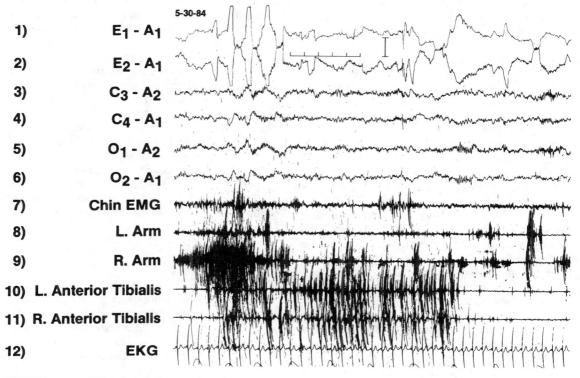

FIGURE 24-7. *REM sleep behavior disorder in man aged 64 years. The polygraph fragment is taken from a sequence that lasted several minutes. It shows REM sleep, indicated by the stage 1 EEG pattern combined with REMs. The chin EMG shows the characteristic sustained muscle tone of this disorder. The four limb EMGs show phasic and tonic increases in muscle tone, the phasic ones being associated with visible myoclonus. (Courtesy of Drs. Carlos Schenck and Mark Mahowald.)*

to 2 mg at bedtime. The mechanisms of its effectiveness are not fully understood, but the drug suppresses both the violent behavior and the intense subjective dream recall. Desipramine, 25 to 50 mg at bedtime, has also been successful in a smaller proportion of cases. Because the clinical attacks occasionally break through drug therapy, dangerous sharp objects should be removed from the sleeping environment and other precautions should be taken against injury. Cessation of medication inevitably leads to recurrence of the attacks.

Sleep paralysis (isolated)

Sleep paralysis[72,73] consists of episodes of inability to perform voluntary movements, either at sleep onset (hypnagogic or predormital form) or upon awakening (hypnapompic or postdormital form). Although sleep paralysis is one of the so-called symptom tetrad of the narcolepsy-cataplexy syndrome, it is considered here in its isolated form. Characteristically, limb, trunk, and head movements are impossible, but the patient can move the eyes and make some degree of respiratory effort. The sufferer is usually conscious of the environment and, combined with the inability to move, feels vulnerable and often frightened. Fragments of dream imagery may be recalled; when present, they are occasionally superimposed on the environment, leading to a form of "double consciousness."[74] Episodes typically last 1 minute to several. Despite efforts to move, the paralysis typically either disappears spontaneously or is aborted by someone else touching or moving part of the person's body.

Isolated sleep paralysis is not infrequently related to irregular sleep-wake patterns in shift workers,[75] in rapid time zone changes,[76] and in medical students and interns.[77,78] It is said to have been experienced at least once during a lifetime by some 30% to 50% of normal subjects.[1] Both sexes are equally affected. Isolated sleep paralysis also takes a rare familial form[79] that tends to be more chronic, affects females more often than males, and appears to have X-linked dominant transmission. No autopsy reports have been published in cases of isolated sleep paralysis, but as patients are neurologically intact on physical examination, any organic cause in chronic cases most likely is microstructural, neurochemical, or neuroimmunologic.

PSG recordings to date have been described only for sleep paralysis in association with the narcolepsy syndrome.[80] They have shown the condition to occur during direct transitions into or out of REM sleep and to consist of absence of muscle tone in submental, other axial, and peripheral EMGs in association with an EEG of wakefulness plus waking ocular movements and blink patterns. Occasionally, drowsy

stage 1 patterns with slow eye movements occur. H-reflex studies during episodes have shown total suppression of this monosynaptic reflex, indicating loss of anterior motorneuron excitability, which normally occurs during full-blown REM sleep. Sleep paralysis is thus considered an incomplete or dissociated REM state in which the motor atonia of REM sleep is present in isolation. Pathophysiologically it thus may be considered the inverse of the REM sleep behavior disorder, in which sleep is preserved but the mechanisms of REM atonia are absent.

Differential diagnosis seldom poses a problem, as the episodes are so characteristic. Narcolepsy syndrome can be excluded by absence of its other features, cataplectic attacks triggered in wakefulness by emotional stimuli; more-or-less irresistible sleep attacks; multiple sleep-onset REM periods on the Multiple Sleep Latency Test; and associated positive histocompatibility testing for HLA-DR2 and -DQw1 antigens. Nocturnal nerve compression palsies must be considered but are usually self-evident and local. Hypokalemic paralysis must be distinguished. It usually occurs in wakefulness, is more common in adolescents, exhibits familial transmission, and, above all, shows characteristic low serum potassium levels during episodes, which can be reversed by taking potassium.

In isolated cases associated with irregular sleep-wake patterns successful treatment may consist of improved sleep hygiene alone. In chronic cases, and especially in the familial ones, medication may be necessary. The usual treatment then is clomipramine hydrochloride, 25 mg at bedtime.[34] Desipramine is less effective, and imipramine has little if any effect. In exceptionally resistant cases, a monoamine oxidase inhibitor such as phenelzine may be indicated, though the risk of serious side effects, and the necessary dietary precautions, with this group of drugs seriously limit its usefulness.

Painful erections

A rare but disturbing parasomnia is painful nocturnal erections[1,81] in males, which are often associated with recall of dreams. If recurrent, they may lead to a form of sleep maintenance insomnia with subsequent daytime sleepiness, anxiety, and irritability. Preoccupation with the symptom may become intense. Penile erections during wakefulness usually are not impaired. In most cases the cause is unknown; however, some are associated with Peyronie's disease or phimosis.

PSG confirms the presence of recurrent awakenings from REM sleep associated with penile erections monitored by strain gauge devices or observation.

Symptomatic cases are treated by surgical correction of the underlying disease. In idiopathic cases, the symptom often disappears spontaneously. A small proportion of patients require REM-suppressant medication.[82]

Light Sleep Stage Disorders (Stages 1, 2, and REM)

Sleep talking

Sleep talking is usually a benign phenomenon and seldom a significant sleep disorder. It consists of speech or sound uttered during sleep without awareness.[83] Sleep talking typically becomes a problem only when it is sufficiently frequent or loud to disturb the sleep of others. It is usually spontaneous (somniloquy); or, more rarely, it can be elicited and the sleeper enters into a dialogue with others.[84] The exceptional occurrence of two sleepers having a dialogue between them, none of which is recalled by either on awakening, has also been reported. Arkin and coworkers[85] have shown that recalled mental activity after awakening, when present, generally shows a reasonable degree of concordance with speech content. This supports the premise that such utterances reflect ongoing mental activity in sleep.

The course is typically benign. Sleep talking may occur only for short intermittent periods, and it often then disappears completely. Chronic sleep talking may be related to significant psychopathology or to intercurrent sleep disturbances. The phenomenon shows no sex preference. Occasionally it appears to be familial.

PSG has shown that sleep talking most commonly occurs in stages 1, 2, and REM sleep[5,83] and only rarely in slow-wave sleep. Speech utterances typically are associated[5] with increase in muscle tone and a transient and incomplete EEG arousal (Figure 24-8). The phenomenon seldom requires treatment, and, in any event, no specific treatment is known.

Bruxism

Bruxism is repeated stereotypical grinding or crunching of the teeth during sleep.[86,87] It often disturbs the bed partner. Bruxism is frequently associated with a preexisting dental, mandibular, or maxillary condition—dental disease, malocclusion, and others.[88] Repeated sleep-related bruxism may itself lead secondarily to excessive tooth wear and decay or to periodontal tissue damage[89]; and it is often associated with jaw pain, including the temporomandibular variety.

Tooth grinding may be seen in otherwise normal persons, when it is typically related to stress, but it is particularly common in children who have some mental deficiency.[90] Tooth grinding in wakefulness—a

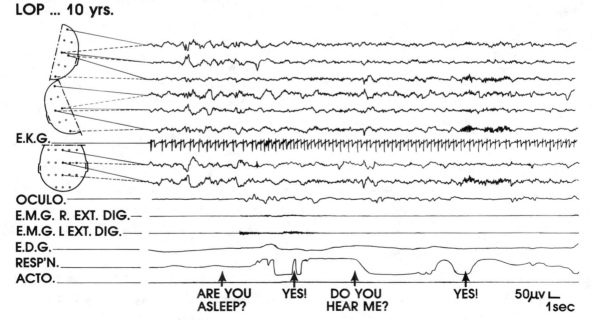

LOP ... 10 yrs.

E.K.G.

OCULO.
E.M.G. R. EXT. DIG.
E.M.G. L EXT. DIG.
E.D.G.
RESP'N.
ACTO.

ARE YOU ASLEEP? YES! DO YOU HEAR ME? YES! 50μv 1sec

FIGURE 24-8. *Sleep talking (dialogue) in NREM sleep. The polygraph fragment begins the stage 2 or 3 sleep. This chronic sleep talker, a 10-year-old boy, was asked, "Are you asleep?" The question evoked a K complex. Transient arousal (return of alpha rhythm) was associated with the answer, Yes. The child heard, understood, and appropriately answered the two questions while remaining asleep, arousing only briefly during answers. A few seconds later he was awakened and recalled nothing.*

habit or tic—is often associated. There is no sex preference. Occasional apparently familial cases have been described.

PSG shows repeated phasic increases of masseter muscle tone that cause artifacts in the EEG (Figure 24-9). These repeat at a frequency of about ½ to 1½ per second in bursts lasting seconds or several dozens of seconds and occur mainly in stages 1, 2, or REM sleep.[5,91,92] Some cases have been described in which it occurs exclusively in REM sleep.

Diagnosis seldom poses a problem. Rhythmic jaw movements in epileptic seizures associated with an ictal EEG discharge are rare but occasionally must be excluded.

Evaluation for treatment[93] includes a comprehensive dental examination and correction of any causal anatomic anomalies. Rare patients have treatable CNS lesions. In most cases, no evident jaw or brain abnormality is found. Stress may be reduced by appropriate counseling or psychotherapy. In some cases relaxation techniques or biofeedback have been useful. A few patients require a rubber "mouth guard" over the teeth to prevent further dental and jaw damage.

Diffuse Sleep Disorders (Those with No Stage Preference)

Enuresis nocturna

Enuresis nocturna or bedwetting consists of involuntary micturition during sleep. It is often classified into primary and secondary types. Primary enuresis patients have never achieved full urinary continence, which they should by age 5 years. Secondary enuresis patients, after learning bladder control for at least 6 months, lose control and become enuretic.[94,95]

Bedwetting is also often divided into idiopathic and symptomatic forms, the latter being associated with genito-urinary or other pathology. Idiopathic primary enuresis is by far the most common type. Bedwetting tends to occur in the first third of the night during a partial or complete arousal. Dreaming may be recalled in association with the enuresis, but it has been shown that dreams that have content about fluids represent postevent incorporation of the wet bed stimuli rather than being causal.[53] Bedwetting often leads to embarrassment and secondary psychological trauma, especially in older children, adolescents, and adults. Bladder control during daytime wakefulness is often normal.

The reasons for the perpetuation or reappearance of bedwetting after age 5 years vary. In some children toilet training is not fully provided or acquired.[96] A small functional bladder[97] or an insensitive bladder[98,99] may be present without actual demonstrable organic disease. Idiopathic enuresis is more common in males, in lower socioeconomic classes, and in institutionalized children.[96] In adults, idiopathic enureis is much more rare, and an organic cause, metabolic or endocrine disorder, or coexisting sleep apnea syndrome is more common. A hereditary factor appears to be present in primary enuresis[100,101] and in certain urogenital malformations of symptomatic cases.

By PSG (Figure 24-10) it has been determined that enuresis episodes can occur in all stages of sleep, with or without concomitant arousal.[102,103] Sleep cystometry[5,104] has shown increased bladder reactivity to environmental stimuli, increased detrusor contractions in sleep prior to onset of micturition, and elevated pressure during sleep at the onset of the enuretic event sufficient to trigger involuntary micturition, at least in wakefulness (Figure 24-11).

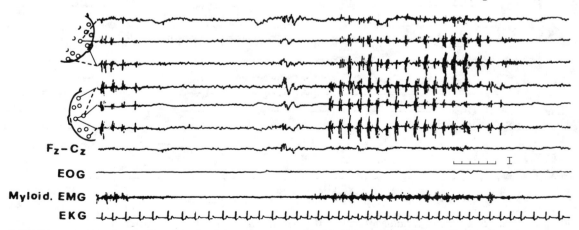

F_z–C_z

EOG

Myloid. EMG

EKG

FIGURE 24-9.   *Tooth grinding (bruxism) in an 18-year-old-girl. One series of four tooth grindings is followed by stage 1 patterns, then stage 2 (K complex), followed by some degree of EEG arousal associated with return of rhythmic EMG artifacts with a frequency of about 0.5 to 1.0 Hz.*

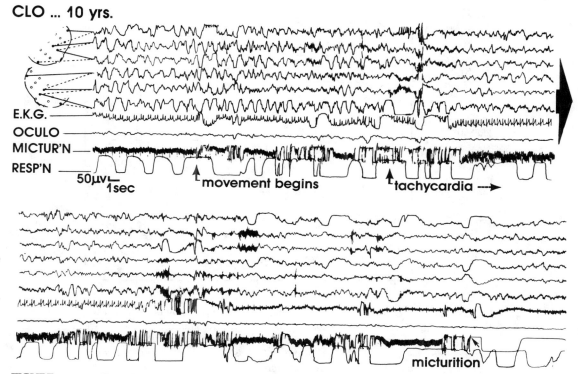

CLO ... 10 yrs.

E.K.G.
OCULO
MICTUR'N
RESP'N

50μv
1sec

movement begins

tachycardia →

micturition

FIGURE 24-10. *Enuresis nocturna. This episode in a 10-year-old girl, a chronic bedwetter, begins in stage 4 sleep. It consists of body movement, tachycardia, EEG desynchronization evolving eventually to stage 1 patterns, and, lower right, micturition indicated by loss of the dark 60-Hz main lines artifact in the relevant channel.*

The diagnosis of idiopathic enuresis requires the exclusion of organic and metabolic causes. Urogenital disease, chronic urinary tract infection, diabetes insipidus, diabetes mellitus, neurologic disease, sleep apnea syndrome, and nocturnal epileptic seizures must all be ruled out by appropriate tests.

The symptomatic form is treated by treating the underlying disease. For idiopathic primary enuresis, a number of approaches are helpful.[105] Avoidance of fluids in late evening may be sufficient. Bladder training exercises during wakefulness, in which the patient is taught to hold increasingly greater amounts of urine in the bladder, may help,[106] as may sphincter training exercises in which the patient repeatedly interrupts the stream of urine while voiding.[105] There may also be a positive response to a conditioning device by which a bell or alarm triggered by the release of urine stimulates the patient, who over time becomes more aware of the enuresis.[107] This apparently leads eventually to learning to sense the detrusor contractions during sleep and, consequently, awakening in time to void. Family support and avoidance of teasing may be crucial.

Particularly for children who are under much social stress and for adults, resort to drug therapy may be necessary. The most effective substance is imipramine hydrochloride, 10 to 75 mg at bedtime.[108] Its effect does not appear to relate to any change in sleep structure, but rather to a direct anticholinergic effect on the bladder myoneural junction. Different tricyclics and other drugs have also been found to be of help in individual cases.

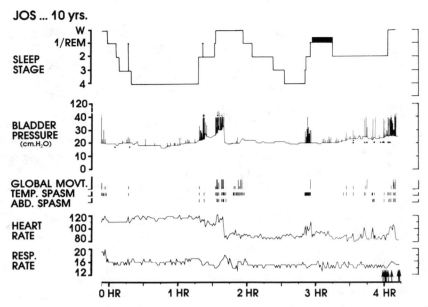

FIGURE 24-11.   *Detailed sleep histogram in a 10-year-old boy bedwetter for the first 4 hours of sleep. The recording included intravesicular bladder pressure as measured by indwelling catheter. Enuresis occurred about 100 minutes after sleep onset. Up to that point there is some degree of sustained tachycardia and tachypnea, as well as increasing bladder pressure with superimposed vesicular contractions (vertical lines). These led to a crescendo during lightening of sleep, from NREM stages 4 to 2 to 1, followed by micturition around the catheter. This movement is associated with abrupt drop of baseline bladder pressure, heart rate, and, to a lesser extent, respiratory rate. With the bladder empty, there are then no further bladder contractions for some 1½ hours, but that is followed by increased bladder pressure and return of contractions. (Note that the baseline pressure is artificially high owing to the location of the manometer head).*

REFERENCES

1. Diagnostic Classification Steering Committee. International Classification of Sleep Disorders: Diagnostic and Coding Manual. Rochester, Minn.: American Sleep Disorders Association, 1990.
2. Mitchell SW. Some disorders of sleep. Int J Med Sci 1890;100:109–127.
3. Roger H. Les Troubles du Sommeil—Hypersomnies, Insomnies, Parasomnies. Paris: Masson, 1932.
4. Oswald I. Sudden body jerks on falling asleep. Brain 1959;82:92–103.
5. Gastaut H, Broughton R. A clinical and polygraphic study of episodic phenomena during sleep. Rec Adv Biol Psychiatry 1965;7:197–222.
6. Broughton R. Pathological fragmentary myoclonus, intensified hypnic jerks and hypnagogic foot tremors: Three unusual sleep-related movement disorders. In: Koella WP, Obal F, Schulz H, et al. eds. Sleep '86. Stuttgart: Gustav Fischer, 1988;240–242.
7. De Lisi L. Su di un fenomeno motorio costanti del sonno normale: Le mioclonie ipniche fisiologiche. Riv Pat Nerv Ment 1932;110:481–503.
8. Loeb C, Massazza G, Sacco G, et al. Etude polygraphique de myoclonies hypniques chez l'homme. Rev Neurol (Paris) 1964;110:258–268.
9. Gastaut H, Villeneuve A. The startle disease or hyperekplexia: Pathological surprise reaction. J Neurol Sci 1967;5:523–542.
10. Gastaut H, Broughton R. Epileptic Seizures: Clinical and Electrographic Features, Diagnosis and Treatment. Springfield, Ill.: Charles C Thomas, 1972.
11. Gastaut H. Séméiologie des myoclonies et nosologie analytique des syndromes myocloniques. Rev Nuerol (Paris) 1968;119:1–30.
12. Coleman RM, Pollak CP, Weitzman ED. Periodic movements in sleep (nocturnal myoclonus): Relation to sleep disorders. Ann Neurol 1980;8:416–421.
13. Ekbom KA. Restless legs. Acta Med Scand Suppl 1944;158:1–123.
14. Zappert J. Uber nachtliche Kopfbewegungen bei Kindern (jactatio capitis nocturna). Jahrbuch Kinderheilk 1905;62:70–83.
15. Cruchet R. Tics et sommeil. Presse Méd 1905;13:33–36.
16. De Lissovoy V. Headbanging in early childhood. Child Dev 1962;13:43–56.

17. Klackenburg G. Rhythmic movements in infancy and early childhood. Acta Paediatr Scand Suppl 1971;224:74–83.

18. Thorpy MJ, Glovinsky P. Jactatio capitis nocturna. In: Kryger M, Roth T, Dement WC, eds. Principles and Practice of Sleep Medicine. Philadelphia: WB Saunders, 1989;648–654.

19. Sallustro F, Atwell CW. Body rocking, head banging and head rolling in normal children. J Pediatr 1978;93:704–708.

20. Freidin MR, Jakowski JJ, Singer WD. Nocturnal head-banging as a sleep disorder: A case report. Am J Psychiatry 1979;136:1469–1470.

21. Baldy-Moulinier M, Levy M, Passouant P. Etude de la jactatio capitis au cours du sommeil de nuit. Rev Neurol (Paris) 1969;120:460–463.

22. Walsh JK, Kramer M, Skinner JE. A case of jactatio capitis nocturna. Am J Psychiatry 1981, 138:524–526.

23. Oswald I. Rocking at night. Electroencephalogr Clin Neurophysiol 1964;16:577.

24. Regenstein RR, Hartman E, Reich P. A head movement disorder occurring in REM sleep. J Nerv Ment Dis 1977;164:432–436.

25. Gagnon P, de Koninck J. Repetitive head movements during REM sleep. Biol Psychiatry 1985;20:176–178.

26. Decatanzaro DA, Baldwin G. Effective treatment of self-injurious behavior through a force arm exercise. Am J Ment Deficiency 1978;82:422–439.

27. Weiher RG, Harman RE. The use of omission training to reduce self-injurious behavior in a retarded child. Behav Res Ther 1975;6:261–268.

28. Marc C. De la Folie. Paris: Baillière, 1840.

29. von Gudden H. Die physiologische und pathologische Schlaftrunkenheit. Arch Psyciatr Nervenkrank 1905; 40:989–1015.

30. Bonkalo A. Impulsive acts and confusional states during incomplete arousal from sleep: Criminological and forensic implications. Psychiatr Q 1974;48:400–409.

31. Ferber RF. In: Kryger M, Roth T, Dement WC, eds. Principles and Practice of Sleep Medicine. Philadelphia: WB Saunders, 1989;640–642.

32. Broughton R. Disorders of sleep: Disorders of arousal? Science 1968;59:1070–1078.

33. Saier J, Regis H, Mano T, et al. Potentiels evoquées visuels pendant les différents phases de sommeil chez l'homme: Études de la réponse visuelle évoqué après le reviel. In: Gastaut H, Lugaresi E, Berti Ceroni G, et al., eds. The abnormalities of sleep in man. Bologna: Aulo Gaggi, 1968;55–66.

34. Roth B. Narcolepsy and Hypersomnia. Basel: Karger, 1980.

35. Cirignotta F, Zucconi M, Mondini S, et al. Enuresis, sleepwalking and nightmares: An epidemiological survey in the Republic of San Marino. In: Guilleminault C, Lugaresi E, eds. Sleep-Wake Disorders: Natural History, Epidemiology and Long-Term Evolution. New York: Raven, 1983;237–241.

36. Abe K, Shimakawa M. Predisposition to sleepwalking. Psychiatr Neurol 1966;152:306–312.

37. Bakwin H. Sleepwalking in twins. Lancet 1970;2:466–467.

38. Kales A, Soldatos CR, Bixler EO, et al. Hereditary factors in sleepwalking and sleep terrors. Br J Psychiatry 1980;137:111–118.

39. Gastaut H, Batini C, Broughton R, et al. Etude électroencepyhalographique des manifestations paroxystique au cours du sommeil nocturne. Rev Neurol (Paris) 1964;110:309.

40. Jacobson A, Kales A, Lehmann D, et al. Somnambulism: All night electroencephalography studies. Science 1965;148:975–977.

41. Kales A, Jacobson A, Paulson M, et al. Somnambulism: Psychophysiological correlates: I. All-night EEG studies. Arch Gen Psychiatry 1966;14:585–594.

42. Broughton R. Phasic and dynamic aspects of sleep: A symposium review and synthesis. In: Terzano MG, Halasz P, Declerck AC, eds. Phasic Events and the Dynamic Organization of Sleep. New York: Raven, 1991;185–205.

43. Jacobson A, Kales A. Somnambulism: All-night EEG and related studies. Res Publ Assoc Res Nerv Ment Dis 1967;45:424–448.

44. Halasz P, Ujszaszi J, Gadorvo P. Are microarousals preceded by electroencephalographic slow-wave synchronization precursors of confusional awakenings? Sleep 1985;8:231–238.

45. Pedley TA, Guilleminault C. Episodic nocturnal wanderings responsive to anticonvulsant drug therapy. Ann Neurol 1977;2:30–35.

46. Guilleminault C. Sleepwalking and night terrors. In: Kryger MH, Roth T, Dement WC, eds. Principles and Practice of Sleep Medicine. Philadelphia: WB Saunders, 1989;379–384.

47. de Villard R, Dalery J, Mouret J. Le somnabulisme de l'enfant: Étude clinique, polygraphique et therapeutique: Á propos de 37 observations. Lyon Méd 1978;240:65–72.

48. Jones E. On the Nightmare. London: Hogarth, 1949.

49. Hallstrom T. Night terror in adults through three generations. Acta Psychiatr Scand 1972;48:350–352.

50. Fisher C, Byrne J, Edwards A, et al. A psychophysiological study of nightmares. J Am Psychoanal Assoc 1970;18:747–782.

51. Fisher C, Kahn E, Edwards A, et al. A psychophysiological study of nightmares and sleep terrors. J Nerv Ment Dis 1973;157:75–98.

52. Fisher C, Kahn E, Edwards A, et al. A psychological study of nightmares and sleep terrors: The suppression of stage 4 sleep terrors with diazepam. Arch Gen Psychiatry 1973;28:252–259.

53. Broughton R. Pathophysiology of enuresis nocturna, sleep terrors and sleepwalking: Current status and the Marseille contribution. In: Broughton RJ, ed. Henri Gastaut and the Marseille School's Contribution to the Neurosciences. Amsterdam: Elsevier, 1982;401–410.

54. Pesikoff RB, Davis PC. Treatment of pavor nocturnus and somnambulism in children. Am J Psychiatry 1971;128:778–781.

55. Marshall JR. The treatment of night terrors associated with the posttraumatic syndrome. Am J psychiatry 1975;132:293–295.

56. Kales JD, Cadieux RJ, Soldatos C, et al. Psychotherapy with night-terror patients. Am J Psychother 1982; 36:399–407.

57. Lugaresi E, Cirignotta F. Hypnogenic paroxysmal dystonia: Epileptic seizure or a new syndrome? Sleep 1981;4:129–138.

58. Cromwell JA, Anders TF. Hypnogenic paroxysmal dystonia. J Am Acad Child Psychiatry 1985;24:353–358.

59. Lugaresi E, Cirignotta F. Two variants of nocturnal paroxysmal dystonia with attacks of short and long duration. In: Degen R, Neidermeyer E, eds. Epilepsy, Sleep and Sleep Deprivation. Amsterdam: Elsevier, 1984;169–175.

60. Godbout R, Montplaisir J, Rouleau J. Hypnogenic paroxysmal dystonia: Epilepsy or sleep disorder? Electroencephalogr Clin Neurophysiol 1985;16:136–142.

61. Hartmann E. The Nightmare: The Psychology and Biology of Terrifying Dreams. New York: Basic Books, 1984.

62. Hartmann E. A preliminary study of the personality of the nightmare sufferer: Relationship to schizophrenia and creativity. Am J Psychiatry 1981;136:794–796.

63. Kales A, Soldatos CR, Caldwell AB, et al. Nightmares: Clinical characteristics and personality patterns. Am J Psychiatry 1980;137:1197–1201.

64. Lavie P, Hefez A, Halpern G, et al. Long-term effects of traumatic war related events on sleep. Am J Psychiatry 1979;136:1175–1178.

65. Kramer M, Schoen LS, Kinney L. Nightmares in Vietnam veterans. J Am Acad Psychoanal 1987;15:67–81.

66. Hartmann E. Normal and abnormal dreams. In: Kryger M, Roth T, Dement WC, eds. Principles and Practice of Sleep Medicine. Philadelphia: WB Saunders, 1989;191–195.

67. Schenck CH, Bundlie SR, Ettinger MC, et al. Chronic behavior disorders of human REM sleep: A new category of parasomnia. Sleep 1986;9:293–308.

68. Schenck CH, Bundlie SR, Patterson AL, et al. Rapid eye movement sleep behavior disorder: A treatable parasomnia affecting older patients. JAMA 1987;257:1786–1789.

69. Mahowald MW, Schenck CH. REM sleep behavior disorder. In: Kryger M, Roth T, Dement WC, eds. Principles and Practice of Sleep Medicine. Philadelphia: WB Saunders, 1989;389–401.

70. Hishikawa Y, Sugita Y, Teshima Y, et al. Sleep disorders in alcoholic patients with delirium tremens. Reevaluation of the REM rebound and intrusion theory. In: Karacan I, ed. Psychophysiological Aspects of Sleep. Park Ridge, N.J.: Noyes Medical, 1981;109–122.

71. Jouvet M, Delorme JF. Locus coeruleus et sommeil paradoxal. CR Soc Biol (Paris) 1965;159:895–899.

72. Goode GB. Sleep paralysis. Arch Neurol 1962;6:228–234.

73. Hishikawa Y. Sleep paralysis. In: Guilleminault C, Dement WC, Passouant P, eds. Narcolepsy. New York: Spectrum, 1976:97–124.

74. Broughton R. Human consciousness and sleep/waking rhythm: A review and some neuropsychological considerations. J Clin Neuropsychol 1982;4:193–218.

75. Folkard S, Condon R, Herbert H. Night sleep paralysis. Experientia 1984,40:510–512.

76. Snyder S. Isolated sleep paralysis after rapid time-zone changes (jet-lag syndrome). Chronobiologica 1983;10:377–379.

77. Everett HC. Sleep paralysis in medical students. J Nerv Ment Dis 1963;136:283–287.

78. Penn NE, Kripke DF, Scharff J. Sleep paralysis among medical students. J Psychol 1981;107:247–252.

79. Roth B, Buhova S, Berkova L. Familial sleep paralysis. Schweiz Arch Neurol Neurochir Psychiatr 1968; 102:321–330.

80. Nan'no H, Hishikawa Y, Koida H, et al. A neurophysiological study of sleep paralysis in narcoleptic patients. Electroencephalogr Clin Neurophysiol 1970;28:382–390.

81. Ware JC. Monitoring erections during sleep. In: Kryger MH, Roth T, Dement WC, eds. Principles and Practice of Sleep Medicine. Philadelphia: WB Saunders, 1989;689–695.

82. Fisher C, Kahn E, Edwards A, et al. Total suppression of REM sleep with the MAO inhibitor Nardil in a subject with painful nocturnal REM erection. Psychophysiology 1972;9:91.

83. Arkin AM. Sleep talking: A review. J Nerv Ment Dis 1966:143:101–122.

84. Aarons L. Evoked sleep talking. Percept Mot Skills 1970;31:27–40.

85. Arkin AM, Toth MF, Baker J, et al. The degree of concordance between the content of sleep talking and mentation recalled in wakefulness. J Nerv Metn Dis 1970;151:375–393.

86. Glaros AG, Rao SM. Bruxism: A critical review. Psychol Bull 1977;84:767–781.

87. Ahmed R. Bruxism in children. J Pedol 1986;10:105–106.

88. Funch DP, Gale EN. Factors associated with nocturnal bruxism and its treatment. J Behav Med 1980;3:385–387.

89. Glaros AG, Rao SM. Effects of bruxism: A review of the literature. J Prosthetet Dent 1977;38:149–157.

90. Richmond G, Rugh JD, Dolfi R, et al. Survey of bruxism in an institutionalized mentally retarded population. Am J Ment Defic 1984;88:418–421.

91. Reding GR, Zepelin H, Robinson JE, et al. Nocturnal tooth-grinding: All-night psychophysiological studies. J Dent Res 1968;47:786–797.

92. Ware JC, Rugh J. Destructive bruxism: Sleep stage relationship. Sleep 1988, 11:172–181.

93. Hartmann E. Bruxism. In: Kryger MH, Roth T, Dement WC, eds. Principles and Practice of Sleep Medicine. Philadelphia: WB Saunders, 1989;385–388.

94. Agarwal A. Enuresis. Acad Fam Pract 1982;May:203–207.

95. Scharf MB. Waking Up Dry: How to End Bedwetting Forever. Cincinatti: Writer's Digest Books, 1986.

96. Ferber R. Sleep-associated enuresis in the child. In: Kryger MH, Roth T, Dement WC, eds. Principles and Practice of Sleep Medicine. Philadelphia: WB Saunders, 1989;643–647.

97. Muellner SR. Development of urinary control in children: A new concept in cause, prevention and treatment in primary enuresis. J Urol 1960;84:714–716.

98. Di Perri R, Meduri MA. A polygraphic approach to the study of enuresis nocturna. In: Levin P, Koella WP, eds. Sleep 1974. Basel: S Karger, 1975;413–416.

99. Bradley WE. Electroencephalography and bladder innervation. J Urol 1977;118:412–414.

100. Hallgren B. Enuresis—a clinical and genetic study. Acta Psychiatr Neurol Scand 1957;32 (suppl 114):1–159.

101. Bakwin H. The genetics of enuresis. In: Kolvin I, MacKeith RC, Meadow SR, eds. Bladder Control and Enuresis. Clin Develop Med 1973;48/49:73–77.

102. Kales A, Kales JD, Jacobson A, et al. Effects of imipramine on enuresis frequency and sleep states. Pediatrics 1977,60:431–436.

103. Mikkelsen EJ, Rapaport JL, Nee L, et al. Childhood enuresis. I. Sleep patterns and psychopathology. Arch Gen Psychiatry 1980;27:1139–1144.

104. Broughton R, Gastaut H. Further polygraphic studies of enuresis nocturna (intra-vesicular pressure). Electroencephalogr Clin Neurophysiol 1964;16:626.

105. Marshall S, Marshall HH, Lyon RP. Enuresis: An analysis of various therapeutic approaches. Pediatrics 1973;52:813–817.

106. Starfield B, Mellits ED. Increase in functional bladder capacity and improvement of enuresis. J Pediatr 1968;72:483–487.

107. Goel KM, Thomson RB, Gibb EM, et al. Evaluation of nine different types of enuresis alarms. Arch Dis Child 1984;59:748–753.

108. Kardash S, Hellman E, Werry J. Efficacy of imipramine in childhood enuresis: A double-blind control study with placebo. Can Med Assoc J 1968;99:236–266.

25

Sleep Disorders in Elderly Persons

Sudhansu Chokroverty

To understand the sleep disorders of elderly persons it is important to know what changes in sleep structure and sleep cycle are normal in aged persons. It is also important to understand the neurology of aging and, in particular, changes in central nervous system (CNS) physiology and morphology in normal healthy older persons.

It is notable that, in 1900, 4% of the American population were older than 65 years; according to the best current estimate, in the year 2000, that figure will be 13%, and by 2050 21%.[1] Older persons are at risk for sleep disturbances, owing to a variety of factors—social and psychosocial problems, increasing prevalence of concurrent medical, psychiatric, and neurologic illnesses, increasing use of medications (often sedative-hypnotics) and alcohol, and alterations in circadian rhythms.

NEUROLOGY OF AGING

Clinical Aspects of Central Nervous System Changes

Before discussing the neurology of aging it is important to define what is meant by aging. No standard definition is available, but for this discussion I arbitrarily define age 65 as the start of old age. Accepting this definition, a variety of changes in mental functions and the general nervous system of healthy elderly persons have been noted. At the outset I must point out certain difficulties in studying the neurology of aging. It is difficult to get a large number of elderly subjects who meet the criteria by being free of neurologic and other systemic disorders. Even if a number of such subjects can be recruited, without many years' subsequent longitudinal study it often remains problematic to decide whether certain abnormal findings are related to a subclinical affection of the nervous system that is expressed in overt manifestations later in life.[2] A large number of elderly persons suffer from general medical and neurologic disorders, particularly dementia of the Alzheimer's type. In addition, there could be subclinical

cerebral infarction, as noted in large series of autopsy examinations,[3] where half the persons who suffered cerebral infarction remained asymptomatic. Therefore, accepting these limitations, I will briefly discuss the neurologic changes of normal aging.

On mental function examination, the most striking changes in old age are in learning new information and in central processing of information.[2] In the Wechsler Adult Intelligence Scale (WAIS),[4] the performance scale declines much more rapidly than the verbal tests.[2,5] This has been confirmed in several cross-sectional and longitudinal studies that compared young and old persons.[5-8] The past and the immediate memory remain relatively intact until about the middle 70s, but recent memory is impaired. There is often forgetfulness and difficulty remembering names and remembering several objects at one time, which suggests impairment of central processing time. Speed of learning is retarded, as is speed of processing new information.[2] The reaction time to simple and complex stimuli is often delayed, and there is impairment of motor speed.[9-13]

In a classic paper in 1931, McDonald Critchley[14] first directed attention to certain changes in the nervous system in the normal healthy elderly persons. Since then, several studies have appeared in the literature that document the presence of abnormal neurologic signs in a small number of such people,[15,16] but these signs may represent asymptomatic subclinical disease,[2] such as cerebrovascular disease or cervical spondylosis, and without longitudinal studies it is impossible to exclude these definitely. Despite this limitation, there is a general consensus about the presence of certain findings in normal elderly persons. There are changes in both somatic and autonomic nervous system.[2,17,17a] In the somatic system an important finding is impairment of the gait and stance.[2,18,19] It is difficult to stand on one leg with the eyes closed.[15,16,19] Also, grip strength declines with age.[16] The ankle reflex may be diminished, which may be related to the loss of the large-diameter nerve fibers.[2] In the sensory examination the striking abnormality is impairment of the vibration sense in the lower extremities.[16]

Many older persons have stooped posture resembling that in the early stage of Parkinson's disease, which may be related to the loss of dopaminergic neurons and striatal dopamine receptors.[2,18] Rowe and Troen[20] stated, "Old age may represent a hyperadrenergic state." Thus, sympathetic overactivity may explain some of the changes noted in elders' cardiovascular reflex, galvanic skin response, erection, maturation, and pupillary response. This overactivity of the sympathetic nervous system may also interfere with cognitive function.

Physiologic Changes in Old Age

EEG changes

Awake EEG. The question remains whether EEG changes seen in old age are maturational changes or are related to pathologic alterations of the CNS. Many elderly persons are afflicted with a variety of dementing illnesses, cerebrovascular disease, or systemic medical disorders that may cause metabolic encephalopathy.[21] Thus it is important to select healthy elderly persons who are free from any of these diseases for EEG study. Such a selection was made in the study of healthy septuagenarians by Katz and Horowitz.[22] The subjects were screened by careful neurologic, psychiatric, and neuropsychological examination to represent normative EEG data. The EEG was quite normal: average alpha frequency was 9.8 Hz, and, so, similar to that of young and middle-aged adults. This study can be contrasted with the report by Torres and colleagues,[23] in which they found that 52% of a group of normal volunteers of mean age of 69 years had mild to moderate EEG abnormalities. Obrist[24] summarized the EEG changes in old age as follows: slowing of the alpha rhythm, an increase of fast activities, diffuse slow activity, and focal slow waves. In an important longitudinal study by Obrist and colleagues[25] alpha frequency fell from 9.4 Hz at age 79 to 8 Hz intermixed with 6- to 7-Hz theta waves at age 89. Spectral analysis by Matejcek[26] and Nakano and coworkers[27] also supported the progressive slowing of the alpha rhythm with aging. Duffy and associates[28] found no significant change in the frequency of the posterior EEG rhythm in a study of 63 men between age 30 and 80 years. Oken and Kaye[29] recently analyzed conventional EEG and computerized EEG frequency in 22 extremely healthy subjects between 84 and 98 years. The posterior peak frequency was above 8 Hz in those younger than 84 but was between 7 and 8 Hz in five of 22 subjects older than 84 years. Alpha slowing appears to be related to the decline in mental function, which may be an early stage of progressive dementia of old age.[30] Alpha blocking and photic driving response to intermittent photic stimulation

are also diminished in old age.[31] These findings may be related to the structural CNS alternations in elderly persons (see below).

An increase of fast activity was noted by Busse and Obrist[32] in elderly volunteer community subjects, especially females. Kugler[33] also reported an increase of fast activity with increasing age. The significance of this is uncertain, but Kugler[33] stated that the presence of fast activity in old age correlates with preserved mental functioning.

Intermittent focal slow waves in the temporal regions (particularly in the middle and anterior temporal regions and greater on the left side) are noted in 17% to 59% of healthy elderly individuals.[23,24,29,34-36] This temporal slow activity may be accompanied by sharp transients, which may be related to cerebral vascular disease causing asymptomatic small infarction of the temporal lobe[30], ventricular enlargement with cerebral atrophy[37] or white matter hyperintensities on magnetic resonance imaging (MRI).[29]

Transient bursts of anteriorly dominant rhythmic delta waves are often noted in elderly subjects in the early stage of sleep. Gibbs and Gibbs[38] used the term *anterior bradyrhythmia* for this finding. Katz and Horowitz[39] obtained sleep-onset frontal intermittent rhythmic delta activity (FIRDA) in normal elderly subjects, which should be differentiated from that associated with a variety of neurologic disorders. These are highly stimulus sensitive and disappear in deeper stages of sleep. In demented elders, however, one can see diffuse slow waves in the delta and theta frequencies.

There is no clear relationship between intellectual deterioration and EEG slowing.[24,29] Whether the EEG changes are correlated with cerebral blood flow study remain controversial. There is, however, no correlation between areas that show the maximum blood flow reduction and those that show prominent EEG slowing, or between the blood flow changes and the alpha frequency changes in normal elderly subjects.[40,41] The other suggestion is that the alpha slowing is related to the loss of choline acetyltransferase, the enzyme for synthesis of acetylcholine.[2]

Sleep EEG changes, including changes in sleep architecture and organization.[42,42a] In addition to awake EEG changes there are also changes during sleep in the elderly. It is interesting to note that Liberson[43] in 1945 described paroxysmal bursts of sleep-like EEG lasting 1 to 10 seconds in the eyes-resting state in elderly subjects, and the incidence of these bursts increases with the age of the subject. Liberson[43] termed these episodes *microsleeps*. Normal elders show normal sleep patterns with certain modifications. The delta waves during slow-wave sleep are reduced in amplitude and incidence.[17,44,45]

The amplitude of delta waves decreases, and thus in the usual Rectschaffen and Kales[46] scoring technique stages III and IV decrease. Feinberg and colleagues[47] discussed this point and suggested that quantification of the amount of time spent in a specified frequency, rather than using an amplitude criterion be utilized for scoring slow-wave sleep in elderly persons. This reduction of amplitude of delta waves could be related to three factors: reduction of neuronal synchronization in the neocortex; alterations in the skull; and changes in the subarachnoid spaces.[17,47]

Sleep spindles may show a variety of changes in old age[48,49]: decreased frequency, amount, and amplitude. The frequency may decrease from 16 to 14 to 12 Hz. The spindles are often poorly formed and poorly developed. Sleep spindle changes thus resemble those noted with alpha frequency in the old age.

Rapid eye movement (REM)–non-REM (NREM) cyclic pattern remains unchanged, but the first cycle may be reduced.[17,50–52] REM density (number of eye movement bursts per minute of REM sleep) and total REM sleep time are reduced, but the percentage of REM in relation to total sleep time remains unaltered.[17,42,53] Sleep fragmentation is due to frequent interruptions at night. Also there are frequent sleep stage shifts, and, thus, frequent awakenings.[17,42] Regarding nocturnal total sleep time (TST), there is discrepancy between subjective report and objective data based on (lights out to lights on) technician's schedule.[17]

Nighttime sleep of elders usually is reported to be decreased (e.g., 5.5 to 6.5 hours, in contrast to the usual 7.5 hour average of TST of young adults).[54,55] This may not be an accurate observation, because elders often take daytime naps, so 24-hour TST probably is no different from the TST of young adults.

Increased fragmentation of sleep and increased numbers of transient arousals accompanied by increased daytime sleepiness have been described in the studies by Carskadon and coworkers.[56,57] Kales[58] and Feinberg[45] in their groups' investigations demonstrated the following changes in sleep with advancing age: state changes, reduction of slow-wave sleep (NREM stages 3 and 4) and a reduction of the EEG amplitude of delta waves, increase stage 1 owing to frequent arousals, decreased total nocturnal sleep, and reduction of total REM sleep time.

Williams and colleagues[59] recruited 120 healthy seniors through advertisements, without mentioning sleep. They tried to carefully screen out sleep disorders by excluding those who had sleep complaints. In their findings they noted that the seniors' sleep quality was poorer than that of young persons. There was a decrease of stage 3 and 4 sleep and an increase in nighttime wakefulness.[59,60] Prinz and Vitiello[61] considered these findings as a benchmark level of sleep change associated with aging per se. In another study involving the Veterans Administration Survey, Cashman and colleagues[62] found that nighttime hypoxemia, which correlated with sleep apena, was worse in several medical disorders—diabetes, cardiovascular disease, history of alcoholism, and vascular headaches. Thus, the data suggest that the disease states may interact with sleep disorders.

Between age 60 and 90 years there are differences in sleep architecture of men and women.[49] Between 60 and 70 years, men have more frequent arousals and more decrements in stage 3 and 4. Between 60 and 80 years women spend 9% of TST in slow-wave stage whereas men spend only 2%. Between 60 and 90 years the percentage of REM and total REM sleep show no difference between the sexes.

Changes in the circadian rhythm.[42a] Circadian rhythm changes result from fundamental changes in social interaction and family demise at this age: alterations of daily routine and activities, mealtime, health needs, and psychosocial factors (e.g., loneliness, divorce).[17] There may also be intrinsic changes in the circadian rhythm that may be related to the pathologic changes noted in apparently normal persons. Animal studies lend support to this conclusion.[63–66] In long-term care facilities circadian rhythm disturbances may be related to alterations of *Zeitgebers* (external time cues): alteration in bedtime, medication time, mealtime, special institutional regulations on lights out and lights on.[17] Wessler and colleagues[67] made an intensive study of 69- to 94-year-old institutionalized patients under strict environmentally controlled conditions and found a remarkable regularity in circadian synchronization. On the other hand, Scheving's group,[68] in a study involving 69- to 86-year-olds subjects, did not find support for the other group's conclusion. In all of these studies involving institutionalized patients the effect of chronic illnesses must be considered to explain circadian rhythm disturbances. Thus, these changes may not be related to "normal" old age.

A study of evolution of sleep shows that the strong monophasic circadian rhythm of youth gives way to a polyphasic ultradian rhythm in old age. Frequent awakenings at night, with reduction of wakefulness, are accompanied by increased daytime naps. These physiologic changes may be related to the structural alterations noted in the suprachiasmatic nucleus and brain stem hypnogenic neurons in experimental studies in several species of animals.[69–72]

There is also phase advance in the elderly; that is, there is a tendency to go to sleep early and awake early. These changes may be related to age-related changes in the core body temperature rhythm.[73,74] In elderly persons the amplitude of the temperature rhythm is attenuated and phase advanced.[74]

Autonomic nervous system changes with age

A number of changes occur in the autonomic nervous system (ANS) in sleep, and there are striking changes in ANS functions in elders.[17,17a] Four most important aspects of ANS changes are (1) thermoregulation, (2) cardiovascular changes (3) respiration, and (4) nocturnal penile tumescence.

Thermoregulation. Thermoregulation is impaired in old age.[17a] In response to passive heating, the sweating response of elders is impaired.[75,76] They are susceptible to hypothermia (both postoperative and in response to low ambient temperature in the environment)[77–79] and hyperthermia.[80,81] There is a clear paucity of studies that show ANS changes during sleep in elders.

Cardiovascular changes. Blood pressure and pulse rate fall at sleep onset, rise on awakening, and fluctuate during the night.[82] The increased incidence of stroke in elders during sleep may be related to these factors.[17]

Respiration. Changes in pulmonary function occur in the aged[17,83]: a reduction of vital capacity, chest wall compliance, diffusion capacity, elastic recoil, and arterial oxygen tension, and mismatch of the ventilation-perfusion ratio. There is a higher incidence of periodic breathing, including Cheyne-Stokes breathing and snoring in elders at night.[82,84–86] Patients with chronic obstructive pulmonary disease, who are often elderly, are at special risk during sleep (both at night and during the day) because of increasing oxygen desaturation, hypercapnia, and apnea during sleep.[87,88]

Nocturnal penile tumescence. Penile erection occurs during REM sleep. This REM-related penile tumescence shows a linear decrease in percentage from youth to old age (from 88% at 20 to 26 years old to 64% to 74% at 60 to 90 years).[89,90]

Endocrine changes with age[17]

Plasma cortisol. The circadian rhythm for plasma cortisol concentration is normal, and the plasma concentration of cortisol does not change in 60- to 95-year-old subjects.[91,92] In depressed patients (both young and old), however, the plasma cortisol level remains high during sleep and wakefulness, and the dexamethasone suppression test does not block secretion of cortisol.[93,94]

Growth hormone. Sleep-related growth hormone release is diminished in old age,[95,96] but the response of the growth hormone secretion to insulin

hypoglycemia is normal.[97] Whether the decreased release of growth hormone is related to reduction of stage IV sleep in the elderly is not known.[17]

Prolactin secretion. Prolactin secretion in old age shows a normal pattern of episodic secretion with a sharp rise just after sleep onset and a sharp fall during morning awakening.[17,98,99] Though older subjects wake up several times during the night and have daytime naps, these episodes are not correlated with the prolactin secretion pattern.[17]

Gonadotropins. (Follicle-stimulating hormone [FSH] and luteinizing hormone [LH]) No good studies correlate sleep changes in the elderly with gonadotropin secretion.[17]

Plasma insulin and glucose. Insulin secretion shows a clear circadian variation in healthy young adults, but there is no adequate study of aged persons.[17]

Thyroid-stimulating hormone. Plasma thyroid-stimulating hormone (TSH) shows a circadian periodicity in adults: high levels are seen just before and just after falling asleep at night.[100] There does not seem to be an adequate study about sleep-related plasma TSH rhythm in elders.[17]

Changes in the cerebral blood flow and cerebral metabolism:

Despite some inconsistent early findings,[2] there is a direct relationship between normal aging, cerebral blood flow (CBF), and cerebral metabolism. Kety,[101] using his own nitrous oxide method, showed a direct relationship between a decrease in CBF and cerebral metabolism and advancing age in normal persons. Others, however, contended that the changes were secondary to associated diseases.[102] Later, introduction of noninvasive and improved technique of xenon-133 inhalation method[103] related a clear-cut decline in the regional blood flow exclusively to advancing age, without the compounding factors of associated diseases.[104–106] This decline with advancing age was noted more in the gray than in the white matter CBF values.[102] Maximal declines were seen in the prefrontal and parietal regions and least in the frontal and frontotemporal regions.[2,102] This decline in old age seems to be related to a progressive decrease in the cerebral metabolic rate,[107,108] and possibly also to the morphologic changes in the neurons in the brains of elderly persons.[102] It should be noted, however, that the decrease of CBF during slow-wave sleep and the increase during REM sleep are similar in normal subjects of all ages.[102] In elderly sleep apnea patients, however, this decrease during slow-wave sleep becomes excessive, which, combined with hypoxemia related to apnea, places elderly persons at increasing risk for sudden death and development of stroke during sleep.[102]

Pathological CNS Changes of "Normal" Aging

Aging represents biologic maturation, which may be accompanied by a variety of pathologic changes in the CNS. The neuropathologic changes of old age can be summarized as follows[2,109]: shrinkage of the brain, alterations in the outline and loss of neurons in various locations, lipofuscin accumulation, collection of corpora amylacea, intraparenchymal vascular changes, loss of dendritic arbor and dendritic spines, presence of senile plaques and amyloid deposits, presence of neurofibrillary tangles and granulovacuolar degeneration, and Hirano bodies. The last three changes are correlated with dementia, but the others are considered nonspecific changes of aging.

From the standpoint of sleep disorders medicine, the cell loss in the locus ceruleus, pontine and midbrain reticular formation, selective hypothalamic regions and the suprachiasmatic neurons as well as accumulation of neurofibrillary tangles, and abnormal pigment in the hypothalamus are important morphologic correlates for widespread sleep disturbances in the elderly.[17] Animal experiments on suprachiasmatic nuclei show the relationship between destruction of these nuclei and alteration of circadian rhythmicity of adrenal cortical secretion, body temperature, activity-rest cycle, and sleep cycle loss.[17]

SLEEP COMPLAINTS IN OLD AGE[42a,110]

In an epidemiologic study, Ford and Kamerow[111] interviewed 7954 subjects and observed that 40% of patients with insomnia and 46.5% of those with hypersomnia had a psychiatric disorder, compared with 16% of those with no sleep complaints. Complaints of persistent insomnia are important late in life. There is a high incidence of depression with insomnia in the elderly persons. Among the 1801 elderly respondents aged 65 and older, the prevalence of insomnia was 12% and the incidence of insomnia was 7.3%.[111] For hypersomnia, the figures for prevalence and incidence were 1.6% and 1.8%, respectively. There was a strong association between persistent insomnia (longer than 1 month) and the risk of major depression. Clayton and coworkers[112] noted that in late-life spousal bereavement there is also a persistent and debilitating complaint of insomnia.

Excessive daytime somnolence (EDS) is often associated with fragmentation of nocturnal sleep, which may have been due to sleep-disordered breathing and periodic leg movements at night.[110] Other factors are changes in the circadian rhythms of temperature, alertness and sleepiness, and social time cues.[110]

Vitiello and Prinz[113] found that CNS degenerative disorders (e.g., dementia of the Alzheimer's type) may cause polyphasic sleep-wake patterns, which constitute a significant problem among old nursing home residents.[110] In demented elderly subjects, nocturnal agitation, night wandering, shouting, and incontinence contribute to a variety of sleep disturbances.[110] There are many factors in the pathogenesis of nocturnal agitation—loss of social *Zeitgebers* and loss of circadian time keeping, sleep apnea, REM-related parasomnias, low ambient light, and cold sensitivity.[114]

An important behavioral disturbance during sleep late in life is snoring.[110] According to Koskenvuo and associates,[115,116] in their study done in Finland habitual snoring was found in 9% of men and 3.6% of women aged 40 to 69 years. Hypertension, ischemic heart disease, and stroke are risk factors for snoring. In an epidemiologic survey Lugaresi and colleagues[117] found that, about 60% of men and 40% of women between age 41 and 64 years were habitual snorers.

Many other factors can disrupt sleep: nocturia, leg cramps, pain, coughing or difficulty breathing, temperature sensitivity, and dreams.[110]

What is the relationship between sleep duration and mortality in elders? In 1989, Ancoli-Israel[118] reexamined the 1979 data of Kripke and coworkers[119] and concluded that 86% of deaths associated with short (less than 7 hours) or long (more than 8 hours) sleep occurred among those older than 60 years. Thus, it could be concluded by extrapolation from these data that older persons who sleep less than 5 hours or more than 9 hours may be at greater risk for death.[110]

The high frequency of sleep complaints in aged persons may be related to the physiologic sleep changes of normal aging as well as to concomitant medical, psychiatric, neurologic, and other disorders that are very prevalent in this group. Subjective sleep complaints are common in older subjects, as many reports attest.[119–122] The subjective complaints were corroborated by objective laboratory data; however, in contrast to the increasing incidence of subjective complaints from women, elderly men had more sleep disturbances than elderly women by objective reports.[123]

CLINICAL ASSESSMENT OF SLEEP DISORDERS

Clinical assessment is discussed under four headings: (1) sleep history, (2) medical history, (3) drug history, and (4) psychiatric history. A general approach was described in Chapter 14; only the points relevant to elders are emphasized in this section.

The Sleep History

Kales and coworkers[124] developed excellent guidelines for taking an adequate sleep history:

1. The specific sleep problem should first be defined from the history. It is important with elders to understand the significance of daytime fatigue, which may result either from insomnia at night or from EDS. The latter condition can be an indirect effect of repeated arousals at night owing to sleep-related respiratory disorders, with or without periodic limb movements in sleep (PLMS). The other important factor to note is that the sleep of elders becomes polyphasic, associated with frequent daytime naps and less sleep at night. Therefore, every daytime nap is not necessarily indicative of EDS.

2. The onset and the clinical course of the condition should be assessed from the history. The course of the illness in some sleep disorders, for example night terrors, nightmares and sleep walking, are different.[125] Nightmares have a chronic course, whereas night terrors may be of recent onset. It should be noted that the relatively sudden onset of sleepwalking or night terror in an elderly person is indicative of an organic CNS disorder, and appropriate investigation should be directed toward that diagnosis.[125]

3. Inquiries should be made into a family history of a sleep disorder. Certain sleep disorders (e.g., narcolepsy, hypersomnia, sleep apnea, sleepwalking, night terrors) may have a family history.[124–126]

4. Various sleep disorders should be distinguished from one another, and any previous diagnosis should be reassessed.

5. It is important to obtain a complete 24-hour sleep-wakefulness pattern. This is important in elderly persons, because in old age the sleep cycle becomes polycyclic, rather than monophasic as in young adults. In elders, because of tendency to take frequent naps, the sleep-wake schedule becomes irregular and may cause circadian rhythm disorders.

6. It might be important to keep a sleep diary or sleep log, and of course it is very important to question the bed partner or other caregivers about sleep disturbances of elders. Keeping a sleep diary may help assess the 24-hour sleep-wake cycle pattern.

7. The bed partner or caregiver should be questioned carefully, as they may have clues to the diagnosis of sleep apnea syndrome. For example, excessively loud snoring, temporary cessation of breathing, or restless movements in the bed are important pointers to the diagnosis of sleep apnea syndrome[126] or PLMS.

8. It is essential to evaluate the impact of the sleep disorder and to determine the presence of other sleep disorders. The history may suggest a diagnosis of sleepwalking, night terror, or REM behavior disorder. A careful sleep history may also suggest nocturnal epilepsy, which is sometimes mistaken for a sleep disorder.

Medical History[127]

Elderly persons often suffer from a variety of medical disorders, such as congestive cardiac failure, hypertension, ischemic heart disease, chronic bronchopulmonary disorders, gastrointestinal disorders, arthritis and muscoloskeletal pain syndromes, cancer, chronic renal disorders, endocrinopathies, and a variety of neurologic disorders. All of these conditions may disrupt sleep by virtue of the uncomfortable symptoms or because of the medications prescribed for them. Therefore, patients often complain of insomnia, but sometimes also of hypersomnia.

Drug History[124]

It is important to obtain drug history, because many medications can cause insomnia[127]: CNS stimulants, bronchodilators, β-blockers, antihypertensives, benzodiazepines (particularly the short-acting ones), steroids, and theophylline. Withdrawal from short and intermediate acting benzodiazepines and withdrawal from nonbenzodiazepine hypnotics causes rebound insomnia. Many CNS depressants, such as hypnotics, sedatives, and antidepressants, may cause EDS. Finally, drinking coffee or cola at night may cause difficulty initiating sleep. Alcohol consumption may cause difficulty maintaining sleep.

Psychiatric History

Psychophysologic and psychiatric problems are the commonest causes of insomnia in elders.[127] They suffer from a variety of psychological and psychiatric problems, such as anxiety, depression, organic psychosis, and obsessive compulsive neurosis. A patient with depression complains of early morning awakenings, whereas a patient with obsessive compulsive neurosis has difficulty initiating sleep. Some drugs (e.g., thioridazine) may increase nightmares.[125] Marital and sexual problems may give rise to interpersonal problems that cause sleep disturbances, particularly insomnia.[127]

SLEEP DISORDERS IN OLD AGE[42a]

It is well-known that the prevalence and intensity of sleep disturbances increase with age.[127-129] Factors that affect the prevalence of sleep disturbances in the elderly are these: (a) physiologic (e.g., age-related changes in sleep patterns), (2) medical, (3) psychiatric, (4) pharmacologic (e.g., use, misuse and abuse of drugs), and (5) social (changing rest-activity schedules, and, thus, changing sleep-wake patterns.[127-131]

The prevalence of sleep-related breathing disorders, periodic limb movements in sleep, and snoring are all greater among elders. The prevalence of sleep apnea increases with age and is greater in men than in women, and in menopausal than in premenopausal women.[118] There is controversy over the exact prevalence of sleep apnea in the older population. In a study in 1971, Webb and Swinburne[132] noted that 75% of healthy volunteer men had periodic apneas. The prevalence rates for sleep apnea in elders in various studies have been estimated to range from 5.6% to 70%.[133-141] The prevalence is greater among the elderly than among younger adults,[142,143] and in men than in women.[144] There is a clear lack of consistency in study methods, so it is very difficult to generalize from these studies.[144]

Reasons for the variation in the prevalence could be sampling of different populations without using a random sampling method, small sample size, or use of different criteria to define sleep apnea.[144] An important problem has been the definition of apnea index (AI) or respiratory disturbance index (RDI).[144] RDI is equivalent to apnea-hypopnea index (AHI). Hypopnea is defined as a 50% decrease in thoracoabdominal effort for at least 10 seconds.[145] Another problem has been the clinical significance of an AI or RDI of 5. According to Ancoli-Israel,[144] an AI of 5 or more may be epidemiologically important but may not be equivalent to the diagnosis of sleep apnea syndrome. Some authors have suggested an AI of 20 or more is related to increased risk of death.[146] In the final results of a survey by Ancoli-Israel and co-workers,[133] among 427 randomly selected community-dwelling people aged 65 years and older in the city of San Diego, California, the prevalence rate of sleep-disordered breathing was 24% for AI greater than 5 and 62% for RDI greater than 10. The prevalence rate was 10% for AI greater than 10, 4% for AI greater than 20, and 1% for AI greater than 40.[133] According to He and coworkers,[146] an AI of 20 or more is related to increased mortality. Another problem has been night-to-night variation of sleep apnea.[133,147-150]

Diagnosis of Sleep Disorders in Old Age

Recognition of a variety of sleep disorders in elders is important for treatment of sleep disturbances and of the associated medical or psychiatric conditions. Some examples of sleep disorders that have been recognized in the aged population[123,151,152] are insomnia, sleep-related respiratory dysfunction with periods of apneas and hypopneas, PLMS, sleep disturbances secondary to a variety of medical or psychiatric illnesses (particularly depression in the elderly), sleep disturbances associated with dementia (particularly of the Alzheimer's type), sleep disturbances related to the abuse of alcohol and sedative-hypnotic drugs, narcolepsy, restless legs syndrome, parasomnias, and circadian rhythm sleep disorders.

Insomnia and EDS are the two most common symptoms that are noted in normal aged persons.[151] There is a high incidence of insomnia in the elderly, particularly elderly women[110,127] (see Chapter 17 for further details about insomnia).

Sleep Apnea Syndrome

For the diagnosis of sleep apnea syndrome (SAS), questioning the bed partner is very important. A history of loud snoring with periods of cessation of breathing at night accompanied by EDS and daytime fatigue suggests SAS.[153] The diagnosis is strongly suspected if the patient is also obese and hypertensive. For a definitive diagnosis, and to quantify the severity, an all-night polysomnographic (PSG) study is essential. The usual type is upper airway obstructive sleep apnea, but often it is mixed with central apnea, giving rise to mixed apnea (see Chapter 16). It is important to diagnose the condition because of possible adverse consequences[153] such as congestive cardiac failure, cardiac arrhythmias, hypertension, neuropsychological impairment,[154] increased risk of traffic accidents,[155,156] and increased mortality related to cardiovascular events.[157] Lugaresi and colleagues[117] reported a high prevalence of snoring in elderly persons, and this can be the forerunner of full-blown sleep apnea syndrome.

Nocturnal Myoclonus or Periodic Limb Movement in Sleep

PLMS is reported more often in older normal subjects than in younger ones.[158-160] According to Coleman and associates,[160] the occurrence of PLMS may be related to disturbance of circadian sleep-wake rhythm in the elderly. In the study by Kripke and coworkers,[159] 20% to 30% of subjects 65 years and older had PLMS, whereas Ancoli-Israel and colleagues[158] reported an incidence of 37% of PLMS in 24 older subjects. This is often associated with sleep apnea syndrome.

Sleep Disturbances Secondary to Medical Illness

A variety of medical disorders may be associated with insomnia—congestive cardiac failure, ischemic heart disease, arthritis and musculoskeletal pain syndrome, chronic respiratory disorder associated with bronchospasm, or dyspnea, which is often worse at night (see Chapter 17). Diabetics with autonomic neuropathy may have sleep apnea syndrome.[161] For medical disorders that cause sleep-disordered breathing, EDS, and other sleep disturbances see Chapter 22. Treatment should be directed toward the primary condition to alleviate secondary sleep disturbances.

Sleep Disturbances Secondary to Psychiatric Illness

An important psychiatric illness that causes sleep disturbances in the elderly is depression,[110,152,162-166] which should be carefully evaluated by a thorough psychiatric history. The condition is treatable; misdiagnosis and prescription of hypnotics for insomnia will lead to a vicious cycle of worsening sleep complaints. An important sleep complaint in these patients is early morning awakening, resembling advanced sleep phase syndrome.[162-164] Anxiety disorders also cause sleep disturbances,[167] and various psychotic disorders may cause both hypersomnolence and insomnia[166] (see Chapter 21).

Sleep Disturbances Secondary to Organic Brain Syndrome

Alzheimer's (AD) and related dementias in the elderly may cause sleep disturbances, including nocturnal confusional episodes (sundowning syndrome), which may require antipsychotic medication (see Chapter 20).

Sleep Disturbances Associated with Drug and Alcohol

A careful drug and alcohol history is important as elderly persons often take a variety of medications, which can include sedative-hypnotics for associated medical conditions, or they use over-the-counter drugs to promote sleep.[123,127,152] These sleeping medications produce secondary drug-related insomnia. Alcohol worsens sleep disturbances and may exacerbate existing sleep apnea syndrome.

Narcolepsy

Narcolepsy is a disease of earlier onset, and the diagnosis would probably have been made much earlier, but it is a lifelong condition. The diagnosis rests on a history of sudden sleep attacks lasting a short time and associated with auxiliary symptoms such as cataplexy, hypnagogic hallucinations, and sleep paralysis. A history of narcoleptic sleep attacks and cataplexy may be sufficient for diagnosis, but for final confirmation an all-night PSG study, followed by the Multiple Sleep Latency Test (MSLT), which will show reduced sleep-onset latency and sleep-onset REM in two out of five recordings will be needed.

Restless Legs Syndrome (see Chapter 19)

Restless legs syndrome is primarily a lifelong condition, though it may be secondary to diabetic or uremic peripheral neuropathy. In addition to the characteristic restless movements during the daytime, nighttime sleep is severely disturbed. The prevalence increases with age, and the symptoms may occur initially in old age.

Parasomnias (see Chapter 24)

The important parasomnias in elderly people are the REM sleep behavior disorder, sleepwalking, and night terrors. The latter two conditions usually present in childhood or adolescence, but if they have a relatively sudden onset in an elderly person an acute neurologic condition should be suspected and excluded by appropriate laboratory investigations.[168,169] REM sleep behavior disorder can be suspected from the history given by the bed partner and by simultaneous video polygraphic evaluation at night.

Disorders of Circadian Function

Morgan and associates[170] reported that occasional sleep complaints are noted by 40% of older persons, and according to Garma and colleagues[171] older persons complain of frequent and prolonged awakenings during the night. It has been speculated by Czeisler and coworkers[172] that these disorders may be due to changes in the human circadian pacemaker with advancing age. Recent work with light by Czeisler and colleagues[173,174] showed that, with appropriately timed exposure to bright light, one can change the temperature cycle—that is, circadian phase—and may be able to correct the circadian sleep disorder. Further research is obviously needed.

In 1962, McGhie and Russell[121] reported that 15% of older persons complained of early morning awakenings, and in 1988 Mant and Eyland[175] reported that 33% of elderly persons woke up early in the morning several times a week. Sleep parameters thus show an advanced phase, which is also noted with other circadian rhythms such as activity rhythm, body temperature rhythm, and timing of REM sleep and the cortisol rhythm.[172] An advance in the circadian phase due to a reduction of the endogenous period of the circadian pacemaker with advancing age is suggested by animal experiments.[176,177] Human data for such studies are lacking, but a cross-sectional study by Weitzman's group[178] documented that the free-running period of the temperature rhythm was significantly shorter in six subjects aged 53 to 60 years than in six healthy young adults. Recent study by Czeisler and colleagues[173] suggested a strong relationship between period reduction and phase advance in the circadian rhythms of older people.

The pathophysiologic mechanism of these changes remains speculative. In 1972,[179,180] a cluster of neurons was discovered in the anterior tip of the hypothalamus on either side of the third ventricle (suprachiasmatic nucleus, SCN). This is the circadian pacemaker. With advancing age the volume of SCN cells shrinks; that is, the number of neurons decreases,[181–183] which may produce functional impairment.

LABORATORY ASSESSMENT

Indications for Diagnostic Evaluation

The diagnostic evaluation should begin with a thorough history of sleep disturbances, which may be EDS, difficulty initiating or maintaining sleep, and intrusions of unusual behavior during sleep. Physical examination may direct attention to appropriate systemic disease. Based on the history and findings of physical examination, a decision should be made regarding referrals to specialized sleep centers for PSG and MSLT studies. Tests should be performed when clinical interview and examination cannot resolve the problems.

Most of the sleep disturbances of elders can be diagnosed by a careful history and physical examination. For some conditions, however, laboratory assessment is important. In sleep apnea syndrome it is important to have an all-night PSG study to determine the severity of and quantify sleep-related respiratory disturbances. Sleep apnea is a treatable condition, so it is important to make this diagnosis correctly. Also, MSLT and PSG studies are important for narcolepsy diagnosis, though in elderly people this diagnosis may have been made many years earlier. All-night video recordings are necessary for some conditions, such as REM behavior disorder and to differentiate from other sleep disorders, such as night terror or partial complex seizures. Finally, appropriate tests should be performed if other medical or neurologic disorders are suspected.

TREATMENT

The objective of treatment is to reduce the risk of mortality and morbidity and improve the quality of life.[184] The first step is accurate assessment and diagnosis.

Indications for Treatment of Obstructive Sleep Apnea

Indications are reviewed briefly here; details are in Chapters 16 and 28. Obstructive sleep apnea is a very important and major cause of hypersomnia in elders, and it is often a reversible condition if appropriately diagnosed and treated. For moderate to severe obstructive sleep apnea treatment is recommended. PSG and MSLT studies should be able to decide the severity when findings are considered with the RDI, the degree of oxygen saturation, and abnormally short sleep latency. Before instituting any specific treatment certain general measures, such as weight loss, avoidance of alcohol, sedatives and hypnotics, avoidance of the supine sleep position, and management of nasopharyngeal disorders are recommended. The majority of patients respond to continuous positive airway pressure (CPAP) treatment. When all measures, including CPAP, fail, surgical measures such as uvulopalatopharyngoplasty (UPP) may be appropriate, particularly if the site of obstruction is in the pharyngeal region. The success rate of UPP is variable, but tracheostomy, which is modified to keep it closed during the day and open at night relieves symptoms of most elderly patients. Major criteria for recommending tracheostomy[185] include severe daytime symptoms that interfere with function, severe hypertension or dangerous cardiac arrhythmias, and the laboratory criteria of an AI of 20 or greater or a decrease in oxygen saturation of more than 10% below average baseline values.

Indications for Treatment of Insomnia (See Chapter 17)

Multiple factors are responsible for insomnia in elders, and, therefore, evaluation and treatment of insomnia should be multidisciplinary.[125,127] Elimination or avoidance of factors that are causing insomnia is the first step in treatment. The next important general measure is paying attention to sleep hygiene.

Insomnia is a very common complaint in the elderly and may be the result of a variety of medical or psychiatric conditions. Insomnia may also result from PLMS, or occasionally from sleep apnea. An important cause is related to the pharmacologic agents (drugs, alcohol), so a careful history and physical examination are important before any treatment is instituted.

PLMS is an important condition in elders, but its incidence and natural history are unknown. Even the relationship between PLMS and insomnia is not clear. Therefore, any pharmacologic treatment for PLMS is subject to controversy, and we also do not know the long-term effect of drug treatment on patients' health. In selected cases where PLMS clearly disrupts sleep therapy may be indicated.

Circadian rhythm disorder, another important cause of insomnia, results from changes in the daily routine or changes in sleep pattern, shift work, or transmeridian travel. Therefore, environmental control and adequate counseling should be the first line of treatment.

When a medial and psychiatric condition causes insomnia, appropriate treatment should be directed toward the primary conditions. In case of depression, appropriate treatment with the tricyclic antidepressants, often those with sedative effect, could be used to advantage.

Medical conditions, such as cardiac failure, hyperthyroidism, respiratory disorders, arthritis and other painful conditions, and esophageal reflux syndrome should be treated appropriately. It should, however, be remembered that medications (theophylline, steroids) themselves may cause sleep disturbance.

For transient or temporary disturbances of sleep, short-term intermittent use of hypnotics and sedative tricyclics may be useful. Long-term use of hypnotics is not indicated. The drug of choice for insomnia in the elderly is a benzodiazepine (see Chapter 17). An intermediate-acting benzodiazepine (e.g., flurazepam, temazepam) in a dose of 15 mg at bedtime is effective as a short-term treatment that produces minimal daytime sedation.[186] A short-acting benzodiazepine (e.g., triazolam) is used with success for short-term treatment.[186] Limiting side effects include behavior disturbances (e.g., confusion, delirium, amnesia), rebound insomnia, and rebound anxiety. These side effects have triggered recent controversy that necessitated suspension of the drug in the United Kingdom and restriction of its use by the United States Food and Drug Administration.

Special Pharmacologic Considerations[152,186]

Vestal and Dawson[187] directed attention to the important factors of alterations of drug metabolism, with its attendant changes in pharmacokinetics in the elderly. It is important to start with a dose smaller than younger subjects require and then gradually to increase the dose, depending on the response. It is also extremely important to obtain a drug history, to prevent drug-drug interactions and exacerbation of sleep disturbances by hypnotics or other agents.

Situational and Life-Style Considerations[152]

Life-style factors are different for elders. Retirement, with disturbance of the sleep-wake schedule (e.g., napping in the daytime and consequent inability to sleep at the scheduled night time), "empty nest syndrome" with children leaving home, bereavement, death of a spouse or close friend, all may lead to loneliness and depression with attendant sleep disturbances. Other causes of sleep disturbances in the elderly include institutionalization, prolonged bed rest, poor sleep hygiene, unsatisfactory bed environment, poor diet habits, and caffeine and alcohol consumption.

Treatment of Sleep Cycle Changes Related to Age

The treatment is to educate the patient about sleep disruptions in old age, discourage multiple naps, and urge participation in special interests and other activities and hobbies.[168] Future research may determine the role of appropriately timed exposure to bright light in treating circadian rhythm sleep disorders in elders.[173,174]

Treatment of Situational Stress

Patients should be given supportive psychotherapy and behavior modification treatment as well as clear explanations, to reduce stress and sleeplessness.[168]

Treatment of Nocturnal Confusional Episodes[188]

Nocturnal confusional episodes are characterized by disorientation, agitation, and wandering at night and often result from acute or chronic organic neurologic dysfunction (see Chapter 20).[168,188] Relatively sudden onset of night terror or sleepwalking indicates an organic brain disorder, and an appropriate investigation should be obtained. This can also be precipitated by other associated medical illnesses. The treatment should be directed toward the precipitating or causal factors for these confusional episodes. Often episodes are precipitated when the patient is transferred from home to an institution. As much as possible, the home environment should be preserved. The darkness of night often precipitates episodes, so a night light is helpful. A careful drug history should be obtained, and gradually medications that are not really needed should be reduced and eliminated. The use of barbiturates or hypnotics may further aggravate the condition. The treatment of choice is high-potency antipsychotics, such as haloperidol and thiothixine, in small doses.[152,188]

Treatment of Medication-Induced Sleep-Wakefulness Disturbances[168]

Some medications cause insomnia while others cause EDS. Elderly persons often take a variety of medications because of the increased prevalence of other illnesses. Furthermore, because of their altered metabolism they are susceptible to the side effects of various medications. The patient should avoid alcohol, caffeine, and cigarettes, and should gradually eliminate drugs that are not essential.

Special environmental considerations

Treatment should be designed and tailored to different environmental situations (e.g., nursing home, hospital, home), as different types of sleep disturbances have been noted in different environments.[42]

REFERENCES

1. Monjan AA. Sleep disorders of older people: Report of a Consensus Conference. Hosp Commun Psychiatry 1990;41:743–744.
2. Katzman R, Terry R. Normal aging of the nervous system. In: Katzman R, Terry R, eds. The Neurology of Aging. Philadelphia: FA Davis, 1983;15–50.
3. Jorgensen L, Torvik A. Ischaemic cerebrovascular diseases in an autopsy series. Part I. Prevalence, location, and predisposing factors in verified thrombo-embolic occlusions, and their significance in the pathogenesis of cerebral infarction. J Neurol Sci 1966;3:490.
4. Wechsler D, ed. Manual for the Wechsler Adult Intelligence Scale. New York: The Psychological Corporation, 1955;75.
5. Wechsler D, ed. The Measurement and Appraisal of Adult Intelligence, ed 4. Baltimore: Williams & Wilkins, 1958;297.
6. Green RF. Age-intelligence relationship between ages sixteen and sixty-four: A rising trend. Develop Psychol 1969;1:618.
7. Schaie KW, Labouvie-Vief G. Generational versus ontogenetic components of change in adult cognitive behavior: A fourteen-year cross-sequential study. Develop Psychol 1974;10:305.
8. Schaie KW, Labouvie GV, Buech BU. Generational- and cohort-specific differences in adult cognitive functioning: A fourteen-year study of independent samples. Develop Psychol 1973;9:151.
9. Birren JE. Age changes in speed of behavior: Its central nature and physiological correlates. In: Welford AT, Birren JE, eds. Behavior, Aging and The Nervous System. Springfield, Ill: Charles C Thomas, 1963;191.
10. Birren JE. Translations in gerontology—from lab to life. Psychophysiology and speed of response. Am Psychol 1974;29:808.
11. Birren JE, Woods AM, Williams MV. Speed of behavior as an indicator of age changes and the integrity of the nervous system. In: Hoffmeister F, Muller C, eds. Brain Function in Old Age. Berlin: Springer-Verlag, 1979;10.
12. Welford At. Motor performance. In: Birren JE, Schaie KW, eds. Handbook of the Psychology of Aging. New York: Van Nostrand Reinhold, 1977;450.
13. Welford AT: Sensory, perceptual, and motor processes in older adults. In: Birren JE, Sloane RB, eds. Handbook of Mental Health and Aging. Englewood Cliffs, N.J.: Prentice-Hall, 1980;192.
14. Critchley M. The neurology of old age. Lancet 1931;i:1119, 1221, 1331.
15. Potvin AR, Syndulko K, Tourellotte WW, et al. Human neurologic function and the aging process. J Am Geriatr Soc 1980;28:1.

16. Potvin AR, Syndulko K, Tourellotte W, et al. Quantitative evaluation of normal age related changes in neurologic function. In: Pirozzolo FJ, Maletta GJ, eds. Advances in Neurogerontology, vol 2. New York: Praeger, 1981;13–57.
17. Weitzman ED. Sleep and aging. In: Katzman R, Terry RD, eds. The Neurology of Aging. Philadelphia: FA Davis, 1983;167–188.
17a. Low PA. The effect of aging on the autonomic nervous system. In: Low PA, ed. Clinical Autonomic Disorders. Boston: Little, Brown, 1993;685–700.
18. Hazzard WR, Bierman EL. Old Age. In: Smith D, Bierman EL, eds. Biological Ages of Man from Conception Through Old Age, ed 2. Philadelphia: WB Saunders, 1978;229.
19. Cowley M: The View from 80. New York: Viking Press, 1976;1.
20. Rowe JW, Troen BR. Sympathetic nervous system and aging in man. Endocr Rev 1980,1:167.
21. Blass JP, Plum F. Metabolic encephalopathies in older adults. In: Katzman R, Terry RD, eds. The Neurology of Aging. Philadelphia: FA Davis, 1983;189–220.
22. Katz RI, Horowitz GR. The septuagenarian EEG: Normative EEG studies in a selected normal ambulatory geriatric population [Abstr]. Electroencephalogr Clin Neurophysiol 1981;51:35p–36p.
23. Torres A, Faoro A, Loewenson R, et al. The electroencephalogram of elderly subjects revisited. Electroencephalogr Clin Neurophysiol 1983;56:391–398.
24. Obrist WD. Problems of aging. In: Remond A, ed. Handbook of Electroencephalography and Clinical Neurophysiology, vol 6A. Amsterdam: Elsevier, 1976;275–292.
25. Obrist WD, Henry CE, Justiss WA. Longitudinal changes in the senescent EEG: A 15-year study. In: Proceedings of the 7th International Congress of Gerontology. Vienna: International Association of Gerontology, 1966;35–38.
26. Matejcek M. The EEG of the aging brain. A spectral analytic study [Abstr]. Electroencephalogr Clin Neurophysiol 1981;51:51p–52p.
27. Nakano T, Miyasaka M, Ohtaka T, et al. A follow up study of automatic EEG analysis and the mental deterioration in the age [Abstr]. Electroencephalogr Clin Neurophysiol 1982;54:27.
28. Duffy FH, Albert MS, McAnulty TG, et al. Age-related differences in brain electrical activity of healthy subjects. Ann Neurol 1984;16:430–438.
29. Oken BS, Kaye JA. Electrophysiologic function in the healthy, extremely old. Neurology 1992;42:519–526.
30. Niedermeyer E. EEG and old age. In: Niedermeyer E, Lopes da Silva F, eds. Electroencephalography. Baltimore: Urban & Schwarzenberg, 1987;301–308.
31. Kelley J, Reilly P, Bellar S. Photic driving and psychogeriatric diagnosis. Clin Electroencephalogr 1983;14:78–81.
32. Busse EW, Obrist WD. Pre-senescent electroencephalographic changes in normal subjects. J Gerontol 1965;20:315–320.
33. Kugler J. Fast EEG activity in normal people of advanced age [Abstr]. Electroencephalogr Clin Neurophysiol 1983;56:67.

34. Arenas AM, Brennar RP, Reynolds CF III. Temporal slowing in the elderly revisited. Am J EEG Technol 1986;26:105–114.

35. Katz RI, Horowitz GR. Electroencephalogram in the septuagenarian: Studies in a normal geriatric population. J Am Geriatr Soc 1982;3:273–275.

36. Hughes JR, Cayafa JJ. The EEG in patients at different ages without organic cerebral disease. Electroencephalogr Clin Neurophysiol 1977;42:776–784.

37. Visser SL, Hooijer C, Jonker C, et al. Anterior temporal focal abnormalities in EEG in normal aged subjects: Correlations with psychopathological and CT brain scan findings. Electroencephalogr Clin Neurophysiol 1987;66:1–7.

38. Gibbs FA, Gibbs EL. Atlas of Electroencephalography, ed 2. Reading, Mass.: Addison-Wesley, 1964:3.

39. Katz RI, Horowitz GR. Sleep-onset frontal rhythmic slowing in a normal geriatric population [Abstr]. Electroencephalogr Clin Neurophysiol 1983;56:27.

40. Libow LS, Obrist WD, Sokoloff L. Cerebral circulatory and electroencephalographic changes in elderly men. In: Granick S, Patterson RD, eds. Human Aging, II. DHEW Publication (HSM) 71-9037, 1971. Rockville, Md: US Department of Health, Education and Welfare.

41. Obrist WD, Sokoloff L, Lassen NA, et al. Relation of EEG to cerebral blood flow and metabolism in old age. Electroencephalogr Clin Neurophysiol 1963;15:610.

42. Miles LE, Dement WC. Sleep and aging. Sleep 1980;3:119–220.

42a. Bliwise DL. Sleep in normal aging and dementia: Review. Sleep 1993;16:40–81.

43. Liberson WT. Functional electroencephalography in mental disorders. Dis Nerv Syst 1945;5:357–364.

44. Feinberg I. Functional implications of changes in sleep physiology with age. In: Terry RD, Gershon S, eds. Neurology of Aging. New York: Raven Press, 1976;23.

45. Feinberg I, Koresko R, Heller N. EEG sleep patterns as a function of normal and pathological aging in man. J Psychiatr Res 1967;5:107–144.

46. Rechtschaffen A, Kales A. A Manual of Standardized Terminology: Techniques and Scoring Stages of Human Subjects. Los Angeles: UCLA Brain Information Service/Brain Research Institute, 1968.

47. Feinberg I, Hibi S, Carlson V. Changes in EEG amplitude during sleep with age. In: Nandy K, Sherwin I, eds. The Aging Brain and Senile Dementia, vol 23. New York: Plenum, 1977;85.

48. Feinberg I. Effects of age on human sleep patterns. In: Kales A, ed. Sleep Physiology and Pathology: A Symposium. Philadelphia: JB Lippincott, 1969;39.

49. Williams R, Karacan I, Hursch C, eds. Electroencephalography of Human Sleep: Clinical Applications. New York: John Wiley & Sons, 1977;49.

50. Kahn E, Fisher C. The sleep characteristics of the normal aged male. J Nerv Ment Dis 1969;148:477.

51. Feinberg I: Changes in sleep cycle patterns with age. J Psychiatr Res 1974;10:283.

52. Brezinova V. Sleep cycle content and sleep cycle durations. Electroencephalogr Clin Neurophysiol 1974;36:275.

53. Kales A, Wilson T, Kales J. Measurements of all night sleep in normal elderly persons. J Am Geriatr Soc 1967;15:405.

54. Tune GS. Sleep and wakefulness in 509 normal human adults. Br J Med Psychol 1969;42:75.

55. Tune GS. The influence of age and temperament on the adult human sleep-wakefulness pattern. Br J Psychol 1969;60:431.

56. Carskadon M, Brown E, Dement W. Sleep fragmentation in the elderly: Relationship to daytime sleep tendency. Neurobiol Aging 1982;3:321–327.

57. Carskadon MA, Dement WC. Sleep loss in elderly volunteers. Sleep 1985;8:207–221.

58. Kales A, Kales J, Jacobson A, et al. All night EEG studies: Children and elderly. Electroencephalogr Clin Neurophysiol 1966;21:415–420.

59. Williams DE, Vitiello MV, Ries RK, et al. Successful recruitment of elderly, community dwelling subjects for Alzheimer's disease research: Cognitively impaired, major depressive disorder, and normal control groups. J Gerontol 1988;43:69–74.

60. Prinz P, Halter J. Sleep disturbances in the elderly: Neurohormonal correlates. In: Chase M, Weitzman E, eds. Sleep Disorders: Basic and Clinical Research, Advances in Sleep Research, vol 8. New York: SP Medical and Scientific, 1983;463–488.

61. Prinz PN, Vitiello M. Sleep in Alzheimer's dementia and in healthy not-complaining seniors. In: Program and Abstracts of NIH Consensus Development Conference on The Treatment of Sleep Disorders in Older People. Bethesda, Md.: National Institutes of Health, 1990;41–42.

62. Cashman MA, Prinz PN, Personius J, et al. Nighttime hypoxemia events in patient groups and in controls. Sleep Res 1989;18:329.

63. Pittendrigh C, Daan S. Circadian oscillations in rodents: A systematic increase of their frequency with age. Science 1974;186:548.

64. Wax T. Effects of age, strain, and illumination intensity on activity and self-selection of light-dark, schedules in mice. J Comp Physiol Psychol 1977;91:51.

65. Wax T. Runwheel activity patterns of mature-young and senescent mice: The effect of constant lighting conditions. J Gerontol 1975;30:22.

66. Samis H. 24-H rhythmic variations in white blood cell counts of the rat with advancing age. Chronobiologia 1977;4:147.

67. Wessler R, Rubin M, Sollberger A. Circadian rhythm of activity and sleep-wakefulness in elderly institutionalized persons. J Interdiscpl Cycle Res 1976;7:333.

68. Scheving L, Roig C, Halberg F, et al. Circadian variations in residents of a "senior citizens" home. In: Scheving L, Halberg F, Pauly J, eds. Chronobiology. Proceedings of the International Society for the Study of Biological Rhythms, Little Rock, Ark. Tokyo: Igaku Shoin, 1974;353.

69. Ibuka N, Kawamura H. Loss of circadian rhythm in sleep-wakefulness cycle in the rat by suprachiasmatic nucleus lesions. Brain Res 1975;96:76.

70. Moore R, Eichler V. Loss of a circadian adrenal corticosterone rhythm following suprachiasmatic lesions in the rat. Brain Res 1972;42:201.

71. Mouret J, Coindet J, Debilly G, et al. Suprachiasmatic nuclei lesions in the rat: Alterations in sleep circadian rhythms. Electroencephalogr Clin Neurophysiol 1978;45:402.

72. Nagai K, Nishio T, Nakagawa H, et al. Effect of bilateral lesions of the suprachiasmatic nuclei on the circadian rhythm of food intake. Brain Res 1978; 142:384.

73. Vitiello MV, Smallwood RG, Avery DH, et al. Circadian temperature rhythms in young and aged men. Neurobiol Aging 1986;72:97–100.

74. Weitzman ED, Molin ML, Czeisler CA, et al. Chronobiology of aging: Temperature, sleep/wake rhythms and entrainment. Neurobiol Aging 1982;3:299–309.

75. Fennell W, Moore R. Responses of aged men to passive heating [Abstr]. J Appl Physiol 1973;231:118.

76. Foster K, Ellis F, Dore C, et al. Sweat responses in the aged. Age Aging 1976;91:91.

77. Fox R, Woodward P, Fry A, et al. Diagnosis of accidental hypothermia of the elderly. Lancet 1971;1:424.

78. Taylor G. The problem of hypothermia in the elderly. Practitioner 1964;193:761.

79. Wollner L, Spalding J. The autonomic nervous system. In: Brockelhurst J, ed. Textbook of Geriatric Medicine and Gerontology. Edinburgh: Churchill-Livingstone, 1973;235.

80. Friedfield L. Heat reaction states in the aged. Geriatrics 1949;4:211.

81. Oechsli F, Buechley R. Excess mortality associated with three Los Angeles September hot spells. Environ Res 1970;3:277.

82. Snyder F, Hobson J, Morrison D, et al. Changes in respiration, heart rate and systolic blood pressure in human sleep. J Appl Physiol 1964;19:417.

83. Klocke R. Influence of aging on the lung. In: Finch C, Hayflick L, eds. Handbook of the Biology of Aging. New York: Van Nostrand Reinhold, 1977;4232.

84. Lugaresi E, Coccaagna C, Parneti P, et al. Snoring. Electroencephalogr Clin Neurophysiol 1975;39:59.

85. Orem J. Breathing during sleep. In: Davies DG, Barnes CD, eds. Regulation of Ventilation and Gas Exchange. New York: Academic Press, 1978;131.

86. Webb P. Periodic breathing during sleep. J Appl Physiol 1974;37:899.

87. Coccagna G, Lugaresi E. Arterial blood gases and pulmonary and systemic arterial pressure during sleep in chronic obstructive pulmonary disease. Sleep 1978;1:117.

88. Wynne J, Block A, Flick M. Disordered breathing and oxygen desaturation during daytime naps. Johns Hopkins Med J 1978;143:3.

89. Karacan I, Hursch C, Williams R. Some characteristics of nocturnal penile tumescence in elderly males. J Gerontol 1972;27:39.

90. Kahn E, Fisher C. REM sleep and sexuality in the aged. J Geriatr Psychiatry 1969;2:181.

91. Colucci CF, D'Alessandro B, Bellastella A, et al. Circadian rhythm of plasma cortisol in the aged (Cosinor method). Gerontologia Clinica (Basel) 1976;17:89.

92. Silverberg A, Rizzo F, Krieger DT, et al. Nycterohemeral periodicity of plasma 17:OHCS levels in elderly subject. J Clin Endocrinol Metab 1968;28:1661.

93. Carroll B, Curtis G, Mendels J. Neuroendocrine regulation in depression. Arch Gen Psychiatry 1976;33: 1039; 1051.

94. Sachar E. Twenty-four hour cortisol secretory patterns in depressed and manic patients. In: Gispen W, van Wimersma Greidanus B, Bohus B, et al., eds. Progress in Brain Research—Hormones, Homeostasis and the Brain, vol 42. Amsterdam: Elsevier, 1975;81.

95. Vidalon C, Khurana C, Chae S, et al. Age related changes in growth hormone in non-diabetic women. J Am Geriatr Soc 1973;21:253.

96. Bazzarre T, Johanson A, Huseman C, et al. Human growth hormone changes with age. Excerpta Medica ICS 1976;381:261.

97. Calderon L, Ryan N, Kovacs K. Human pituitary growth hormone cells in old age. Gerontology 1978;24:441.

98. Sassin J, Frantz A, Kapen S, et al. The nocturnal rise of human prolactin is dependent on sleep. In: Chase MH, Stern WC, Walter PL, eds. Sleep Research, vol 2. Los Angeles: Brain Research Institute, 1973;199.

99. Sassin J, Frantz A, Weitzman E, et al. Human prolactin: 24-hour pattern with increased release during sleep. Science 1972;177:1205.

100. Weitzman ED. Circadian rhythms and episodic hormone secretion in man. Ann Rev Med 1976;27:225.

101. Kety SS. Human cerebral blood flow and oxygen consumption as related to aging. J Chron Dis 1956;8:478–486.

102. Meyer JS. Cerebral blood flow in aging. AAN Course #142. Minneapolis, Minn.: American Academy of Neurology, 1992;65–91.

103. Meyer JS. Improved method for non-invasive measurement for regional cerebral blood flow by ^{133}xenon inhalation. Part II: Measurements in health and disease. Stroke 1978;9:205–210.

104. Naritomi H, Meyer JS, Sakai F, et al. Effects of advancing age on regional cerebral blood flow. Studies in normal subjects and subjects with risk factors for atherothrombotic stroke. Arch Neurol 1979;36:410–416.

105. Malamed E, Lavy S, Bentin S, et al. Reduction in regional cerebral blood flow during normal aging in man. Stroke 1980;11:31–35.

106. Imai A, Meyer JS, Kobari M, et al. LCBF values decline while Lk values increase during normal human aging measured by stable xenon enhanced computed tomography. Neuroradiology 1988;30:463–472.

107. Pantano P, Baron JC, Lebrun-Grandie P, et al. Regional cerebral blood flow and oxygen consumption in human aging. Stroke 1984;15:635–641.

108. Sokoloff L. Effects of normal aging on cerebral circulation and energy metabolism. In: Hoffmeister F, Muller C, eds. Brain Function in Old Age. New York: Springer Verlag, 1979;367–380.

109. Foncin JF. Classical and ultrastructural neuropathology of aging processes in the human: A critical review [Abstr]. Electroencephalogr Clin Neurophysiol 1981; 52:30.

110. Reynolds CF III. Subjective and objective sleep complaints in late life. In: Program and Abstracts of NIH Consensus Development Conference on The Treatment

of Sleep Disorders of Older People. Bethesda, Md.: National Institutes of Health, 1990;21–24.

111. Ford DE, Kamerow DB. Epidemiological studies of sleep disturbances and psychiatric disorders: An opportunity for prevention. JAMA 1979;262(1):1479–1484.

112. Clayton PJ, Halikas JA, Mauria WL. The depression of widowhood. Br J Psychiatry 1972;120:71–78.

113. Vitiello MV, Prinz PN. Alzheimer's disease: Sleep and sleep/wake patterns. Clin Geriatr Med 1989;5:289–300.

114. Reynolds CF, Hoch CC, Monk TH. Sleep and chronobiologic disturbances in late life. In: Busse EW, Blazer DG, eds. Geriatric Psychiatry. Washington, D.C.: American Psychiatric Press, 1989;475–488.

115. Koskenvuo M, Kaprio J, Partinen M, et al. Snoring as a risk factor for hypertension and angina pectoris. Lancet 1985;1:893–896.

116. Koskenvuo M, Kaprio J, Telaviki T, et al. Snoring as a risk factor for ischemic heart disease and stroke in men. Br Med J 1987;294:16–19.

117. Lugaresi E, Cirignotta F, Coccagna G, et al. Some epidemiological data on snoring and cardiocirculatory disturbances. Sleep 1980;3:221–224.

118. Ancoli-Israel S. Epidemiology of sleep disorders. Clin Geriatr Med 1989;5:347–362.

119. Kripke DF, Simons RN, Garfinkel L, et al. Short and long sleep and sleeping pills: Is increased mortality associated? Arch Gen Psychiatry 1979;36:103–116.

120. Karacan I, Thornby J, Anch M, et al. Prevalence of sleep disturbance in a primarily urban Florida county. Social Sci Med 1976;10:239.

121. McGhie A, Russell S. The subjective assessment of normal sleep patterns. J Ment Sci 1962;108:642–654.

122. Thornby J, Karacan I, Searle R, et al. Subjective reports of sleep disturbance in a Houston metropolitan health survey. In: Chase MH, Mitler MM, Walter PL, eds: Sleep Research, vol 6. Los Angeles: BIS/BRI, 1977;181.

123. Vitiello MV, Prinz PN. Aging and sleep disorders. In: Williams RL, Karacan I, Moore CA, eds. New York: John Wiley & Sons, 1988;293–312.

124. Kales A, Soldatos CR, Kales JD. Taking a sleep history. Am Fam Physician 1980;22:101–108.

125. Kales A, Soldatos Cr, Kales JD. Sleep disorders: Insomnia, sleep-walking, night terrors, nightmares, and enuresis. Ann Intern Med 1987;106:582–592.

126. Kales A, Vela-Bueno A, Kales JD. Sleep disorders: Sleep apnea and narcolepsy. Ann Intern Med 1987; 106:434–443.

127. Kales A, Kales JD. Evaluation and Treatment of Insomnia. New York: Oxford University Press, 1984.

128. Bixler EO, Kales A, Soldatos CR, et al. Prevalence of sleep disorders in the Los Angeles metropolitan area. Am J Psychiatry 1979;136:1257–1262.

129. Dement WC, Miles LE, Carskadon MA. "White paper" on sleep and aging. J Am Geriatr Soc 1982;30:25–50.

130. Cadieux RJ, Voolley D, Kales JD. Sleep disorders in the elderly. In: Berlin RM, Soldatos CR, eds. Psychiatric Medicine. Sleep Disorders in Psychiatric Practice, 1986.

131. Prinz PN. Sleep patterns in the healthy aged: Relationship with intellectual function. J Gerontol 1977; 32:179–186.

132. Webb W, Swinburne H. An observational study of sleep in the aged. Percept Mot Skills 1971;32:895–898.

133. Ancoli-Israel S, Kripke DF, Klauber MR, et al. Sleep-disordered breathing in community-dwelling elderly. Sleep 1991;14:486–495.

134. Coleman RM, Miles LE, Guilleminault CC, et al. Sleep-wake disorders in the elderly: A polysomnographic analysis. J Am Geriatr Soc 1981;29:289–296.

135. Hoch CC, Reynolds CF III, Kupfer DJ, et al. Sleep-disordered breathing in normal and pathologic aging. J Clin Psychiatry 1986;47:499–503.

136. Krieger J, Mangin P, Kurtz D. Respiration changes during sleep in healthy elderly subjects (French). Rev EEG Neurophysiol 1980;10:177–185.

137. McGinty DJ, Littner M, Beahm E, et al. Sleep-related breathing disorders in older men: A search for underlying mechanisms. Neurobiol Aging 1982;3:337–350.

138. Roehrs T, Zorick F, Sicklesteel J, et al. Age-related sleep-wake disorders at a sleep disorder center. J Am Geriatr Soc 1983;31:364–370.

139. Smallwood RG, Vitiello MV, Giblin EC, et al. Sleep apnea: Relationship to age, sex, and Alzheimer's dementia. Sleep 1983;6:16–22.

140. Kreis P, Kripke DF, Ancoli-Israel S. Sleep apnea: A prospective study. West J Med 1983;139:171–173.

141. Ancoli-Israel S. Epidemiology of sleep disorders. Clin Geriatr Med 1989;5:347–362.

142. Block AJ, Boysen PG, Wynne JW, et al. Sleep apnea, hypopnea and oxygen desaturation in normal subjects. A strong male predominance. N Engl J Med 1979;300:513–517.

143. Bixler EO, Kales A, Soldatos CR, et al. Sleep apneic activity in a normal population. Res Commun Chem Pathol Pharmacol 1982;36:141–152.

144. Ancoli-Israel S. Critical review of epidemiological studies on sleep apnea. Program and Abstracts of NIH Consensus Development Conference on The Treatment of Sleep Disorders of Older People. National Institute of Health, Bethesda, Md.: 1990;47–49.

145. Gould GA, Whyte KF, Rhind GB, et al. The sleep hypopnea syndrome. Am Rev Respir Dis 1988;137:895–898.

146. He J, Kryger MH, Zorick FJ, et al. Mortality and apnea index in obstructive sleep apnea: Experience in 385 male patients. Chest 1988;94:9–14.

147. Bliwise DL, Benkert RE, Ingham RH. Factors associated with nightly variability in sleep-disordered breathing in the elderly. Chest 1991;100:973–976.

148. Mason WJ, Ancoli-Israel S, Kripke DF. Apnea revisited: A longitudinal follow-up. Sleep 1989;12:423–429.

149. Mosko SS, Dickel MJ, Ashurst J. Night-to-night variability in sleep apnea and sleep in sleep-related periodic leg movements in the elderly. Sleep 1988;11:340–348.

150. Wittig RM, Romaker A, Zorick E, et al. Night to night consistency of apneas during sleep. Am Rev Respir Dis 1984;129:244–246.

151. Prinz PN, Vitiello MV, Raskind MA, et al. Geriatrics: Sleep disorders and aging. N Engl J Med 1990;323:520–526.

152. Vitiello MV, Prinz PN. Sleep and sleep disorders in normal aging. In: Thorpy MJ, ed. Handbook of Sleep Disorders. New York: Marcel Dekker, 1990,139–151.

153. Guilleminault C, Dement WC. Sleep apnea syndromes and related sleep disorders. In: Williams RL, Karacan I, Moore CA, eds. Sleep Disorders: Diagnosis and Treatment, ed 2. New York: John Wiley & Sons, 1988;47–71.

154. Bliwise DL. Neuropsychological function and sleep. Clin Geriatr Med 1989;5:381–394.

155. Aldrich MS. Automobile accidents in patients with sleep disorders. Sleep 1989;12:487–494.

156. Findley LJ, Fabrizio M, Thommi G, et al. Severity of sleep apnea and automobile crashes. N Engl J Med 1989;320:868–869.

157. Ancoli-Israel S, Klauber MR, Kripke DF, et al. Sleep apnea in female patients in a nursing home: Increased risk of mortality. Chest 1989;96:1054–1058.

158. Ancoli-Israel S, Kripke DR, Mason W, et al. Sleep apnea and nocturnal myoclonus in a senior population. Sleep 1981;4:349–358.

159. Kripke DF, Ancoli-Israel S, Okudaira N. Sleep apnea and nocturnal myoclonus in the elderly. Neurobiol Aging 1982;3:329–336.

160. Coleman RM, Pollak CP, Weitzman ED. Periodic movements in sleep (nocturnal myoclonus): Relation to sleep-wake disorders. Ann Neurol 1980;8:416–421.

161. Rees PJ, Cochrane GM, Prior JG, et al. Sleep apnoea in diabetic patients with autonomic neuropathy. JR Soc Med 1981;74:192–195.

162. Rodin J, McAvay G, Timko C. Depressed mood and sleep disturbance in the elderly: A longitudinal study. J Gerontol 1988;43:45–52.

163. Reynolds CF, Kupfer DJ, Taska LS, et al. EEG sleep in elderly depressed, demented, and healthy subjects. Biol Psychiatry 1985;20:431–442.

164. Reynolds CF, Kupfer DJ, Houck PR, et al. Reliable discrimination of elderly depressed and demented patients by EEG sleep data. Arch Gen Psychiatry 1987;44:982–990.

165. Ulrich RF, Shaw DH, Kupfer DJ. Effects of aging on sleep in depression. Sleep 1980;3:31–40.

166. Vogel G, Reynolds CF III, Akiskal HS, et al. Psychiatric disorders. In: Kryger MH, Roth T, Dement WC, eds. Principles and Practice of Sleep Medicine. Philadelphia: WB Saunders, 1989;413–430.

167. Ware JC. Sleep and anxiety. In: Williams RL, Karacan I, Moore CA, eds. Sleep Disorders: Diagnosis and Treatment, ed 2. New York: John Wiley & Sons, 1988;189–214.

168. Cadieux RJ, Woolley D, Kales JD. Sleep disorders in the elderly. In: Berlin RM, Soldatos CR, eds. Psychiatric Medicine. Sleep Disorders in Psychiatric Practice, 1986. Longwood, Fla.: Ryandic Publishing, 1987;165–180.

169. Culebras A, Magana R. Neurologic disorders and sleep disturbances. Semin Neurol 1987;7:277–285.

170. Morgan K, Dalloso H, Ebrahim S, et al. Characteristics of subjective insomnia in the elderly living at home. Age Aging 1988;17:1–7.

171. Garma L, Bouard G, Benoit O. Age and intervening wakefulness in chronic insomnia. In: Koella WP, ed. Sleep 1980. Basel: S Karger, 1981;391–393.

172. Czeisler CA, Dumont M, Richardson GS, et al. Disorders of circadian function: Clinical consequences and treatment. Program and Abstracts of NIH Consensus Development Conference on The Treatment of Sleep Disorders of Older People. Bethesda, Md.: National Institutes of Health, 1990; pp95–101.

173. Czeisler CA, Allan JS, Strogatz SH, et al. Bright light resets the human circadian pacemaker independent of the timing of the sleep-wake cycle. Science 1986;233:667–671.

174. Czeisler CA, Allan S. Acute circadian phase reversal in man via bright light exposure. Application of jet lag. Sleep Res 1987;16:605.

175. Mant A, Eyland EA. Sleep patterns and problems in elderly general practice attenders: An Australian survey. Community Health Study 1988;12:192–199.

176. Pittendrigh CS, Daan S. Circadian oscillations in rodents: A systematic increase of their frequency with age. Science 1974;186:548–550.

177. Morin LP. Age-related changes in hamster circadian period, entrainment, and rhythm splitting. J Biol Rhythms 1988;3:237–248.

178. Weitzman ED, Moline ML. Czeisler CA, et al. Chronobiology of aging: Temperature, sleep-wake rhythms and entrainment. Neurobiol Aging 1982;3:299–309.

179. Moore RY, Eichler VB. Loss of circadian adrenal corticosterone rhythm following suprachiasmatic lesions in the rat. Brain Res 1972;42:201–206.

180. Stephan FK, Zucker I. Circadian rhythms in drinking behavior and locomotor activity of rats are eliminated by hypothalamic lesions. Proc Natl Acad Sci USA 1972;69:1583–1586.

181. Hofman MA, Fliers E, Goudsmit E, et al. Morphometric analysis of the suprachiasmatic and paraventricular nuclei in the human brain: sex differences and age-dependent changes. J Anat 1988;160:127–143.

182. Swaab DF, Fliers E, Partiman TS. The suprachiasmatic nucleus of the human brain in relation to sex, age, and senile dementia. Brain Res 1985;342:37–44.

183. Swaab DF, Fisser B, Kempherst W, Troost D. The human suprachiasmatic nucleus: Neuropeptide changes in serium and Alzheimer's disease. Basic Appl Histochem 1988;2:43–54.

184. Remmers JE, Issa FG. Indications and rationale for treatment of sleep-disordered breathing in older people. Program and Abstracts of NIH Consensus Development Conference on The Treatment of Sleep Disorders of Older People. Bethesda, Md.: National Institutes of Health, 1990;55–57.

185. Kales A, Vela-Bueno A, Kales JD. Sleep disorders: Sleep apnea and narcolepsy. Ann Intern Med 1987;106:434–443.

186. Gottlieb GL. Sleep disorders and their management: Special considerations in the elderly. Am J Med 1990;88 (suppl 3A):29S–33S.

187. Vestal R, Dawson G. Pharmacology and aging. In: Finch CE, Schneider EL, eds. Handbook of the Biology of Aging, ed 2. New York: Van Nostrand Reinhold, 1985;744–819.

188. Kales JD, Carvell M, Kales A. Sleep and sleep disorders. In: Cassell CK, Riesenberg DE, Sorensen LB, et al. eds. Geriatric Medicine. New York: Springer-Verlag, 1990;562–578.

26

Sleep Disorders of Childhood

Richard Ferber

The same types of sleep disorders that occur in adults also occur in children: sleep apnea, narcolepsy, parasomnias, circadian rhythm disorders, and insomnia. All, however, have presentations that are peculiar to children, a fact that much affects proper evaluation and treatment. For example, narcolepsy in children may present initially as a form of hypersomnolence with a single prolonged sleep period, and only later as more classical daytime sleepiness with short, refreshing naps. Sleep apnea in children often looks more like an upper airway resistance syndrome than the typical pattern of clear-cut apneas and desaturations. Bedwetting at age 3 years reflects normal function, not the disorder of enuresis. Confusional arousals are much more frequent in children than sleepwalking or sleep terrors. But, the class of childhood sleep disorders that are most different from the adult presentations are insomnias, or sleeplessness, particularly the forms seen in young children (especially if one is willing to include relevant circadian problems).[1-4] For this reason, this chapter focuses primarily on a discussion of factors that need to be considered when dealing with a young child who has difficulty falling asleep or remaining asleep.

Newborns enter the world already able to sleep. They have rapid eye movement (REM) and non-rapid eye movement (NREM) sleep. But, at birth, NREM sleep is not fully developed and is not yet divisible into four substages.[5-9] The pattern of sleep cycling itself is also immature, not yet being well-organized into a circadian pattern.[8,10-12] Periods of sleeping and waking are almost randomly spread across the 24-hour day.

Changes occur rapidly—both in the electrophysiologic aspects of sleep and in its circadian control. The trace alternant electroencephalographic (EEG) pattern of NREM sleep in the newborn (2- to 6-second bursts of high-amplitude slow waves separated by 4 to 8 seconds of low-voltage mixed activity) disappears within a few weeks and is replaced by a more continuous pattern.[5,8] Division of NREM into four stages is quite clear by age 6 months. Sleep spindles appear by age 4 to 6 weeks and are extremely prominent by 2 months.[7] Vertex waves suggestive of K complexes are usually seen by about 4 months, and are quite clearly defined by 6 months.[6]

There is some evidence that the circadian clock is already functioning at birth but that it does not become linked to the sleep rhythm it controls until age 6 to 12 weeks.[13] By 3 months of age there is consolidation of the major sleep period into the night and beginning organization of daytime sleep into a regular pattern of naps.[8-12] These changes progress rapidly, along with the decrease in the need for nighttime feedings, after 5 to 6 months. By the second half of the first year of life, sleep should be well-organized, with good nighttime sleep and about two daytime naps. The morning nap is usually dropped around the first birthday; the final nap is most often given up in the third year of life.

Largely because of these facts, one would not expect a youngster to begin sleeping through the night much before age 3 months. On the other hand, it is reasonable to expect (and surveys confirm) that full-term, appropriately developing, and normally growing infants should be (at least close to) sleeping through the night by age 5 to 6 months.[14,15] If bedtime problems or nighttime awaking continues to be a significant problem after that, reasons can usually be identified and corrected, most often by behavioral means.[1,2,4,16-19]

PROBLEM VERSUS DISORDER; PROBLEM VERSUS NO PROBLEM

Youngsters are very plastic, in terms of their ability to vary their sleep patterns, change habits associated with sleep, sleep at different times, and divide their sleep into different numbers of segments. This is especially true during the months that a youngster normally naps more than once a day. Much of what is seen, therefore, only represents a variation on a theme. Certain of these variations, though not technically *disorders*, may still present a significant problem for family members. The bulk of the complaints of sleeplessness in young children seen in practice fall into this category.

For a sleep problem to truly represent a disorder the sleep of the child should be interrupted inappropriately (i.e., should not be part of the normal sleep cycling), total sleep time should be reduced below the sleep requirements of that child, or daytime functioning should be affected. The last symptom is often difficult to assess. A 1-year-old who sleeps only 7 hours a night but naps 5 hours during the day could be viewed as getting a normal amount of sleep though in a manner that is difficult for the family to accommodate. He could also be viewed as a youngster who gets insufficient sleep at night and so, is excessively sleepy during the day. Usually, the former interpretation is best, as the cause of such a presentation generally is not related to any underlying disorder—and, it is easily corrected. It is also difficult to evaluate the consequences of insufficient sleep in a child, because children frequently do not show obvious signs (yawning, dozing) of (at least mild) sleepiness. Behavioral symptoms such as irritability and decreased attention are more common but may not be recognized if they are mild or long standing. Their existence is often inferred only after the fact, when behavior improves following adjustment of the sleep pattern.

Even before discussing the specific causes of sleeplessness in young children, certain points should be emphasized. Unlike adults, children generally do not deal with their sleep problems by themselves. There is an interaction between child and parent (or caretaker), one that determines whether or not a specific sleep pattern is viewed as a problem.[1,2,17,18,20,21] If parents must get up at night to help a youngster return to sleep after awaking (wherever the child may be sleeping), they may consider this a problem. And what is a problem for one family may not be for the next. Often what determines the existence or severity of a complaint is the ability of the parent who gets up at night to go back to sleep after intervening. Thus, even a brief intervention required only once a night (perhaps covering a child at 1:00 A.M.) may represent a major problem to a parent who cannot go back to sleep for 2 hours.

Nighttime awakings occur as part of the normal pattern of sleep cycling from the day a child enters this world. Many problems exist because parents, misinterpreting these wakings as abnormal, develop habitual patterns of intervention that only ensure continued difficulties.

Finally, what works for one family may not work at all for the next. This reflects individual differences and varied temperaments.[22] Although two children may be managed exactly the same way at bedtime and (if they should occur) at nighttime awakings, one may go down quickly and sleep through the night and the other may protest loudly at bedtime and be up three times a night, unable (or unwilling)

to go back to sleep by himself. Management of the first child requires no changes; management of the second child does. Although that may seem simplistic, it is actually quite important and frequently overlooked. The decision for parents to change their approach usually should be dictated by their youngster's actual sleep pattern.

GENERAL CONSIDERATIONS

A major advance in the treatment of insomnia in adults came with the realization that many factors were involved, that a differential diagnosis was possible, and that specific treatment could be designed to fit the specific cause of the patient's complaint.[23,24] No longer was it appropriate to treat insomnia as a single diagnosis with a single treatment, barbiturates. The same considerations must be applied to children. By assuming that all sleepless youngsters need the same treatment, a practitioner is sure to treat many children inappropriately and unsuccessfully.

When dealing with an insomniac adult, one must take the history directly from the patient. For children, this history is usually obtained from the parent or caretaker. In the adult situation, it is the degree with which the patient is unhappy with the sleep pattern that determines the severity of the complaint. For a child, it is the impact on the family that determines it. It is uncommon for a young sleepless child to act like an insomniac adult, frustrated by an inability to sleep despite a desire to do so. It is much more common to see a youngster not wanting to sleep at an hour that the parents wish he would.

In most cases a very careful history from the family provides enough diagnostic information to decide on therapy.[3] A physical exam should not be neglected, but it only rarely provides the answers. The history itself cannot be rushed, and it should be all inclusive, as multiple factors often contribute to a child's sleep difficulties.

It is helpful to obtain the history in a circadian format, finding out what happens and at what time, around the clock.[3] Of course, there must be emphasis on the times of sleep (bedtime, actual time of falling asleep, nap times) and awakings, and the exact circumstances under which all sleep transitions take place (even after nighttime awaking). If there are variations from night-to-night, relative incidences of the various patterns should be determined (often this requires great effort on the part of the examiner). Weekend versus weekday schedules (even differences at the respective homes of a child's divorced parents) should be clarified. Parents often forget to mention short periods of sleep (such as in the car or stroller) that may have much impact on the rest of the sleep pattern. The timing and pattern of daytime events is also important: day care, other structured activities, peer interactions, and television viewing. A careful description of the sleeping environment may be crucial: the organization of the house, where the bedrooms are located, who sleeps where, whether there is a nightlight (and how bright it is), if the child's bedroom door is open or closed, if there is a transitional object, if other children share the room, if the child sleeps with the parents, and if the parents are on the same floor of the house at bedtime and during the night. External stimulation, such as a parent or sibling coming home and making noise just as a youngster is about to go to sleep or a parent getting up and showering to leave for work very early in the morning, may also be relevant.

A complete social history should be obtained.[3] The makeup of the family should be known, marital discord should be probed, alcohol or drug abuse should be ascertained, and any other factors that could lead to stress in the home should be investigated.

SPECIFIC DISORDERS

Although intrinsic and extrinsic sleep disorders[25] are both possible in young children, the vast majority of those encountered would be classified as extrinsic. These are discussed next.

Sleep-Onset Association Disorder

When sleep-onset association disorder is the only problem, the youngster's inherent ability to fall asleep at the desired time and to sleep the desired number of hours is not affected.[1,18,26] The youngster has come to associate falling asleep with some behavioral pattern that is partially outside his control.[1,2,16–19,21,25,27–32] It is generally necessary for the parents to establish this routine at bedtime and then to reestablish it at times of (normal) nighttime awaking.

Although the associated routines may be the same at bedtime as at nighttime awakings, they might not be considered a problem then, as interventions at that hour are not usually disruptive to the family (who are still awake anyway) and because interactive bedtime rituals are desirable. *Bedtime* may really not be a problem; a youngster who goes to sleep quickly by himself may still need help several times during the night. To be a problem at bedtime, the process of sleep transition must be extended, for example, 45 minutes of rocking before a child can be transferred to the crib.

A pattern of specific associations with sleep transitions is common at all ages, but after a certain age most persons are able to take on the responsibility for generating these patterns completely by themselves (whether it means sleeping on their back or side, under a heavy or light blanket, with or without music, a light, or a transitional object, and with a fat or a thin pillow). Whether by necessity or choice, parents of young children often become entangled in this routine. Such parent-assisted patterns may truly be necessary to help a very young infant smoothly negotiate the transition from wakefulness to sleep at bedtimes and following spontaneous interruptions of sleep (particularly from the unstable state of REM sleep). A youngster who is colicky in the early months may also need special help. By age 3 or 4 months most youngsters have passed the age of colic and, in any case, have matured sufficiently to be able to handle these transitions by themselves if desired or required. As discussed above, sleep-onset associations that require parental intervention are not, in and of themselves, problematic. Some youngsters are rocked to sleep quickly at bedtime, then are transferred to the crib easily without waking and sleep through the night. Though they continue to associate rocking with the initial sleep transition, they do not have to have it repeated at nighttime awakings. For these youngsters and their families, no problem exists and no changes need be made.

Similar bedtime routines may lead to major problems in other children if these routines have to be repeated during the night. Rocking and back patting or rubbing are perhaps the most common. Youngsters may require a bottle or cup of water, juice, or milk. They may be handed a pacifier, walked about, or driven in the car. They may fall asleep quickly and transfer easily to the crib, or they may fall asleep slowly and be difficult to move from arms to mattress until they reach stage 4 sleep (in this case there would be a complaint of a bedtime problem). Once asleep, children generally do well for several hours (the initial delta sleep epochs). Though awakings may begin earlier, they typically start 3 to 4 hours after the child first falls asleep (at, or shortly after, the time the parents go to bed themselves). This middle third of the night is when sleep is lightest, as youngsters change back and forth between stage 2, REM, and brief periods of waking. If they wake sufficiently to realize that the patterns associated with sleep transitions are no longer present, they are aroused more completely and let the parents know of their dissatisfaction by crying or calling. We have here an unusual situation, one rarely seen in adults: youngsters fall asleep under one set of conditions but awake during the night finding them to be completely changed. (Perhaps some adults do the same when falling asleep with the television on and waking up during the night in a totally silent environment.) Often this means a youngster falls asleep in the parent's arms, in the living room, and with the lights and television on, only to wake during the night alone, in a crib, in a dark, quiet room. It is not surprising that a youngster in such a situation would have difficulty returning to sleep (perhaps it is only surprising that some do not).

The key diagnostic feature comes from the description of the nighttime awakings.[1,3,17,18,27] The youngster goes back to sleep promptly when the parents respond quickly, reinstituting conditions that have become associated with sleep transitions. If simply rocking a child at this point lets him go back to sleep quickly, most other causes of sleeplessness, including pain and schedule disorders, can be ruled out. There certainly can be no problem with the youngster's inherent ability to sleep if he falls back asleep with such minimal intervention. A truly frightened youngster may behave similarly, but usually parents can make this distinction. When associations are at fault, a youngster may seem angry at the parents if they do not do what he wants, but he does not appear frightened.

There usually are one to three awakings per night. Often the last several hours of the night are quiet again, reflecting the tendency of young children to return to delta sleep toward morning.

Once sleep-onset associations have been identified as the cause of a child's problem (i.e. interfering with return to sleep after normal nighttime wakings) and if the parents want to take steps to improve matters an appropriate pattern of intervention can be designed. Typically, this involves giving the youngster a chance to learn to make the transition from waking to sleep under the conditions that will be present at the time of spontaneous nighttime awakings.[1,17,18,21,33-38] If this means in the crib, alone, in a relatively dark and quiet room, then this should be the environment in which the youngster learns to go to sleep. Though some workers begin the training at naptime,[33] it seems reasonable to start at bedtime, when the drive to sleep is greater. If there is any question about when the youngster is ready to fall asleep, the chosen time should be somewhat on the late side, to be sure. The youngster simply needs to be put down awake after an appropriate bedtime ritual and given increasing amounts of time to fall asleep, interrupted by brief parental visits for reassurance. The same patterns should be used at times of nighttime wakings, increasing the waiting times as needed on successive nights.

Although some recommendations suggest starting before 2 months of age,[33] it seems appropriate to wait until it is clear that the youngster has the neurologic capability to manage these transitions smoothly. As, ordinarily, children sleep through the night by age 5 or 6 months, this seems a reasonable time to start. Though some have recommended starting the training process from the beginning (i.e.,

always putting a youngster down awake) in an effort to avoid problems, it does not seem clear why trying to teach a neonate to negotiate the transitions to sleep alone is of any particular value. Parental closeness is much more important at that age and, if necessary, new patterns can be learned later on without much difficulty. The learning process takes only 1 to 3 nights.

Another approach is scheduled awakenings.[39-42] Here, the child is awakened during the night, before the expected time of natural awaking. The assumption is that the child is quite sleepy at that point (instead of waking out of lighter sleep), can go to sleep more quickly with less parental intervention, will learn new habits at that time, and will sleep through subsequent times of usual awakings.

In some situations it is best to have the parents sleep in the child's room for 1 or 2 weeks, to be present at times of awaking but not to reinstitute rocking or other learned associations. This is particularly useful for a child with separation (or other) anxiety. In this case, the reassurance of having a parent in the room is enough to let the child return to sleep. This differs from the situation of a youngster for whom the habitual nighttime interventions themselves, not parental reassurance, is desired. In fact, such a child often finds it more frustrating to have a parent nearby if the parent refuses to rock or pat him.

Nocturnal Eating (Drinking) Disorder

A youngster with nocturnal eating disorder is fed at times of nighttime awaking (and usually also at bedtime).[1,14,20,25,32,43-46] To some degree, this is analogous to the problem just discussed, sleep-onset associations, at least if the youngster falls asleep at the breast or while taking a bottle. The difference is that the child has more awakings at night because of excessive feedings.

To make this diagnosis, one must be sure that the number of nighttime awakings is more than is required for nutritional purposes. Though many children continue to be fed at night beyond age 5 or 6 months, this is generally the result of habit, not need. Again, continued nighttime feeding after 6 months does not define the existence of a problem; this depends on the frequency of awakings at night and the effect they have on family members who have to deal with them. On the other hand, an 8-month-old who is fed six times a night has his sleep disrupted to a degree that is not likely in his best interests, regardless of whether or not the parents see the awakings as a problem for themselves.

Besides the factor of associations, the feedings themselves have a major impact. With intake of food there is stimulation of digestive processes, increased body temperature and other disruptions of circadian cycling, and increased urine output, all factors that may lead to increased wakings. In addition, a youngster who learns to expect feeding during the night learns to get hungry at those times.[1,2,15,16,27] The associated gastric contractions and central signals can also stimulate arousal. The effect on the circadian system should not be underestimated. A youngster who continues to feed multiple times during the night remains on a pattern typical of early infancy, when sleeping, waking, and feeding are all distributed across the 24-hour day.[16,27]

If the nighttime feedings take place through nursing, this must be carefully explored with the mother before changes are made. It must be clear what her desires are regarding nighttime nursing, when she plans or desires to wean, and what she would consider ideal. Though most nursing is done for appropriate reasons (the mother's desire to care for and nurture her child), some psychosocial settings have pathologic overtones (marital discord with parents looking for excuses to be apart during the night, self-image difficulties with the mother needing to be nurtured herself, nonparticipation of the father, depression). A youngster who is fed at night by bottle often does not even require the presence of a parent during the process of returning to sleep; he just needs someone to hand him another bottle (in this case it is obvious that neither separation nor social nurturance issues are key).

The amount of milk or juice taken during the night is frequently extraordinary, up to a quart (four bottles) or more. It is easy to understand how such intake can disrupt sleep.

If the family decides to decrease or eliminate the nighttime feedings, there are different ways it can be accomplished and these should be discussed with the family so that one is chosen that they feel best suits them. Perhaps the easiest is simply to progressively lengthen the interval between feedings, for example increasing by 30 minutes each night, eliminating the nighttime feedings over 1 week or so. Decreasing the amount of milk or juice per bottle may also help. Some families prefer to water down the formula or juice progressively; once only pure water is given the nutritional aspects of nighttime feedings are eliminated, and then the water may be stopped. The association problems that may be part of the difficulty can be dealt with at the same time or after the feedings stop.

It is not always necessary to eliminate the bedtime feeding. If it is kept, the youngster should be fed and put into the crib. He should not be allowed back to the breast or given another bottle after that (even if he wakes at time of transition) to prevent an extended associational problem from persisting. Occasionally, a parent wants to decrease nighttime feedings from several to one. This can be attempted by

spacing out the minimum time between feedings then stopping at a preselected time (such as 5 hours). This is often, but not always, successful.

Limit-Setting Sleep Disorders

Limit-setting sleep disorder is usually seen in youngsters somewhat older than those discussed in the previous section, typically those 3 to 6 years old. Problems often start the day a youngster learns how to climb out of a crib or is moved to a bed for other reasons. With the loss of the control of the bars of the crib, the locus of nocturnal control is shifted from the parents to the youngster. He is now requested to control his own urges—urges to stall, to make endless requests, and to leave his bed and room. The same thing may occur even if the youngster sleeps in the parents' bed. If the parents are unable to enforce controls by setting appropriate limits, the youngster becomes increasingly anxious,[47,48] there is further testing of limits, tension increases, and the nighttime becomes more difficult.

A typical scenario has a youngster stalling at bedtime with multiple requests for an extra story, another glass of water, to watch more television, or to make extra trips to the bathroom. The more the parents give in to these requests, the more the child continues to make them (often searching for the point at which a limit will be set). If the parents are not nearby, the child may get out of bed and search for them, possibly going back downstairs.

Many factors have to be considered in these situations. A parent may not understand the importance of limit setting: that it is actually part of appropriate nurturing and not punishment. This point must be made clear. The tension that exists in the home when parents are obviously distraught at the youngster's continued demands is certainly not in the youngster's best interest, even if the parents are continuing to give in. A little boy who climbs into his parents' bed and kicks his father until his father goes to another room to sleep is made to feel inappropriately powerful and should feel frightened by that power rather than happy at getting what he wanted. Parents may have no idea how to set limits. They may describe their 2-year-old getting up and walking right past them into the livingroom at bedtime, and helplessly ask, what can I do?

Another consideration is secondary gain. Though parents may not like their child getting up in the middle of the night, they may enjoy cuddling with him in front of the television in the late evening. If they allow this, they give the youngster mixed messages.

The issue of guilt is a complicated one. It is very difficult to set limits on a youngster who has, or had, significant medical problems (prematurity, chronic illness, deafness). It may be impossible (and often is contraindicated) to set firm limits in a home where there is ongoing psychosocial stress—owing to marital discord, depression, alcoholism, fighting, financial difficulties, or a recent move. In this setting, a child who is not being appropriately nurtured during the day may use the struggles at night as a way of ensuring some type of interaction with the parents, negative though its tone.

Finally, to make a diagnosis of a limit-setting disorder one assumes that the youngster is ready to fall asleep at the designated bedtime. If circadian factors speak to the contrary, then what appears to be a limit-setting disorder may actually be something quite different.[49] A careful history is usually sufficient to make this distinction.

Management must take into account why this disorder exists. If the need is clearly to replace limits that have been lost (or were never present), then considerable time must be spent working with the family. First is the process of education: helping them understand that setting limits is important to a youngster's development. Then a concrete plan must be devised that the family can follow to accomplish this.[43,50,51] Often this can be done quite easily, for example replacing the bars of the crib with gates at the doorway. Parents can respond in a progressive manner, coming back to the gates (as outlined for an association problem). A youngster who can knock gates over or climb over even a double gate may have to be kept in the room with a closed door,[1,4] though it is never reasonable to leave a youngster behind a locked door. The idea of door closure is to use the door as a passive limit setter, to avoid major confrontation between parents and child while enforcing the parents' rules. This should be done with the parent by the door and starting with *very* short closure time (say, 30 seconds). The objective is not to frighten the youngster, only to set and enforce rules.

Older children (at least age 3) may be motivated with a star chart–reward system.[1,18] If the child is motivated and is willing to follow through with such a program, that is preferred; a positive reinforcement system is always better than a negative one.

Often, to the parents' surprise, once limits are firmly set anxiety decreases markedly[2,48] and the youngster becomes much happier in the evening as nighttime tensions disappear. In fact, such children frequently remind their parents to close the gate before they leave, to be sure the parents remain in control.

In situations involving guilt, secondary gain, or psychosocial difficulties, there must be careful evaluation and discussion before proceeding.[2,3] Parents who feel guilty may need to have more gradual limit-setting measures outlined for them; those who get secondary gain from the nighttime experience may have to understand it and be willing to give it up; and families with psychosocial difficulties may require very individualized care. In this last setting, a child may actually need more access to the parents at night (as well as during the day), and it may be best to hold off on a strict limit-setting program until the psychosocial issues themselves can be better addressed. Counseling is often indicated.[2,3]

Food Allergy Insomnia

Kahn and associates have described a condition of food allergy insomnia in which young children with documented allergy to cow's milk protein have severely disrupted sleep.[52–54] Typically, they have delayed sleep initiation and frequent and prolonged nighttime awakings. Symptoms begin whenever cow's milk is introduced into the diet. Total sleep time is often significantly reduced. In addition, more typical systemic signs of milk allergy, such as excema, wheezing, or gastrointestinal disturbances, may be minimal or absent. Regardless of treatment, there is generally spontaneous resolution by age 2 to 4 years.

In these youngsters, radioallergosorbent testing (RAST) shows elevated immunoglobulin E (IgE) against β-lactoglobulin. Eosinophil count, IgE titer, and skin reactivity may be normal, especially before the first birthday. There may be some cross-reactivity with soy-based products.

Switching to a hypoallergenic hydrolyzed formula is followed by resolution of symptoms within days to weeks. A challenge with even small amounts of cow's milk protein causes a return of symptoms until the apparent allergy is outgrown.

For some reason, this disorder has not frequently been described in the United States. Perhaps this is because of the tendency of U.S. pediatricians to switch formulas empirically when things are not going well.

Circadian Rhythm Sleep Disorders

Delayed or advanced sleep phase

Circadian rhythm disorders have been well-described in adults (see Chapter 23).[13,55] The syndromes are conceptually the same in young children, except that it is the parents' dissatisfaction with the schedule that generates the complaint. Strictly speaking, these are situations in which a youngster gets (or is capable of getting) a normal amount of sleep at night but it does not occur during the desired hours (neither the start nor end of the spontaneous sleep period is at a preferred time, at least when the full nocturnal sleep requirement is taken into account).[13,49,55,56]

A youngster with an advanced sleep phase may fall asleep by 7:00 at night but wake at 4:00 or 5:00

in the morning. The complaint is early morning awakings. The parents of a youngster with a delayed sleep phase may complain that it takes him several hours to fall asleep (perhaps not until 9:00 or 10:00 P.M. or later) but that the time of spontaneous morning awaking is at or later than the desired hour (perhaps anywhere from 7:00 to 10:00 A.M.).

A careful history of a child with an advanced sleep phase usually shows advance of other aspects of the daytime schedule, including meals and naptimes.[1,49] The child who wakes at 5:00 A.M. may be fed shortly after that and nap as early as 7:00 A.M. Both the early feeding and early nap may contribute to persistence of this syndrome.[1] The bedtime behavior of a child with a delayed sleep phase may resemble that of a youngster with limit-setting difficulties. There is a major difference, however. In the situation of a phase delay, the youngster is completely unable to fall asleep, even if the parents set very firm limits. Instead of calling and coming out of bed, some youngsters try to "be good" and lie in bed each night for hours, waiting for sleepiness (and sleep) to arrive. During that time they are generally not allowed to read, listen to the radio, or watch television. They must lie in the dark room, and they have nothing to do but think. Thinking in a dark room may lead to fantasy, and fantasy may lead to scary thoughts. Some of these youngsters end up scaring themselves, and nighttime fears may be the presenting complaint.

The diagnosis should come from a careful history.[3] The youngster with an advanced sleep phase falls asleep easily and sleeps normally. Though he wakes early, it is after a normal amount of sleep, especially when the amount of daytime sleep is taken into account.

The youngster with a delayed sleep phase must be distinguished from one with a limit-setting disorder or true nighttime fears. Typically, the time of sleep onset is fairly independent of the bedtime. A youngster who falls asleep at 10:00 P.M. usually does so regardless of what hour he is put to bed, only the sleep latency changes. If a history can be obtained of occasional late bedtimes, much shorter sleep latencies should be reported. On a night when the family does not get home until after the child's usual hour of sleep onset, the child likely falls asleep in the car. Weekend and vacation schedules may be similarly helpful in recognizing this syndrome. Also, a child who scares himself because of long sleep latency will not experience nighttime fears on nights that he goes to bed late.

Often these children are allowed to (or want to) sleep late in the morning. If they are attending school or day care, late morning sleep may be limited to weekends. Waking them earlier during the week may be accomplished only with great difficulty. Though later sleep is expected on weekends, this is not always the case with children old enough to watch television by themselves. A 5-year-old may "get up" early on the weekends (despite having to be wakened at that hour during the week) only to creep into a dark room to watch television for several hours. He probably dozes by the television; he certainly is not fully awake. To determine the true end of the sleep phase, it is more important to find out when the youngster climbs out from under the blanket on the sofa, asks for breakfast, and appears to be wide awake.

In young children, a delayed sleep phase can usually be corrected easily by controlling morning awaking.[1,49] It is best to start with a late bedtime, at the time the youngster actually has been falling asleep, to remove the stresses that have been present during the presleep hours and to help the youngster become accustomed to falling asleep quickly. If he is awakened for school or day care 5 days a week, this schedule should be enforced on weekends as well. If he usually sleeps late, the time of waking can be advanced gradually, perhaps by 15 minutes a day. Once awaking is better-controlled, bedtime can be slowly advanced in a similar manner.

It is best to ensure that the youngster is up, fed, and moving about in the morning, preferably exposed to as much light as possible. Formal use of light boxes[57] or around-the-clock progressive phase delay[58] is not usually necessary at this age.

For a youngster with an advanced sleep phase, ensuring plenty of light in the evening, progressively delaying bedtime, and progressively delaying the early morning meal and naptimes should lead to resolution. Control of early morning light exposure may also be helpful.

Regular but inappropriate schedule

Inappropriately timed meal or nap. It is quite well-known that a regular nap in the late afternoon may delay the onset of sleep in the evening. What is less well-known is that a very early meal or naptime may reinforce early morning awaking.[1,49] Youngsters who nap very early, say, at 6:00 or 7:00 P.M., may wake at 5:00 A.M. only to return to sleep after 1 or 2 hours. The youngster acts as if the last sleep cycle was broken off from the night and moved 1 or 2 hours later. An early feeding, such as 5:00 A.M. (usually given "because" the youngster has awakened at that hour), may only reinforce continued early awaking, because the youngster learns to get hungry at that hour and hunger may trigger arousal. In these cases, gradually delaying the morning nap to an appropriate time, such as 10 A.M., moving it into the afternoon as a single nap (if the child is older than a year), or eliminating it altogether (depending on age) may allow later sleep in the morning. Delaying the first feeding to an appropriate breakfast time may be similarly useful.

Time in bed is more than sleep requirement. The syndrome of spending too much time in bed is similar to one sometimes seen in elderly persons, though, here, too, it is not the child's own decision to do so but the parents'. It is not at all uncommon for parents to incorrectly estimate the amount of sleep their youngster needs.[59] Their estimate is often based on desire rather than reason. Thus, parents may decide that their 18-month-old should get 11 hours' sleep at night, and they keep him in the crib from 7:00 P.M. to 6:00 A.M. In fact, this child may need and get 11 hours' sleep, but it is 11 hours per 24 hours. He may get 2 hours as part of a regular afternoon nap, leaving only 9 hours to sleep at night. These hours of nighttime sleep might run from 7:00 P.M. to 4:00 A.M., or (more commonly) from 9:00 P.M. to 6:00 A.M In both cases the parents inappropriately leave an unhappy wakeful youngster in the crib for 2 hours. In the first case it is from 4:00 A.M. (when the child finished sleeping) until 6:00 A.M. (when the parents are willing to take him out of the crib). In the second case it is from 7:00 P.M. (when they insist on putting him to bed) until 9:00 P.M. (when he is finally ready to, and does, fall asleep).

Older children may be forced to spend too much time in bed as well, but at least sometimes they are allowed to read or play quietly (if they can do this).

Finally, some youngsters split their sleep time into two segments, separated by an extended period of nighttime wakefulness: in the example above, this child might sleep from 7:00 P.M. to 1:00 A.M. and from 3:00 A.M. to 6:00 A.M. (and still get 9 hours at night). In this case, no type of parental intervention during the period of nighttime wakefulness will get the youngster back to sleep. He is wide awake, just wants to play, and is usually allowed to do so (though young children are sometimes simply left crying in the crib).

The solution to all of these problems is the same: the time in bed should be limited to the sleep requirement.[1,49,59,60] In the cases described above, bedtime and waking should be made 9 hours apart, whichever 9 hours the parents find most workable (perhaps 9:00 to 6:00 or even 10:00 to 7:00). Middle-of-the-night play should not be allowed. Daytime naps should continue but should not be extended. All these problems generally resolve quite quickly.

Sometimes the total sleep time is inappropriately divided into nighttime sleep that is too short and daytime sleep that is too long. A 15-month-old may be taking a 3- or 4-hour nap (or two 2-hour naps), leaving him time for only 7 to 8 hours of sleep at night. In this case, of course, part of the treatment involves limiting the nap time to that appropriate for age.

Medical/Psychiatric Sleep Disorders

Sleep disorders associated with mental disorders

In young children the most common "psychiatric" disorder affecting sleep is anxiety. Fears and worries of various kinds are common in young childhood, and many would be considered normal, especially if they are transient. In some cases the fears are more pronounced, passing beyond the bounds of what might be called a normal developmental stage.[37,47]

It is common for youngsters to pass through a period of separation anxiety. Also, as they go through other developmental hurdles, such as toilet training, the start of school, and accepting a new sibling into the home, transient regression and anxiety commonly return. Other problems may reflect more general psychosocial issues in the home, such as marital strife, divorce, alcoholism, depression, parental fighting, abuse, drug use, and lack of appropriate nurturance. A child who has handicaps or undergoes frequent medical or surgical procedures may have good reason for increased needs or worries.

In terms of sleep, anxiety usually causes a child to be unwilling to separate from parents at night. If this is the only problem, the child is able to fall asleep without difficulty as long as parents are close by, either in the child's room or with the child in theirs. This fact—that such a youngster falls asleep quickly when sleeping with or close to the parents—helps rule out many other causes of sleeplessness, such as the circadian issues described above. Even a child who is using a complaint of fears as an excuse to be back in the livingroom watching television can be differentiated from one who is truly afraid. A manipulative youngster is not happy simply having a parent nearby even in his own room; he is happy only if he is in the livingroom (and there, the parents may not even have to be present).

Youngsters who are truly frightened appear so, and most often the parents are able to recognize this and describe it in a convincing manner (they similarly can identify a youngster who is just "demanding"). Such youngsters may become quite panicky as bedtime approaches. They usually do not enjoy the bedtime routines because they are fearful of the separation that will follow, and they become progressively more upset. Those that are sufficiently frightened are willing to accept any punishment simply to be allowed to be near the parents.

The main challenge, for diagnostic and treatment decisions, is to identify the severity of the anxiety. If it is very mild, firm reassurance is often all that is necessary. Sometimes in these settings, part of the anxiety stems from a lack of limit setting, and firmer limits are even helpful. On the other hand, a child who is truly frightened at night will not be helped by increased limits, it only makes matters worse. Such a child needs help. Whatever is necessary to make this youngster feel safe and comfortable at night should be provided. This may temporarily require a parent sleeping in the child's room or the child sleeping in the parent's room or bed. If the child is old enough, a sleeping bag on the floor of the parents' bedroom is often sufficient.

A child who is sufficiently verbal is usually able to discuss his or her concerns with the examiner in a manner that allows appropriate planning. Sometimes the youngster only needs the reassurance of having a parent on the same floor of the house when he goes to sleep (being on the second floor of a house alone at bedtime may be quite frightening, even to a youngster without major fears). A youngster may also state that having someone upstairs, checking on him every 5 minutes until he goes to sleep, is sufficient. Or, the youngster may make it quite clear that even that degree of separation cannot be tolerated.

If the anxiety is relatively mild, this often can be dealt with by providing the supports necessary, perhaps adding a reward system, and gradually, with the youngster's approval, decreasing the degree of support. Each time the youngster is successful, he feels more confident, is able to take the next step, and is reassured. When the fears are long standing and significant, professional counselling (family or individual) is usually required.

Sleep disorders associated with neurologic disorders

The list of disorders that fit in this category is almost endless, including epilepsy and the associated drug therapy. Youngsters with central nervous system dysfunction are subject to the same type of sleep disorders as other youngsters, perhaps more so because of parents' guilt feelings, which affect the pattern of nighttime intervention. When the disorders are severe and psychomotor retardation is marked, normal interaction with family members may not be possible, sleep may become inappropriately distributed across the day, and nighttime sleep may be severely disrupted.[61] Much more careful control of the timing and regularity of sleep may be an important consideration.

Certain children, however, do have severe sleep disorders that do not fit into other categories. Their function suggests that the sleep abnormalities are due to dysfunction of the central systems that control sleep. This is seen with some frequency in youngsters with pervasive developmental delay (autism) and in those with severe malformations or injury of the central nervous system. In these cases, total (day plus night) sleep time may be severely limited.[62] Though the electrophysiologic aspects of

sleep in an autistic youngster are generally normal, they certainly may not be in youngsters with more obvious structural abnormalities.

In any case, behavioral intervention may not be sufficient to manage these children. One must keep in mind that managing such a child at home may be extremely difficult for even the most caring of families. Such a child may require a great deal of attention throughout the day. Then if he gets only 5 hours of sleep, the parents are not afforded sufficient time to recuperate. Because of this (and with the assumption of central dysfunction), pharmacologic intervention may have to be considered. There are few formal studies of such drug interventions in young children (and it would be difficult to generalize from these studies anyway, since many of these youngsters differ significantly one to the next in terms of their structural abnormalities). Anecdotally, from work in our center, we can report that the types of medication generally used for adult insomnia (such as benzodiazepines) usually are not effective in these youngsters. And, one would probably be correct in assuming that if a mild sedative such as an antihistamine were able to get such a youngster to sleep, then behavioral methods probably would also.

The drug with which we have had the best and most consistent results is chloral hydrate (a drug that has been useful in pediatrics for many years). The physician must be prepared to give larger than usual doses. Small doses that only make a child drowsy may actually worsen his behavior and not improve sleep. We have found that doses from 500 to 3000 mg sometimes are necessary. The aim is to increase nighttime sleep while (hopefully) improving daytime function, or at least not worsening it. The smallest effective does should be used, and periodically the dose should be tapered to see if it is still needed. Often a satisfactory dose can be found and maintained for months to years, increasing only to adjust for growth. It is reasonable to obtain periodic blood screens, though hematopoietic or hepatic side effects are not common. One problem with chloral hydrate is its taste: it is very bitter, and the taste cannot be covered up with chocolate, sugar, or honey. It does come in a gelcap form for youngsters who can take that. It is preferable to avoid nightly use of suppositories (often they are only expelled). One alternative medication is promethazine, which is sometimes successful in these settings.

Although generally one should approach use of such levels of medication in children with great hesitancy, one should also be willing to treat when indicated. Helping such a youngster increase sleep from 5 to 7 or 8 hours may have a tremendous impact on the family and may make the difference between a family's being willing to keep the youngster at home or place him in an institution. With more sleep, parents often do report some improvement in daytime function, a definite extra benefit.

Sleep disorders associated with other medical disorders

Almost any medical problem may be associated with a sleep disorder because of direct effects on the sleep system, associated fever, pain, medication, or parental concern. These are obvious in short-term situations and usually do not demand intervention.

Certain medical problems may be more chronic and problematic. Asthma, with nighttime wheezing (and associated fear), may certainly prove quite disruptive[63,64] and is usually treated by medication, and, if necessary, counseling. On the other hand, the stimulant medications used to treat asthma (such as theophylline) may be directly responsible for sleep disruption. Changing the dosage or switching to an inhaled preparation is sometimes helpful.

Gastroesophageal reflux or chronic middle ear disease may be associated with poor sleep as well. Often in these settings there is nighttime awaking, the child seems in discomfort, and parental interventions are slow to aid return to sleep. Treating the underlying condition, medically or surgically, is usually curative.

Colic is the most common cause of sleep difficulties in the early months. Typical symptoms include irritability and inconsolable crying, especially in the late afternoon and evening.[65-68] Colic usually resolves by 3 months of age, and since nighttime sleep is not expected to consolidate before then, it is actually the consequences of patterns developed during the colicky period that are most relevant. These youngsters often must be held, walked, rocked, placed in a swing, or patted to try to help them calm and fall asleep. The patterns may persist as simple habits once the colic disappears, and it is these habits that need treatment.

Finally, every medication must be considered a potential sleep disrupter in a given youngster. Probably even certain of the additives in liquid preparations affect youngsters in undesirable ways. Youngsters who take medications routinely do so for a reason, and the underlying medical problem, as well as the associated psychosocial effects, must all be considered. For example, a young leukemia patient taking chemotherapy has many reasons for sleeping poorly: the effects of the illness itself, the medication, concerns about the illness, family concerns about the illness, and altered patterns of parent-child interaction. Separating these variables and designing appropriate therapy represents one of the greatest challenges to the sleep clinician, but success in this setting may bring the greatest rewards.

REFERENCES

1. Ferber RA. Solve Your Child's Sleep Problem. New York: Simon and Schuster, 1985.
2. Ferber RA. Behavioral "insomnia" in the child. Psychiatr Clin North Am 1988;10:641–653.
3. Ferber RA. Assessment procedures for diagnosis of sleep disorders in children. In: Noshpitz JD, ed. Basic Handbook of Child Psychiatry, vol V. New York: Basic Books, 1987;185–193.
4. Ferber R. Sleeplessness in the child. In: Kryger MH, Roth T, Dement WC, eds. Principles and Practice of Sleep Medicine. Philadelphia: WB Saunders, 1989; 633–639.
5. Ellingson RJ. Ontogenesis of sleep in the human. In: Lairy GC, Salzarulo R, eds. Experimental Study of Human Sleep: Methodological Problems. Amsterdam: Elsevier, 1975;120–140.
6. Metcalf D, Mondale J, Butler F. Ontogenesis of spontaneous K-complexes. Psychophysiology 1971;8:340–347.
7. Metcalf D. Sleep spindle ontogenesis in normal children. In: Smith W, ed. Drugs, Development, and Cerebral Function. Springfield, Ill.: Charles C Thomas, 1972;125–144.
8. Parmelee AH. Ontogeny of sleep patterns and associated periodicities in infants. In: Faulkner E, Kretchmer N, Ross E, eds. Pre-and Postnatal Development of the Human Brain. Basel: S Karger, 1974;298–311.
9. Lenard HG. Sleep studies in infancy. Acta Paediatr Scand 1970;59:572–581.
10. Stern E, Parmelee AH, Harris MA. Sleep state periodicity in prematures and young infants. Dev Psychobiol 1973;6:357–365.
11. Stern E, Parmelee AH, Akiyama Y, et al. Sleep cycle characteristics in infants. Pediatrics 1969;43:65–70.
12. Coons S, Guilleminault C. Development of consolidated sleep and wakeful periods in relation to the day/night cycle in infancy. Dev Med Child Neurol 1984;26:169–176.
13. Moore-Ede MC, Sulzman FM, Fuller CA. The Clocks That Time Us. Cambridge: Harvard University Press, 1982.
14. Moore T, Ucko LE. Nightwaking in early infancy: Part 1. Arch Dis Child 1957;32:333–342.
15. Ragins N, Schachter S. A study of sleep behavior in two-year-old children. J Am Acad Child Psychiatry 1971;10:464–480.
16. Ferber R. The sleepless child. In: Guilleminault C, ed. Sleep and Its Disorders in Children. New York: Raven Press, 1987;141–163.
17. Douglas J, Richman N. My Child Won't Sleep: A Handbook of Management for Parents. London: Penguin, 1984.
18. Douglas J, Richman N. Sleep Management Manual. London: Department of Psychological Medicine, Hospital for Sick Children, 1982.
19. Ferber R. Sleep, sleeplessness, and sleep disruptions in infants and young children. Ann Clin Res 1985;17:227–237.

20. Richman N. A community survey of characteristics of one- to two-year-olds with sleep disruptions. J Am Acad Child Psychiatry 1981;20:281–291.

21. Richman N. Sleep problems in young children. Arch Dis Child 1984;56:491–493.

22. Carey W. Night waking and temperament in infancy. J Pediatr 1974;84:756–758.

23. Zorick FJ, Roth T, Hartse K, et al. Evaluation and diagnosis of persistent insomnia. Am J Psychiatry 1981;138:769–773.

24. Kripke DF, Simons RN, Garfinkle L, et al. Short and long sleep and sleeping pills: Is increased mortality associated? Arch Gen Psychiatry 1970;36:103–116.

25. Diagnostic Classification Steering Committee. International Classification of Sleep Disorders: Diagnostic and Coding Manual. Rochester, Minn.: American Sleep Disorders Association, 1990.

26. Ferber R, Boyle MP. Sleeplessness in infants and toddlers: Sleep initiation difficulty masquerading as a sleep maintenance insomnia. Sleep Res 1983;12:240.

27. Ferber R. Sleeplessness, night awakening, and night crying in the infant and toddler. Pediatrics Rev 1987;9:1–14.

28. Illingworth R. The child who won't sleep and whose parents won't let him. Mims Mag 1976;November 71–77.

29. Illingworth RS. Sleep problems in the first three years. Br Med J 1951;1:722–728.

30. Bax MCO. Sleep disturbance in the young child. Br Med J 1980;280:1177–1179.

31. Bax M. Sleep (editorial). Dev Med Child Neurol 1983; 25:281–282.

32. Ferber R. Childhood insomnia. In: Thorpy M, ed. Handbook of Sleep Disorders. New York: Marcel Dekker, 1990;435–455.

33. Cutherbertson J, Schevill S. Helping Your Child Sleep Through the Night. Garden City, N.Y.: Doubleday, 1985.

34. Jones DPH, Verduyn CM. Behavioral management of sleep problems. Arch Dis Child 1983;58:442–444.

35. Younger JB. The management of night waking in older infants. Pediatr Nurs 1982;8:155–158.

36. Largo RH, Hunziker UA. A developmental approach to the management of children with sleep disturbances in the first three years of life. Eur J Pediatr 1984;142:170–173.

37. Leach P. Babyhood. New York: Alfred A Knopf, 1976.

38. Valman HB. Sleep problems. Br Med J 1981;283:422–423.

39. Johnson CM, Bradley-Johnson S, Stack JM. Decreasing the frequency of infants' nocturnal crying with the use of scheduled awakenings. Fam Pract Res J 1981;1:98–104.

40. Johnson CM, Lerner M. Amelioration of infant sleep disturbances: II. Effects of scheduled awakenings by compliant parents. Infant Ment Health J 1985;6:21–30.

41. McGarr RJ, Hovell MF. In search of the sand man: Shaping an infant to sleep. Ed Treatment Child 1980;3:173–182.

42. Rickert VI, Johnson CM. Reducing nocturnal awakening and crying episodes in infants and young children:

A comparison between scheduled awakenings and systematic ignoring. Pediatrics 1988;81:203–212.

43. Ferber R, Boyle MP. Nocturnal fluid intake: A cause of, not treatment for, sleep disruption in infants and toddlers. Sleep Res 1983;12:243.

44. Osterholm P, Lindeke LL, Amidon D. Sleep disturbance in infants aged 6 to 12 months. Pediatr Nurs 1983;9:269–271.

45. Van Tassel EB. The relative influence of child and environmental characteristics on sleep disturbances in the first and second years of life. J Dev Behav Pediatr 1985;6:81–86.

46. Wright P, MacLeod HA, Cooper MJ. Waking at night: The effect of early feeding experience. Child Care Health Dev 1983;9:309–319.

47. Fraiberg, SH. The Magic Years. New York: Scribner's, 1959.

48. Leach P. Your Baby and Child, from Birth to Age Five. New York: Alfred A Knopf, 1978.

49. Ferber R, Circadian and schedule disturbances. In: Guilleminault C, ed. Sleep and Its Disorders in Children. New York: Raven Press, 1987;165–175.

50. Jackson H, Rawlins MD. The sleepless child. Br Med J 1979;2:509.

51. Kleitman N. Sleep and Wakefulness. Chicago: University of Chicago Press, 1939.

52. Kahn A, Mozin MJ, Casimir G, et al. Insomnia and cow's milk allergy in infants. Pediatrics 1985;76:880–884.

53. Kahn A, Rebuffat E, Blum D, et al. Difficulty in initiating and maintaining sleep associated with cow's milk allergy in infants. Sleep 1987;10:116–121.

54. Kahn A, Francois G, Sottiaux M, et al. Sleep characteristics in milk-intolerant infants. Sleep 1988;11:291–297.

55. Weitzman ED, Czeisler CA, Coleman RM, et al. Delayed sleep phase syndrome: A chronobiologic disorder with sleep onset insomnia. Arch Gen Psychiatry 1981;38:737–746.

56. Ferber R, Boyle MP. Phase shift dyssomnia in early childhood. Sleep Res 1983;12:242.

57. Lewy AJ, Sack RL. Light therapy and psychiatry. Proc Soc Exp Biol Med 1986;183:11–18.

58. Czeisler CA, Richardson GS, Coleman RM, et al. Chronotherapy: Resetting the circadian clocks of patients with delayed sleep phase insomnia. Sleep 1981;4:1–21.

59. Galofre I, Santacana P, Ferber R. The "TIB > TST" syndrome. A cause of wakefulness in children. Sleep Res 1992;21:199.

60. Hauri P. Behavioral treatment of insomnia. Med Times 1979;107:36–47.

61. Okawa M, Sasaki H. Sleep disorders in mentally retarded and brain-impaired children. In: C. Guilleminault, ed. Sleep and Its Disorders in Children. New York: Raven Press, 1987;269–290.

62. Ferber R. Unpublished data.

63. Gaultier C. Respiration during sleep in children with chronic obstructive pulmonary disease and asthma. In: C. Guilleminault, ed. Sleep and Its Disorders in Children. New York: Raven Press, 1987;225–230.

64. Kales A, Kales JD, Sly RM, et al. Sleep pattern of asthmatic children: All-night electro-encephalographic studies. J Allergy 1970;46:301–308.

65. Weissbluth M. Sleep and the colicky infant. In: Guilleminault C, ed. Sleep and Its Disorders in Children. New York: Raven Press, 1987;129–140.

66. Illingworth RS. "Three months" colic. Arch Dis Child 1954;29:167–174.

67. Wiessbluth M. Infant colic. In: Gellis SS, Kagan BM, eds. Current Pediatric Therapy, ed 12. Philadelphia: WB Saunders, 1986.

68. Weissbluth M. Crybabies: Coping with Colic: What To Do When Baby Won't Stop Crying. New York: Arbor House, 1984.

27

Sleep and Epilepsy

Sudhansu Chokroverty

The relationship between sleep and epilepsy has intrigued researchers and thinkers since antiquity. Passouant[1] mentioned about Hippocrates' description of "fears, rages, deliria, leaps out of bed and seizures during the night." Aristotle observed that in many cases epilepsy began during sleep. Despite this early description this intriguing relationship between seizure and sleep has been neglected by the medical profession until the end of the last century. Echeverria (1879),[2] Fere[3] (1890), Gowers (1885),[4] gave clear description of relationship of epilepsy to sleep-wake cycle. Fere[3] in a study of the hospitalized epileptics noted that in more than 2/3rds of 1985 patients the attacks occurred between 8 P.M. and 8 A.M. It is interesting to note that even in those days Fere mentioned the effect of epilepsy on sleep in the form of difficulties of falling asleep or impairment of sleep efficiency. He apparently mentioned the facilitation of seizures by sleep deprivation.

In the beginning of this century Turner,[5] Gallus,[6] and Amann[7] emphasized that many seizures were nocturnal with occurrence at certain times at night. These reports are followed by those of Langdon-Down and Brain,[8] Patry,[9] Buscaino[10] and Magnusson.[11]

All of above observations have been made on the basis of the clinical features only without the benefit of the electroencephalograph which was not described until 1929. The modern era combining the clinical and the EEG observations to show a distinct relationship between epilepsy and sleep began with the observations of Gibbs and Gibbs[12] in 1947 of occurrence of paroxysmal discharges in the EEG twice as often during sleep as during the waking state. This report was followed by many original observations, notably those of Janz,[13] Passouant,[14] Gastaut et al,[15] Cadilhac,[16] Niedermeyer,[17] Montplaisir,[18] Broughton,[19] Billiard[20] and Kellaway[21] and co-workers and other workers.

In this chapter I will give an overview of the effect of sleep on epilepsy as well as the effect of epilepsy on sleep. I will also discuss usefulness of sleep in the diagnosis of epilepsy and the practical relevance to understanding the relationship between sleep and epilepsy.

INTERRELATIONSHIP BETWEEN SLEEP AND EPILEPSY: PHYSIOLOGIC MECHANISMS

There is a reciprocal relationship between sleep and epilepsy: Sleep affects epilepsy and epilepsy in turn affects sleep. To understand this interrelationship it is important to review briefly the mechanism which generates paroxysmal EEG discharges and clinical seizures as well as the mechanism of initiation of sleep.

Basic Mechanism of Epilepsy

An understanding of the basic mechanism of epilepsy is derived primarily from studies of the animal models and later from the studies on the human clinical epilepsy.[22] Experimental animal models of epilepsy are produced by topical application of agents or focal electrical stimulation to the neocortex and limbic cortex for producing partial seizures while electric shock or systemic injection of convulsants and penicillin have been utilized for generalized epilepsy model.[22] Neuronal synchronization and neuronal excitability are two fundamental physiological factors that may transform interictal to an ictal state.[22] Factors enhancing synchronization are conducive to active ictal precipitation in susceptible individuals. These factors include nonspecific influences, such as, sleep, sleep deprivation, etc. In addition, seizure itself may produce sleep disturbance. A fundamental mechanism in the epileptic neurons is a paroxysmal depolarization shift (PDS) in the epileptic neurons as originally described by Matsumoto and Ajmone-Marsan[23] followed by after-hyperpolarization.[24]

Nonspecific thalamic reticular nuclei are responsible for recruiting and specific thalamic nuclei are responsible for augmenting responses; these are also responsible for triggering generalized seizure by synchronizing afferent inputs to the cortex from these nuclei.[25,26] This thalamocortical interaction is responsible for changing the name of centrencephalic epilepsy to corticoreticular epilepsy for petit mal absence type of seizure.[27] The generalized tonic-clonic seizure is initiated in the cortex but the pontine reticular formation participates in the tonic phase.[22]

Epileptogenesis of the neurons is dependent on factors (genetic and acquired) which maintain increased neuronal hyperexcitability and increased neuronal synchronization.[22] Examples of some of these factors are:[22] decreased dendritic spines and decreased number of dendritic branches; cortical sprouting of surviving axons to cause increased synchronization; altered ionic microenvironment in and around the epileptic neurons; attenuation of inhibitory influences causing enhanced synchronization; and alteration of calcium and chloride ion channel distribution.

It is important to understand the interictal state and precipitation of ictus as well as the mechanism of ictal termination and postictal state. The hallmark of an interictal state from physiological point of view is focal or diffuse interictal EEG spike and wave discharge.[22] The epileptic neuronal aggregates show increased synchronization but with a decrease in firing rates which may explain hypometabolism of the interictal focus as noted on positron emission tomography (PET) using ^{18}F-fluorodeoxyglucose (FDG) scans.[22] Prevention of ictal spread and maintenance of interictal state are determined by strong inhibitory influences which also keep the neuron in an excessively synchronous state.[22]

The ictal onset is determined by a combination of a failure of inhibitory interictal mechanism and enhancement of excitatory synaptic activities which may be initiated by an excess of subcortical synchronizing afferent input as in generalized seizure or focal hypersynchronous discharge.[22] The true ictus in generalized seizure is initiated in the cortex and may depend on a failure of inhibitory mechanism coupled with synchronizing thalamocortical input, as well as the influence of the reticular formation of the brain stem, particularly in the pontine region for the tonic phase.[22] A combination of diminution of synaptic inhibition, nonspecific excitation, propagation along the efferent projection pathways and transsynaptic alteration in excitation determine the appearance of partial ictus.[22] For the ictal termination the 2 most important mechanisms are active inhibition and the failure of synchronization.[22] If these mechanisms fail, then the patient may develop status epilepticus. Postictal phenomena (neuronal depression, neuronal deficit, EEG slowing, etc.) are sequela to events that cause termination of the ictus.

Mechanism of Sleep

In humans there are 2 sleep states: synchronized or non-rapid eye movement (NREM) and desynchronized or rapid eye movement (REM) sleep. These 2 sleep states are determined by 2 different mechanisms.[28]

NREM or synchronized sleep seems to act as a convulsant because this state is characterized physiologically by an excessive diffuse cortical synchronization mediated by the thalamocortical input.[29] This predisposes to activation to seizure in an already hyperexcitable cortex.

In REM or desynchronized sleep there is inhibition of thalamocortical synchronizing influence as evidenced by depression of recruiting rhythms generated by low frequency electrical stimulation of the nonspecific thalamic nuclei.[29] Thus, there is attenuation of bilaterally synchronous epileptiform discharges at this stage of sleep. During REM sleep there is also a tonic reduction in the interhemispheric impulse traffic through the corpus callosum.[30] This also contributes to the limitation of the propagation of the generalized epileptiform discharges.

Cortical excitability for epileptogenesis is higher during sleep than during wakefulness.[29] This factor coupled with the fact that the inhibitory mechanism (e.g., postspike hyperpolarization and afferent inhibition) may be less effective during sleep favors activation of focal cortical epileptiform discharge.

According to Steriade[31] physiological synchronization may be defined as a state during which there is appearance of the same frequency in 2 or more oscillators due to coactivation of a large number of neurons. In NREM sleep spindles and slow waves result from synchronization. The nonspecific thalamic reticular nucleus is the synchronizing pacemaker of EEG spindle rhythmicity.[31] In athalamic animals spindles disappear but slow waves persist suggesting extrathalamic origin for sleep slow waves.[32] It has recently been suggested that subcortical white matter participates in the production of EEG slow waves[33] (see also Chapter 3).

Lesions and stimulation experiments have shown the existence of structures responsible for cortical synchrony in the forebrain as well as in the hindbrain.[31,34] Fifty years ago Morison and Dempsey[35] showed an intimate thalamocortical relationship by observing recruiting synchronizing cortical responses following low frequency electrical stimulation of the midline thalamic nuclei. In 1944 Hess[36] even suggested the existence of a thalamic sleep center. Later studies, however, have shown that thalamus is responsible for the genesis of spindles and not for sleep slow waves or behavioral aspect of sleep.[34]

The recent theory about REM or desynchronized sleep suggests that there are anatomically distributed and neurochemically interpenetrated REM "on" and REM "off" cells in the brain stem[28,37] (see also Chapter 3). REM Sleep is dependent upon an interaction between the REM "on" cells and the REM "off" cells in the brain stem. During REM sleep there is maximum cholinergic hyperactivity and aminergic hypoactivity.[28,37] Thus the interaction and oscillation between the cholinergic REM promoting and aminergic

REM inhibiting neurons generate REM-NREM cycle. The various chemical mechanisms participating in NREM and REM sleep may also be responsible for activation or inhibition of epileptiform discharges during sleep.

Thus, an understanding of the basic mechanism of epilepsy and sleep may help us understand the mechanism of activation and suppression of seizure discharges during sleep and in particular during different stages of sleep. The activation of ictal and interictal seizures during NREM sleep seems to be related to the existence of thalamocortical synchronizing mechanism while suppression during REM sleep is due to depression of thalamic synchronizing mechanism and a tonic reduction of interhemispheric transmission during REM sleep.[29,30]

Interrelationship between epilepsy and sleep

The activation of 3 Hz spike and wave discharges during NREM sleep is supported by the hypothesis of corticoreticular epilepsy of Kostopoulos and Gloor[38] and Gloor.[27] Kostopoulos and Gloor[38] presented evidence which showed that the 3 Hz spike and wave discharges of primary generalized corticoreticular ("centrencephalic?") or petit mal epilepsy resulted from an excessive response of cortical neurons to those thalamocortical volleys which are responsible for production of normal sleep spindles. In 1942 Morrison and Dempsey[35] produced recruiting responses following intralaminar thalamic stimulation. Later in 1947 Jasper and Droogleever-Fortuyn[39] succeeded in producing 3 Hz spike and wave discharges following similar stimulation in presence of cortical hyperexcitability. Spencer and Brookhart[40,41] showed similarities between recruiting responses and cortical sleep spindles in the cat. Both of these waves resulted from summated postsynaptic potentials of cortical neurons due to low frequency thalamocortical volleys. Gloor[42] confirmed and extended these observations based on the feline model of generalized epilepsy induced by intramuscular penicillin and concluded that spike and wave discharges resulted from summated postsynaptic potentials of the cortical neurons as a result of the thalamocortical volleys which would normally produce sleep spindles and recruiting responses. Penicillin obviously caused cortical hyperexcitability. In this connection it is important to note that Niedermeyer[43] was the first to suggest that generalized synchronous spike and wave discharges originated from the physiological K complex.

Wyler[44] studied epileptic neurons during sleep and wakefulness in 14 normal and 17 abnormal neurons recorded from alumina gel-induced chronic neocortical epileptic foci in 4 male Macaca mulatta monkeys during transition between sleep and wakefulness. During sleep the neurons which were mildly epileptic during wakefulness changed their firing pattern drastically and behaved like neurons which were grossly epileptic during wakefulness. During sleep, normal neurons and those neurons which were grossly epileptic during wakefulness did not change the firing pattern significantly. The author concluded that the neurons may represent the "critical mass" for initiation of seizure activity during synchronized sleep which is characterized by burst-synchronizing events such as sleep spindles.

Shouse et al[45] studied the mechanism of seizure suppression during REM sleep in cats. They produced 2 seizure models in 20 cats: systemic penicillin epilepsy and electroconvulsive shock. They produced 2 types of lesions: bilateral electrolytic lesions in the medial-lateral pontine tegmentum producing a syndrome of REM sleep without atonia; and systemic atropine injection to produce REM sleep without thalamocortical EEG desynchronization. They made the following conclusions based on these experiments: (1) REM sleep retarded the spread of epileptiform discharges in the EEG. (2) The descending brain stem pathways responsible for lower motor neuron inhibition during REM sleep also protected against generalized motor seizure during REM sleep. (3) The mechanism to prevent spread of seizure discharge utilized a separate pathway in the ascending brain stem structures which caused thalamocortical EEG desynchronization during REM sleep. (4) Their data thus suggested a cholinergic mechanism for thalamocortical EEG desynchronization and for retardation of EEG discharges during wakefulness and REM sleep. They further concluded that for generalized epilepsy REM sleep was the most potent antiepileptic state in the sleep-wake cycle. It is important to note that Cohen et al[46] found lowered convulsive threshold during REM deprivation in the cats. REM deprivation thus may exacerbate epilepsy.

EFFECT OF SLEEP ON EPILEPSY

General Description

Because of the awareness of an intimate relationship between sleep and epilepsy in the past various authors tried to classify seizures according to the time of occurrence of the seizures (clinical and electrical) during certain times in the sleep-wake cycle. Thus, seizures have been classified as waking epilepsy, sleep epilepsy, diffuse epilepsies (both diurnal and nocturnal) as well as circadian, ultradian and infradian epilepsies.

As early as 1885 Gowers[4] analyzed 840 institutionalized patients with a variety of seizure disorders and observed 21% of seizures occurring exclusively at night, 42% exclusively in daytime and 37% at random both during day and night. According to Gowers[4] the two most susceptible periods were the onset of sleep and the end of sleep. Langdon-Down and Brain[8] and later Patry[9] made somewhat similar observations. In all these 3 series the analysis was based on institutionalized patients. Langdon-Down and Brain[8] observed that 24% had sleep epilepsies, 43% had diurnal and 33% diffuse epilepsies in a series of 66 patients. In a sample size of 31 Patry[9] found 19% sleep epilepsies, 45% diurnal and 36% diffuse epilepsies. Taking the average of these 3 groups of institutionalized epileptics the incidence of 3 types of seizures in relation to sleep-wake cycle is found to be as follows: 22% sleep epilepsies; 44% diurnal epilepsies; and 34% diffuse epilepsies. Thus, the incidence is fairly similar in these 3 series. Langdon-Down and Brain[8] found the peak incidence of waking epilepsies 1–2 hours after awakening, i.e., about 7:00 to 8:00 A.M.; smaller peaks were found at around 3:00 P.M. and 6:00 to 8:00 P.M. Sleep epilepsies had 2 peaks: 10:00–11:00 P.M. and 4:00–5:00 A.M., i.e., early and late at night similar to that noted by Gowers.[4]

Amongst the contemporary epileptologists, Janz[13,47] contributed most towards classification of seizure based on sleep-wake cycle. Janz[13,47] analyzed 2 large series of outpatients with tonic-clonic generalized seizures. In the first series of 2110 patients[13] he found 45% sleep epilepsies, 34% diurnal and 21% diffuse epilepsies. In the second series of 2825 similar patients[47] the incidence was 44% sleep epilepsies, 33% diurnal and 23% diffuse epilepsies. Therefore, the 2 series were quite similar. Janz[13] called diurnal seizure awakening epilepsies because of high prevalence of seizure during awakening from sleep. Billiard[20] in a sample size of 314 outpatient seizure patients found 15% sleep, 53% diurnal and 32% diffuse epilepsies. It should be noted that Billiard[20] included a variety of types of epilepsies in his analysis. Earlier Hopkins[48] analyzed a series of outpatient tonic-clonic generalized seizures and found 51% sleep epilepsies, 30% diurnal and 19% diffuse epilepsies. Janz[13,47] also noted increased frequency at the beginning and end of the night in sleep epilepsies similar to that observed by Gowers[4] in the last century. It is important to note that the earlier classification was based only on clinical studies and no night time EEGs were obtained. The contemporary epileptologists and neurologists had the benefit of obtaining the EEG and all night polysomnographic studies utilizing the standard sleep scoring criteria. As regards stability of the type Janz[13] reported that 10% of awakening epilepsies later became sleep epilepsies while only 6% became diffuse epilepsies in course of time. According to Janz[13,47] and Hopkins[48] sleep and diffuse epilepsies lasting for 2 years rarely become awakening epilepsies.

The differences in the incidence of the 3 types of seizures may be due to the selection of patients (i.e., outpatient, institutionalized, generalized or partial seizures). The importance of classification based on sleep-wake cycle is that this classification may shed light on the prognosis and etiology. Patients with diffuse epilepsies often have intractable seizures, have structural neurological deficits with poor prognosis as against patients with awakening or sleep epilepsies.[49] Analyzing the various data Shouse[49] stated that idiopathic type is generally awakening type, those associated with organic structural lesions are of the diffuse type and the sleep epilepsies are intermediate in terms of organicity. D'Alessandro et al[50] analyzed 1200 patients visiting the epilepsy center during a 5 year period (1974–1979). They found that 90 out of 1200 (7.5%) had sleep epilepsy, i.e., had 1 or more seizures exclusively during sleep. This frequency is lower than that found by Janz[13] and Kajtor[51] but similar to that noted by Gibberd and Bateson.[52] The authors concluded that pure sleep epilepsies have a good prognosis. They rarely have waking seizures during the first few years after the onset of epilepsy.

The question I would like to discuss next is whether epilepsy manifests biorhythmicity. Specifically are there circadian, ultradian, or even infradian epilepsies? Kellaway et al[21,53] cited the specific relationship of epileptic phenomenon to the sleep-wake cycle as an example of a circadian rhythm. It should, however, be noted that Autret et al[54] noted an increase in the focal discharges during NREM stages I and II and of generalized discharges during NREM stages III and IV and a reduction or disappearance of the discharges in REM sleep during any time of the day and night. This is against a circadian rhythmicity. Kellaway and co-workers[21,53,55] thought that epileptiform actively may be linked to 2 rhythms: Circadian and ultradian related to NREM-REM cycle at 90–100 minutes. Stevens et al[56] suggested in adults that focal EEG discharges may at times show an ultradian 90–100 minutes periodicity in phase with prior NREM-REM sleep cycles throughout the day and night. Binnie,[57] Martins da Silva and Binnie[58] also noted periodicities of interictal discharges both during diurnal waking and nocturnal sleep EEG recordings. In most of their patients periodicities were longer or shorter than the typical 90–100 minutes REM-NREM cycle. However, Kellaway et al[53] failed to document waking ultradian rhythmicity in petit mal spike wave discharges. In one case of petit mal absence Broughton et al[59] provided strong evidence for ultradian daytime variations of spike-wave discharges mainly at the REM cycle rate. However, these observations have been made based only on one case study.

There are clear methodological problems in studying the biorhythmicity in epilepsy.[57] The classical methods include temporal isolation to observe the free running rhythms (entrainment) or by shifting the time zone. However, such studies in epilepsy have not been performed in detail.[57]

Finally, the question of infradian rhythmicity in epilepsy as exemplified by the catamenial epilepsy (i.e., menstrual-related epilepsy) remains controversial. Almqvst[60] found a periodicity in 47 out of 146 long-stay patients with epilepsy. The author noted that in some of the female patients the interval of the attack was equal to the period of the menstrual cycle. However, as mentioned by Newmark and Penry[61] the concept of catamenial epilepsy, although generally accepted, remains questionable as far as published evidence is concerned.

In conclusion, epilepsy in some patients may show a circadian temporal periodicity and an association with sleep periodicity, but it is not known if this periodicity is "state" linked (sleep vs. wakefulness) or "time" (nocturnal vs diurnal) linked.[62] Epileptic events are thought to be "state-dependent" by Webb[62] but "time-dependent" by Martins da Silva and Binnie.[58] Little is thus known why a seizure occurs at a particular time of the day or night. This understanding may be important for effective control of epilepsy by optimization of the drug regimen. Binnie[57] aptly raised the question without an answer: Can we improve patient care if we learn about biorhythms in epilepsy? Because of inconsistencies and contradictions in terms of classification related to biorhythms the modern epileptologists use the International classification of epilepsy.[63]

SPECIFIC DESCRIPTION IN RELATION TO SEIZURE TYPES:

In this section I will briefly describe the effect of sleep on the clinical seizures as well as on the interictal EEG epileptiform discharges in both the generalized and partial seizures.

Clinical Seizures

Generalized epilepsies

These commonly include generalized tonic-clonic (Grand Mal) epilepsy, Petit Mal (absence epilepsy), juvenile myoclonic epilepsy, infantile spasms (West syndrome) and Lennox-Gastaut syndrome. Awakening epilepsy or epilepsy on waking, a term introduced by Janz[64] to separate this from sleep and diffuse epilepsies, also belongs to the category of generalized epilepsies which include generalized tonic-clonic, absence and benign juvenile myoclonic seizure. Some varieties of diffuse epilepsies (e.g.,

Lennox-Gastaut and West syndrome, progressive myoclonic epilepsies) also belong to generalized seizures.

Primary generalized grand mal seizure. Primary generalized "grand mal" seizure occurs almost exclusively in non-REM sleep[65] and is most frequently seen 1–2 hours after sleep onset and at 5–6 a.m. as noted originally in 1985 by Gowers[4] and later by others.[8,9,13] Grand mal seizure may occur only during sleep, only during daytime or randomly distributed. In a study of 171 patients Billiard et al[66] found exclusively nocturnal seizures in only 8%. This study also confirmed the observations of Passouant et al[67] and Bessett[65] that primary generalized seizure occurs exclusively in non-REM sleep. Passouant[68] called the seizure occurring exclusively during sleep "L'Épilepsie morphéique" and this is considered a benign form of epilepsy. These patients rarely go on to develop waking epilepsies and only after the first 2 years of onset.[50]

Petit mal (absence) epilepsy. Absence seizures occurring during sleep are difficult to diagnose and clinical absence seizures are observed in the waking state. According to Niedermeyer[17] there may be fluttering of the eyelids during the spike and wave discharges in sleep. Gastaut and colleagues[69,70] and Patry et al[71] described occasional cases of petit mal status in REM sleep.

Juvenile myoclonic epilepsy. Meier-Ewert and Broughton[72] noted increased myoclonic seizures shortly after awakening in the morning and the duration of the attack is longer on awakening from non-REM than from REM sleep. Occasionally these attacks may occur on awakening in the middle of the night or later in the afternoon.[9,13,73]

Lennox-Gastaut syndrome. In this syndrome the clinical seizures consist of tonic, myoclonic, generalized tonic-clonic, atonic and atypical absences.[74] Information regarding the effect of sleep on the clinical seizures in this syndrome is lacking in the literature.[75] Tonic seizures, however, are typically activated by sleep[76] and are much more frequent during NREM sleep than during wakefulness and are never seen during REM sleep.[77]

West syndrome (infantile spasms). Maximum clinical seizures, often spasms in series, are seen on arousal from sleep or prior to going to sleep.[21,78] Less than 3% of spasms are obtained in sleep.

Partial epilepsies

Clinical seizures in simple and complex partial seizures are more frequent during the day.[20,50] In Billiard's[20] study of 156 patients, 61.5% had daytime and 11.5% had nocturnal seizures only. According to Montplaisir and co-workers[79-82] and Rossi et al[83] REM sleep did not facilitate temporal lobe seizure. However, other authors[67,84-86] observed ictal phenomena during both stages of sleep. In fact Epstein and Hill[86] described a case of temporal lobe seizure with unpleasant dreams during REM sleep associated with increased epileptiform activities in the EEG in the temporal region.

Pure sleep epilepsies mostly present as focal seizures with or without secondary generalization.[13,20] Benign Rolandic epilepsy and electrical status epilepticus during sleep (ESES) are also typical examples of sleep epilepsies which will be described in the next sections.

Interictal Epileptiform Discharges

Generalized seizures

Primary generalized "Grand Mal" tonic-clonic seizures. Interictal EEG discharges (Fig. 27-1) generally increase in NREM sleep and disappear in REM sleep.[18,20,54,70,87-89] Mostly the discharges are prominent at sleep onset and during the first part of the night. Sometimes the discharges are activated

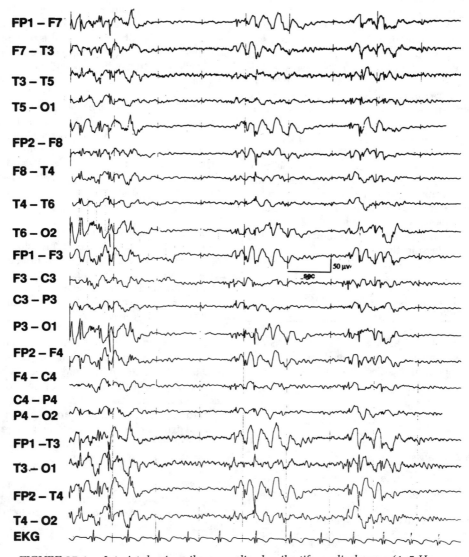

FIGURE 27-1. *Interictal primarily generalized epileptiform discharges (4–5 Hz spike-wave and multiple spike-wave discharges) seen synchronously and symmetrically with frontal dominance of amplitude in a patient with generalized tonic-clonic seizures.*

during non-REM sleep in the late part of the night which may have resulted from reduced serum levels of antiepileptic medications.[18] Interictal discharges may be fragmented or may appear as polyspikes or focal spikes during NREM sleep. According to Billiard[20] interictal discharges are more frequent during NREM than during REM sleep (41% vs 9%) in pure sleep epilepsy but in waking or random epilepsy interictal discharges are seen throughout the day and night. In patients with nocturnal epilepsies daytime EEG remains normal in high percentage of patients.[90]

Petit Mal (absence epilepsy) According to Sato et al,[91] Tassinari et al,[92] and Billiard et al[66] interictal EEG discharges (Fig. 27-2) in absence attacks are present during all stages of non-REM sleep. These are more marked during first sleep cycle[91] but generally absent in REM sleep. The pattern during REM sleep is similar to that during wakefulness with reduced duration.[91,92] Sato et al[91] described alterations of morphology of spike and wave discharges during different sleep stages: regular or irregular spike wave discharges in NREM stages I and II, and irregular polyspikes and slow waves during NREM

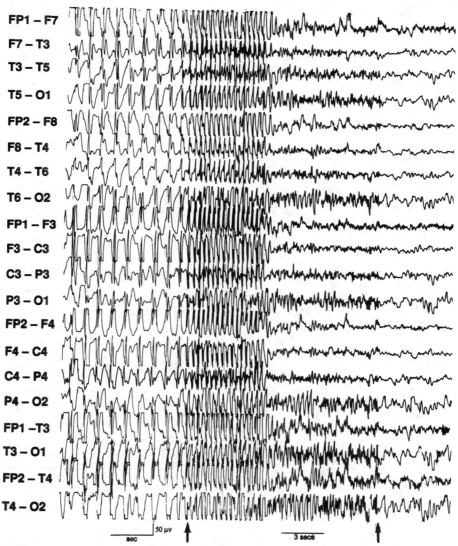

FIGURE 27-2. *3 Hz spike and wave discharges noted synchronously and symmetrically with dominance of the amplitude anteriorly in a patient with absence spells (Petit Mal). Note the paper speed on the left-hand panel at 30 mm/sec (sec) and on the right-hand panel at 10 mm/sec (3 secs; between the arrows).*

stages III and IV. In addition, fragmentation focalization of spikes can be seen over the frontal regions during NREM sleep.

Juvenile myoclonic epilepsy Interictal discharges (Fig. 27-3) in these patients are prominent at sleep onset and on awakening but are virtually nonexistent during rest of the sleep cycle.[18] According to Touchon[73] induced awakening is a better facilitator than spontaneous awakening in these patients.

Lennox-Gastaut syndrome. The typical EEG (Fig. 27-4) finding in this syndrome is slow spike and wave (1.5–2.5 Hz). In sleep this may be intermixed with trains of fast spikes of 10–25 Hz lasting for 2 to 10 seconds (so called Grand Mal discharges) as interictal abnormalities. The spike and waves charac-

teristically increase in NREM sleep.[75] Sometimes bursts of electrodecremental activity may alternate with bursts of polyspikes giving rise to a burst-suppression-like pattern.[75] According to Markand[93] prognosis is better in those patients with significant increase of interictal EEG abnormalities during sleep.

West syndrome (infantile spasm). The characteristic EEG finding (Fig. 27-5) is hypsarrhythmia (high amplitude slow waves and spike or sharp waves occurring irregularly) which may show progressive changes during sleep. The characteristic pattern seen during wakefulness may increase in non-REM sleep. The hypsarrhythmic EEG of wakefulness may change during non-REM sleep into periodic bilaterally synchronous diffuse pattern interspersed with flattening resembling "burst suppression" pattern[67]

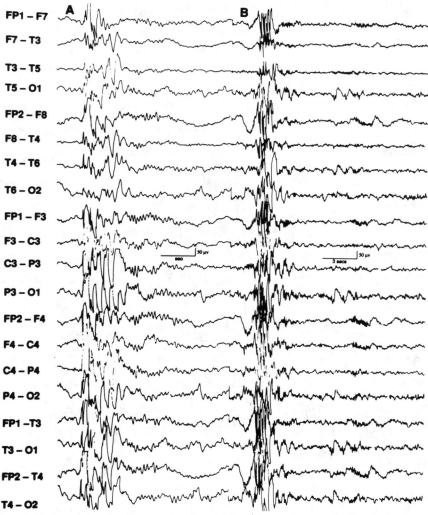

FIGURE 27-3.   *Interictal generalized multiple spike and wave discharges in the EEG of a patient with myoclonic epilepsy. Note the recording at 30 mm/sec (sec) on the left (A) and at 10 mm/sec (3 secs) on the right (B) side.*

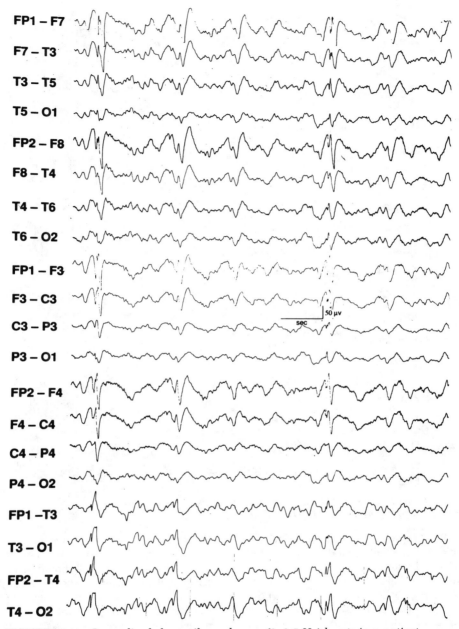

FIGURE 27-4. *Generalized slow spike and wave (2–2.5 Hz) bursts in a patient with Lennox-Gastaut syndrome.*

and may even normalize during REM sleep. Occasionally waking EEG may be normal but NREM sleep EEG may show the irregular high voltage slow waves and spikes.[94]

Partial epilepsies. An increase of interictal EEG discharges (Fig. 27-6) during non-REM and diminution or disappearance during REM sleep have been found both on surface and depth electrode studies as well as in animal studies.[85,95–97] On the other hand, Touchon,[73] Passouant et al,[98] Mayersdorf and Wilder[99] and Epstein and Hill[86] found an increase of focal temporal discharges during REM sleep. An important point to note is that during NREM sleep the discharges spread ipsilaterally and contralaterally from the primary focus while during REM sleep the discharges seem to focalize maximally.[80,88,100] Activation of discharges during REM sleep were also found by Frank and Pegram[101] in alumina cream monkey models of temporal lobe

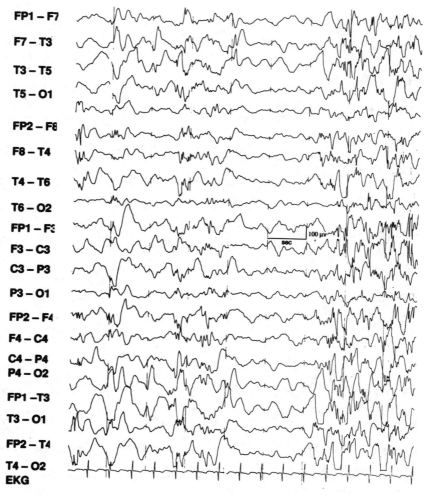

FIGURE 27-5.   *EEG showing hypsarrhythmic EEG pattern (for description see text) in a 9 month old girl with infantile spasms.*

epilepsies. But Mayanagi[102] did not confirm these findings in a similar monkey model.

Depth electrode studies in human by Montplaisir et al[82] and Lieb et al[100] showed increased spike discharges during NREM sleep and a reduction of the discharges during REM sleep. Depth electrode studies also showed that during REM sleep the spike discharges became maximally focalized.[82,83,100]

Autret et al[89] reviewed 236 adult epileptics attending outpatient clinics and they classified the seizures in 2 ways: 1. According to the time of onset of seizures by history, e.g., diurnal, nocturnal, waking and diffuse epilepsies; and 2. according to the interictal activation during all night polysomnographic study. They found more frequent myoclonic attacks and increased seizure frequency in patients with diurnal epilepsy. Patients with increased incidence of interictal activities during sleep have less generalized motor seizure but more frequent partial complex seizures, a higher seizure frequency and the

appearance of new interictal activities during sleep. They did not find a significant relationship between these two classifications. It should be noted that these data are at variance with the results of Janz.[13,47]

Lieb et al[100] performed all night depth electrode recordings in 10 patients with medically refractory partial complex seizures and used computer spike recognition technique for depth spike activities arising from medial temporal lobe sites. They found most frequent depth spike activity during deep sleep in 6 and light sleep in 3 patients and equal number during sleep and light sleep in 1 patient. They did not find a strong relationship between temporal lobe epilepsy and sleep pattern. Their findings that the discharge rates are greatest during non-REM sleep and are suppressed during REM sleep are in agreement with the previous reports of temporal lobe epileptics. Similar depth electrode findings in temporal lobe epilepsies have also been reported by Montplaisir and co-workers[79–82,103] and Passouant.[104] The only differ-

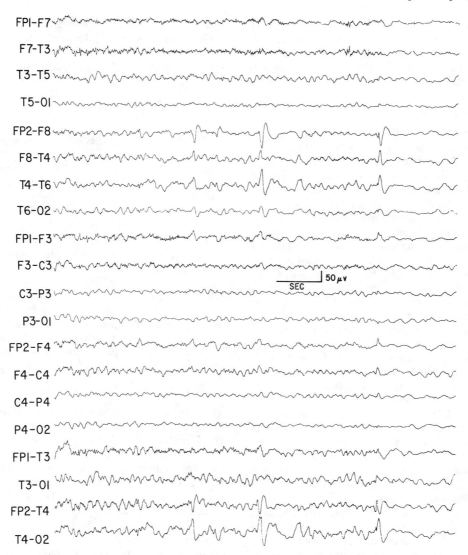

FPI-F7

F7-T3

T3-T5

T5-OI

FP2-F8

F8-T4

T4-T6

T6-O2

FPI-F3

F3-C3

C3-P3

P3-OI

FP2-F4

F4-C4

C4-P4

P4-O2

FPI-T3

T3-OI

FP2-T4

T4-O2

50 μν

SEC

FIGURE 27-6. *Focal right anterior and midtemporal sharp and slow waves showing phase reversal at F8-T4 electrodes in a patient with partial complex seizure.*

ence is that in some previous studies[85,105] maximal spike activity was seen during light sleep. In the study by Lieb et al[100] the side showing maximal spike activity did not necessarily correspond to the site chosen for temporal lobectomy. This suggests that the interictal spikes and seizure generating capacity may not bear a close relationship to underlying pathology.

Rossi et al[83] obtained direct cerebral recordings (Stereo EEG) by stereotactic implantation of stainless steel electrodes on preselected brain sites in 19 patients suffering from medically refractory partial epilepsy and were potential candidates for surgery. They found that interictal spiking increased at the onset of sleep reaching maximum during deep non-REM sleep and returned to a lower level during REM sleep. The level in REM sleep was slightly lower as compared with the activity during wakefulness. They further noted that the spike rate was not influenced by spike location and the rate of spiking was affected by the local level of epileptogenicity, i.e., higher the epileptogenicity lower was the variation. They further noted that the interictal spiking across sleep and wakefulness showed wide variation in different patients and in the different regions of the same patients.

In conclusion, NREM sleep is the stage of augmentation of interictal focal and generalized EEG discharges. In REM sleep generalized discharges are usually suppressed but focal discharges may persist.

In order to explain the variation in spiking during sleep and wakefulness, three factors may be cited:[83] (1) Subcortical-cortical interplay of mechanism for sleep and wakefulness as well as EEG synchronization;

(2) Alteration in the cortical excitability during sleep and wakefulness; and (3) Location of the epileptic lesion. The first factor may play a role in the generalized seizure and the second and the third factors may play in a role in the genesis of the partial seizures.

Status Epilepticus

The information regarding effect of sleep on status epilepticus is limited as this is a neurological emergency and the first priority is treatment of the patients rather than spending time on prolonged recording. Therefore, limited information is available in certain types of status epilepticus. Gastaut[106] defined status as a condition in which seizure persists for a sufficient length of time or is repeated frequently enough to produce a fixed and enduring epileptic condition. An arbitrary time of 30–60 minutes has been accepted as a time to justify the term. Gastaut[106] classified status into three types: (1) Generalized status epilepticus consisting of convulsive and nonconvulsive types; (2) simple and partial complex status epilepticus; and (3) unilateral status epilepticus.

Generalized tonic-clonic (Grand Mal) status epilepticus recurs during early part of the night.[107] Tonic status as may be seen in patients with Lennox-Gastaut syndrome occurs almost exclusively during sleep and is seen mostly during NREM sleep.[108] Myoclonic status epilepticus may arise in two forms:[106] as part of the primary generalized status epilepticus and the type associated with acute or subacute encephalopathies. In both the conditions the myoclonic status epilepticus is markedly attenuated during sleep.[108] Petit mal status or absence status epilepticus may be terminated during sleep.[108] Gastaut and Tassinari[109] demonstrated that non-REM sleep disrupts the EEG discharges which are replaced by polyspikes or polyspike-wave complexes or even isolated bursts of spikes. According to several authors[110–112] there may be recurrence of absence status on awakening during the night or in the morning. Occasionally the spike and wave discharges of petit mal status epilepticus may persist during NREM and REM sleep throughout the night.[110] In simple partial, status epilepticus both improvement and activation during sleep have been noted.[108] According to Froscher[108] the role of nocturnal sleep in partial complex status epilepticus has remained unknown. The entity of electrical status epilepticus in sleep will be discussed below.

SPECIAL SEIZURE TYPES RELATED TO SLEEP-WAKE CYCLE

Certain varieties of epilepsy are seen during specific periods of human sleep-wake cycle: (1) Benign focal epilepsy of childhood with rolandic spikes (BERS); (2) Juvenile myoclonic epilepsy of Janz; (3) Epileptic syndrome with generalized tonic-clonic seizure on awakening, and (4) Electrical status epilepticus during sleep (ESES).

Benign Focal Epilepsy of Childhood with Rolandic Spikes (BERS)

A clear description of this electroclinical syndrome was given by Nayrac and Beaussart in 1958.[113] Later Beaussart[114] drew attention to the benign nature of the condition. This is a childhood seizure seen mostly during drowsiness and sleep. The clinical seizures are characterized by focal clonic facial seizures often preceded by perioral numbness. In many cases the patients have generalized tonic-clonic seizures which appear to be secondary generalization. There is sometimes speech arrest. The consciousness is preserved. The EEG shows centrotemporal or rolandic spikes or sharp waves (Fig. 27-7). These discharges are present throughout the night in all stages of sleep. The prognosis is excellent with cessation of seizures by the age of 15 to 20 and without any neurological sequelae. The patients respond to anticonvulsants satisfactorily.

Juvenile Myoclonic Epilepsy of Janz

This electroclinical syndrome was described by Janz and Mathes[115] and later published in detail by Janz and Christian.[116] The onset of the syndrome is usually between 13 and 19 years and is manifested by massive bilaterally synchronous myoclonic jerks which are most commonly seen in the morning shortly after awakening.[116,117] The EEG is characterized by generalized spike and wave and typically polyspike and wave discharges (Fig. 27-3) seen in a synchronous and symmetrical manner. The response to anticonvulsant is excellent and in this respect it is benign and easily distinguishable from the malignant syndrome of progressive myoclonus epilepsies.

Epileptic Syndrome with Generalized Tonic-Clonic Seizure on Awakening[117,118]

This syndrome is manifested by the occurrence in the second decade of generalized tonic-clonic seizures on awakening from sleep. This is a rare syndrome and clinically there may be occasional absence or myoclonic manifestations and photosensitivity resembling juvenile myoclonic epilepsy.

Electrical Status Epilepticus During Sleep (ESES) or Continuous Spike and Waves During Sleep (CSWS)

This is a disease of childhood characterized by generalized continuous spike and wave EEG discharges during slow wave sleep. All night polysomnographic

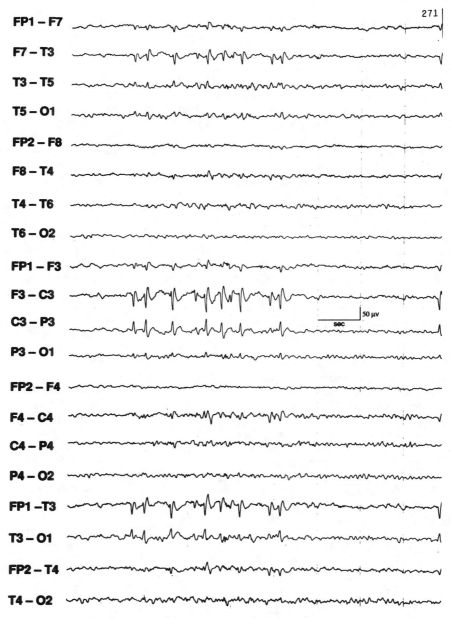

FIGURE 27-7. *Left centrotemporal spikes and sharp waves in a patient with benign focal epilepsy of childhood with rolandic spikes.*

study is necessary for diagnosis. The patients display progressive behavioral disturbances, although the seizures disappear within months or years. This entity is rare and found in children between 5–15 years. This was first described by Patry et al[71] in 1971 in 6 children and later Tassinari et al[119] reviewed the literature and described 19 cases of their own. Most of the patients had a prior history of epilepsy. The characteristic EEG finding consists of 2 to 2.5 cycle per second generalized spike and wave discharges seen during at least 85% of NREM sleep

and suppressed during REM sleep. Occasional bursts of spike and waves or focal frontal spikes were noted during REM sleep. During wakefulness there were a few bursts of generalized spike and wave discharges seen in the EEG. These EEG discharges disrupted the different stages of NREM sleep and in particular the vertex sharp waves, K-complexes and spindles could not be well recognized. However, the cyclic pattern of REM-NREM persisted normally. Usually, there were no sleep disturbances but some children had difficulty awakening in the morning.

EFFECT OF SLEEP DEPRIVATION ON EPILEPSY

The diagnostic value of sleep deprived EEG has been well documented.[95,120–123] What is the mechanism of activation during sleep deprivation? This is probably not a sampling effect and not related to sleep alone.[120,121,123] Sleep deprivation increases the epileptiform discharges mostly in the transition period between waking and light sleep and it also has a localizing value.[121,123] Although the original study by Rodin et al[124] in 1962 found epileptiform discharges in healthy subjects after sleep deprivation, later studies[123,125] failed to confirm these observations.

Rowan et al[121] studied consecutive 43 patients using two types of activation: sleep deprivation (24 hrs in adults and partial deprivation in children) and sedated sleep (after oral secobarbital). They obtained useful information in 44% of sleep deprived as against 14% of sedated sleep records. The patients were referred because of doubtful diagnosis of epilepsy or because seizure types could not be determined. They also found sleep deprivation superior to sedated sleep for differentiating those with a final diagnosis of true seizure. It should be noted that sleep alone does not explain the activating effect of sleep deprivation. The mechanism remains largely unknown. Rowan et al[121] suggested increased cerebral excitability following sleep deprivation in normal individuals.

Degen[122] studied 127 waking and sleep EEGs after sleep deprivation in 120 epileptic patients on anticonvulsant medication. He found seizure activity in 63% of the patients while in the previous EEG records of these patients only 19% had shown seizure activity; thus sleep deprivation increased the incidence of seizure activity. Approximately 48% of discharges occurred during slow wave and 25% during REM sleep.

It is interesting to note that in 1896 Patrick and Gilbert[126] apparently used sleep deprivation study in human beings, however, the studies by Bennett[127] in 1963 and Mattson et al[128] in 1965 established the value of sleep deprivation as a diagnostic tool in patients with seizure disorders. Rodin[129] computed the incidence of activation following sleep deprivation from an analysis of the literature and the figure appears to be around 45%.

PHENOMENA DURING SLEEP WHICH MAY BE MISTAKEN FOR EPILEPSY (NONEPILEPTIFORM DISORDERS)

Certain parasomnias in NREM sleep which are paroxysmal arousal disorders may be mistaken for seizures, particularly for partial complex seizures. Some examples of these disorders are the following:

night terror (pavor nocturnus), somnambulism (sleep walking), somniloquy (sleep talking), tooth grinding (bruxism), head banging (jactatio capitis nocturnas), nocturnal enuresis. There are two other parasomnias, namely, REM behavior disorder and nightmares (dream-anxiety attacks) which are considered as parasomnias usually associated with REM sleep. These conditions are described in chapter 24 by Broughton.

Paroxysmal nocturnal dystonia and periodic limb movements in sleep are two other nocturnal events which may be mistaken for seizures and these are described in chapter 19.

Episodic nocturnal wanderings as described by Pedley and Guilleminault[130] may represent special types of nocturnal seizures. However, whether these are true nocturnal seizures or a type of parasomnias can not be definitely ascertained although the patients showed interictal EEG epileptiform abnormalities and responded to anticonvulsant. Finally, small sharp spikes or benign epileptiform transients of sleep as noted in the EEG (Fig. 27-8) in stages I and II NREM sleep may resemble true epileptiform spikes but the distribution, morphology and the occurrence during particular stages of sleep without any clinical accompaniments differentiate these from the true epileptiform spikes.[131]

The above nocturnal events (clinical and electrographic) of nonepileptiform significance must be differentiated from true epileptic attacks otherwise unnecessary medications and tests will be used. Characteristic clinical features combined with EEG and polysomnographic recordings are important to differentiate these conditions. It should be noted that presence of EEG epileptiform discharges independent of nocturnal attacks may not be proof sine qua non that the attacks are of epileptic nature.[19] However, video-EEG recordings to correlate behavior with EEG manifestations may establish or exclude the diagnosis. Sometimes the two conditions (epileptic and nonepileptic attacks) may coexist. Finally, an improvement after empirical treatment with the anticonvulsant medication does not necessarily prove the epileptic nature of the condition.[19]

EFFECT OF EPILEPSY ON SLEEP

An objective evaluation of the states of sleep in epileptic patients reveals that they are altered in a large percentage of patients studied. Although the utility of sleep in the diagnosis of epilepsy is well established, the altered sleep characteristics in epileptics are not well known. One of the difficulties has been that most of the studies have been conducted in patients who have been on anticonvulsants thus adding the confounding factors of the effect of anticonvulsants on sleep architecture. Furthermore,

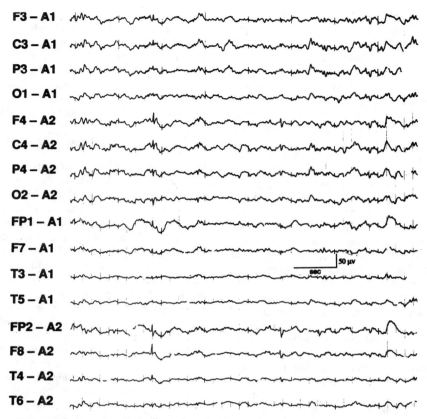

FIGURE 27-8. *Small sharp spikes (benign epileptiform transients of sleep) seen in channels 5–8 and 13–16 from the top.*

there have not been good longitudinal studies to determine the effect of epilepsy on sleep in the early versus late stage of the illness. Despite this limitation there have been several studies and a general consensus has arisen regarding the effect of epilepsy on sleep and sleep structure. A variety of sleep disturbances have been observed in epileptics and can be summarized as follows:[85,87,98,132,133] a reduction in REM sleep; an increase in WASO (wake after sleep onset); increased instability of sleep states, such as unclassifiable sleep epochs; an increase in NREM stages I and II; a decrease in NREM sleep stages III and IV; a reduction in the density of sleep spindles; and an increase of sleep onset latency.

Three questions may be asked regarding the effect of epilepsy on sleep: (1) Is it related to the duration and type of seizures? (2) Is it related to repeated episodes of seizures or poorly controlled seizures? (3) Can epilepsy lead to a sleep disorder? These questions will be discussed below.

Relationship Between Seizure Type and Sleep

WASO, sleep stage shifts and sleep fragmentation are found in all seizure types.[65,132,134–137] Reduction of REM sleep and an increase in NREM stages I

and II are in part dependent on the type of epilepsy. Declerck et al[132] found an increase of NREM stages I and II and a reduction of REM sleep in 258 patients with primary generalized or partial seizure with secondary generalization as compared with 223 nonepileptic subjects. Similar findings are obtained by Bessett et al.[65] Baldy-Moulinier[134] noted a decrease of REM sleep in patients with partial complex seizures occurring during sleep. It is interesting to note that Bessett[65] in human epileptics and Baldy-Moulinier[134] in temporal lobe epilepsy models found no rebound REM sleep in subsequent recordings following REM sleep loss which is contrary to the usual findings of REM rebound following REM deprivation. In summary, WASO and sleep fragmentation are found in all types of epilepsy; generalized seizures are associated with reduction of NREM stages I and II and REM sleep. In partial complex seizure there is often REM reduction only.

Hoeppner et al[138] studied self-reported sleep disorders symptoms in epilepsy. They gave a questionnaire on sleep relating to 6 aspects of sleep: delayed sleep onset; night awakenings; dreams; night terrors; sleep walking and fatigue on awakening. They evaluated four groups of subjects: (1) Four patients with simple partial seizures; (2) Eighteen patients with partial complex seizure; (3) Eight patients with generalized seizures; and (4) Twenty-three controls (14 females and 9 men aged 16–53 years). They found significantly more sleep disorders symptoms (particularly frequent awakenings at night) in patients with simple and partial complex seizures. The generalized group behaved like the control group. Patients with most frequent seizures irrespective of the type, had the most sleep disturbances.

Roder-Wanner et al[139] obtained polygraphic sleep recordings in 43 patients with different types of epilepsies. They found that patients with generalized epilepsy had higher percentage of deeper stages of sleep (NREM III and IV) than in patients with focal epilepsy. These observations are correlated with the factor of photosensitivity which was noted in a subgroup of these patients. The authors concluded that there was no real relationship between sleep structure and the type of epilepsy. Thus there is some controversy regarding the relationship between seizure type and sleep. In previous studies sleep structure abnormalities may have been related to clinical or subclinical seizure activity preceding the polysomnographic investigation or may have been related to the medication received during the study.

Regarding REM sleep disturbance there are contradictory reports.[87] On seizure free nights REM sleep is usually normal, but REM decrement is noted when there are primary or secondary generalized seizures during the night. There is no REM suppression during partial seizure without secondary generalization.[65,134] Bowersox and Drucker-Colin[140] stated that increased cortical neuronal excitability and reduced seizure threshold may result from chronic REM sleep deprivation secondary to repeated and frequent nocturnal generalized seizures.

Touchon et al[141] in a series of 15 patients with temporal lobe seizure disorders found increased WASO, shifting of the sleep stages and an increase of NREM sleep stages I and II. The site of the primary focus may determine the type of the sleep disturbances.[18] Foci in the amygdalo-hippocampal region may lead to increased WASO, and decreased sleep efficiency. On the other hand, frontal lobe epileptics may show a specific reduction in stages III and IV NREM sleep.

Severity of Seizure and Extent of Sleep Deficits

Seizure occurrence during sleep accentuates sleep deficits which are more marked in primary generalized and partial seizures with secondary generalization than in other types. In 25% of epileptics Declerck et al[132] could not evaluate polysomnographic recording because of severe encephalopathies associated with seizures. Bessett[65] could not discriminate NREM stages in the EEG and even REM sleep

because of disruption of sleep architecture due to the seizures (ictal and interictal). On the other hand, Baldy-Moulinier[134] found marked reduction of REM sleep in patients having only one attack of secondary generalized seizure during the night. However, it can be concluded that the severity of sleep deficits is in part correlated with severity of the seizure disorder. Animal studies support such conclusions.[142,143]

Can Epilepsy Lead to a Sleep Disorder?

It is generally thought that sleep deficits in seizure disorders are secondary to the severity of seizure disorder and a direct result of seizures during sleep. However, studies by Tanaka and Naquet[144] demonstrated progressive sleep deficits in amygdala kindling model. Also the sleep deficits persisted after one month following discontinuation of kindling procedures.

Shouse and Sterman[142] produced amygdala kindling in 10 adult cats and studied their sleep and waking patterns chronically. They found a progressive sleep disturbance and retention of the deficit over a prolonged period following termination of amygdala stimulation. These findings suggest the "kindling" of a sleep disorder in addition to a seizure disturbance. The authors further stated that sleep abnormalities can not be viewed as a simple or temporary side effect of epileptiform activity. It appears that a permanent change in sleep physiology occurs in epilepsy. These observations of Shouse and Sterman[142] partially answer the question posed by Passouant:[1] "Can epilepsy lead to a sleep disorder?" Effective treatment of epilepsy with anticonvulsant medications or surgical methods normalizes sleep disturbances in human epilepsy.[136]

EFFECT OF ANTICONVULSANTS ON SLEEP IN EPILEPTICS

There is a dearth of well controlled careful studies to document the effects of anticonvulsant medications on the sleep architecture separating the effects of seizures on sleep. Only limited data are available. Johnson[136] reviewed the literature on acute and chronic exposure to anticonvulsant drugs in relation to the sleep pattern. Acute exposure to anticonvulsants may reduce REM and NREM stages III and IV and increase stage II NREM sleep. However, acute and chronic drug trials in epileptics suggest that the main effects of anticonvulsants consist of sleep stabilization which includes a reduction in WASO, an increase in NREM stages II, III and IV along with sleep spindle density. These improvements are concomitant with the reduction of seizures. The bulk of the evidence in the literature points to the fact that effective anticonvulsant treatment and control of seizure result in reduction of sleep disturbance. Thus, the effects are due to the reduction of seizures and not due to any specific effect of the anticonvulsants on sleep architecture.

In a survey in the experimental epilepsy in animals Wauquier et al[145] observed that sleep fragmentation as obtained in epileptic animals as well as in humans may be the consequence of microarousals. Anticonvulsants may suppress microarousals because of their sedative properties and hence lead to stabilization of sleep fragmentation and normalization of sleep. On the other hand, anticonvulsants may normalize sleep because of a specific action on particular abnormal EEG patterns. Thus, despite the suggestion that anticonvulsants themselves may be responsible in part for the fragmentation and disruption of sleep architecture the general consensus is that the anticonvulsant medications normalize the sleep architecture most probably by reduction of the seizures.

Touchon et al[146] studied sleep architecture in epileptic patients with partial complex seizures before and after treatment by carbamazepine. Initially, they studied 80 patients with partial complex seizures and found an increase in WASO and awakenings. These effects were not related to the seizure itself but may be related to the duration of seizure or to the anticonvulsants. They also found a decrement of sleep efficiency. In a later study they prospectively studied 10 patients with partial complex seizures and compared with a group of normal age-matched subjects. Seizure patients were on 800 milligram carbamazepine daily. Polysomnographic studies were made on two consecutive nights: two nights before and two nights after the patient had been on carbamazepine treatment for one month. Before instituting carbamazepine they found that the percentage of stage I NREM sleep, number of awakenings and WASO were increased. After carbamazepine treatment these sleep characteristics were partially modified and controlled by the treatment. They concluded that the length of seizure and drug treatment were not responsible for abnormal sleep architecture. The abnormal sleep structure may be related to seizure itself. Carbamazepine treatment improves sleep architecture to an extent.

Wolf et al[147] reviewed the literature to assess the effect of barbiturates, phenytoin, carbamazepine and valproic acid treatment on sleep. They noted significant reduction of REM sleep, a reduction in total awake time and an increase in NREM stage II sleep as the short-term effects of barbiturates. The long-term effects of barbiturates are somewhat similar or in some cases the sleep pattern returned to the premedication level.

Wolf et al[147] performed a prospective polygraphic study of sleep in epileptic patients before and after medications using a cross over design. They studied phenobarbital, phenytoin, ethosuximide, valproic acid and carbamazepine. They included 40 unmedicated patients to study the effect of phenobarbital

and phenytoin. The short-term effects of phenobarbital included reduction of WASO and REM sleep and increase of stage II NREM sleep. There was no relationship with the serum drug levels. The short-term effects of phenytoin included no change in the percentage of WASO but there was a decrease in NREM sleep stages I and II with an increase in sleep stages III and IV; REM sleep remained unaltered. Again there was no relationship with the serum drug levels.

In 12 patients Wolf et al[147] studied the long-term effects of phenytoin. The long-term effects were in general a reversal of the short-term effects and consisted of an increase of NREM sleep stages I and II with a decrease of stages III and IV. REM sleep, however, remained unaltered. The effects of ethosuximide included an increase in stage I, a decrease in stages III and IV sleep and increased awakenings.[147] Valproic acid similarly increased stage I but did not decrease the stages III and IV NREM sleep.[147]

Long-term phenytoin treatment by Hartmann[148] revealed a shortened sleep onset and an increase of light sleep in some subjects. Roder-Wanner et al[149] noted a temporary increase of slow wave sleep following phenytoin treatment.

Baldy-Moulinier[150] reported normalization of disturbed sleep pattern in temporal lobe epileptics after carbamazepine treatment. Following acute carbamazepine administration in cats Gigli et al[151] reported an increase of NREM stage I sleep and total sleep time, a decrease of REM sleep, and reduced duration of awakenings.

Findji et al[152] reported an improvement of sleep organization and an increase of deep NREM sleep in epileptic children after treatment with valproic acid. At high dosage, however, Harding et al[153] observed a decrease of delta and REM sleep.

A survey of the literature thus reveals that we need more studies to understand the interactions of the anticonvulsants, sleep and epilepsy. Based on the literature search and their own investigations, Declerck and Wauquier[154] emphasized the importance of the use and development of automatic methods to assess antiepileptic-induced sleep changes in patients with epilepsy. It may be that the anticonvulsants disrupt the circadian distribution of interictal discharges during the night and this may have practical relevance in terms of treatment.

SLEEP, EPILEPSY, AND AUTONOMIC DYSFUNCTION

There are a number of autonomic nervous system changes involving particularly the respiratory and the cardiovascular systems during sleep[155] (see also Chapter 5). Furthermore, epilepsy itself may cause changes in the autonomic nervous system and thus there is a close interrelationship between sleep, epilepsy, and the autonomic nervous system.

Autonomic nervous system (ANS) changes involving the cardiovascular system during sleep consist of reduction of the blood pressure and heart rate during NREM sleep and wide fluctuation of these during REM sleep.[155] Respiration shows considerable changes during NREM and REM in particular during REM sleep.[28] Sleep, adversely affects breathing even in normal individuals and sleep, of course, often triggers seizures in epileptic patients. A knowledge of the central autonomic network makes it easily understandable why such a relationship between ANS, sleep, circulation and respiration exists.[156] Nucleus tractus solitarius (NTS), an important structure in the region of the medulla, for controlling sleep, cardiovascular and respiratory regulation, is reciprocally connected with the limbic-hypothalamic and other forebrain structures[156] (see chapter 5). It is easy to understand then why epileptic seizures triggered by the limbic-hypothalamic or other forebrain structures may interact with the cardiovascular and respiratory regulation during sleep. Respiratory dysrhythmia during generalized seizures in man and following seizure discharges in the limbic system, and experimental stimulation of the limbic areas is known to occur.[157] However, the combination of sleep apnea and epilepsy is rare. There have been occasional reports[158-160] of upper airway obstructive, mixed and central sleep apneas in patients with epilepsy (Fig. 27-9).

It is well known that in generalized tonic-clonic and many patients with partial complex seizures transient abnormalities of ANS functions may occur and may consists of alterations in cardiac rhythms, blood pressure and respiration.[161] Also it is well known that epileptiform discharges without any clinical accompaniments may produce a variety of autonomic abnormalities. In patients after electroconvulsive[162] treatment and in animal models after pentylenetetrazol[163] injection there are intense changes in the blood pressure and cardiac rhythms. Similar changes have been observed in patients with focal temporal lobe discharges. Also the phenomenon of unexpected sudden death in patients with epilepsy[164] which may account for up to 15% may be the result of some unexplained autonomic dysfunction affecting the cardiac rhythm.

UTILITY OF SLEEP IN THE DIAGNOSIS OF EPILEPSY

Utility of sleep in the diagnosis of epilepsy is well established since the landmark paper by Gibbs and Gibbs[12] in 1947 showing activation of epileptiform discharges in the sleep EEG. For the diagnosis of

epilepsy a variety of sleep recordings are recommended: (1) standard sleep EEG recording; (2) EEG recording after sleep deprivation; (3) all night polysomnographic (PSG) study; (4) Video-polysomnographic (Video-PSG) study; (5) multiple sleep latency test; and (6) 24-hour ambulatory EEG and sleep recording. Table outlines a suggested protocol for EEG recording in patients suspected to have epilepsy.

Sleep EEG Recording and Sleep Deprivation Study

The usefulness of these two types of recordings have been discussed in detail in the above paragraphs. For such recordings a full complement of electrodes should be used and various montages have been suggested (see Chapter 6). Broughton[19] listed some of the main indications and objectives of the daytime sleep EEG recording as follows: (1) Normal EEGs in patients suspected of epilepsy in order to establish the diagnosis of true epilepsy; (2) Normal waking EEGs in patients with known epilepsy in order to clarify the type of epilepsy; (3) Patients with febrile convulsions showing normal waking EEGs; (4) An assessment of the familial predisposition to epilepsy in family members; and (5) an assessment of the degree of drug control, for example in patients with hypsarrhythmia.

TABLE 27-1. A Suggested Protocol for EEG Recording in Patients Suspected of Epilepsy

1. Routine EEG recording with hyperventilation and photic stimulation.
2. If negative for interictal epileptiform activity (IEA), EEG with sleep (natural or induced) recording
3. If negative for IEA, EEG study with partial (at least 4 hours) or total (24 hours) sleep deprivation
4. If negative for IEA after three to four EEGs, prolonged (4-6 hours) daytime EEG with sleep recording
5. If negative for IEA, overnight polysomnographic (PSG) study, preferably video-PSG study for electroclinical correlation

   Use paper speed of 30 mm/sec as used during standard EEG recording instead of the usual PSG recording speed of 10 mm/sec, particularly during suspicious behavioral episodes.

   Use appropriately devised seizure montage with full complement of electrodes (see Chapter 6) or special electrode placements (e.g., T1 and T2 electrodes).
6. If still negative for IEA, cassette ambulatory EEG recording
7. Finally, if still negative for IEA, long-term video-EEG monitoring for 24-72 hours or longer if necessary.

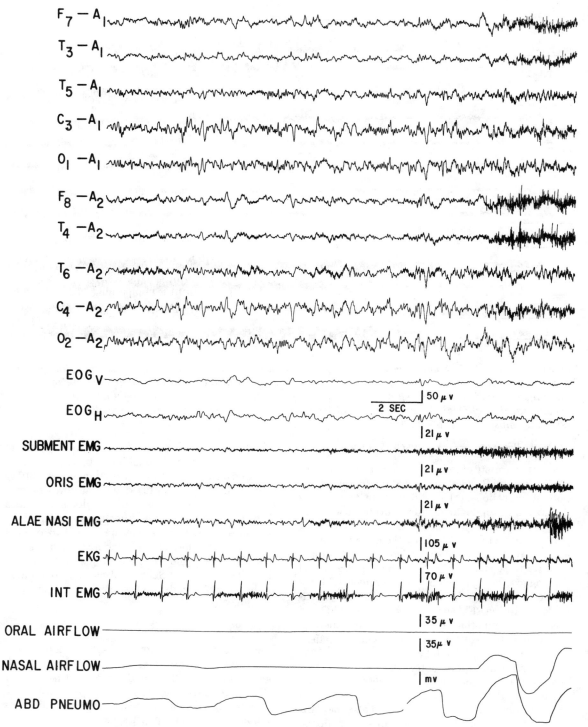

FIGURE 27-9. *Polysomnographic recording in a patient with partial complex seizure and sleep apnea showing EEG (Top 10 channels), vertical (EOGv) and horizontal (EOG_H) electrooculograms, submental (SUBMENT), orbicularis oris (ORIS), alae nasi and intercostal (INT) electromyograms (EMG), electrocardiogram (ECG), oral and nasal airflow, and abdominal pneumogram (ABD PNEUMO). Note upper airway obstructive apnea during NREM stage II sleep. No epileptiform discharges are seen in the EEG during the episodes. Paper speed = 15 mm/sec.*

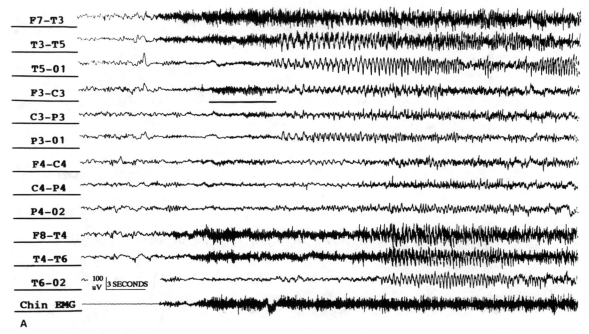

A

FIGURE 27-10.   *A. Portion of a polysomnographic recording using 12 channels of EEG showing the onset of a partial seizure recorded at 10 mm/sec paper speed. The underlined activity represents rhythmic ictal discharges beginning over the left hemisphere (F3-C3) and spreading rapidly to the right hemisphere, and is accompanied by clinical seizure. Although at 10 mm/sec paper speed the underlined activity superficially resembles muscle artifacts, at 30 mm/sec*

All Night Polysomnographic (PSG) Recording

There are a variety of indications to perform all night PSG study and Broughton[19] listed the following important indications: (1) To differentiate between epileptic and nonepileptic nocturnal events, e.g., pseudoseizures, syncope due to cardiac arrhythmias, parasomnias, etc.; (2) To clarify the classification in patients with known sleep epilepsies; (3) To diagnose electrical status epilepticus in sleep (ESES); (4) To diagnose benign epilepsy of childhood with rolandic spikes; (5) To lateralize or localize the principal focus during REM sleep by use of stereo-EEG and this may be important before surgical treatment is considered; (6) To unmask primary focus in a patient with secondary bilateral synchrony during REM sleep by causing suppression of the generalized discharges; (7) In patients with hypsarrhythmia where the waking EEGs rarely may be normal but sleep EEG may reveal the abnormalities and also for clarification of the focal abnormalities in such patients; (8) To diagnose tonic seizures in patients with Lennox-Gastaut syndrome; (9) To diagnose sleep apnea or other primary sleep disorder which may be mistaken for epilepsy or which may be associated with epilepsy; and (10) For investigation of patients complaining of excessive daytime somnolence

which cannot be explained by the anticonvulsant medication. Two additional indications are: to document cardiac arrhythmias which may arise during sleep and may be confused with seizures or may even give rise to seizures and to document sleep disturbances and sleep architecture in epileptics so that these disturbances may be treated to prevent chronic sleep deprivation which may have deleterious effects on epilepsy itself. In suspected seizure disorder all night PSG recording should include multiple EEG leads and special montages (see Chapter 6).

Video-PSG Study

The value of this study for the diagnosis of parasomnias and seizure disorders has been well-documented by Aldrich and Jahnke[165] (see Chapter 14). Figure 27-10 is a polysomnograph showing the onset of a partial seizure recorded at 10 mm/sec as well as at 30 mm/sec paper speed.

Multiple Sleep Latency Test (MSLT)[166]

This test is indicated in patients complaining of excessive daytime somnolence which may not be explained on the basis of anticonvulsant medication. Furthermore, seizure during sleep may lead to

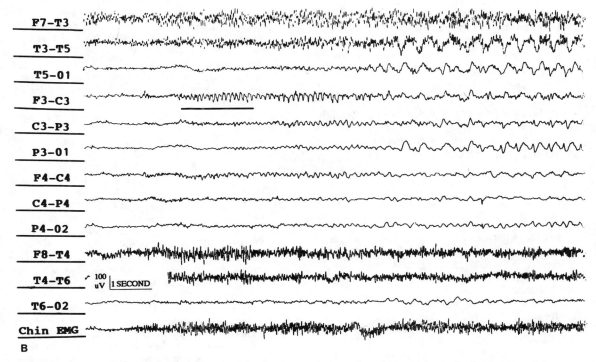

FIGURE 27-10. *(continued) (B) paper speed it becomes obvious that this activity is the beginning of the rhythmic epileptiform discharges in the EEG. (Reprinted with permission[165] from Aldrich M, Jahnke B. Diagnostic value of video-EEG polysomnography. Neurology 1991;41:1060–1066.)*

repeated arousals causing excessive daytime somnolence with further increase of seizure frequency thus creating a vicious cycle. Sometimes patients with narcolepsy may be mistaken for epilepsy and an important diagnostic test in narcolepsy is MSLT. And finally, as stated above, patients with epilepsy may have sleep apnea, which may cause excessive daytime somnolence and this could be diagnosed by showing reduced sleep onset latency on MSLT.

Ambulatory 24-Hour EEG Recording and Sleep Scoring

This test is important to record the EEG discharges throughout the day to understand the circadian and ultradian rhythmicity and the effects of sleep on the interictal discharges. The question of epilepsy and biorhythmicity has been discussed above.

PRACTICAL RELEVANCE TO UNDERSTAND RELATIONSHIP BETWEEN SLEEP AND EPILEPSY

An understanding of the relationship between sleep and epilepsy is important for three main purposes:

1. For the diagnosis of seizure and for the purpose of differential diagnosis between epileptic and nonepileptic events and between different types of seizures.
2. For understanding the pathogenesis of triggering mechanisms of seizures during sleep and for understanding the mechanism and the nature of sleep disturbances induced by epilepsy.
3. For therapeutic manipulation. It may be possible to adjust the timing of the drug dose but this really has not been useful from a practical point of view. An understanding of the biorhythmicity and the relationship between sleep and epilepsy may be important to choose the type of anticonvulsant so that one may avoid those with marked hypnotic effects in nocturnal seizure patients and use drugs with less sedative effects (e.g., carbamazepine, valproic acid, felbamate). Finally, one may manipulate sleep stages, that is, give anticonvulsants which may increase REM or NREM stages III and IV to reduce the ictal or interictal discharges.

Finally, as Broughton[19] stated that because of the deleterious effects of the epilepsy on sleep and sleep on epilepsy it may be important in some patients to follow a strict program of sleep hygiene (see Table 17-3) or even to treat the sleep disturbances by pharmacologic agents. Such patients may be advised to avoid sleep deprivation, avoid alcohol in the evening, avoid taking late evening exercises but continue exercise in the afternoon and continue with regular sleep and waking hours. Broughton[19] suggested that the improvement of nocturnal sleep following such a regime may be associated with definite reduction of the seizure frequency and overall improvement in their general well-being.

REFERENCES

1. Passouant P. Historical aspects of sleep and epilepsy. In: Degen R, Niedermeyer E, eds. Epilepsy, Sleep Deprivation. Amsterdam: Elsevier, 1984;67–73.
2. Echeverria MC. De l'epilepsie nocturne. Ann Med Psychol 1879;5:177–197.
3. Fere L. Les Epilepsies et les Epileptiques. Paris: Alcan, 1890.
4. Gowers WR. Epilepsy and Other Chronic Convulsive Diseases, vol 1. London: Williams Wood, 1885.
5. Turner WA. Epilepsy: A Study of the Idiopathic Disease. London: MacMillan, 1907.
6. Gallus R. Die allgemeinen Ursachen der Anfallshaufungen innerhalb grobgerer Gruppen von Kranken. Epilepsi (Leipzig) 1911;3:46.
7. Amann R. Untersuchungen über die Veränderungen in der Häufigkiet der epileptischen Anfälle und deren Ursachen. Z ges Neurol Psychiatr 1914;24:5.
8. Langdon-Down M, Brain WR. Time of day in relation to convulsions in epilepsy. Lancet 1929;2:1029–1032.
9. Patry FL. The relation of time of day, sleep and other factors to the incidence of epileptic seizures. Am J. Psychiatry 1931;87:789–813.
10. Busciano VM. Etiologia dell'accesso epilettica. Osped Psychiatr 1936;4:33.
11. Magnussen G. Eighteen cases of epilepsy with fits in relation to sleep. Acta Psychol (Amst) 1936;11:289–321.
12. Gibbs EL, Gibbs FA. Diagnostic and localizing value of electroencephalographic studies in sleep. Res Publ Assoc Res Nerv Ment Dis 1947;26:366–376.
13. Janz D. The grand mal epilepsies and the sleep-waking cycle. Epilepsia 1962;3:69–109.
14. Passouant P. Influence des etats de vigilance sur les epilepsies. In: Koella WP, ed. Sleep, vol 3. Basel: S Karger, 1977;57–65.
15. Gastaut H, Batini C, Fressy J, et al. Etude electroencephalographique des phenomenes episodiques course du sommeil. In: Fischgold H, ed. Le Sommeil de Nuit Normal et Pathologique. Paris: Masson, 1965;239:254.
16. Cadilhac JC. Le Sommeil Nocturne des Epileptiques. Etude polygraphique. These de Medecine, Monsieur 1967;150.
17. Niedermeyer E. Sleep electroencephalograms in petit mal. Arch Neurol 1965;12:625–630.
18. Montplaisir J. Epilepsy and sleep: Reciprocal interactions and diagnostic procedures involving sleep. In: Thorpy MJ, ed. Handbook of Sleep Disorder. NY: Marcel Dekker, 1990;643–661.
19. Broughton RJ. Epilepsy and sleep: A synopsis and prospectus. In: Degin R, Niedermeyer E, eds. Epilepsy, Sleep and Sleep Deprivation. Amsterdam: Elsevier, 1984:317–356.
20. Billiard M. Epilepsy and the sleep-wake cycle. In: Sterman MB, Shouse MN, Passouant P, eds. Sleep and Epilepsy. New York: Academic Press, 1982;269–286.
21. Kellaway P. Sleep and epilepsy. Epilepsia 1985;26 (suppl 1):S15–S30.
22. Engel J Jr. Seizures and Epilepsy. Philadelphia: FA Davis, 1989;71–111.
23. Matsumoto H, Ajmone-Marsan C. Cortical cellular phenomena in experimental epilepsy: Interictal manifestations. Exp Neurol 1964;9:286–304.
24. Margerison JH, Corsellis JA. Epilepsy and the temporal lobes; a clinical, electroencephalographic and neuropathological study of the brain in epilepsy, with particular reference to the temporal lobes. Brain 1966;89:499–530.
25. Gloor P, Quesney LF, Zumstein H. Pathophysiology of generalized penicillin epilepsy in the cat: The role of cortical and subcortical structures. II. Topical applications of penicillin to the cerebral cortex and to subcortical structures. Electroencephalogr Clin Neurophysiol 1977;43:79–94.
26. Quesney LF, Gloor P, Kratzenberg E, et al. Pathophysiology of generalized penicillin epilepsy in the cat: The role of cortical and subcortical structures. I. Systematic application of penicillin. Electroencephalogr Clin Neurophysiol 1977;42:640–655.
27. Gloor P. Generalized cortico-reticular epilepsy: Some considerations on the pathophysiology of generalized bilaterally synchronous spike and wave discharge. Epilepsia 1968;9:249–263.
28. Chokroverty S. The assessment of sleep disturbances in autonomic failure. In: Bannister R, Mathias CJ, eds. Autonomic Failure. Oxford: Oxford University Press, 1992;442–461.
29. Pompeiano O. Sleep mechanism. In: Jasper HH, Ward AA Jr., Pope A, eds. Basic Mechanisms of the Epilepsies. Boston: Little Brown, 1969;453–473.
30. Berlucchi G. Callosal activity in unrestrained, unanesthetized cats. Arch Ital Biol 1965;103:623.
31. Steriade M. Brain electrical activity and sensory processing during waking and sleep states. In: Kryger MH, Roth T, Dement WC, eds. Principles and Practice of Sleep Medicine. Philadelphia: WB Saunders, 1989;86–103.
32. Villablanca J. Role of the thalamus in sleep control: Sleep-wakefulness studies in chronic diencephalic and athalamic cats. In: Petre-Quadens O, Schlag J, eds. Basic Sleep Mechanisms. New York: Academic Press, 1974;51–81.
33. Ball GJ, Gloor P, Schaul N. The cortical electromicrophysiology of pathological delta waves in the electroencephalogram of cats. Electroencephalogr Clin Neurophysiol 1977;43:346–361.

34. Jones BE. Basic mechanisms of sleep-wake states. In: Kryger MN, Roth T, Dement WC, eds. Principles and Practice of Sleep Medicine. Philadelphia: WB Saunders, 1989;121–138.

35. Morison RS, Dempsey EW. A study of thalamocortical relations. Am J Physiol 1942;135:281–292.

36. Hess WR. Das schlafsyndrom als folge diencephaler reizung. Healv Physiol Pharmacol Acta 1944;2:305–344.

37. Hobson JA, Lydic R, Baghdoyan HA. Evolving concepts of sleep cycle generation: From brain centers to neuronal populations. Behav Brain Sci 1986;9:371–448.

38. Kostopoulos G, Gloor P. A mechanism for spike-wave discharge in feline penicillin epilepsy and its relationship to spindle generation. In: Sterman MB, Shouse MM, Passouant P, eds. Sleep and Epilepsy. New York: Academic Press, 1982; 11–27.

39. Jasper H, Droogleever-Fortuyn J. Experimental studies on the functional anatomy of petit mal epilepsy. Res Publ Assoc Res Nerv Ment Dis 1947;26:272.

40. Spencer WA, Brookhart JM. A study of spontaneous spindle waves in sensorimotor cortex of cats. J Neurophysiol 1961;24:50–65.

41. Spencer WA, Kandel ER. Synaptic inhibition in seizures. In: Jasper HH, Ward AA Jr., Pope A, eds. Basic Mechanisms of the Epilepsies. Boston: Little, Brown, 1969;575–603.

42. Gloor P. Evolution of the concept of the mechanism of generalized epilepsy with bilateral spike and wave discharge. In: Wada JA, ed. Modern Prospectives in Epilepsy. Montreal: Eden Press, 1978;99–137.

43. Niedermeyer E. The Generalized Epilepsies. Springfield: Charles C Thomas, 1972.

44. Wyler AR. Epileptic neurons during sleep and wakefulness. Exp Neurol 1974;42:593–608.

45. Shoulse MN, Siegel JM, Wu MF, et al. Mechanism of seizure suppression during rapid-eye movement (REM) sleep in cats. Brain Res 1989;505:271–282.

46. Cohen HB, Thomas J, Dement WC. Sleep stages, REM deprivation and electroconvulsive threshold in the cat. Brain Res 1970;19:317–321.

47. Janz D. Epilepsy and the sleeping-waking cycle. In: Vinken PJ, Bruyn GW, eds. Handbook of Clinical Neurology: The Epilepsies. Amsterdam: North-Holland Publishing Company, 1974;457–490.

48. Hopkins H. The time of appearance of epileptic seizures in relation to age, duration and type of syndrome. J Nerv Ment Dis 1933;77:153–162.

49. Shouse MN. Epilepsy and seizures during sleep. In: Kryger MH, Roth T, Dement WC, eds. Principles and Practices of sleep medicine. Philadelphia: WB Saunders, 1989;364–376.

50. D'Allesandro R, Santini M, Pazzagli P, et al. Pure sleep epilepsies: Prognostic features. In: Nistico G, DiPerri R, Meinardi H, eds. New York: Alan R Liss, 1983;235–239.

51. Kajtor F. The influence of sleep and the waking state on the epileptic activity of different cerebral structures. Epilepsia 1962;3:274.

52. Gibberd FB, Bateson HC. Sleep epilepsy: Its pattern and prognosis. Br Med J 1974;2:403.

53. Kellaway P, Frost JD Jr, Crawley JM. Time modulation of spike-and-wave activity in generalized epilepsy. Ann Neurol 1980;8:491–500.

54. Autret A, Laffont F, Roux S. Influence of waking and sleep stages on the interictal paroxysmal activity in partial epilepsy with complex seizures. Electroencephalogr Clin Neurophysiol 1983;55:406–410.

55. Kellaway P, Frost JD Jr. Biorhythmic modulation of epileptic events. In: Pedley TA, Meldrum BS, eds. Recent Advances in Epilepsy. London: Churchill-Livingstone, 1983;139–154.

56. Stevens JR, Lonsbury BL, Goel SL. Seizure occurrence and interspike interval. Arch Neurol 1972;26:409–419.

57. Binnie CD. Are biological rhythms of importance in epilepsy? In: Martins de Silva A, Binnie CD, Meinardi H, eds. Biorhythms and Epilepsy. New York: Raven Press, 1985;1–9.

58. Martins da Silva A, Binnie CD. Ultradian variations of epileptiform EEG activity. In: Martins da Silva, Binnie CD, Meinardi H, eds. Biorhythms and Epilepsy. New York: Raven Press, 1985;69–77.

59. Broughton R, Stampi C, Romano S, et al. Do waking ultradian rhythms exist for Petit Mal absences? A case report. In: Martins da Silva, Binnie CD, Meinardi H, eds. Biorhythms and Epilepsy. New York: Raven Press, 1985;95–105.

60. Almqvist R. The rhythm of epileptic attacks and its relationship to the menstrual cycle. Tryckeriaktiebolaget Smaland, Jönköping, 1955.

61. Newmark ME, Penry JK. Catamenial epilepsy: A review. Epilepsia 1980;21:281–300.

62. Webb WB. Circadian biological rhythm aspects of sleep and epilepsy. In: Martins da Silva A, Binnie CD, Meinardi H, eds. Biorhythms and Epilepsy. New York: Raven Press, 1985;13–24.

63. Commission on Classification and Terminology of the International League Against Epilepsy. Proposal for classification of epilepsies and epileptic syndromes. Epilepsia 1985;26:268–278.

64. Janz D. "Aufwach-Epilepsien." Arch Psychaitr Nervenkr 1953;191:73–98.

65. Besset A. Influence of generalized seizures on sleep organization. In: Sterman MB, Shouse MN, Passouant P, eds. Sleep and Epilepsy. New York: Academic Press, 1982;339–346.

66. Billiard M, Besset A, Zachariev Z, et al. Relation of seizures and seizure discharged to sleep stages. In: Wolf P, Dam M, Janz F, et al. Advances in Epileptology. New York: Raven Press, 1987;665–670.

67. Passouant P, Besset A, Carrier A, et al. Night sleep and generalized epilepsies. In: Koella WP, Levin P, eds. Sleep 1974. Besel: S. Karger, 1975;185–196.

68. Passouant P, Latour H, Cadilhac J. L'Épilepsie morphéique. Ann Med Psychol 1951;109:526–540.

69. Gastaut H, Batini C, Broughton R, et al. An electroencephalographic study of nocturnal sleep in epileptic patients [Abstr]. Electroencephalogr Clin Neurophysiol 1965;18:96.

70. Gastaut H, Broughton R. A clinical and polygraphic study of episodic phenomenon during sleep. In: Wortis J,

ed. Recent Advances in Biological Psychiatry, vol 7. New York: Plenum Press, 1965;197–221.

71. Patry G, Lyagoubi S, Tassinari CA. Subclinical electrical status epilepticus induced by sleep in children. Ann Neurol 1971;24:242–252.

72. Meier-Ewert K, Broughton R. Photomyoclonic response of epileptic subjects during wakefulness, sleep and arousal. Electroencephalogr Clin Neurophysiol 1967;23:142–151.

73. Touchon J. Effect of awakening on epileptic activity in primary generalized myoclonic epilepsy. In: Sterman MB, Shouse MN, Passouant P, eds. Sleep and Epilepsy. New York: Academic Press, 1982;239–248.

74. Gastaut H, Roger J, Soulayrol R, et al. Childhood Epileptic encephalopathy with diffuse slow spike-waves (otherwise known as Petit Mal variant) or Lennox syndrome. Epilepsia 1966;7:139–179.

75. Dinner DS. Sleep and Pediatric Epilepsy. Cleve Clin J Med 1989;56:S234–S239.

76. Gastaut H, Broughton R, Roger J, et al. Generalized convulsive seizures without local onset. In: Vinken PJ, Bruyn GW, eds. Handbook of Clinical Neurology, vol 15. The Epilepsies. Amsterdam: Elsevier, 1974;107–129.

77. Erba G, Moschen R, Ferber R. Sleep-related changes in EEG discharge activity and seizure risk in patients with Lennox-Gastaut syndrome. Sleep Res 1981;10:247.

78. Gomez MR, Klass DW. Epilepsies of infancy and childhood. Ann Neurol 1983;13:113–124.

79. Montplaisir J, Laverdiere M, Saint-Hilaire JM, et al. Sleep and temporal lobe epilepsy: A case study with depth electrodes. Neurology (Minneap) 1981;31:1352–1356.

80. Montplaisir J, Laverdiere M, Saint-Hilaire JM. Sleep and focal epilepsy: Contribution of depth recording. In: Sterman MB, Shouse MN, Passouant P, eds. Sleep and Epilepsy. New York: Academic Press, 1982;301–314.

81. Laverdiere M, Montplaisir J. Frequency of epileptic spike activity and sleep disturbances in temporal lobe epilepsy. Sleep Res 1984;13:177.

82. Montplaisir J, Laverdiere M, Rouleau I, et al. Nocturnal sleep recording in partial epilepsy: A study with depth electrodes. J Clin Neurophysiol 1987;4(4):383–388.

83. Rossi GF, Colicchio G, Polla P. Interictal epileptic activity during sleep: A stereo-EEG study in patients with partial epilepsy. Electroencephalogr Clin Neurophysiol 1984;58:97–106.

84. Cadilhac J. Complex partial seizures and REM sleep. In: Sterman MB, Shouse MN, Passouant P, eds. Sleep and Epilepsy. New York: Academic Press, 1982;315–324.

85. Kikuchi S. An electroencephalographic study of nocturnal sleep in temporal lobe epilepsy. Foli Psychiatr Neurol Jpn 1969;23:59–81.

86. Epstein AW, Hill W. Ictal phenomena during REM sleep of a temporal lobe epileptic. Ann Neurol 1966; 15:3767–375.

87. Montplaisir J, Laverdiere M, Saint-Hiliare JM. Sleep and epilepsy. In: Gotman J, Ives JR, Gloor P, eds. Long-Term Monitoring in Epilepsy (EEG suppl No 37). Amsterdam: Elsevier, 1985;215–239.

88. Ross JJ, Johnson LC, Walter RD. Spike and wave discharges during stages of sleep. Ann Neurol 1966; 14:399–407.

89. Autret A, Lucas B, Laffont F, et al. Two distinct classifications of adult epilepsies: By time of seizures and by sensitivity of the interictal paroxysmal activities to sleep and waking. Electroencephalogr Clin Neurophysiol 1987;66:211–218.

90. Bittner-Manicka M. Investigations on the mechanism of nocturnal epilepsy. J Neurol 1976;211:169–181.

91. Sato S, Dreifuss F, Penry JK. The effect of sleep on spike-wave discharges in absence seizures. Neurology (Minneap) 1973;23:1335–1345.

92. Tassinari CA. Bureau-Paillas M, Dalla-Bernardina B, et al. Generalized epilepsies and seizures during sleep. A polygraphic study. In: Van Praag HM, Meinardi H, eds. Brain and Sleep. Amsterdam: De Erven Bohn, 1974;154–166.

93. Markand ON. Slow spike-wave activity in EEG and associated clinical features : Often called "Lennox" or "Lennox-Gastaut" syndrome. Neurology 1977; 27:746–757.

94. Jeavons PM, Bower BD. The natural history of infantile spasms. Arch Dis Child 1961;36:17–21.

95. Niedermeyer E, Rocca U. The diagnostic significance of sleep electroencephalographs in temporal lobe epilepsy. A comparison of scalp and depth tracings. Eur Neurol 1972;7:119–129.

96. Frank G. Epileptiform discharges during various stages of sleep. Electroencephalogr Clin Neurophysiol 1970;28:95.

97. Angelieri F. Partial epilepsies and nocturnal sleep. In: Levin P, Koella WP, eds. Sleep 1974. Basel: S Karger 1975;196–203.

98. Passouant P, Cadilhac J, Delange M. Indications apportees par l'etude du dommeil du nuit sur la physiopathologie des epilepsies. Int J Neurol 1965;5:207–216.

99. Mayersdorf A, Wilder BJ. Focal epileptic discharges during all night sleep studies. Clin Electroencephalogr 1974;5:73–87.

100. Lieb J, Joseph JP, Engel J, et al. Sleep state and seizure foci related to depth spike activity in patients with temporal lobe epilepsy. Electroencephalogr Clin Neurophysiol 1980;49:538–557.

101. Frank GS, Pegram GV. Interrelations of Sleep and Focal Epileptiform Discharge in Monkeys with Alumina Cream Lesions. Aeromed Res Lab Publ 1974:27.

102. Mayanagi Y. The influence of natural sleep on focal spiking in experimental temporal lobe epilepsy in the monkey. Electroencephalogr Clin Neurophysiol 1977;43:813–824.

103. Montplaisir J, Laverdiere M, Walsh J, et al. Influence of nocturnal sleep on the epileptic spike activity recorded with multiple depth electrodes [Abstr]. Electroencephalogr Clin Neurophysiol 1980;49:85P–86P.

104. Passouant P. Epilepsie temporale et sommeil. Rev Roum Neurol 1967;4:151–163.

105. Giaquinto S. Sleep recordings from limbic structures in man. Confin Neurol (Basel) 1973;35:285–303.

106. Gastaut H. Classification of status epilepticus. In: Delgado-Escueta A, ed. Status Epilepticus. New York: Raven Press, 1982.

107. Janz D. Die Epilepsien. Stuttgart: Georg Thieme, 1969.

108. Froscher W. Sleep and prolonged epileptic activity (status epilepticus). In: Degen R, Rodin EA, eds. Epilepsy, Sleep and Sleep Deprivation, ed 2. Amsterdam: Elsevier, 1991;165–176.

109. Gastaut H, Tassinari C. Status epilepticus. In: Remond A, ed. Handbook of Electroencephalography and Clinical Neurophysiology, vol 13A. Amsterdam: Elsevier, 1975.

110. Passouant P. Influence des états de vigilance sur les épilepsies. In: Koella W, Levin P, eds. Sleep 1976. Basel: S Karger, 1977;57:69.

111. Roger J, Lob H, Tassinari CA. Status epilepticus. In: Vinken PJ, Bruyn GW, eds. Handbook of Clinical Neurology, vol 15. Amsterdam: Elsevier North-Holland, 1974.

112. Tassinari CA, Terzano G, Capocchi G, et al. Epileptic seizures during sleep in children. In: Penry JK, ed. Epilepsy the Eighth International Symposium. New York: Raven Press, 1977.

113. Nayrac P, Beaussart M. Les pointes-ondes prerolandiques: expression EEG très particulière. Etude electroclinique de 21 cas. Rev Neurol 1958;99:201–206.

114. Beaussard M. Benign epilepsy of children with rolandic (centrotemporal) paroxysmal foci. A clinical entity. Study of 221 cases. Epilepsia 1973;13:795–811.

115. Janz D, Mathes A. Die propulsiv-petit-mal-epilepsie. Klinik and Verlauf der sog. Blitz-, Nick-und Salaamkrampfe. Basel: S Karger, 1955.

116. Janz D, Christian W. Impulsive petit mal. Dtsch Z Nervenheilkd 1957;176:346–386.

117. Janz D. Epilepsy with impulsive petit mal (juvenile myoclinic epilepsy). Acta Neurol Scand, 1985;72:449–459.

118. Wolf P. Epilepsy with grand mal on awakening. In: Roger J, Dravet C, Bureau M, et al., eds. Epileptic Syndromes in Infancy, Childhood, and Adolescence. London: John Libbey, 1985;259:270.

119. Tassinari CA, Bureau M, Dravet C, et al. Electrical status epilepticus during sleep in children (ESES). In: Sterman MB, Shouse MN, Passouant P, eds. Sleep and epilepsy. New York: Academic Press, 1982;465–479.

120. Pratt KL, Mattson RH, Weikers NJ, et al. EEG activation of epileptics following sleep deprivation: A prospective study of 114 cases. Electroencephalogr Clin Neurophysiol 1968;24:11–15.

121. Rowan AJ, Veldhuisen RJ, Nagelkerke NJD. Comparative evaluation of sleep deprivation and sedated sleep EEGs as diagnostic aids in epilepsy. Electroencephalogr Clin Neurophysiol 1982;54:357–364.

122. Degen R. A study of the diagnostic value of waking and sleep EEGs after sleep deprivation in epileptic patients on anticonvulsive therapy. Electroencephalogr Clin Neurophysiol 1980;49:577–584.

123. Arne-Bes MC, Calvet U, Thiberge M, et al. Effects of sleep deprivation in an EEG study of epileptics. In: Sterman MB, Passouant P, eds. Sleep and Epilepsy. New York: Academic Press, 1982;339–346.

124. Rodin ES, Luby ED, Gottlieb JS. The electroencephalogram during prolonged experimental sleep deprivation. Electroencephalogr Clin Neurophysiol 1962;14:544–551.

125. Declerck AC. Interaction Epilepsy, Sleep and Antiepileptics. Lisse: Swets and Zeitlinger, 1983.

126. Patrick GTW, Gilbert JA. On the effects of loss of sleep. Psychol Rev 1896;3:469–483. Cited in Kleitman N. Sleep and Wakefulness. Chicago: University of Chicago Press, 1963;219.

127. Bennett DR. Sleep deprivation and major motor convulsions. Neurology 1963;13:983–988.

128. Mattson RH, Pratt KL, Calverley JR. Electroencephalograms of epileptics following sleep deprivation. Ann Neurol 1965;13:310–315.

129. Rodin E. Sleep deprivation and epileptological implications. In: Degen R, Rodin EA, eds. Epilepsy, Sleep and Sleep Deprivation, ed 2. (Epilepsy Res Suppl 2) Amsterdam: Elsevier, 1991;265–273.

130. Pedley TA, Guilleminault C. Episodic nocturnal wanderings responsive to anticonvulsant drug therapy. Ann Neurol 1977;2:30–35.

131. Niedermeyer E, Lopes da Silva F. Electroencephalography: Basic Principles, Clinical Applications and Related Fields. Baltimore: Urban and Schwarzenberg, 1987.

132. Declerck AC, Wauquier A, Sijben-Kiggen R, et al. A normative study of sleep in different forms of epilepsy. In: Sterman MB, Shouse MN, Passouant P, eds. Sleep and Epilepsy. New York: Academic Press, 1982;329–337.

133. Delange D, Castan P, Cadilhac J, et al. Study of night sleep during centrencephalic and temporal epilepsies [Abstr]. Electroencephalogr Clin Neurophysiol 1962;14:777.

134. Baldy-Moulinier M. Temporal lobe epilepsy and sleep organization. In: Sterman MB, Passouant P, eds. Sleep and Epilepsy. New York: Academic Press, 1982;347–359.

135. Hamel AR, Sterman MB. Sleep and epileptic abnormalities during sleep. In: Sterman MB, Shouse MN, Passcount P, eds. Sleep and Epilepsy. New York: Academic Press, 1982;361–377.

136. Johnson LC. Effects of anticonvulsant medication on sleep patterns. In: Sterman MB, Shouse MN, Passouant P, eds. Sleep and Epilepsy. New York: Academic Press, 1982;381–384.

137. Landau-Ferey J. A contribution to the study of nocturnal sleep in patients suspected of having epilepsy. In: Sterman MB, Shouse MN, Passouant P, eds. Sleep and Epilepsy. New York: Academic Press, 1982;421–429.

138. Hoeppner J, Garron DC, Cartwright RD. Self-reported sleep disorder symptoms in epilepsy. Epilepsia 1984;25:434–437.

139. Roder-Wanner U, Wolf P, Danninger T. Are sleep patterns in epileptic patients correlated with their type of epilepsy? In: Martins da Silva A, Binnie CD, Meinardi H, eds. Biorhythms and Epilepsy. New York: Raven Press, 1985;109–119.

140. Bowersox SS, Drucker-Colin R. Seizure modification by sleep deprivation: A possible protein synthesis mechanism. In: Sterman MB, Shouse MN, Passouant P, eds. Sleep and Epilepsy. New York: Academic Press, 1982;91–104.

141. Touchon J, Baldy-Moulinier M, Billiard M, et al. Organization du sommeil dans l'epilepsie recente du lobe temporal avant et apres traitement par carbamazepine. Rev Neurol (Paris) 1987;5:462–467.

142. Shouse MN, Sterman MP. Sleep pathology in experimental epilepsy: amygdala kindling. In: Sterman MB, Shouse MN, Passouant P, eds. Sleep and Epilepsy. New York: Academic Press, 1982;151–164.

143. Cepeda C, Tanaka T. Limbic status epilepticus and sleep in baboons. In: Sterman MB, Shouse MN, Passouant P, eds. Sleep and Epilepsy. New York: Academic Press, 1982;165–172.

144. Tanaka T, Naquet R. Kindling effect and sleep organization in cats. Electroencephalogr Clin Neurophysiol 1975;39:449–454.

145. Wauquier A, Clincake GHC, Declerck AC. Sleep alterations by seizures and anticonvulsants. In: Martins da Silva A, Binnie CD, Meinardi H, eds. Biorhythms and Epilepsy. New York: Raven Press, 1985;123–133.

146. Touchon J, Baldy-Moulinier M, Billiard M, et al. Sleep architecture in epileptic patients with complex partial seizures before and after treatment by carbamazepine [Abstr]. Epilepsia 1986;27:640.

147. Wolf P, Roder-Wanner UU, Brede M, et al. Influences of antiepileptic drugs on sleep. In: Martins da Silva A, Binnie CD, Meinardi H, eds. Biorhythms and Epilepsy. New York: Raven Press, 1985;137–148.

148. Hartmann E. The effects of diphenylhydantoin (DPH) on sleep in man. Psychophysiology 1970;7:316.

149. Roder-Wanner VV, Noachtar S, Wolf P. Response of polygraphic sleep to phenytoin treatment of epilepsy. A longitudinal study of immediate, short- and long-term effects. Acta Neurol Scand 1987;76:157–167.

150. Baldy-Moulinier M. In: Sterman MB, Shouse MN, Passouant P, eds. Sleep and Epilepsy. New York: Academic Press, 1982;347–359.

151. Gigli GL, Gotman J, Thomas ST. Sleep alterations after acute administration of carbamazepine in cats. Epilepsia 1988;29:748–752.

152. Findji F, Catani P. Readjustment des therapeutiques anticonvulsives chez l'enfant. L'Encephale 1982;8:595–613.

153. Harding GFA, Alford CA, Powell TE. The effect of sodium valproate on sleep, reaction times and visual evoked potential in normal subjects. Epilepsia 1985;26:597–601.

154. Declerck AC, Wauquier A. Influence of antiepileptic drugs on sleep patterns. In: Degen R, Rodin EA, eds. Epilepsy, Sleep and Sleep Deprivation. Amsterdam: Elsevier, 1991;153–163.

155. Parmeggiani PL, Morrison AR. Alterations in autonomic functions during sleep. In: Loewy AD, Spyer KM, eds. Central Regulation of Autonomic Functions. Oxford: Oxford University Press, 1990;366–386.

156. Chokroverty S. Functional anatomy of the autonomic nervous system: Correlated with symptomatology of neurological disease. AAN Course No. 246, San Diego, 1992.

157. Nelson DA, Ray CD. Respiratory arrest from seizure discharges in limbic system. Ann Neurol 1968;19:199–207.

158. Wyler AR, Weymuller EA. Epilepsy complicated by sleep apnea. Ann Neurol 1981;9:403–404.

159. Chokroverty S, Sachdeo R, Goldhammer T, et al. Epilepsy and sleep apnea [Abstr]. Electroencephalogr Clin Neurophysiol 1985;61:26P.

160. Vashista S, Ehrenberg B. Benefits of treating sleep-apnea in complex partial epilepsy [Abstr]. Electroencephalogr Clin Neurophysiol 1988;70:41P.

161. Van Buren JM. Some autonomic concomitants of ictal automatisms. Brain 1958;81:505–528.

162. Brown ML. Cardiovascular changes associated with electroconvulsant therapy in man. Arch Neurol Psychiatry 1953;69:601–608.

163. Lathers CM, Schrader PL. Autonomic dysfunction in epilepsy. Characterization of cardiac neural discharge associated with pentylenetetrazol-induced seizures. Epilepsia 1982;23:633–647.

164. Jay GW, Leestma JE. Sudden death in epilepsy. Acta Neurol Scand Suppl 1981;82:1–66.

165. Aldrich M, Jahnke B. Diagnostic value of video-EEG polysomnography. Neurology 1991;41:1060–1066.

166. Carskadon MA, Dement WC, Mitler MM, et al. Guidelines for the multiple sleep latency test (MSLT): A standard measure of sleepiness. Sleep 1986;9:519–524.

28

Positive Airway Pressure in the Treatment of Sleep-Related Breathing Disorders

Mark H. Sanders
Ronald A. Stiller

NASAL POSITIVE AIRWAY PRESSURE FOR SLEEP APNEA

The application of nasal continuous positive airway pressure (CPAP) for the treatment of obstructive sleep apnea (OSA) in adults was first described in 1981.[1] Since then, it has become the medical therapy of choice for OSA.

In essence, nasal CPAP systems consist of a blower unit that generates and directs airflow downstream to the patient. Positive pressure is generated by variations in delivered airflow and resistance within the system. This positive pressure, delivered to the patient through one of several types of interfaces (discussed later), pressurizes the upper airway. Thus, the collapsible region of the upper airway is pneumatically splinted open, an effect that represents the primary mechanism of therapeutic action. Some authors have speculated that nasal CPAP maintains upper airway patency during sleep by virtue of a reflex mediated through the increase in end-expiratory lung volume that usually accompanies its administration.[2-4] Alternately, a direct relationship between lung volume and upper airway patency could be due to traction created on mediastinal and upper airway structures.[5,6] However, although upper airway resistance does vary directly with lung volume, this effect is relatively small.[7] Furthermore, Series and coworkers have demonstrated that there is no significant reduction of CPAP's impact on upper airway resistance when the increase in lung volume is prevented by the concomitant application of positive extrathoracic pressure.[8] Reinforcing the findings of this study is the observation that, with comparable augmentation of lung volume, CPAP eliminates obstructive apnea whereas application of continuous negative extrathoracic pressure does not.[9] Finally, several investigators

have demonstrated that the administration of nasal CPAP depresses electromyographic activity of the upper airway dilator muscles, which is evidence against a reflex-mediated reduction in upper airway resistance.[10-12] Regardless of the mechanism, nasal CPAP has documented effectiveness in eliminating mixed and obstructive apneas.[13] Some "central" apneas, particularly those observed in patients with predominantly obstructive events, are also eliminated by nasal CPAP.[13,14] This finding strongly supports the contention of Sanders and coworkers[15] that the central portion of mixed apneas and many central apneas may actually represent delayed inspiratory effort due to prolongation of the preceding expiration. These investigators hypothesized that this increase in expiratory time is related to expiratory upper airway instability with augmented upper airway resistance and slowing of expiratory airflow.[15,16]

Shortly after the initiation of nasal CPAP therapy, most OSA patients report increased daytime alertness, relief of morning headaches, decreased nocturnal awakenings, improved temperament, and a sense of well-being. Reduced daytime sleepiness has been reported just after one night of nasal CPAP therapy,[17] though further increases in daytime alertness, as assessed by multiple sleep latency testing, may occur over the ensuing 2 weeks.[18] This progressive improvement in symptoms highlights the importance of recognizing that patients may not be maximally, or even sufficiently, alert to resume full activities (especially those that require particular vigilance, such as operating vehicles or potentially dangerous tasks) within the first several days of

Supported in part by VA Merit Review Funding, and NHLBI Training Grant #5T32HL07563-07.

treatment. Similarly, it should be emphasized to patients that subjective reduction in daytime sleepiness immediately after beginning nasal CPAP therapy does not invariably indicate normalization of daytime alertness, nor does it obviate the necessity for ongoing compliance with therapy.

Clinical experience indicates that nasal CPAP can maintain upper airway patency and acceptable oxygenation during sleep in the overwhelming majority of patients with OSA. Some, however, continue to have alveolar hypoventilation and oxyhemoglobin desaturation on the basis of persistent partial upper airway obstruction, despite maximal achievable or tolerable levels of CPAP. Under these circumstances, supplemental oxygen can be added to the CPAP system, either directly into the mask or into the tubing that leads to the mask.[19-22] Other patients, however, continue to have episodic reductions in oxyhemoglobin saturation or reset their baseline saturation to unacceptably low levels despite elimination of discrete apneas and hypopneas by nasal CPAP. These persons often have underlying lung or chest wall abnormalities that impair gas exchange during wakefulness. Such abnormalities take on greater physiologic significance during sleep, when there is a reduction in ventilatory chemosensitivity and alteration of ventilatory muscle function.[23-28]

Like most therapies, nasal CPAP is variably associated with a variety of generally minor but nonetheless troublesome side effects (Table 28-1). These are most often attributable to either the patient-device interface or the sensation of high airflow or pressure. Some patients simply find that nasal CPAP is too cumbersome and unacceptably interferes with their lifestyle. These are generally younger patients who

are unable to envision using nasal CPAP for an indefinite period, potentially a lifetime. On the other hand, most clinicians have patients for whom nasal CPAP is an inconvenience worth enduring. Indeed, some of our patients have taken their devices on camping or business trips to places as remote as Mongolia. The major complaints of such travelers revolve about the difficulty of getting their CPAP units through airport security screening stations.

Problems with skin abrasion or leakage of air directed into the eyes, with or without consequent conjunctivitis[29] as a result of a poor mask fit, can generally be overcome by trying different sizes of commercially available masks or by having a mask custom made. Mask leaks have been reported to increase in prevalence once CPAP exceeds 12 cm H_2O.[30] Other complaints include nasal dryness, congestion, and rhinorrhea, the prevalence of such effects is approximately 10%.[30] The former can often be treated with either administration of saline nasal spray at bedtime or a room vaporizer. Occasionally, difficult cases require the addition of a low-resistance humidifying unit to the CPAP system. Whereas nasal dryness is rarely a serious problem, a case of massive epistaxis was reported in a patient with sleep apnea, right ventricular dysfunction, and a coagulopathy.[30] The authors believed that mucosal dryness contributed to the epistaxis, which did not recur after placement of an in-line humidifier. In light of this report, it is probably prudent to follow with particular care patients with bleeding tendencies who are on nasal CPAP, and to consider humidifying the delivered air from the outset of their therapy. Although routine use is to be discouraged, occasional administration of a vasoconstrictive nasal spray may be beneficial when nasal congestion is related to a self-limited condition such as an upper respiratory tract infection. We have found rhinorrhea to be a more difficult problem to solve, though it is a significant complaint in only about 5% of our patients. The cause of this untoward effect is uncertain. While it may be related to drying of the airways, we have not found humidification to be of noteworthy benefit. Another suggestion that has been offered is that this problem is related to stimulation of pressure-sensitive nasal mucosal receptors.[31] We have found the administration of chromoglycate or anticholinergic nasal sprays such as ipratropium bromide to be only variably effective among patients with rhinorrhea. Nasal steroids, on the other hand, have been observed to provide more consistent benefit.

Surprisingly, pneumomediastinum and pneumothorax have not proven to be prevalent in patients receiving CPAP for OSA, at least as assessed by review of the literature. Pneumoencephalus has been reported in one sleep apnea patient with a

TABLE 28-1. Side Effects of Nasal CPAP

Mask-related
    Skin abrasion or rash
    Conjunctivitis from air leak
Pressure or airflow-related
    Chest discomfort
    Aerophagia
    Sinus discomfort
    Smothering sensation
    Difficulty exhaling
    Difficulty initiating and/or maintaining sleep
    Rhinorrhea*
    Nasal congestion or dryness*
    Massive epistaxis‡
    Pneumothorax or pneumomediastinum‡
    Pneumoencephalus‡
Other
    Cumbersomeness or inconvenience
    Noise
    Spousal intolerance

*Thought to be related to pressure or airflow.
‡Uncommon but potential side effect.

cerebrospinal fluid leak who was placed on nasal CPAP.[32] This is a well-described complication of CPAP application via face mask in patients with head trauma and should be considered when any patient using CPAP therapy develops a nasal discharge and neurologic signs and symptoms including headache, seizures, dizziness, or evidence of cranial nerve palsy.

A number of patients also complain of chest discomfort on nasal CPAP,[13,31,33] which is probably related to increased end-expiratory pressure and the consequent elevation of resting lung volume during therapy.[12] This stretches the chest wall muscles and cartilaginous structures, creating a sensation of chest wall pressure that persists through the hours of wakefulness. Although chest discomfort should be taken seriously and evaluated completely in any patient, if cardiac work-up in the OSA patient on CPAP is not diagnostic, efforts should be made to reduce the expiratory pressure, if necessary using bilevel positive airway pressure, or BiPAP. Similarly, a certain proportion of patients feel sufficiently uncomfortable exhaling against expiratory pressure as to preclude their using nasal CPAP. Here also, if the level of CPAP cannot be minimized, a trial of BiPAP should be considered.

While it is usually beneficial to patients with OSA, administration of nasal CPAP may also be associated with untoward effects on arterial blood gases and oxyhemoglobin saturation. Krieger and colleagues[34] reported severe oxyhemoglobin desaturation in a hypercapnic OSA patient with cor pulmonale during nasal CPAP therapy. Though the cause of this desaturation is not certain, it may be due to worsening hypoventilation related to the added mechanical impedance to ventilation associated with exhalation against increased pressure. Alternatively, it is conceivable that the CPAP resulted in sufficient elevation of intrathoracic pressure to decrease venous return in this patient with already impaired right ventricular function. This sequence of events may have further compromised cardiac output, with resultant deterioration in oxygenation. Though situations such as this are not common, exacerbation of hypoventilation during nasal CPAP has occasionally been noted in clinical situations, and it highlights the need to conduct nasal CPAP trials under monitored conditions.

In contrast, nasal CPAP administration has also been reported to improve awake arterial blood gases in sleep apnea patients with hypercapnia and cor pulmonale.[35,36] The mechanism responsible for augmented alveolar ventilation during wakefulness in these persons has not been clearly defined. Some authors have reported a leftward shift in the ventilatory response to carbon dioxide without a change in the slope of the line describing the relationship.[37]

This suggests a reduction in the chemoreceptor(s) set point to arterial carbon dioxide tension following initiation of therapy. Though the question was not specifically addressed by these investigators, this alteration in the relationship between ventilation and carbon dioxide stimulation might be related to reduced serum buffering capacity accompanying CPAP-associated relief of apnea and carbon dioxide retention during sleep. Alternatively, improved ventilation during wakefulness could be due to improved ventilatory muscle function, relief of hypoxic depression of central nervous system respiratory centers, or elimination of sleep fragmentation. Further studies are needed before conclusions can be made with confidence.

The most significant disadvantage to nasal CPAP therapy is its volitional nature. In other words, patients must actively participate in their own treatment, as without conscientious use, nasal CPAP will not provide effective therapy. Several studies have examined patient compliance with nasal CPAP therapy. Sullivan and associates[38] reported starting nasal CPAP therapy on 35 of 50 patients with OSA with good compliance over periods of 3 to 30 months. Frith and Cant[19] found that 72% of patients used nasal CPAP from 3 to 22 months. McEvoy and Thornton[20] reported that seven of 11 patients consented to use nasal CPAP at home and of these, one discontinued therapy. The importance of considering the frequency of nasal CPAP use when defining compliance is illustrated by the study of Nino-Murcia's group,[39] who reported compliance with therapy—defined simply as continued use of the device—by 83% of patients. When compliance was defined as nightly or nearly nightly use, only 67% of patients were found to be compliant. None of these studies evaluated the number of hours of nasal CPAP use per night.

Sanders and coworkers[40] found that 85% of patients undergoing a therapeutic trial of nasal CPAP in the laboratory were suitable candidates for home therapy when candidacy was defined as (1) satisfactory amelioration of sleep-disordered breathing (SDB) by CPAP and (2) patient willingness to use the device on a long-term basis. In addition, these investigators defined adequate compliance as nightly use of CPAP, and patients were deemed compliant if they did not sleep without CPAP therapy more than 1 hour per night. Employing this definition, they found that 75% of patients who were sent home on therapy were compliant over 10.3 ± 8 months (mean ± SD) of follow-up. These findings are supported by the recent investigation of Waldhorn and colleagues,[33] which also found that 85% of patients tolerated a laboratory trial of nasal CPAP and 76% of patients sent home on the device were still using it after 14.5 ± 10.7 months. A potential methodologic problem inherent in all these studies is that patient compliance was determined from questionnaire or interview data. Only a few studies have employed objective techniques, such as timers on the CPAP device, to measure compliance. Those that are available, however, also suggest less than total therapeutic compliance. One such study[41] reported that the mean duration of use was 5.1 ± 2.6 hours per night and that 40% of patients used the device more than 6 hours per night. Another study reported an average of 6 hours' CPAP use per night by patients.[42] Even if timers are used to assess the duration of machine use per night, uncertainties persist regarding the proportion of *total sleep time* during which the machine is actually in use. This information, while difficult to obtain in an objective fashion, is essential for optimal interpretation of the data. For example, if CPAP is used by a patient during 4 of 5 hours' sleep overnight, compliance might be considered to be relatively good. On the other hand, if CPAP is used for the same 4 hours but the patient is asleep for 8 hours, compliance is significantly poorer.

Complicating the evaluation of patient compliance is variability among the definitions of clinically adequate compliance. Should the percentage of compliant patients be calculated from the total population of individuals undergoing a therapeutic trial, or just from those patients who are sent home to use this therapy? Using the former population in the denominator includes patients who reject CPAP therapy outright and are not sent home to use it. On the other hand, evaluating only compliance of those for whom this modality is prescribed as long-term treatment assesses use only in those who are thought to be using it as such by their health care providers. Even if the definition of compliance is standardized, its significance remains unclear, as clinicians do not at present know the level of severity at which OSA has adverse impact on the quality or quantity of life.[43] In the same vein, compliance goals of CPAP therapy are currently difficult to establish, as the minimal degree of CPAP use that prevents the adverse consequences of OSA is also unclear. There is some suggestion, however, that optimal results are obtained only by consistent nightly use of this device. One study reported an increase in objectively determined daytime sleepiness following only one night without nasal CPAP,[44] and another indicated progressive improvement in daytime sleepiness over several weeks of consistent use.[18]

Not only do the techniques for assessing CPAP compliance require refinement, but the determinants of patient compliance remain unclear. Some data suggest that compliance improves with increased severity of daytime sleepiness.[33,45] The frequency or variety of side effects to CPAP therapy, initial apnea plus hypopnea frequency, gender, weight, or prescribed level of CPAP do not appear to discriminate compliant groups of patients from noncompliant ones.[33,42]

A great deal remains to be learned about the factors that influence compliance. To conclude that side effects to treatment have no impact on acceptance of therapy because of similar prevalence in both compliant and noncompliant populations ignores the likelihood that any given side effect of CPAP may be perceived differently by different persons and thus may have a different degree of impact. Thus, a simple comparison of prevalence may be misleading and can obscure the impact of a particular side effect on the compliance of individual patients. From our perspective, every effort should be made to minimize the side effects of positive-pressure therapy, in order to enhance the quality of the patient's life and to increase the likelihood of good therapeutic compliance. In summary, when all things are considered, compliance with nasal CPAP, which entails the presence of a relatively cumbersome box at or near the bedside, with an equally cumbersome (if not unappealing) interface over the nose, is surprisingly good. Undoubtedly, this relates to the remarkable symptomatic improvement experienced by the majority of users.

In addition to minimizing side effects of CPAP, several other practices may enhance patient acceptance. Compliance is almost certainly enhanced by appropriate patient selection. It is intuitively obvious that any patient who requires coercion to take a nasal CPAP unit home, even after efforts have been made to explain the need for the device and the manner in which it operates, is unlikely to use it conscientiously on a long-term basis. Therefore, nasal CPAP should be provided only to patients who are receptive to using it or who are sufficiently open minded to give it a reasonable home trial. Though a recent study has suggested that positive reinforcement by periodic telephone contact with sleep apnea patients using nasal CPAP does not favorably influence therapeutic compliance,[42] it is possible that such an impersonal medium as the telephone is inadequate to have a motivating effect. It is also essential that the physician and staff of the sleep laboratory or center act as a continuing educational resource for patients who seek answers to questions and reassurance when uncertainties arise. At our center and others, patient support groups serve a very important function in fostering a climate of openness and sharing of information as well as providing a forum for discussion of issues relevant to SDB and overall health. Group meetings provide patients with the realization that they are not alone with their disorder. This is crucial, as many have been labeled by society as obese, lazy, or malingering, resulting in social ostracism and low self-esteem. Many of these consequences of OSA are reversible by nasal CPAP therapy, with remarkable and gratifying results for all concerned. In our experience, there is no doubt that important benefits are obtained form support groups, judging from the excellent attendance and favorable patient comments.

As noted earlier, all patients should undergo a monitored trial of nasal CPAP to establish therapeutic levels of pressure before being sent home for long-term therapy. Because the requisite level of CPAP may vary according to body position during sleep, clinicians should be certain that the delivered pressure is effective in maintaining adequate upper airway patency and oxygenation during sleep in all positions. Patient tolerance can be reasonably assessed and patients can become acclimatized to CPAP in the presence of health care professionals who may answer questions and allay fears during such a monitored trial. In addition, the device should be explained at this time and an opportunity provided for a hands-on examination of the CPAP unit before the patient retires to sleep on positive pressure. The patient should also be allowed to determine the most comfortable and leak-free interface with the device (i.e. nasal mask, prongs, or a full-face mask). Following this, while the patient is still awake, positive pressure should be administered across a wide range of pressures, to permit familiarization with the associated sensations. Another advantage of monitored evaluation of the patient on CPAP is the immediate availability of knowledgeable and caring health care professionals. When wearing nasal CPAP for the first time, patients occasionally awaken in the middle of the night disoriented and terrified by the apparatus. Under these circumstances, reassurance is readily supplied by the laboratory personnel conducting the trial.

Several other benefits have also been attributed to monitored trials of CPAP therapy. Fry and coworkers[46] recently demonstrated that the number of periodic leg movements during sleep (PLMS), with and without accompanying arousals, increased significantly during nasal CPAP therapy. These investigators hypothesized that improved sleep quality and architecture associated with relief of SDB by nasal CPAP can reveal underlying PLMS. It is therefore conceivable that a patient will experience physiologic relief of OSA with maintenance of acceptable oxygenation on nasal CPAP but not obtain symptomatic relief of daytime sleepiness or fatigue because of persistent sleep fragmentation attributable to the emergence of PLMS.

Thus, a monitored initial trial of CPAP addresses many issues and concerns that, if not considered, may lead to dismissal of this form of therapy as a viable therapeutic option. Attention to these factors at the outset of therapy will maximize the opportunity for a successful outcome.

PATIENT–POSITIVE-PRESSURE DEVICE INTERFACE OPTIONS

Nasal Prong Systems

In the initial report by Sullivan's group,[1] CPAP was applied via nasal prongs sealed within the nares by medical-grade silicon rubber. Subsequently, self-sealing nasal masks and nasal prongs have been employed as interfaces between the patient and the positive-pressure device.[35,47–49] A preliminary study has suggested that there is roughly equal initial acceptance of the two interfaces.[50] Importantly, in that study a relatively large number of patients changed their preference after using one particular interface for a period of time. Thus, since the requisite pressures do not seem to vary,[50,51] patients should be made aware that this choice remains open to them at all times during their treatment. At the present time, clinicians and patients have the option of using either custom-made or commercially available nasal masks and prongs. The former type have the advantage of providing individualized and optimal fit, whereas the latter offer the convenience of an off-the-shelf product. Clinicians also have the option to employ a full-face mask to deliver positive pressure to patients who are unable, or unwilling, to use a nasal interface.

Positive Airway Pressure Delivered by Full Face Mask

Patients are occasionally encountered who are either intolerant of nasal masks or prongs or unable to keep their mouth sufficiently closed during sleep to permit maintenance of adequate positive intrapharyngeal pressure. In our experience, a chin strap is rarely helpful, and, under these circumstances, the delivery of positive pressure via a full face mask should be considered. This interface has been successful in a substantial majority of the patients in whom it has been applied (MH Sanders, unpublished data). Some patients are equally intolerant of the full face mask, and on rare occasion, application of positive pressure via this interface fails to alleviate upper airway obstruction. In our experience, however, these patients represent a definite minority.

Particular care must be taken when employing a full face mask, owing to the potential risk of aspiration of gastric contents if the patient vomits. Though this complication has not been encountered in more than 25 OSA patients and patients with neuromuscular disease who have received nocturnal positive-pressure ventilatory support via full face mask, experience must still be considered limited. It is reassuring, however, that the use of prophylactic nasogastric tubes has not been recommended by other investigators as a routine precaution for critically ill patients receiving CPAP via full face mask who did not have risk factors for vomiting.[52,53] Accordingly, patients for whom a full face mask is prescribed as an interface for chronic nocturnal positive-pressure therapy should be instructed not to take anything by mouth for at least 3 hours before applying the positive pressure. Furthermore, patients should be instructed to notify their physician if they are experiencing nausea or vomiting from any cause before using the positive pressure via face mask during sleep.

Coverage of both the nose and mouth by a full face mask also raises theoretical concerns about the potential consequences of machine failure when airflow entrained through a nonfunctional or dysfunctional CPAP or BiPAP device is limited. Safety valves should be incorporated in the circuit, close to the patient, to facilitate inhalation of fresh air and to minimize dead space in the event of machine malfunction. Optimally, an alarm should also be present to signal power failure.

VARIATIONS OF POSITIVE AIRWAY PRESSURE THERAPY FOR SLEEP-DISORDERED BREATHING

Some patients find the administration of positive pressure sufficiently bothersome to precipitate complete intolerance of therapy or at least result in unsatisfactory compliance. To minimize the adverse or potentially adverse consequences associated with the delivery of positive pressure, several modifications of CPAP recently became available.

Pressure Ramping

For some patients, the sensation of positive pressure is unpleasant enough to cause difficulty in initiating sleep. The pressure-ramping feature of CPAP allows adjustment of the rate of rise in delivered pressure over time, from a negligible level to that required to maintain upper airway patency during sleep. This modification provides a window during which it may be easier for the patient to fall asleep (Figure 28-1). Because the level of positive pressure may be transiently below that required to maintain upper airway patency during sleep, pressure ramping may allow apnea and oxyhemoglobin desaturation to occur for a variable period of time, until the pressure reaches the prescribed, optimal value. At the present time, no published studies address the level of risk that the delay in optimal pressure delivery may present to patients, nor are any data available on the effectiveness of pressure ramping in improving patient compliance with CPAP therapy. Thus, although conceptually pressure ramping is an attractive feature, its degree of effectiveness and safety remain to be documented, and the specific patient populations for which it might provide maximal benefit have yet to be identified.

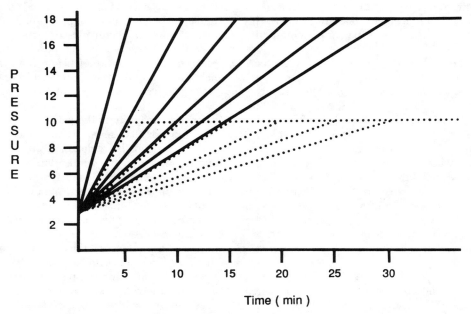

FIGURE 28-1.   *Graph depicts pressure "ramping." Pressure can be gradually increased over prescribed periods to reach maximum required pressures (here illustrated as 18 cm H_2O and 10 cm H_2O).*

Bilevel Positive Airway Pressure

As noted previously, a number of troublesome side effects associated with positive pressure can preclude adequate therapeutic tolerance or safety of CPAP administration. These untoward consequences include a smothering sensation associated with exhalation against positive pressure, chest wall discomfort, and bothersome nasal or sinus pressure. Additionally, some patients may be at increased risk for barotrauma by virtue of emphysema or bullous lung disease (though a review of the literature suggests that this is not a prevalent complication of CPAP therapy for OSA), while in others, elevated expiratory pressure may be associated with a tendency toward alveolar hypoventilation. For many patients, the only way to avoid these side effects while ensuring the success and safety of positive-pressure therapy for OSA may lie in reducing the required pressure to a minimal effective value delivered to the patient during wakefulness and sleep.

Recent studies of the pathogenesis of OSA have indicated that upper airway resistance increases during expiration despite the absence of negative intrapharyngeal pressure.[15,16,54,55] Along these lines, Sanders and associates speculated that instability of the upper airway during expiration is the initial event in the sequence leading to obstructive apnea.[15] This was reinforced by the study of Mahadevia and colleagues,[56] which indicated that expiratory positive airway pressure was associated with a reduction in apnea frequency. Sanders' group[21] further hypothesized that the splinting action of positive pressure in the upper airway, during both inspiration and expiration, was necessary to eliminate obstructive events, and that less pressure would be required to maintain upper airway patency during expiration than during inspiration. This was based on the assumption that, during expiration, inherent upper airway instability represents the primary factor that favors airway closure, whereas during inspiration inadequate upper airway patency is related to two factors: the collapsing influence of negative intraluminal pressure and the inherent instability of the airway. This hypothesis cannot be tested using CPAP, because this modality requires equal pressure during inspiration and expiration. Independent adjustment of inspiratory and expiratory pressure is possible, however, with bilevel positive airway pressure (BiPAP) which provides inspiratory positive airway pressure (IPAP) and expiratory positive airway pressure (EPAP). IPAP delivery is initiated in response to low-level, patient-generated inspiratory airflow ($\sim$ 40 ml per second). Pressure falls to the set EPAP level when inspiratory airflow falls below a threshold value. Sanders' group[21] speculated that, in patients with OSA, BiPAP can deliver EPAP at a level

that is sufficient to prevent the upper airway from being occluded during expiration. Then, at the initiation of inspiratory effort, minimal inspiratory airflow would trigger the delivery of a predetermined level of IPAP before the airway can be collapsed by the developing negative intrapharyngeal pressure. In this manner, IPAP would prevent generation of negative intraluminal pressure and subsequent upper airway collapse throughout inspiration. Over and above simply preventing complete upper airway occlusion, delivery of a sufficient level of IPAP would augment airway patency, thus eliminating partial obstructions (hypopneas) with desaturation or arousals from sleep. If the airway were to become occluded during expiration, IPAP would not be triggered and the apnea would become apparent.

With BiPAP, patients can determine their own inspiratory airflow as well as frequency and, in general, can maintain a more physiologic breathing pattern. IPAP is similar to the inspiratory pressure support that is available on larger, more complex mechanical ventilators used as life-support systems. Importantly, inspiratory-expiratory pressure cycling by the patient can be achieved in BiPAP, even in the presence of mild to moderate leaks at the mask-patient interface or in the event of a partially open mouth when positive pressure is delivered via the nasal route. Since larger, conventional mechanical ventilators are not "leak tolerant" in delivering inspiratory pressure support, they necessitate use of a cuffed endotracheal tube or tracheotomy tube.

In a preliminary investigation of 13 patients with obstructive SDB (12 with sleep apnea syndrome, one with sleep hypopnea syndrome) in which optimal settings of nasal CPAP and BiPAP were compared, Sanders' group[21] noted that in each patient the EPAP delivered during BiPAP was significantly lower than the level of CPAP, and the mean value of EPAP for the group was 37% lower than the required level of CPAP ($P<0.001$). On the other hand, there was no difference between the level of IPAP during BiPAP administration and the level of CPAP. Thus, comparable relief of SDB was achieved in the two modalities, despite the lower mean pressure during the BiPAP trial. In all patients, apnea was not relieved until a critical level of EPAP was reached, whereas persistent obstructive hypopneas were eliminated by increasing the IPAP alone. All patients found BiPAP more comfortable than conventional CPAP, a feature attributed to greater comfort associated with exhaling against lower pressure. These data support the importance of expiratory upper airway obstruction in the pathogenesis of OSA.

There are three modes by which BiPAP can be delivered. In the spontaneous or s mode, IPAP is delivered in response to a patient "trigger," in the form of spontaneously generated, low-level airflow.

In the spontaneous/timed or S/T mode, the patient may also trigger the delivery of IPAP as above, but in addition the physician may set the device so that IPAP is delivered at prescribed intervals if a spontaneously triggered delivery does not occur within that interval. This back-up feature is uncommonly needed in the treatment of patients with OSA, though it has been helpful in providing nocturnal ventilatory assistance to other patient groups such as those with ventilatory muscle dysfunction on the basis of neuromuscular disease and to patients with nocturnal hypoventilation attributable to chest wall deformities such as kyphoscoliosis (see later). Another potential use for the S/T mode is in patients with central sleep apnea. In these patients the capability for spontaneous triggering facilitates tolerance of the device by the awake patient, whereas during sleep the timed BiPAP "breaths" delivered at prescribed intervals prevent the long breathing pauses between lung inflations that are characteristic of central sleep apnea.[57] Finally, the TIMED mode on BiPAP is similar to controlled ventilation on conventional mechanical ventilators in that the patient cannot spontaneously trigger the delivery of IPAP, as it is administered only at the intervals prescribed by the health care professional. In this mode, the duration of IPAP delivery is set by the clinician who prescribes it for a specific percentage of the total cycle time. For example, if the frequency of time-delivered IPAP is 10 per minute (every 6 seconds), the clinician might establish that the IPAP duration should be 30% of the total cycle time, or 2 seconds.

Thus, BiPAP may be a therapeutic alternative for patients who find conventional nasal CPAP uncomfortable or for those in whom the delivery of positive airway pressure represents an unacceptable degree of risk (i.e., patients with bullous lung disease). Because average mask pressures are lower on BiPAP, air leakage around the skin-mask interface may be less of a problem, as might nasal congestion and rhinorrhea (especially if these sequelae are related to stimulation of pressure-sensitive nasal mucosal receptors). The lower respiratory pressure also tends to minimize chest discomfort, as end-expiratory lung volume is not increased as much when the expiratory pressure is lower. In addition, the risk of hypoventilation due to augmented mechanical impedance, which was described earlier, is probably also reduced with the lower expiratory pressures. This may be a particular advantage to patients with ventilatory muscle weakness or chest wall abnormalities and to those with OSA (see later). Though it is clear that many patients prefer nasal BiPAP to CPAP, whether the theoretical advantages of the former modality translate into uniformly better long-term

patient compliance awaits completion of controlled, prospective studies.

Algorithm for Adjusting Positive Pressure

The goal of positive-pressure therapy for SDB is to eliminate apneas and hypopneas. In addition, therapy should abolish arousals from sleep and episodes of oxyhemoglobin desaturation that are associated with SDB events. Finally, if possible, it is desirable to eliminate snoring, as this phenomenon reflects upper airway instability and the tendency to occlude with minimal provocation. Along these lines, recent reports have described the upper airway resistance syndrome, in which patients do not have discrete apneas or hypopneas but exhibit snoring associated with repetitive arousals and consequent excessive daytime sleepiness.[58,59] It has been speculated that the generation of large negative pleural pressure swings with elevated upper airway resistance and decreased airflow precipitates the arousals that fragment sleep. With these factors in mind, the clinician should adjust the level of positive pressure to abolish discrete SDB events, maintain satisfactory oxyhemoglobin saturation, eliminate arousals, and if possible, eliminate snoring. It is appropriate to increase the level of pressure enough to accomplish these therapeutic goals but no higher, as excessive pressure may increase the likelihood of side effects and poor patient tolerance without adding to (if not actually reducing) physiologic benefit.

Description of proper polysomnographic procedure is beyond the scope of this chapter, but specific clinical circumstances may require particular consideration and decision making with regard to therapeutic trials of positive airway pressure therapy for OSA. For example, it is well-established that alcohol augments upper airway instability and suppresses the arousal response, thus enhancing the frequency and duration of SDB events.[60-62] On this basis, it is generally accepted that OSA patients should abstain from alcohol. Clinical experience indicates that this advice is often incompletely heeded by some patients. Given the adverse but transient impact of alcohol on upper airway stability, it is possible that the pressures required to maintain airway patency during sleep vary with the patient's alcohol consumption immediately prior to the application of the positive-pressure trial. Some reassurance, however, may be obtained from a recent report indicating that moderate alcohol consumption (1.5 to 2 mg/kg) does not significantly alter the level of positive pressure required to maintain upper airway patency during sleep in OSA patients.[63] This does not obviate the need to advocate abstinence, however. Nonetheless, it is important to establish an honest relationship with patients, and if it is clear that an individual is not going to alter his or her alcohol consumption habits, it is reasonable to conduct the evaluation of positive-pressure therapy under the prevailing, rather than artificially enforced and temporary, life circumstances. Similarly, patients who regularly use medication that may potentially increase the likelihood of upper airway obstruction during sleep should be allowed to maintain their usual regimen at the time of polysomnographic evaluation.

In conducting a therapeutic trial of nasal CPAP, the patient is allowed to go to bed at the usual retiring time while wearing the nasal CPAP, which is initially set at levels of 2.5 to 5 cm H_2O. The pressure is incrementally raised to eliminate apneas, hypopneas, desaturation events, arousals associated with abnormal breathing events, and, if feasible, snoring (Figure 28-2). The specific magnitude of the prescribed pressure increments is a matter of choice. In the author's laboratory, CPAP is increased by 2.5-cm H_2O increments. This represents a sufficiently small change to provide good resolution of the required pressure while allowing a sufficiently rapid increase in pressure to allow determination of optimal levels during the finite period of the study. We and others[64] have noted that the pressure required to alleviate snoring is generally higher than that that ameliorates obstructive apnea.

As with nasal CPAP, it is critically important to familiarize the patient with BiPAP before he or she retires to sleep. We have found that patients may still be given the choice of nasal mask, prongs, or full face mask. Although the starting pressures are selected by

the sleep disorders physician, we employ initial settings of 5 cm H_2O for IPAP and 2.5 cm H_2O for EPAP. When occlusive apnea is observed, EPAP is raised by 2.5 cm H_2O, so that the patient is getting 5 cm H_2O of IPAP and 5 cm H_2O of EPAP (functionally representing 5 cm H_2O of CPAP). With further apneic episodes, both the IPAP and EPAP are raised concomitantly, in 2.5-cm H_2O increments, until these events no longer occur. IPAP alone is increased in response to nonapneic desaturation (generally due to obstructive hypopnea) or snoring. If apneas recur when the level of IPAP is greater than EPAP, the latter is progressively raised in 2.5-cm H_2O increments, until either the apneas are no longer present or EPAP equals IPAP. If apneas still persist, then again both IPAP and EPAP are increased concomitantly. In this algorithm, schematically presented in Figure 28-3, the difference between the optimal level of IPAP and the optimal level of EPAP represents the pressure required to prevent nonapneic desaturation and snoring over and above the pressure that was needed to prevent apneas.

When To Consider BiPAP

A trial of BiPAP therapy for OSA should be considered in patients who are intolerant of the pressure sensation of CPAP. This includes patients who complain of difficulty exhaling, smothering, or chest wall discomfort. In addition, BiPAP should be considered for patients who are at particular risk for barotrauma. Finally, because BiPAP provides inspiratory pressure support, it can be used to provide nocturnal

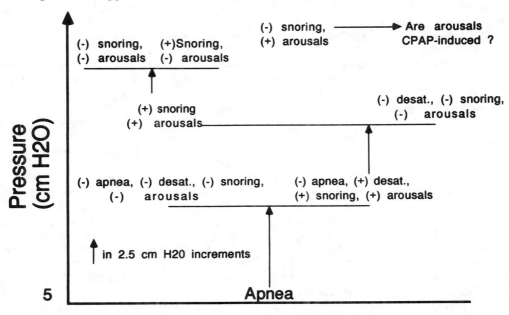

FIGURE 28-2. *Algorithm for establishing proper level of CPAP.*

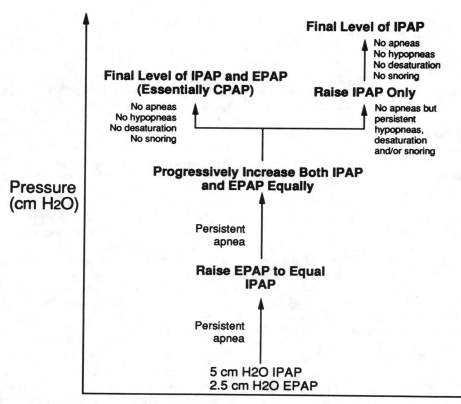

FIGURE 28-3.   *Algorithm for establishing proper levels of BiPAP.*

ventilatory assistance as well as maintenance of upper airway patency during sleep. Thus, it should be considered an alternative to CPAP for patients with neuromuscular disease or chest wall disorders and associated OSA who might benefit from nocturnal ventilatory assistance. Along these lines, as discussed below, even in the absence of overt OSA, nocturnal BiPAP therapy can reduce the arterial carbon dioxide tension during wakefulness and improve daytime function in hypercapnic patients with neuromuscular and chest wall disorders.[65]

Other Uses for Positive Airway Pressure in Treating Sleep-Disordered Breathing

Positive airway pressure may be useful for diagnostic as well as therapeutic purposes in patients with clinical signs and symptoms consistent with OSA. Occasionally patients have multiple sleep disorders, such as PLMS as well as OSA, both of which may contribute to sleep fragmentation and excessive daytime sleepiness. In individual patients it is desirable to direct the initial therapeutic effort toward the disorder that is primarily responsible for the clinical and physiologic sequelae and then to reevaluate the need for additional intervention. Positive airway pressure therapy provides a noninvasive means of

eliminating the OSA component of the patient's disorder complex and permits assessment of any residual clinical and physiologic abnormalities. Similarly, some patients suffer from intercurrent narcolepsy and OSA, either or both of which may contribute to excessive daytime sleepiness. In patients for whom relief of excessive daytime sleepiness, rather than nocturnal oxyhemoglobin desaturation, is the primary therapeutic objective, distinguishing which, if any, is the principal causative disorder directs and simplifies treatment. For example, if elimination of OSA adequately relieves excessive daytime sleepiness despite coexisting narcolepsy, the latter disorder may not warrant specific pharmacologic intervention.

As public awareness of sleep-disordered breathing increases, more patients are brought to medical attention because of concern for snoring or observed apnea during sleep. Many of these patients do not report symptoms that classically are associated with OSA. Indeed, many such persons have "low-level" abnormalities of sleep-related breathing and oxygenation that are of uncertain clinical significance. Because there are, as yet, no accepted guidelines that establish the minimal level of OSA that mandates treatment, it is important to document that patients with minimal OSA and no evident physiologic sequelae are truly asymptomatic before dismissing the need for active therapeutic intervention. Not infrequently, patients do not realize their level of impairment and believe themselves to be asymptomatic until OSA is relieved. Thus, a trial of nocturnal positive-pressure therapy, perhaps in conjunction with multiple sleep latency or wakefulness testing, may help determine the effect of OSA in this regard. Failure of positive-pressure therapy to favorably influence the patient's clinical condition or improve daytime alertness following relief of OSA suggests that, in fact, the nocturnal disordered breathing had no physiologic impact. Unfortunately, the usefulness of positive airway pressure therapy in this context may be limited by the inability of some "asymptomatic" persons with minimal OSA to tolerate any of the available therapeutic devices. Care must also be taken to ensure that the positive-pressure therapy does not itself induce sleep fragmentation and increase daytime sleepiness by virtue of poor patient tolerance.

On the other end of the clinical spectrum from the putatively asymptomatic individual with OSA, a trial of positive airway pressure therapy may also be informative in patients whose symptoms are disproportionately severe relative to the severity of objectively documented OSA (i.e., those who are very symptomatic despite relatively mild OSA). Such a trial may establish or mitigate against a cause-and-effect relationship between OSA and the patient's complaints. Persistence of symptoms despite relief of OSA suggests the need to consider the presence of a non-pulmonary sleep-wakefulness disorder.

NASAL POSITIVE AIRWAY PRESSURE THERAPY OF NONAPNEIC SLEEP-DISORDERED BREATHING

In recent decades, it has become increasingly recognized that patients with compromised lung or chest wall function are also susceptible to significant SDB, which results in substantial nocturnal hypoxemia and hypercapnia.[65-71] SDB in this patient population is often nonapneic, however. Health care professionals have also become increasingly cognizant of the benefits of providing nocturnal ventilatory support for such patients. Clinicians have the option of choosing negative-pressure ventilation, using a tank-type ventilator, cuirass, or poncho, or supporting ventilation during sleep with a positive-pressure device. Although these measures are successful for many patients with neuromuscular and chest wall disorders,[72-78] the data on the application of negative-pressure ventilatory support in sleeping patients with

chronic airflow obstruction are somewhat contradictory.[79,80] To some degree the inconsistent results are related to the inability of these patients to sleep with this modality. In addition, negative-pressure ventilation during sleep has been associated with upper airway obstruction and oxyhemoglobin desaturation.[81-83] On the other hand, until recently positive-pressure ventilation could be applied only via tracheotomy,[74,84] although now noninvasive delivery of ventilatory support via nasal or face mask is available virtually universally.

A growing number of reports attest to the success of nocturnal positive-pressure ventilatory assistance via nasal mask in reducing the awake arterial carbon dioxide tension (Pa_{CO_2} in hypercapnic patients with neuromuscular and chest wall disorders (Table 28-2).[85-92] Ventilatory support may be delivered using a conventional, portable volume-cycled or pressure-cycled device in either an assisted or fully controlled mode of ventilation. The ideal device for providing nocturnal positive-pressure ventilatory assistance in the home should be small and portable, easy to operate, unencumbered by unnecessary alarms, and affordable. In addition, the ventilator should be capable of matching the airflow demanded

TABLE 28-2.   Effect of Nocturnal Positive Pressure Ventilatory Assistance Via Mask on Awake Arterial Carbon Dioxide Tension in Patients with Neuromuscular or Chest Wall Disorders

Study	Pre–Nocturnal Ventilation P_aCO_2 (mmHg)*	Post–Nocturnal Ventilation P_aCO_2 (mmHg)*
Leger et al.[92]‡	51 ± 16	40 ± 4
Leger et al.[92]‡	55 ± 3	40 ± 3
Ellis et al.[87]§	61 ± 14	46 ± 7
Ellis et al.[89]‖	62 ± 6	49 ± 5
Goldstein et al.[91]¶	62 ± 13	52 ± 9
Gay et al.[90]#	64 ± 13	51 ± 7
Sanders et al.[95]**	61 ± 17	49 ± 10

*P_aCO_2 expressed as mean ± SD.
‡Used nocturnal volume-cycled ventilator in control mode (patients with neuromuscular disease).
‡Used nocturnal volume-cycled ventilator in control mode (patients with kyphoscoliosis).
§Used nocturnal volume-cycled ventilator (patients with neuromuscular disease).
‖Used nocturnal volume-cycled ventilator (patients with kyphoscoliosis).
¶Used nocturnal volume-cycled ventilator (patients with kyphoscoliosis and/or neuromuscular disease).
#Used nocturnal volume-cycled ventilator (patients with brain stem disease, kyphoscoliosis, neuromuscular disease, or chronic obstructive pulmonary disease).
**Used BiPAP (patients with kyphoscoliosis and/or neuromuscular disease).

by the patient and permit maintenance of a physiologic breathing pattern to facilitate synchronization between patient and ventilator. Finally, a back-up mechanism should be available on the device to ensure a satisfactory level of ventilation in the event of apnea. These requirements have been nicely outlined by Branthwaite.[93]

In this context, BiPAP has been used to provide nocturnal ventilatory assistance to patients with neuromuscular and chest wall disorders.[94-97] Nocturnal use of this device has been shown to reduce $PaCO_2$ during wakefulness in hypercapnic patients and to relieve symptoms indicative of nocturnal hypoxemia, hypercapnia, and disturbed sleep (e.g., morning headaches, foggy-headedness, personality change, and hypersomnolence). Though many authors have described the need for in-hospital acclimatization to nocturnal ventilation with conventional volume- and pressure-cycled ventilators,[86,90,98,99] we have not found this to be necessary with BiPAP. This may be explained by the fact that patients can determine their own breathing pattern, including inspiratory time, flow rate, and total cycle time while on BiPAP, which may maximize comfort and synchrony with the device. It should be noted, however, that systematic, comparative studies of BiPAP and conventional portable ventilators with respect to time required for acclimatization have yet to be performed.

Though it is evident that positive-pressure ventilatory assistance tends to normalize the $PaCO_2$ in hypercapnic patients with neuromuscular and chest wall disorders (see Table 28-2), what mechanism is responsible for this improvement is unclear. One possibility is that there is a reduction in $PaCO_2$ while the patient sleeps with positive-pressure therapy and this results in reduced blood-buffering capacity (i.e., lower serum bicarbonate), so that ventilatory chemoresponsiveness to carbon dioxide is augmented. Arguing against this, however, is our observation, as well as that of others, that awake $PaCO_2$ falls even in persons for whom positive pressure does not reduce the $PaCO_2$ during sleep.[90,95,99] Alternatively, it is possible that nocturnal ventilatory assistance "rests" fatigued ventilatory muscles which consequently grow stronger. In this regard, several studies have suggested that positive-pressure ventilatory assistance via mask reduces the work performed by inspiratory muscles in patients with neuromuscular or chest wall disorders and chronic obstructive airways disease and that it may be more effective in doing so than negative-pressure ventilation.[100-102] Our own data indicate that the application of positive-pressure ventilatory support during sleep in some of these patients results in a variable degree of central apnea, even in the absence of respiratory alkalosis,

which can be relieved by the timed-delivery application of positive inspiratory pressure support.[95] This observation supports the concept proposed by Rochester and colleagues[103] that the application of external ventilatory assistance to patients with increased work of breathing (or increased workload relative to the maximum capacity of the inspiratory muscles) is in some way perceived by the patient as a signal to reduce, or even cease, the activity of the inspiratory muscles, thus permitting "rest." On the other hand, there is only equivocal evidence to suggest that ventilatory muscle *strength* is increased by nocturnal ventilatory assistance. Though some investigators have observed an increase in forced vital capacity and augmented maximal inspiratory pressure[86,89] following initiation of therapy, others have reported no increase in these variables or in the maximal voluntary ventilation, despite a reduction in awake $PaCO_2$.[90-92,95,98] Ventilatory muscle *endurance*, however, may be a more relevant factor to consider than ventilatory muscle strength as a mechanism to explain the reduction in awake $PaCO_2$ following initiation of nocturnal positive-pressure ventilatory support. Importantly, Goldstein and coworkers[91] observed a significant increase in inspiratory muscle endurance after 3 months' nocturnal therapy but no change in respiratory muscle strength as measured by maximal inspiratory and expiratory pressures or by maximal voluntary ventilation.

In addition to central apnea, some patients with neuromuscular or chest wall disorders develop obstructive apnea during sleep on positive-pressure ventilation.[87,94,95] Unlike negative-pressure ventilation, positive-pressure support is not associated with the generation of negative intrapharyngeal pressure, which could contribute to the development of upper airway obstruction. The pathogenesis of these events during positive pressure therapy is uncertain, but it is intriguing to speculate that the upper airway dilator muscles behave in a fashion similar to the chest wall inspiratory muscles during positive-pressure ventilatory support, so that there is a loss of inspiratory activity or tone (i.e., rest). This could make the upper airway susceptible to closure even in the absence of negative intrapharyngeal pressure.[15,16,54,55] Whatever the mechanism, it is, of course, essential to maintain upper airway patency during sleep. To this end, positive pressure may be delivered during expiration, either as positive end-expiratory pressure when using a conventional portable ventilator[85] or, if using BiPAP, as EPAP,[94,95] in conjunction with IPAP to maintain upper airway patency and support the patient. In this way, treating obstructive apneas that occur during nocturnal ventilatory support is similar to treating them in OSA patients. In both patient populations, success in eliminating obstructive apnea by the addition of positive pressure, particularly during expiration, reinforces the importance of pathophysiologic events during this phase of the breathing cycle.[15,16]

Interfaces Between Positive-Pressure Devices and Patients

Maintenance of a comfortable and leak free interface in patients with neuromuscular or chest wall disorders who are receiving nocturnal positive-pressure ventilatory support is as important as it is in OSA patients receiving poisitive-pressure therapy. For OSA patients the overriding therapeutic concern is maintenance of a patent upper airway, whereas in non-OSA patients with neuromuscular or chest wall disorders who are receiving nocturnal ventilatory support, providing adequate minute ventilation is the critical goal (though reestablishing upper airway patency when necessary in these patients is, obviously, also important). Leaks can confound the attainment of this objective and may necessitate increasing the tidal volume delivered by conventional ventilators as a compensatory maneuver. In addition, it has been shown that mask leaks may have a very disruptive impact on sleep quality and architecture.[104] Thus, it is essential to provide patients with the best-fitting and most leak-free mask available. We have found that many patients obtain excellent results using commercially available nasal masks. A number of others, however, particularly those with neuromuscular disorders, have a great deal of difficulty keeping the mouth closed enough to prevent substantial air leakage, which can compromise therapeutic efficacy. For these patients we have successfully delivered long-term nocturnal positive-pressure therapy via a full face mask.[95] We have employed either a large nasal mask for this purpose, a custom-made full face mask (oral-nasal), or a prototype total face mask. A strapless oral-nasal interface has also been described.[105] Of course the same precautions described in the previous section on the delivery of CPAP to OSA patients via full face mask apply to the use of such an interface for any patient who requires nocturnal ventilatory support.

Another approach to the problem of providing a noninvasive interface to patients using positive-pressure devices is the use of mouthpieces.[105-107] Bach and coworkers have had substantial experience using this type of interface in postpolio and quadriplegic patients with ventilatory insufficiency. Loss of air is minimized by holding the mouthpiece in place with a lip seal. This technique is ineffective,

however, for those with incompetent buccopharyngeal muscles. In addition, positive-pressure ventilatory support via mouthpiece may be associated with increased risk of aspiration of gastric contents, development of bite deformities, and dry mouth.[105,106]

Establishing Proper Ventilatory Support Settings

Given the uncertainty about the exact mechanism(s) that reduce awake $PaCO_2$ following initiation of nocturnal ventilatory support, the diversity of approaches to determine the "correct" ventilator settings is not surprising.

Several authors adjust tidal volume and inspiratory flow on conventional portable ventilators according to patient comfort,[99] whereas others report adjusting tidal volume by monitoring end-tidal or arterial carbon dioxide, with the goal of maintaining values during sleep that approximate those during wakefulness.[86] Still others have monitored transcutaneous carbon dioxide ($PtcCO_2$) together with diaphragm and sternocleidomastoid electromyograms using surface electrodes. In these studies adequate ventilatory support during sleep is defined as a reduction in electromyogram activity by 50% with an accompanying increase in oxyhemoglobin saturation and decrease in $PtcCO_2$. Unfortunately, all of the methods described thus far are imperfect. Adjusting settings to the awake patient's comfort may not ensure satisfactory support during sleep. End-tidal carbon dioxide may not be an accurate or consistent reflection of $PaCO_2$ during sleep, as there may be changes in dead space on the basis of delivered tidal volume, changing cardiac output, or variation in the position of the capnograph catheter in the mask. Technically adequate electromyograms may be difficult to obtain in certain patients, and indeed, as we and others have found, one can silence the activity of the ventilatory muscles without appreciably changing the $PaCO_2$ (though, as previously noted, the necessity of reducing the $PaCO_2$ during sleep has yet to be established). There is, nevertheless, intuitive attractiveness to employing the $PaCO_2$ as a parameter by which ventilator settings may be determined during sleep. Monitoring this value helps the clinician avoid the development of additional respiratory acidosis over and above that that exists during wakefulness as well as excessive respiratory alkalosis during nocturnal ventilatory support, which can alter cerebral blood flow and enhance the likelihood of cardiac dysrhythmias. Unfortunately, peripheral arterial catheterization is the only way to sample $PaCO_2$ during sleep, and even then the information provided is not continuous. An alternative that has been proposed is $PtcCO_2$ monitoring. Though this technique provides a continuous data readout, there are conflicting data in the literature regarding its accuracy in adults. Several studies have reported a good correlation between $PtcCO_2$ and $PaCO_2$ in hemodynamically stable adults and children,[108-111] though some of the data reflect substantial scatter in the relationship between the two variables.[109] Along these lines, one study indicated that there may be greater overestimation of $PaCO_2$ by $PtcCO_2$ as the former value increases,[112] and observations from our laboratory in six sleeping patients with neuromuscular or chest wall disorders support this finding (MH Sanders, unpublished data). In any event, in view of the inconsistencies that exist, it seems clear that further studies are needed before there is general, unqualified use of the $PtcCO_2$ to monitor the safety and efficacy of nocturnal mechanical ventilatory assistance. At the least, it may be prudent to establish that there is satisfactory accuracy of the $PtcCO_2$ as a reflection of $PaCO_2$ in individual patients before the former variable is employed as a parameter by which ventilator settings are established.

In our laboratory, when nocturnal ventilatory support via mask is provided by BiPAP or by a conventional portable ventilator, the initial settings are determined both by patient comfort during wakefulness and by monitoring the $PaCO_2$ during sleep, which ensures that unacceptable hyperventilation has not developed. During BiPAP therapy, IPAP is increased to keep the $PaCO_2$ within a range between the awake $PaCO_2$ and 10 mm Hg below that value, provided the pH remains no higher than 7.49. On those infrequent occasions when, owing to concerns about barotrauma or patient discomfort, the IPAP level is higher than desirable, the timed back-up rate is raised, to increase the patient's ventilation while minimizing the applied inspiratory pressure. For patients who develop central apnea in the absence of respiratory alkalosis, a timed back-up rate is instituted to provide acceptable ventilatory frequency. Finally, in the event that obstructive apneas are observed, the EPAP is increased as described above for OSA patients.

SUMMARY

Positive-pressure ventilation via mask during sleep constitutes a safe and effective treatment for OSA and, at the same time, represents a new and exciting technique that can reduce the $PaCO_2$ in hypercapnic patients with neuromuscular and chest wall disorders. This modality is generally accepted as the medical therapy of choice for OSA. Long-term patient compliance is good, though not optimal. Further studies are needed to better define the factors that determine compliance.

Among patients with neuromuscular respiratory failure, early studies suggest that the improvement in ventilation during wakefulness is related to increased endurance of the ventilatory muscles, though other mechanisms have not been excluded. These studies also suggest that nocturnal positive-pressure ventilation is tolerated well by the majority of patients, and that it relieves symptoms and improves quality of life. At the present time, large, systematic, longitudinal studies of these potential benefits have yet to be reported.

REFERENCES

1. Sullivan CE, Issa FG, Berthon-Jones M, et al. Reversal of obstructive sleep apnoea by continuous positive airway pressure applied through the nares. Lancet 1981;1:862–865.
2. Hoffstein V, Zamel N, Phillipson EA. Lung volume dependence of pharyngeal cross-sectional area in patients with obstructive sleep apnea. Am Rev Respir Dis 1984;130:175–178.
3. Brown I, Taylor R, Hoffstein V. Obstructive sleep apnea reversed by increased lung volume? Eur J Respir Dis 1986;68:375–380.
4. Series F, Cormier Y, Lampron N, et al. Increasing the functional residual capacity may reverse obstructive sleep apnea. Sleep 1988;11:349–353.
5. Van de Graaf WB. Thoracic influence on upper airway patency. J Appl Physiol 1988;65:2124–2131.
6. Begle RL, Sadr S, Skatrud JB, et al. Effect of lung inflation on pulmonary resistance during NREM sleep. Am Rev Respir Dis 1990;141:854–860.
7. Series F, Cormier Y, Desmeules M. Influence of passive changes of lung volume on upper airways. J Appl Physiol 1990;68:2159–2164.
8. Series F, Cormier Y, Couture J, et al. Changes in upper airway resistance with lung inflation and positive airway pressure. J Appl Physiol 1990;68:1075–1079.
9. Abbey NC, Cooper KR, Kwentus JA. Benefit of nasal CPAP in obstructive sleep apnea is due to positive pharyngeal pressure. Sleep 1989;12:420–422.
10. Rapoport DM, Garay SM, Goldring RM. Nasal CPAP in obstructive sleep apnea: Mechanisms of action. Bull Eur Physiopathol Respir 1983;19:616–620.
11. Strohl KP, Redline S. Nasal CPAP therapy, upper airway activation, and obstructive sleep apnea. Am Rev Respir Dis 1986;134:555–558.
12. Alex CG, Aronson RM, Onal E, et al. Effects of continuous positive airway pressure on upper airway and respiratory muscle activity. J Appl Physiol 1987;62:2026–2030.
13. Sanders MH. Nasal CPAP effect on patterns of sleep apnea. Chest 1984;86:839–844.
14. Issa FG, Sullivan CE. Reversal of central sleep apnea using nasal CPAP. Chest 1986;90:165–171.
15. Sanders MH, Rogers RM, Pennock BE. Prolonged expiratory phase in sleep apnea: A unifying hypothesis. Am Rev Respir Dis 1985;131:401–408.

16. Sanders MH, Moore SE. Inspiratory and expiratory partitioning of airway resistance during sleep in patients with sleep apnea. Am Rev Respir Dis 1983;127: 554–558.

17. Rajagopal KR, Bennett LL, Dillard TA, et al. Overnight nasal CPAP improves hypersomnolence in sleep apnea. Chest 1986;90:172–176.

18. Lamphere J, Roehrs T, Wittig R, et al. Recovery of alertness after CPAP in apnea. Chest 1989;96:1364–1367.

19. Frith RW, Cant BR. Severe obstructive sleep apnoea treated with long term nasal continuous positive airway pressure. Thorax 1985;40:45–50.

20. McEvoy RD, Thornton AT. Treatment of obstructive sleep apnea syndrome with nasal continuous positive airway pressure. Sleep 1984;7:313–325.

21. Sanders MH, Kern N. Obstructive sleep apnea treated by independently adjusted inspiratory and expiratory positive airway pressures via nasal mask. Physiologic and clinical implications. Chest 1990;98:317–324.

22. Demirozu MC, Steinberg N, Kiel M, et al. The effect of positive end expiratory pressure and site of oxygen entrainment on inspiratory oxygen concentration when using supplemental oxygen with nasal continuous positive airway pressure. Sleep Res 1990;19:321.

23. Douglas NJ, White DP, Weil JV, et al. Hypercapnic ventilatory response in sleeping adults. Am Rev Respir Dis 1982;126:758–762.

24. Douglas NJ, White DP, Weil JV, et al. Hypoxic ventilatory response decreases during sleep in normal men. Am Rev Respir Dis 1982;125:286–289.

25. White DP. Occlusion pressure and ventilation during sleep in normal humans. J Appl Physiol 1986;61:1279–1287.

26. Skatrud JB, Dempsey JA. Interaction of sleep state and chemical stimuli in sustaining rhythmic ventilation. J Appl Physiol 1983;55:813–822.

27. Henke KG, Dempsey JA, Kowitz JM, et al. Effects of sleep-induced increases in upper airway resistance on ventilation. J Appl Physiol 1990;69:617–624.

28. Tabachnik E, Muller NL, Bryan AC, et al. Changes in ventilation and chest wall mechanics during sleep in normal adolescents. J Appl Physiol 1981;51:557–564.

29. Stauffer JL, Fayter NA, McClure BJ. Conjunctivitis from nasal CPAP apparatus. Chest 1984;86:802.

30. Strumpf DA, Harrop P, Dobbin J, et al. Massive epistaxis from nasal CPAP therapy. Chest 1989;95:1141.

31. Sullivan CE, Grunstein RR. Continuous positive airways pressure in sleep-disordered breathing. In: Kryger MH, Roth T, Dement WC, eds. Principles and Practice of Sleep Medicine. Philadelphia: WB Saunders, 1989; 559–570.

32. Jarjour NN, Wilson P. Pneumoencephalus associated with nasal continuous positive airway pressure in a patient with sleep apnea syndrome. Chest 1989;96: 1425–1426.

33. Waldhorn RE, Herrick TW, Nguyen MC, et al. Long-term compliance with nasal continuous positive airway pressure therapy of obstructive sleep apnea. Chest 1990;97:33–38.

34. Krieger J, Weitzenblum E, Monassier J-P, et al. Dangerous hypoxaemia during continuous positive airway

pressure treatment of obstructive sleep apnoea. Lancet 1983;2:1429–1430.

35. Rapoport DM, Sorkin B, Garay SM, et al. Reversal of the "pickwickian syndrome" by long-term use of nocturnal airway pressure. N Engl J Med 1982;307:931–933.

36. Sullivan CE, Berthon-Jones M, Issa FG. Remission of severe obesity-hypoventilation syndrome after short-term treatment during sleep with nasal continuous positive airway pressure. Am Rev Respir Dis 1982;128: 177–181.

37. Berthon-Jones M, Sullivan CE. Time course of change in ventilatory response to CO_2 with long-term CPAP therapy for obstructive sleep apnea. Am Rev Respir Dis 1987;135:144–147.

38. Sullivan CE, Issa FG, Berthon-Jones M, et al. Home treatment of obstructive sleep apnoea with continuous positive airway pressure applied through a nose mask. Bull Eur Physiopathol Respir 1984;20:49–54.

39. Nino-Murcia G, McCann CC, Bliwise DL, et al. Compliance and side effects in sleep apnea patients treated with continuous positive airway pressure. West J Med 1989;150:165–169.

40. Sanders MH, Gruendl CA, Rogers RM. Patient compliance with nasal CPAP therapy for sleep apnea. Chest 1986;90:330–333.

41. ANTADIR. A multicenter survey of long term compliance with nasal CPAP treatment in patients with obstructive sleep apnea syndrome. Am Rev Respir Dis 1990;141:A863.

42. Fletcher EC, Luckett RA. The effect of positive reinforcement on hourly compliance in continuous positive airway pressure users with obstructive sleep apnea. Am Rev Respir Dis 1991;143:936–941.

43. Sanders MH, Rogers RM. Sleep apnea: When does better become benefit? Chest 1985;88:320–321.

44. Sanders MH, Holzer BC. Does sleep apnea beget sleep apnea? Clin Res 1984;32:436A.

45. Olson LG, Rolfe IE, Saunders NA. Tolerance of nasal CPAP treatment of obstructive sleep apnea, and its effect on disease severity. Am Rev Respir Dis 1990; 141:A866.

46. Fry JM, DiPhillipo MA, Pressman MR. Periodic leg movements in sleep following treatment of obstructive sleep apnea with nasal continuous positive airway pressure. Chest 1989;96:89–91.

47. Sanders MH, Moore SE, Eveslage J. CPAP via nasal mask: A treatment for occlusive sleep apnea. Chest 1983;83:144–145.

48. Remmers JE, Sterling JA, Thorasinsson B, et al. Nasal airway positive pressure in patients with occlusive sleep apnea: Methods and feasibility. Am Rev Respir Dis 1984;130:1152–1155.

49. Mayer LS, Kerby GR, Whitman RA, et al. Continued evaluation of a new nasal device for administration of continuous positive airway pressure. Am Rev Respir Dis 1990;141:A684.

50. Harris C, Daniels B, Herold D, et al. Comparison of cannula and mask systems for administration of nasal continuous positive airway pressure for treatment of obstructive sleep apnea. Sleep Res 1990;19:233.

51. Mayer LS, Kerby GR, Whitman RA. Evaluation of a new nasal device for administration of continuous

positive airway pressure for obstructive sleep apnea. Am Rev Respir Dis 1989;139:A114.

52. Covelli HD, Weled BJ, Beekman JF. Efficacy of continuous positive airway pressure administered by mask. Chest 1982;2:147–150.

53. Branson RD, Hurst JM, DeHaven CB. Mask CPAP: State of the art. Respir Care 1985;30:846–857.

54. Smith PL, Wise RA, Gold AR, et al. Upper airway pressure-flow relationships in obstructive sleep apnea. J Appl Physiol 1988;64:789–795.

55. Schwartz AR, Smith PL, Wise RA, et al. Induction of upper airway occlusion in sleeping individuals with subatmospheric nasal pressure. J Appl Physiol 1988;64:535–542.

56. Mahadevia AK, Onal E, Lopata M. Effects of expiratory positive airway pressure on sleep-induced abnormalities in patients with hypersomnia– sleep apnea syndrome. Am Rev Respir Dis 1983;128:708–711.

57. Parisi RA, England SJ, Santiago TV. Treatment of central sleep apnea with respiratory-cycled variable nasal positive pressure (BiPAP). Am Rev Respir Dis 1991;143:A586.

58. Guilleminault C, Stoohs R. Upper airway resistance syndrome. Am Rev Respir Dis 1991;143:A589.

59. Duncan S, Guilleminault C, Stoohs R, et al. Snoring (1): Daytime sleepiness in regular heavy snorers. Chest 1991;99:40–48.

60. Issa FG, Sullivan CE. Upper airway closing pressures in snorers. J Appl Physiol 1984;57:528–535.

61. Block AJ, Hellard DH, Slayton PC. Effect of alcohol ingestion on breathing and oxygenation during sleep. Am J Med 1986;80:595–600.

62. Issa FG, Sullivan CE. Alcohol, snoring and sleep apnea. J Neurol Neurosurg Psychiatr 1982;5:353–359.

63. Berry RB, Desa MM, Light RW. Effect of ethanol on the efficacy of nasal continuous positive airway pressure as a treatment for obstructive sleep apnea. Chest 1991;99:339–343.

64. Berry RB, Block AJ. Positive nasal airway pressure eliminates snoring as well as obstructive sleep apnea. Chest 1984;85:15–20.

65. Smith PEM, Calverly PMA, Edwards RHT. Hypoxemia during sleep in Duchenne muscular dystrophy. Am Rev Respir Dis 1988;137:884–888.

66. Bye PTP, Issa F, Berthon-Jones M, et al. Studies of oxygenation during sleep in patients with interstitial lung disease. Am Rev Respir Dis 1984;129:27–32.

67. Perez-Padilla R, West P, Lertzman M, et al. Breathing during sleep in patients with interstitial lung disease. Am Rev Respir Dis 1985;132:224–229.

68. Steljes DG, Kryger MH, Kirk BW, et al. Sleep in postpolio syndrome. Chest 1990;98:133–140.

69. Bye PTP, Ellis ER, Issa FQ, et al. Respiratory failure and sleep in neuromuscular disease. Thorax 1990;45:241–247.

70. Gay PC, Westbrook PR, Daube JR, et al. Effects of alterations in pulmonary function and sleep variables on survival in patients with amyotrophic lateral sclerosis. Mayo Clin Proc 1991;66:686–694.

71. Douglas NJ. Breathing during sleep in patients with respiratory disease. Semin Respir Med 1988;9:586–593.

72. Wiers PWJ, Le Coultre R, Dallinga OT, et al. Cuirass respirator treatment of chronic respiratory failure in scoliotic patients. Thorax 1977;32:221–228.

73. Curran FJ. Night ventilation by body respirators for patients in chronic respiratory failure due to late stage Duchenne muscular dystrophy. Arch Phys Med Rehabil 1981;62:270–274.

74. Garay SM, Turino GM, Goldring RM. Sustained reversal of chronic hypercapnia in patients with alveolar hypoventilation syndromes. Long-term maintenance with noninvasive nocturnal mechanical ventilation. Am J Med 1981;70:269–274.

75. Goldstein RS, Molotiu, Skrastins R, et al. Reversal of sleep-induced hypoventilation and chronic respiratory failure by nocturnal negative pressure ventilation in patients with restrictive ventilatory impairment. Am Rev Respir Dis 1987;135:1049–1055.

76. Kinnear W, Hockley S, Harvey J, et al. The effects of one year of nocturnal cuirass assisted ventilation in chest wall disease. Eur Respir J 1988;1:204–208.

77. Splaingard ML, Frates RC, Jefferson LS, et al. Home negative pressure ventilation: Report of 20 years of experience in patients with neuromuscular disease. Arch Phys Med Rehabil 1985;66:239–242.

78. Mohr CH, Hill NS. Long-term follow-up of nocturnal ventilatory assistance in patients with respiratory failure due to Duchenne-type muscular dystrophy. Chest 1990;97:91–96.

79. Zibrak JD, Hill NS, Federman EC, et al. Evaluation of intermittent long-term negative pressure ventilation in patients with severe chronic obstructive pulmonary disease. Am Rev Respir Dis 1988;138:1515–1518.

80. Celli B, Lee H, Criner G, et al. Controlled trial of negative pressure ventilation in patients with severe chronic airflow obstruction. Am Rev Respir Dis 1989;140:1251–1256.

81. Scharf SM, Feldman NT, Goldman MD, et al. Vocal cord closure. Incidence of upper airway obstruction during controlled ventilation. Am Rev Respir Dis 1978;117:391–397.

82. Levy RD, Bradley TD, Newman S, et al. Negative pressure ventilation. Effects on ventilation during sleep in normal subjects. Chest 1989;95:95–99.

83. Hill NS. Clinical applications of body ventilators. Chest 1986;90:897–905.

84. Hoeppner VH, Cockcroft DW, Dosman JA, et al. Night-time ventilation improves respiratory failure in secondary kyphoscoliosis. Am Rev Respir Dis 1984;129:240–243.

85. Ellis ER, Bye PTP, Bruderer JW, et al. Treatment of respiratory failure during sleep in patients with neuromuscular disease. Positive-pressure ventilation through a nose mask. Am Rev Respir Dis 1987;135:148–152.

86. Kerby GR, Mayer LS, Pingleton SK. Nocturnal positive pressure ventilation via nasal mask. Am Rev Respir Dis 1987;135:738–740.

87. Ellis ER, McCauley VB, Mellis C, et al. Treatment of alveolar hypoventilation in a six-year-old girl with intermittent positive pressure ventilation through a nose mask. Am Rev Respir Dis 1987;136:188–191.

88. Segall D. Noninvasive nasal mask-assisted ventilation in respiratory failure of Duchenne muscular dystrophy. Chest 1988;93:1298–1300.

89. Ellis ER, Grunstein RR, Chan S, et al. Noninvasive ventilatory support during sleep improves respiratory failure in kyphoscoliosis. Chest 1988;94:811–815.

90. Gay PC, Patel AM, Viggiano RW, et al. Nocturnal nasal ventilation for treatment of patients with hypercapnic respiratory failure. Mayo Clin Proc 1991;66:695–703.

91. Goldstein RS, De Rosie JA, Avendano MA, et al. Influence of noninvasive positive pressure ventilation on inspiratory muscles. Chest 1991;99:408–415.

92. Leger P, Jennequin J, Gerard M, et al. Home positive pressure ventilation via nasal mask for patients with neuromuscular weakness or restrictive lung or chest-wall disease. Respir Care 1989;34:73–79.

93. Branthwaite MA. Home mechanical ventilation. Eur Respir J 1990;3:743–745.

94. Sanders MH, Black J, Stiller RA, et al. Nocturnal ventilatory assistance with bi-level positive airway pressure. Operative Tech Otolaryngol Head Neck Surgery 1991;2:56–62.

95. Sanders MH, Kern NB. Long-term experience with BiPAP in neuromuscular disease patients: Clinical and physiologic implications. Presented at III World Congress for Sleep Apnea and Rhonchopathy. Tokyo Japan, September 1991. In: Abstracts of the III World Congress for Sleep Apnea and Rhonchopathy, Tokyo Japan, September 1991;22.

96. Hill NS, Eveloff SE, Carlisle CC, et al. Efficacy of nocturnal nasal ventilation administered by the Bi-PAP ventilator in restrictive pulmonary diseases. Am Rev Respir Dis 1991;143:A602.

97. Herold DL, Staats BA. Symptomatic nasal CPAP treatment of bilateral diaphragm paralysis. Sleep Res 1991;20:256.

98. Carroll N, Branthwaite MA. Control of nocturnal hypoventilation by nasal intermittent positive pressure ventilation. Thorax 1988;43:349–353.

99. Rodenstein DO, Stanescu DC, Delguste PM, et al. Adaptation to intermittent positive pressure ventilation applied through the nose during day and night. Eur Respir J 1989;2:473–478.

100. Levine S, Henson D, Levy S. Respiratory muscle rest therapy. Clin Chest Med 1988;9:297–309.

101. Carrey Z, Gottfried SB, Levy RD. Ventilatory muscle support in respiratory failure with nasal positive pressure ventilation. Chest 1990;97:150–158.

102. Belman MJ, Soo Hoo GW, Kuei JH, et al. Efficacy of positive vs. negative pressure ventilation in unloading the respiratory muscles. Chest 1990;98:850–856.

103. Rochester DF, Braun NMT, Laine S. Diaphragmatic energy expenditure in chronic respiratory failure. Am J Med 1977;63:223–232.

104. Robert D, Langevin B, Leger P. Mouth air leaks during noninvasive nasal intermittent positive pressure ventilation. Am Rev Respir Dis 1991;143:A587.

105. Bach JR, Alba AS, Shin D. Management of alternatives for post-polio respiratory insufficiency. Am J Phys Med Rehabil 1989;68:264–271.

106. Bach JR, Alba AS, Bohatiuk G, et al. Mouth intermittent positive pressure ventilation in the management of postpolio respiratory insufficiency. Chest 1987;91:859–864.

107. Bach JR, Alba AS. Noninvasive options for ventilatory support of the traumatic high level quadriplegic patient. Chest 1990;98:613–619.

108. McLellan PA, Goldstein RS, Ramacharan V, et al. Transcutaneous carbon dioxide monitoring. Am Rev Respir Dis 1981;124:199–201.

109. Mahutte CK, Michiels TM, Hassel KT, et al. Evaluation of a single transcutaneous Po_2-Pco_2 sensor in adult patients. Crit Care Med 1984;12:1063–1066.

110. Martin RJ. Transcutaneous monitoring: Instrumentation and clinical applications. Respir Care 1990;35:577–582.

111. Shacter EN, Rafferty TD, Knight C, et al. Transcutaneous oxygen and carbon dioxide monitoring. Uses in adult surgical patients in an intensive care unit. Arch Surg 1981;116:1193–1196.

112. Martin RJ, Beoglos A, Miller MJ, et al. Increasing arterial carbon dioxide tension: Influence on transcutaneous carbon dioxide tension measurements. Pediatrics 1988;81:684–687.

Glossary of Terms Used in Sleep Disorders Medicine*

Actigraph: A biomedical instrument for the measurement of body movement.

Active Sleep: A term used in the phylogenetic and ontogenetic literature for the stage of sleep that is considered to be equivalent to rapid eye movement (REM) sleep (*see REM Sleep*).

Alpha activity: An alpha electroencephalogram (EEG) wave or sequence of waves with a frequency of 8–13 Hz.

Alpha-Delta Sleep: Sleep in which alpha activity occurs during slow-wave sleep. Because alpha-delta sleep is rarely seen without alpha occurring in other sleep stages the term *alpha sleep* is preferred.

Alpha Intrusion (-Infiltration, -Insertion, -Interruption): A brief superimposition of EEG alpha activity on sleep activities during a stage of sleep.

Alpha Rhythm: An EEG rhythm with a frequency of 8 to 13 Hz in human adults that is most prominent over the parietooccipital cortex when the eyes are closed. The rhythm is blocked by eye opening or other arousing stimuli. It is indicative of the awake state in most normal individuals. It is most consistent and predominant during relaxed wakefulness, particularly with reduction of visual input. The amplitude is variable but typically is below 50 μV in adults. The alpha rhythm of an individual usually slows by 0.5 to 1.5 Hz and becomes more diffuse during drowsiness. The frequency range also varies with age; it is slower in children and older age groups than in young to middle-aged adults.

Alpha Sleep: Sleep in which alpha activity occurs during most, if not all, sleep stages.

Apnea: Cessation of airflow at the nostrils and mouth lasting at least 10 seconds. There are three types of apnea: obstructive, central, and mixed. Obstructive apnea is secondary to upper airway obstruction; central apnea is associated with a cessation of all respiratory movements; mixed apnea has both central and obstructive components.

Apnea-Hypopnea Index: The number of apneic episodes (obstructive, central, and mixed) plus hypopneas per hour of sleep as determined by all-night polysomnography.

Apnea Index: The number of apneic episodes (obstructive, central and mixed) per hour of sleep as determined during all-night polysomnography.

Sometimes a separate obstructive apnea index or central apnea index is stated.

Arise Time: The clock time that an individual gets out of bed after the final awakening of the major sleep episode (distinguished from final wake-up).

Arousal: An abrupt change from a deeper stage of non-REM (NREM) sleep to a lighter stage, or from REM sleep toward wakefulness, with the possibility of awakening as the final outcome. Arousal may be accompanied by increased tonic electromyographic (EMG) activity and heart rate as well as body movements.

Arousal Disorder: A parasomnia disorder presumed to be due to an abnormal arousal mechanism. Forced arousal from sleep can induce episodes. The "classical" arousal disorders are sleepwalking, sleep terrors, and confusional arousals.

Awakening: The return to the polysomnographically defined awake state from any NREM or REM sleep stage. It is characterized by alpha and beta EEG activity, a rise in tonic EMG, voluntary REMs, and eye blinks. This definition of awakenings is valid only insofar as the polysomnogram is paralleled by a resumption of a reasonably alert state of awareness of the environment.

Axial System: A means of stating different types of information in a systematic manner by listing on several "axes," to ensure that important information is not overlooked by the statement of a single major diagnosis. The International Classification of Sleep Disorders (ICSD) utilizes a three-axis system: axes A, B, and C.

Axis A: The first level of the ICSD axial system, on which the sleep disorder diagnoses, modifiers and associated code numbers are stated.

Axis B: The second level of the ICSD axial system, on which the sleep-related procedures and procedure features, and associated code numbers, are stated.

Axis C: The third level of the ICSD axial system, on which ICD nonsleep diagnoses and associated code numbers are stated.

Baseline: The typical or normal state of an individual or of an investigative variable prior to an experimental manipulation.

---

*Reprinted with the permission of the American Sleep Disorders Association, Rochester, MN

Bedtime: The clock time at which one attempts to fall asleep, as differentiated from the clock time when one gets into bed.

Beta Activity: A beta EEG wave or sequence of waves with frequency greater than 13 Hz.

Beta Rhythm: An EEG rhythm in the range of 13 to 35 Hz, when the predominant frequency, beta rhythm, is usually associated with alert wakefulness or vigilance and is accompanied by a high tonic EMG. The amplitude of beta rhythm is variable but usually is below 30 μV. This rhythm may be drug induced.

Brain Wave: Use of this term is discouraged. The preferred term is *EEG wave.*

Cataplexy: A sudden decrement in muscle tone and loss of deep tendon reflexes leading to muscle weakness, paralysis, or postural collapse. Cataplexy usually is precipitated by an outburst of emotional expression, notably laughter, anger, or startle. One of the symptom tetrad of narcolepsy. During cataplexy, respiration and voluntary eye movements are not compromised.

Cheyne-Stokes Respiration: A breathing pattern characterized by regular "crescendo-decrescendo" fluctuations in respiratory rate and tidal volume.

Chronobiology: The science of temporal, primarily rhythmic, processes in biology.

Circadian Rhythm: An innate daily fluctuation of physiologic or behavioral functions, including sleep-wake states generally tied to the 24-hour daily dark-light cycle. Sometimes occurs at a measurably different periodicity (e.g., 23 or 25 hours) when light-dark and other time cues are removed.

Circasemidian Rhythm: A biologic rhythm that has a period length of about half a day.

Conditional Insomnia: Insomnia produced by the development, during an earlier experience of sleeplessness, of conditioned arousal. Causes of the conditioned stimulus can include the customary sleep environment or thoughts of disturbed sleep. A conditional insomnia is one component of psychophysiologic insomnia.

Constant Routine: A chronobiologic test of the endogenous pacemaker that involves a 36-hour baseline monitoring period followed by a 40-hour waking episode of monitoring with the individual on a constant routine of food intake, position, activity, and light exposure.

Cycle: Characteristic of an event exhibiting rhythmic fluctuations. One cycle is defined as the activity from one maximum or minimum to the next.

Deep Sleep: Common term for combined NREM stage 3 and 4 sleep. In some sleep literature, deep sleep is applied to REM sleep because of its high awakening threshold to nonsignificant stimuli (see *"Intermediary" Sleep Stage; Light Sleep*).

Delayed Sleep Phase: A condition that occurs when the clock hour at which sleep normally occurs is moved ahead in time within a given 24-hour sleep-wake cycle. This results in a temporarily displaced, that is delayed, occurrence of sleep within the 24-hour cycle. The same term denotes a circadian rhythm sleep disturbance, called the delayed sleep phase syndrome.

Delta Activity: EEG activity with a frequency of less than 4 Hz (usually 0.1 to 3.5 Hz). In human sleep scoring, the minimum characteristics for scoring delta waves is conventionally 75 μV (peak-to-peak) amplitude, and 0.5 seconds' duration (2 Hz) or less.

Delta Sleep Stage: The stage of sleep in which EEG delta waves are prevalent or predominant (sleep stages 3 and 4, respectively, see *Slow-Wave Sleep*).

Diagnostic Criteria: Specific criteria established in the ICSD to aid in determining the unequivocal presence of a particular sleep disorder.

Diurnal: Pertaining to daytime.

Drowsiness: A stage of quiet wakefulness that typically occurs prior to sleep onset. If the eyes are closed, diffuse and slowed alpha activity usually is present, which then gives way to early features of stage 1 sleep.

Duration Criteria: Criteria (acute, subacute, chronic) established in the ICSD for determining the duration of a particular disorder.

Dyssomnia: A primary disorder of initiating and maintaining sleep or of excessive sleepiness. The dyssomnias are disorders of sleep or wakefulness per se; not a parasomnia.

Early Morning Arousal (Early A.M. Arousal): Premature morning awakening.

Electroencephalogram (EEG): A recording of the electrical activity of the brain by means of electrodes placed on the surface of the head. With the EMG and electrooculogram (EOG), the EEG is one of the three basic variables used to score sleep stages and waking. Sleep recording in humans utilizes surface electrodes to record potential differences between brain regions and a neutral reference point, or simply between brain regions. Either the C_3 or C_4 (central region) placement, according to the International 10-20 System, is referentially (referred to an earlobe) recorded as the standard electrode derivation from which state scoring is done.

Electromyogram (EMG): A recording of electrical activity from the muscular system; in sleep recording, synonymous with resting muscle activity or potential. The chin EMG, along with EEG and EOG, is one of the three basic variables used to score sleep stages and waking. Sleep recording in humans typically utilizes surface electrodes to measure activity from the submental muscles. These reflect maximally the changes in resting activity of axial body muscles. The submental muscle EMG is tonically inhibited during REM sleep.

Electrooculogram (EOG): A recording of voltage changes resulting from shifts in position of the ocular gloves, as each glove is a positive (anterior) and negative (posterior) dipole; along with the EEG and EMG, one of the three basic variables used to score sleep stages and waking. Sleep recording in humans utilizes surface electrodes placed near the eyes to record the movement (incidence, direction, and velocity) of the eyeballs. Rapid eye movements in sleep form one part of the characteristics of REM sleep state.

End-Tidal Carbon Dioxide: Carbon dioxide value usually determined at the nares by an infrared carbon dioxide gas analyzer. The value reflects the alveolar or pulmonary arterial blood carbon dioxide level.

Entrainment: Synchronization of a biologic rhythm by a forcing stimulus such as an environmental time cue (see *Zeitgeber*). During entrainment, the frequencies of the two cycles are the same or are integral multiples of each other.

Epoch: A measure of duration of the sleep recording, typically 20 or 30 seconds in duration, depending on the paper speed of the polysomnograph. An epoch corresponds to one page of the polysomnogram.

Excessive Sleepiness (-Somnolence, Hypersomnia, Excessive Daytime Sleepiness): A subjective report of difficulty in maintaining the alert awake state, usually accompanied by a rapid entrance into sleep when the person is sedentary. May be due to an excessively deep or prolonged major sleep episode. Can be quantitatively measured by use of subjectively defined rating scales of sleepiness, or physiologically measured by electrophysiologic tests such as the Multiple Sleep Latency Test (see *MSLT*). Most commonly occurs during the daytime; however, excessive sleepiness may be present at night in a person whose major sleep episode occurs during daytime, such as a shift worker.

Extrinsic Sleep Disorders: Disorders that originate, develop, or arise from causes outside of the body. The extrinsic sleep disorders are a subgroup of the dyssomnias.

Final Awakening: The duration of wakefulness after the final wake-up time until the arise time (lights on).

Final Wake-Up: The clock time at which an individual awakens for the last time before the arise time.

First-Night Effect: The effect of the environment and polysomnographic recording apparatus on the quality of the subject's sleep during the first night of recording. Sleep is usually of reduced quality compared to what would be expected in the subject's usual sleeping environment, without electrodes and other recording procedure stimuli. The subject usually is habituated to the laboratory by the time of the second night of recording.

Fragmentation (of Sleep Architecture): The interruption of any stage of sleep owing to the appearance of another stage or to wakefulness, leading to disrupted NREM–REM sleep cycles; often used to refer to the interruption of REM sleep by movement arousals or stage 2 activity. Sleep fragmentation connotes repetitive interruptions of sleep by arousals and awakenings.

Free-Running: A chronobiologic term that refers to the natural endogenous period of a rhythm when *Zeitgebers* are removed. In humans, it most commonly is seen in the tendency to delay some circadian rhythms, such as the sleep-wake cycle, by approximately 1 hour every day, when a person has an impaired ability to entrain or is without time cues.

Hertz (Hz): A unit of frequency; preferred to the synonymous expression *cycles per second* (cps).

Hypercapnia: Elevated level of carbon dioxide in blood.

Hypersomnia (Excessive Sleepiness): Excessively deep or prolonged major sleep period. May be associated with difficulty in awakening. Hypersomnia is primarily a diagnostic term (e.g., idiopathic hypersomnia); *excessive sleepiness* is preferred to describe the symptom.

Hypnagogic: Descriptor for events that occur during the transition from wakefulness to sleep.

Hypnagogic Imagery (-Hallucinations): Vivid sensory images occurring at sleep onset, but particularly vivid with sleep-onset REM periods. A feature of narcoleptic naps, when the onset occurs with REM sleep.

Hypnagogic Startle: A "sleep start" or sudden body jerk (hypnic jerk), observed normally just at sleep onset and usually resulting, at least momentarily, in awakening.

Hypnopompic (Hypnopomic): Descriptor of an occurrence during the transition from sleep to wakefulness at the termination of a sleep episode.

Hypopnea: An episode of shallow breathing (airflow reduced by at least 50%) during sleep lasting 10 seconds or longer, usually associated with a fall in blood oxygen saturation.

ICSD Sleep Code: A code number of the International Classification of the Sleep Disorders that refers to modifying information of a diagnosis, such as associated symptom, severity, or duration of a sleep disorder.

Insomnia: Difficulty in initiating and/or maintaining sleep. A term that is employed ubiquitously to indicate any and all gradations and types of sleep loss.

"Intermediary" Sleep Stage: A term sometimes used for NREM stage 2 sleep (see *Deep Sleep; Light Sleep*). Often used, especially in the French literature, for stages combining elements of stage 2 and REM sleep.

Into-Bed Time: The clock time at which a person gets into bed. The into-bed time is the same as bedtime for many people, but not for those who spend time in wakeful activities in bed, such as reading, before attempting to sleep.

Intrinsic Sleep Disorders: Disorders that either originate or develop from or arise from causes within the body. The intrinsic sleep disorders are a subgroup of the dyssomnias.

K-Alpha: A K complex followed by several seconds of alpha rhythm; a type of microarousal.

K Complex: A sharp, negative EEG wave followed by a high-voltage slow wave. The complex duration is at least 0.5 second, and may be accompanied by a sleep spindle. K complexes occur spontaneously during NREM sleep, and begin and define stage 2 sleep. They are thought to be evoked responses to internal stimuli. They can also be elicited during sleep by external (particularly auditory) stimuli.

Light-Dark Cycle: The periodic pattern of light (artificial or natural) alternating with darkness.

Light Sleep: A common term for NREM sleep stage 1, and sometimes stage 2.

Maintenance of Wakefulness Test (MWT): A series of measurements of the interval from "lights out" to sleep onset that is utilized in the assessment of the ability to remain awake. Subjects are instructed to try to remain awake in a darkened room when in a semireclined position. Long latencies to sleep are indicative of the ability to remain awake. This test is most useful for assessing the effects of medication on the ability to remain awake.

Major Sleep Episode: The longest sleep episode that occurs on a daily basis. Typically the sleep episode dictated by the circadian rhythm of sleep and wakefulness; the conventional or habitual time for sleeping.

Microsleep: An episode that lasts up to 30 seconds during which external stimuli are not perceived. The polysomnogram suddenly shifts from waking characteristics to sleep. Microsleeps are associated with excessive sleepiness and automatic behavior.

Minimal Criteria: Criteria of the ICSD derived from the diagnostic criteria that provide the minimum features necessary for making a particular sleep disorder diagnosis.

Montage: The particular arrangement by which a number of derivations are displayed simultaneously in a polysomnogram.

Movement Arousal: A body movement associated with an EEG pattern of arousal or a full awakening; a sleep-scoring variable.

Movement Time: The term used in sleep record scoring to denote when EEG and EOG tracings are obscured for more than half the scoring epoch because of movement. It is scored only when the preceding and subsequent epochs are in sleep.

Multiple Sleep Latency Test (MSLT): A series of measurements of the interval from "lights out" to sleep onset that is utilized in the assessment of excessive sleepiness. Subjects are allowed a fixed number of opportunities to fall asleep during their customary awake period. Excessive sleepiness is characterized by short latencies. Long latencies are helpful in distinguishing physical tiredness or fatigue from true sleepiness.

Muscle Tone: A term sometimes used for resting muscle potential or resting muscle activity (see *Electromyogram*).

Myoclonus: Muscle contractions in the form of abrupt jerks or twitches generally lasting less than 100 milliseconds. The term should not be applied to the periodic leg movements of sleep that characteristically have a duration of 0.5 to 5 seconds.

Nap: A short sleep episode that may be intentionally or unintentionally taken during the period of habitual wakefulness.

Nightmare: An unpleasant and frightening dream that usually occurs in REM sleep. Occasionally called a dream anxiety attack, it is not a sleep (night) terror. Nightmare in the past has been used to indicate both sleep terror and anxiety dream attacks.

Nocturnal Confusion: Episodes of delirium and disorientation close to or during nighttime sleep; often seen in the elderly and indicative of organic central nervous system deterioration.

Nocturnal Dyspnea: Respiratory distress that may be minimal during the day but becomes quite pronounced during sleep.

Nocturnal Penile Tumescence (NPT): The natural periodic cycle of penile erections that occur during sleep, typically associated with REM sleep. The preferred term is sleep-related erections.

Nocturnal Sleep: The typical "nighttime" or major sleep episode related to the circadian rhythm of sleep and wakefulness; the conventional or habitual time for sleeping.

Non–Rapid Eye Movement (NREM) Sleep: See *Sleep Stages*.

NREM–REM Sleep Cycle (Synonymous with Sleep Cycle): A period during sleep composed of an NREM sleep episode and the subsequent REM sleep episode; each NREM–REM sleep couplet is equal to one cycle. Any NREM sleep stage suffices as the NREM sleep portion of a cycle. An adult sleep period of 6.5 to 8.5 hours generally consists of four to six cycles. The cycle duration increases from infancy to young adulthood.

NREM Sleep Intrusion: An interposition of NREM sleep, or a component of NREM sleep physiology (e.g., elevated EMG, K complex, sleep spindle, delta waves) in REM sleep; a portion of NREM sleep not appearing in its usual sleep cycle position.

NREM Sleep Period: The NREM sleep portion of NREM–REM sleep cycle; such an episode consists primarily of sleep stages 3 and 4 early in the night and of sleep stage 2 later (see *Sleep Cycle, Sleep Stages*).

Obesity-Hypoventilation Syndrome: A condition of obese persons who hypoventilate during wakefulness. Because the term can apply to several different disorders, its use is discouraged.

Paradoxical Sleep: Synonymous with REM sleep, which is the preferred term.

Parasomnia: Disorder of arousal, partial arousal, or sleep stage transition, not a dyssomnia. It represents an episodic disorder in sleep (such as sleepwalking) rather than a disorder of sleep or wakefulness per se. May be induced or exacerbated by sleep.

Paroxysm: Phenomenon of abrupt onset that rapidly attains maximum intensity and terminates suddenly; distinguished from background activity. Commonly refers to an epileptiform discharge on the EEG.

Paroxysmal Nocturnal Dyspnea (PND): Respiratory distress and shortness of breath due to pulmonary edema, which appears suddenly and often awakens the sleeper.

Penile Buckling Pressure: The amount of force applied to the glans of the penis sufficient to produce at least a 30-degree bend in the shaft.

Penile Rigidity: The firmness of the penis as measured by the penile buckling pressure. Normally, the fully erect penis has maximum rigidity.

Period: The interval between the recurrence of a defined phase or moment of a rhythmic or regularly recurring event; that is, the interval between one peak or trough and the next.

Periodic Leg Movement (PLM): Rapid partial flexion of the foot at the ankle, extension of the big toe, and partial flexion of the knee and hip that occurs during sleep. The movements occur with a periodicity of 20 to 60 seconds in a stereotyped pattern lasting 0.5 to 5.0 seconds and are a characteristic feature of the periodic limb movement disorder.

Periodic Movements of Sleep (PMS): See Periodic Leg Movement.

Phase Advance: The shift of an episode of sleep or wake or an earlier position in the 24-hour sleepwake cycle. A shift of sleep from 11 P.M.–7 A.M. to 8 P.M.–4 A.M. represents a 3-hour phase advance (see *Phase Delay*).

Phase Delay: A shift of an episode of sleep or wake to a later time of the 24-hour sleep-wake cycle. It is the exact opposite of phase advance. These terms differ from common concepts of change in clock time; to effect a phase delay, the clock is moved ahead or advanced. In contrast, to effect a phase advance, the clock moves backward (see *Phase Advance*).

Phase Transition: One of the two junctures of the major sleep and wake phases in the 24-hour sleepwake cycle.

Phasic Event (-Activity): Brain, muscle, or autonomic event of a brief and episodic nature occurring in sleep; characteristic of REM sleep, such as eye movements, or muscle twitches. Usually the duration is milliseconds to 1 or 2 seconds.

Photoperiod: The period of light in a light-dark cycle.

Pickwickian: Descriptor for an obese person who snores, is sleepy, and has alveolar hypoventilation. The term has been applied to many different disorders and therefore its use is discouraged.

PLM-Arousal Index: The number of sleep-related periodic leg movements per hour of sleep that are associated with an EEG arousal (see *Periodic Leg Movement*).

PLM Index: The number of periodic leg movements per hour of total sleep time as determined by all-night polysomnography. Sometimes expressed as the number of movements per hour of NREM sleep because the movements are usually inhibited during REM sleep (see *Periodic Leg Movement*).

PLM Percentage: The percentage of total sleep time occupied with recurrent episodes of periodic leg movements.

Polysomnogram: The continuous and simultaneous recording of multiple physiologic variables during sleep (i.e., EEG, EOG, EMG—the three basic stage scoring parameters—electrocardiogram (ECG), respiratory airflow, respiratory movements, leg movements, and other electrophysiologic variables.

Polysomnograph: A biomedical instrument for the measurement of physiologic variables of sleep.

Polysomnographic (as in -Recording, -Monitoring, -Registration, or -Tracings): Describes a recording on paper, computer disc, or tape of a polysomnogram.

Premature Morning Awakening: Early termination of the sleep episode, with inability to return to sleep, sometimes after the last of several awakenings. It reflects interference at the end, rather than at the commencement, of the sleep episode. A characteristic sleep disturbance of some people with depression.

Proposed Sleep Disorder: A disorder in which insufficient information is available in the medical literature to confirm the unequivocal existence of the disorder. A category of the ICSD.

Quiet Sleep: A term used to describe NREM sleep in infants and animals when specific NREM sleep stages 1 to 4 cannot be determined.

Rapid Eye Movement (REM) Sleep: See *Sleep Stages.*

Record: The end product of the polysomnograph recording process.

Recording: The process of obtaining a polysomnographic record. The term is also applied to the end product of the polysomnograph recording process.

REM Density (-Intensity):   A function that expresses the frequency of eye movements per unit time during sleep stage REM.

REM Sleep Episode: The REM sleep portion of a NREM–REM sleep cycle. Early in the night it may be as short as a half minute, in later cycles longer than an hour (see *Sleep Stage REM*).

REM Sleep Intrusion: A brief interval of REM sleep appearing out of its usual position in the NREM–REM sleep cycle; an interposition of REM sleep in NREM sleep; sometimes appearance of a single, dissociated component of REM sleep (e.g., eye movements, "drop out" of muscle tone) rather than all REM sleep parameters.

REM Sleep Latency: The interval from sleep onset to the first appearance of stage REM sleep in the sleep episode.

REM Sleep Onset: The designation for commencement of a REM sleep episode. Sometimes also used as a shorthand term for a sleep-onset REM sleep episode (see *Sleep Onset; Sleep-Onset REM Period (SOREMP).*

REM Sleep Percent: The proportion of total sleep time constituted by REM stage of sleep.

REM Sleep Rebound (Recovery):   Lengthening and increase in frequency and density of REM sleep episodes, which results in an increase in REM sleep percent above baseline. REM sleep rebound follows REM sleep deprivation once the depriving influence is removed.

Respiratory Disturbance Index (RDI; Apnea-Hypopnea Index):   The number of apneas (obstructive, central, or mixed) plus hypopneas per hour of total sleep time as determined by all-night polysomnography.

Restlessness: Referring to quality of sleep, persistent or recurrent body movements, arousals, and brief awakenings in the course of sleep.

Rhythm: An event occurring with approximately constant periodicity.

Sawtooth Waves: A form of theta rhythm that occurs during REM sleep and is characterized by a notched waveform. Occurs in bursts lasting up to 10 seconds.

Severity Criteria: Criteria for establishing the severity of a particular sleep disorder according to categories: mild, moderate, or severe.

Sleep Architecture: The NREM–REM sleep stage and cycle infrastructure of sleep understood from the vantage point of the quantitative relationship of these components to each other. Often plotted in the form of a histogram.

Sleep Cycle: Synonymous with the NREM–REM sleep cycle.

Sleep Efficiency (Sleep Efficiency Index):   The proportion of sleep in the episode potentially filled by sleep (i.e., the ratio of total sleep time to time in bed).

Sleep Episode: An interval of sleep that may be voluntary or involuntary. In the sleep laboratory, the sleep episode occurs from the time of "lights out" to the time of "lights on." The major sleep episode is usually the longest one.

Sleep Hygiene: Conditions and practices that promote continuous and effective sleep. These include regularity of bedtime and arise time; conformity of time spent in bed to the time necessary for sustained and individually adequate sleep (i.e., the total sleep time sufficient to avoid sleepiness when awake); restriction of alcohol and caffeine beverages prior to bedtime; and employment of exercise, nutrition, and environmental factors so that they enhance, rather than disturb, restful sleep.

Sleepiness (Somnolence, Drowsiness):   Difficulty in maintaining alert wakefulness so that a person falls asleep if not actively aroused. This is not simply a feeling of physical tiredness or listlessness. When sleepiness occurs in inappropriate circumstances, it is considered excessive sleepiness.

Sleep Interruption: Breaks in sleep resulting in arousal and wakefulness (see *Fragmentation; Restlessness*).

Sleep Latency: The duration of time from "lights out," or bedtime, to the onset of sleep.

Sleep Log (-Diary):   A daily, written record of a person's sleep-wake pattern containing such information as time of retiring and arising, time in bed, estimated total sleep time, number and duration of sleep interruptions quality of sleep, daytime naps, use of medications or caffeine beverages, nature of waking activities.

Sleep-Maintenance DIMS (Insomnia):   A disturbance in maintaining sleep, once achieved; persistently interrupted sleep without difficulty falling asleep. Synonymous with sleep continuity disturbance.

Sleep Mentation: The imagery and thinking experienced during sleep. Sleep mentation usually consists of combinations of images and thoughts during REM sleep. Imagery is vividly expressed in dreams involving all the senses in approximate proportion to their waking representations. Mentation is experienced generally less distinctly in

NREM sleep, but it may be quite vivid in stage 2 sleep, especially toward the end of the sleep episode. Mentation at sleep onset (hypnagogic reverie) can be as vivid, as in REM sleep.

Sleep Onset: The transition from awake to sleep, normally to NREM stage 1 sleep but in certain conditions such as infancy and narcolepsy into stage REM sleep. Most polysomnographers accept EEG slowing, reduction, and eventual disappearance of alpha activity, presence of EEG vertex sharp transients, and slow, rolling eye movements (the components of NREM stage 1) as sufficient criteria for sleep onset; others require appearance of stage 2 patterns (see Sleep Latency; Sleep Stages).

Sleep-Onset REM Period (SOREMP): The beginning of sleep by entrance directly into stage REM sleep. The onset of REM occurs within 10 minutes of sleep onset.

Sleep Paralysis: Immobility of the body that occurs in the transition from sleep to wakefulness that is a partial manifestation of REM sleep.

Sleep Pattern (24-Hour Sleep-Wake Pattern): A person's clock hour schedule of bedtime and arise time as well as nap behavior; may also include time and duration of sleep interruptions (see *Sleep-Wake Cycle; Circadian Rhythm; Sleep Log*).

Sleep-Related Erections: The natural periodic cycle of penile erections that occur during sleep, typically associated with REM sleep. Sleep-related erectile activity can be characterized as four phases: T-up (ascending tumescence), T-max (plateau maximal tumescence), T-down (detumescence), and T-zero (no tumescence). Polysomnographic assessment of sleep-related erections is useful for differentiating organic from nonorganic erectile dysfunction.

Sleep Spindle: Spindle-shaped bursts of 11.5- to 15-Hz waves lasting 0.5 to 1.5 seconds. Generally diffuse, but of highest voltage over the central regions of the head. The amplitude is generally less than 50 μV in the adult. One of the identifying EEG features of NREM stage 2 sleep, it may persist into NREM stages 3 and 4 but is generally not seen in REM sleep.

Sleep Stage Demarcation: The significant polysomnographic characteristics that distinguish the boundaries of the sleep stages. In certain conditions and with drugs, sleep stage demarcations may be blurred or lost, making it difficult to identify certain stages with certainty or to distinguish the temporal limits of sleep stage lengths.

Sleep Stage Episode: A sleep stage interval that represents the stage in an NREM–REM sleep cycle; easiest to comprehend in relation to REM sleep, which is a homogeneous stage (i.e., the fourth REM sleep episode is in the fourth sleep cycle unless a previous REM episode was skipped). If one interval of REM sleep is separated from another by more than 20 minutes, they constitute separate REM sleep episodes (and are in separate sleep cycles); a sleep stage episode may be of any duration.

Sleep Stage NREM: The other major sleep state apart from REM sleep, it comprises sleep stages 1 to 4, which constitute levels in the spectrum of NREM sleep "depth" or physiologic intensity.

Sleep Stage REM: The stage of sleep with highest brain activity, characterized by enhanced brain metabolism and vivid hallucinatory imagery or dreaming. There are spontaneous rapid eye movements, resting muscle activity is suppressed, and awakening threshold to nonsignificant stimuli is high. The EEG is a low-voltage, mixed-frequency, non-alpha record. REM sleep is usually 20% to 25% of total sleep time. It is also called *paradoxical sleep*.

Sleep Stages: Distinctive stages of sleep best demonstrated by polysomnographic recordings of the EEG, EOG, and EMG.

Sleep Stage 1 (NREM Stage 1): A stage of NREM sleep that occurs at sleep onset or that follows arousal from sleep stages 2, 3, 4, or REM. It consists of a relatively low-voltage EEG with mixed frequency, mainly theta activity and alpha activity of less than 50% of the scoring epoch. It contains EEG vertex waves and slow, rolling eye movements; no sleep spindles, K complexes, or REMs. Stage 1 normally represent 4% to 5% of the major sleep episode.

Sleep Stage 2 (NREM Stage 2): A stage of NREM sleep characterized by the presence of sleep spindles and K complexes present in a relatively low-voltage, mixed-frequency EEG background. High-voltage delta waves may comprise up to 20% of stage 2 epochs; usually accounts for 45% to 55% of the major sleep episode.

Sleep Stage 3 (NREM Stage 3): A stage of NREM sleep defined by at least 20%—and not more than 50%—of the episode consisting of EEG waves less than 2 Hz and more than 75 μV (high amplitude delta waves). A delta sleep stage, with stage 4 it constitutes "deep" NREM sleep, so-called slow-wave sleep (SWS). It is often combined with stage 4 into NREM sleep stage 3/4 because of the lack of documented physiologic differences between the two. It appears usually only in the first third of the sleep episode; usually comprises 4% to 6% of total sleep time.

Sleep Stage 4 (NREM Stage 4): All statements concerning NREM sleep stage 3 apply to stage 4 except that high-voltage, EEG slow waves persist during 50% or more of the epoch. NREM sleep stage 4 usually represents 12% to 15% of total sleep time.

Sleepwalking, night terrors, and confusional arousal episodes generally start in stage 4 or during arousals from this stage (see *Sleep Stage 3*).

Sleep Structure: Similar to sleep architecture, sleep structure, in addition to encompassing sleep stages and sleep cycle relationships, assesses the within-stage qualities of the EEG and other physiologic attributes.

Sleep Talking: Talking in sleep that usually occurs in the course of transitory arousals from NREM sleep. It can occur during stage REM sleep, at which time it represents a motor breakthrough of dream speech. Full consciousness is not achieved and no memory of the event remains.

Sleep-Wake Cycle: Basically, the clock hour relationships of the major sleep and wake episodes in the 24-hour cycle (see *Phase Transition; Circadian Rhythm*).

Sleep-Wake Shift (-Change, -Reversal): Displacement of sleep, entirely or in part, to a time of customary waking activity, and of waking activity to the time of the major sleep episode. Common in jet lag and shift work.

Sleep-Wake Transition Disorder: A disorder that occurs during the transition from wakefulness to sleep or from one sleep stage to another. A parasomnia; not a dyssomnia.

Slow-Wave Sleep (SWS): Sleep characterized by EEG waves of duration slower than 4 Hz. Synonymous with sleep stages 3 plus 4 combined (see *Delta Sleep Stage*).

Snoring: A noise produced primarily with inspiratory respiration during sleep owing to vibration of the soft palate and the pillars of the oropharyngeal inlet. All snorers have incomplete obstruction of the upper airway, and many habitual snorers have complete episodes of upper airway obstruction.

Spindle REM Sleep: A condition in which sleep spindles persist atypically during REM sleep seen in chronic insomnia conditions, and occasionally in the first REM period.

Synchronized: A chronobiologic term used to indicate that two or more rhythms recur with the same phase relationship. In EEG it is used to indicate increased amplitude—and usually decreased frequency—of the dominant activities.

Theta Activity: EEG activity with a frequency of 4 to 8 Hz, generally maximal over the central and temporal cortex.

Total Recording Time (TRT): The interval from sleep onset to final awakening. In addition to total sleep time, it is comprised of the time taken up by wake periods and movement time until wake-up (see *Sleep Efficiency*).

Total Sleep Episode: The total time available for sleep during an attempt to sleep. It comprises NREM and REM sleep as well as wakefulness. Synonymous with (and preferred to) *total sleep period.*

Total Sleep Time (TST): The amount of actual sleep time in a sleep episode; equal to total sleep episode minus awake time. Total sleep time is the total of all REM and NREM sleep in a sleep episode.

Tracé Alternant: EEG pattern of sleeping newborns, characterized by bursts of slow waves, at times intermixed with sharp waves, and intervening periods of relative quiescence with extreme low-amplitude activity.

Tumescence (Penile): Hardening and expansion of the penis (penile erection). When associated with REM sleep, it is referred to as a sleep-related erection.

Twitch (Body Twitch): A very small body movement, such as a local foot or finger jerk; not usually associated with arousal.

Vertex Sharp Transient: Sharp negative potential, maximal at the vertex, occurring spontaneously during sleep or in response to a sensory stimulus during sleep or wakefulness. Amplitude varies but rarely exceeds 250 μV. Use of the term *vertex sharp wave* is discouraged.

Wake Time: The total time scored as wakefulness in a polysomnogram occurring between sleep onset and final wake-up.

Waxing and Waning: A crescendo-decrescendo pattern of activity, usually EEG activity.

Zeitgeber: German term for an environmental time cue that usually helps entrainment to the 24-hour day, such as sunlight, noise, social interaction, alarm clock.

LIST OF ABBREVIATIONS

AHI	Apnea-hypopnea index
AI	Apnea index
ASDA	American Sleep Disorders Association
CNS	Central nervous system
cps	Cycles per second (Hertz is preferred)
DIMS	Disorder of initiating and maintaining sleep
DOES	Disorder of excessive somnolence
DSM	Diagnostic and statistical manual
EEG	Electroencephalogram
EMG	Electromyogram
EOG	Electrooculogram
Hz	Hertz (cycles per second)
ICD	International Classification of Diseases
ICSD	International Classification of Sleep Disorders
MSLT	Multiple Sleep Latency Test
MWT	Maintenance of Wakefulness Test
NPT	Nocturnal penile tumescence
NREM	Non–rapid eye movement (sleep)
PLM	Periodic leg movement
PND	Paroxysmal nocturnal dystonia
PSG	Polysomnogram
RDI	Respiratory disturbance index
REM	Rapid eye movement (sleep)
REMs	Rapid eye movements
RLS	Restless legs syndrome
SDB	Sleep-disordered breathing
SOREMP	Sleep-onset REM period
SWS	Slow-wave sleep
TST	Total sleep time

Index

Page numbers followed by *t* and *f* denote tables and figures, respectively.